UNDERSTANDING THE COMPLEXITIES OF KIDNEY TRANSPLANTATION

Edited by **Jorge Ortiz** and **Jason André**

Understanding the Complexities of Kidney Transplantation
Edited by Jorge Ortiz and Jason André

Published by InTech
Janeza Trdine 9, 51000 Rijeka, Croatia

Publishing Process Manager Davor Vidic

Technical Editor Teodora Smiljanic

Cover Designer InTech Design Team

Additional hard copies can be obtained from orders@intechopen.com

Understanding the Complexities of Kidney Transplantation, Edited by Jorge Ortiz and Jason André
p. cm.
ISBN 978-953-307-819-9

For EU product safety concerns:
IN TECH d.o.o., Prolaz Marije Krucifikse Kozulić 3, 51000 Rijeka, Croatia,
info@intechopen.com or visit our website at intechopen.com.

Meet the editors

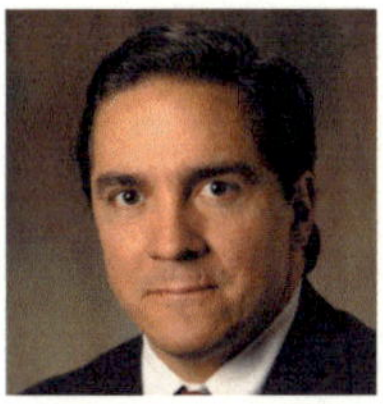

Dr. Jorge Ortiz completed the General Surgery Residency Program at North Shore University Hospital in New York, NY from 1991-1996. Following the completion of his residency he completed an Organ Transplant Fellowship at University of Miami Medical Center from 1996 – 1998 following which he joined the staff in the Division of Transplantation at UC Irvine Medical Center at the University of California and was appointed Director, Renal Transplant Program from 1998-2000 when he left to join the medical staff at Einstein. Today, Dr. Ortiz is the Director of Liver Transplantation and Hepatobiliary Surgery and the Director of Surgical Transplant Fellowship at Albert Einstein Medical Center and has over ten years experience in liver transplantation and research.

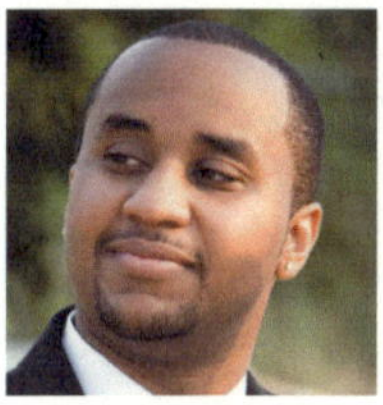

Dr. Jason André is currently a surgery resident at Albert Einstein Medical Center. Raised in Virginia, Dr. André began his path to become a surgeon at the University of Virginia (UVA) where he majored in Psychology. During his time at UVA, Dr. André spent time working with inner city kids and educating men about the effects of sexual abuse on women. Once he completed his training at UVA, Dr. André received his doctorate of medicine at Howard University College of Medicine where his passion for surgery grew. Dr. André is now completing his training at Albert Einstein Medical Center.

Contents

Preface

Kidney failure is a major financial burden throughout the world. Renal failure and dialysis in particular are associated with an increased mortality risk and high medical costs. According to an article published in USA Today in 2009, dialysis cost the US $8.6 billion in 2007 and in 2006 20.1% of dialysis patients died. The only alternative that is available to dialysis at this time is kidney transplantation, a way to give patients with renal failure a new beginning.

Kidney transplantation is a complex field that incorporates several different specialties to manage the transplant patient. Because patients with kidney failure frequently have other significant comorbidities, the workup for a potential transplant recipient can be quite involved. A potential transplant recipient often has significant exposure to blood borne infections like hepatitis, HIV, and many other potential pathogens. Patients often have severe hypertension or poorly controlled diabetes that has lead to their renal failure and yet others still have a history of heart problems.

This book was created because of the importance of kidney transplantation. This particular volume focuses on the complexities of the transplant patient. In particular, there is a focus on the comorbidities and special considerations for a transplant patient and how they affect kidney transplant outcomes.

In this book you will also find a brief history on the field of kidney transplantation as well as the ethical considerations in the field of transplantation. Next, the reader will find a section dedicated to special potential transplant recipients who require specialized considerations when contemplating transplantation. There is a discussion on the actual transplant procedure and potential for newer and innovative methods to completing a kidney transplantation.

Contributors to this book are from all over the world and are experts in their individual fields. They were all individually approached to add a chapter to this book and with their efforts this book was formed. *Understanding the Complexities of Kidney Transplantation* gives the reader an excellent foundation to build upon to truly understand kidney transplantation.

Dr. Jorge Ortiz and Dr. Jason André
Albert Einstein Medical Center
Philadelphia, PA

Part 1

Pretransplant Considerations

1

The History of Kidney Transplantation: Past, Present and Future (with Special References to the Belgian History)

Squifflet Jean-Paul
University of Liege
Belgium

1. Introduction

The history of kidney transplantation is thought to have originated at the early beginning of the previous century with several attempts of Xenografting, and experimental works on vascular sutures (Küss & Bourget, 1992)[1]. But it really started more than 60 years ago with first attempts of deceased donor transplantation (DCD) and the first successful kidney transplantation of homozygote twins in Boston (Toledo-Pereyra et al, 2008)[2]. Belgian surgeons contributed to that field of medicine by performing in the early sixties the first ever organ procurement on a brain dead heart beating donor (DBD) (June 1963) (Squifflet, 2003)[3]. Later on, in the eighties, they published a first series of living unrelated donor (LURD) transplantations, as well as ABO-Incompatible living donor (ABO-Inc LD) transplantations. With the advent of Cyclosporine A, and later other calcineurin inhibitors such as Tacrolimus, with the advent of more potent immunosuppressive drugs (IS), the gap between the number of renal transplant candidates and the number of transplanted recipients was and is continuously increasing in Belgium and most countries. It opened the search for other sources of organs such as donors after cardiac death (DCD) defined with the Maastricht conference and the extended criteria donors (ECD) compared to standard criteria donors (SCD). In Belgium another source of DCD was identified after the promulgation in 2002 of a law on euthanasia. The Belgian example and all its historical measures could help others to fight against organ shortage and its consequences, organ trafficking, commercialization and tourism.

2. The prehistory of transplantation

Already in old civilizations, the Egyptians, the Greeks, the Romans, were dreaming and expecting morphological changes in the structure and behavior of the human body. Old mythologies with their sculptures and art offer many examples such as gods, heroes, sirens, tritons, centaurs which are "prefiguration" of the xenotransplantation era (Küss & Bourget, 1992)[1].

The real transplantation story started with Saints COSMAS and DAMIAN during the fourth century: the extraordinary influence of these physicians extended far beyond the Middle Ages and even into modern times (Squifflet, 2003)[4]. After learning the medical art, these legendary early Christian brothers were said to have earned so much grace through the

Holy Spirit that they were able to banish all diseases from man and beast. Therefore, in the fourth century, they transplanted a Moor's leg to their Sacristan (Fig. 1). In Rome, the healing brothers were venerated, but they were also martyred under Diocletian (Fig. 2) and subsequently canonized. Today, they are acknowledged as the patron Saints of Surgery.

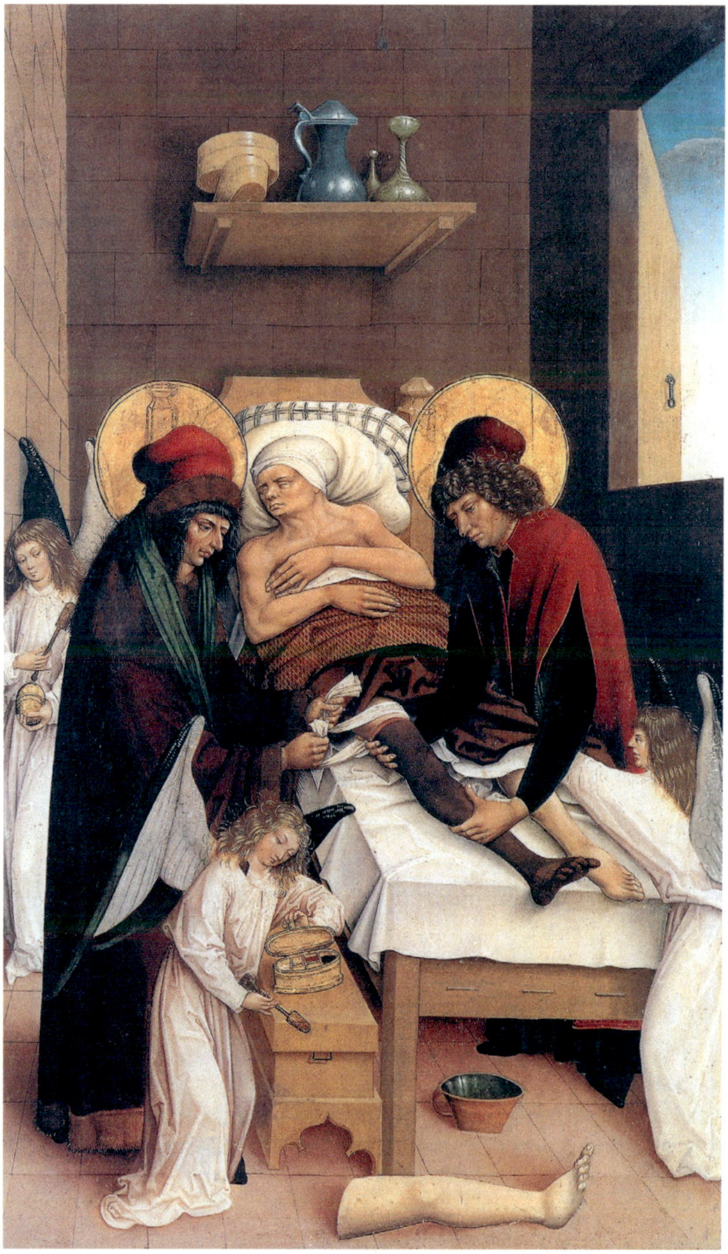

Oil on wood. Wüttembergisches Landesmuseum, Stuttgart, Germany.
Fig. 1. Transplantation of the Moor's leg by the brothers Cosmas and Damian.

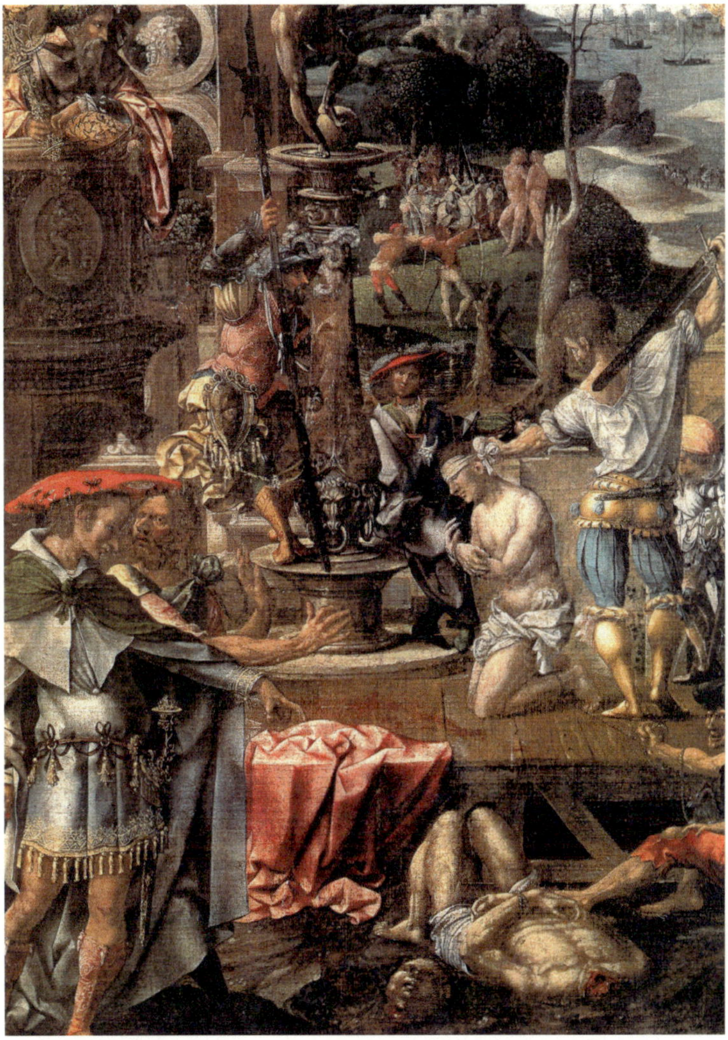

Sint-Jacobskerk, Brugge, Belgium.
Fig. 2. Lancelot Blondeel'stritych on canvas. The martyrdom of the twin brothers Cosmas and Damian.

At the beginning of the twentieth century (Table 1), the kidney became the pilot organ in the field of transplantation development with Emerich Ullmann (Vienna, Austria, 1902) who successfully transplanted a dog kidney into the animal neck. In parallel, the Lyon School with Mathieu Jaboulay described the circular suture of the arteries, a first step towards transplanting in 1906 a pig kidney and shortly after, a goat kidney in the inner elbow of end-stage renal failure patients. Both kidneys rapidly thrombosed, while Mathieu Jaboulay was erroneously blaming his suture technique!

An indelible mark on the pages of the transplantation history was made by one of Jaboulay's pupil, Alexis Carrel who immigrated to the United States and got, later on, the 1912 Nobel price. For vascular sutures, he moved to another technique, the so-called "triangulation" while using and exchanging dog legs in order to prove its efficiency (Fig. 3). Even if the procedure was effective for vascular anastomosis and organ revascularization, Carrel mis-recognized that transplanted organ allografts were not permanently accepted. Indeed he did not recognize the immunological reaction and the existence of the immune system. Nevertheless, his surgical technique for vascular suturing is still valid and persists today, with several modifications introduced for microsurgery like the eccentric biangulation technique proposed by Cobett in the Sixties (Fig. 4) (Squifflet et al. 1993)[5].

Year	Author	Dicovery or application
1902	Ullmann	Dog kidney into the neck
1902	Carrel	Developed vascular anastomotic techniques
1906	Jaboulay	Pig and goat kidneys to the elbow
1909	Unger	En bloc Maccacus kidneys
1912	Carrel	Nobel price
1928	Voronoff	Testis transplantation
1936	Voronoy	First deceased donor kidney transplantation
1951	Küss	Free kidneys from guillotined donors transplanted with surgical techniques still in use today
1952	Hamburger	First use of living related donor kidney (mother to son)
1954	Hume Murray Merril	First transplantation of identical twin kidney (+ first post-transplant pregnancy) (+ TBI: total body irradiation)
1962	Hamburger	Successful transplantations of two living related but non-twin kidney allografts (TBI-Steroids)
1962	Küss	Successful transplantations of two non-related kidney Allografts (TBI-Steroids-6-Mercaptopurine)
1962	to 1964 Remtsma Starzl Hume	Xenograft period: 5 en-bloc kidneys from chimpanzees 6 baboon kidneys and 1 liver 1 baboon kidney (54 Liters of urine)
1963	Starzl	First three attempts at orthotopic liver transplantation in humans 25/27 successful renal transplantations with 6-MP
1966	Kelly Lillehei Barnard	First human pancreas transplantation at the University of Minnesota
1967		First transplantation of a human heart in Cape Town

Table 1. A timeline in organ transplantation.

In 1909, Ernst Unger used en-bloc Macaccus kidneys in humans which rapidly failed, due to the unknown hyperacute vascular rejection. By contrast, the success of dog autografts at the Mayo Clinic in Rochester helped the transplant physicians to suspect the rejection phenomena; it was also the open door for human kidney homografting.
In 1928, Serge Voronoff at the Collège de France in Paris, who was well-known for his monkey to human testis transplantations, was ready to transplant a young girl with renal tuberculosis. The candidate for the organ donation was a murderer condemned to be beheaded, but willing to offer his organs after death. Unfortunately, the Prosecutor of the Republic took a wrong decision and opposed his veto. That's why, only 5 years later, in 1933, another Russian Surgeon, Voronoy, underwent in Kherson, the first ever renal

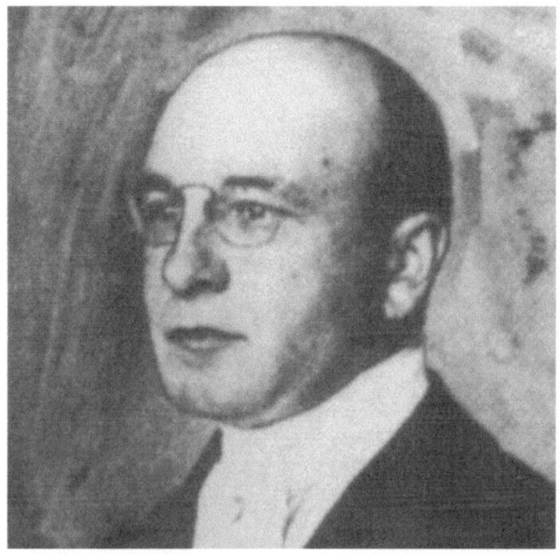

a.

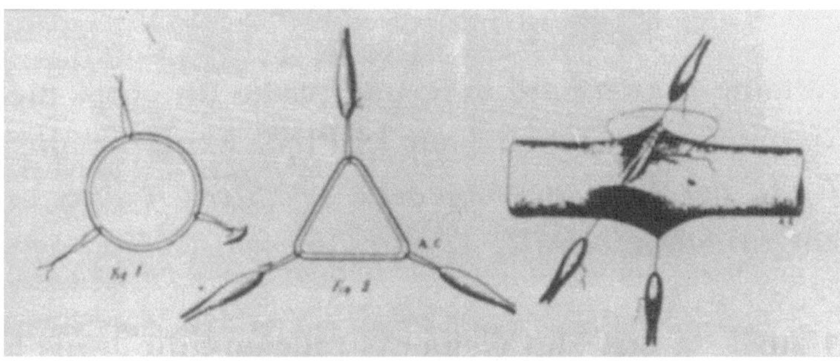

b.

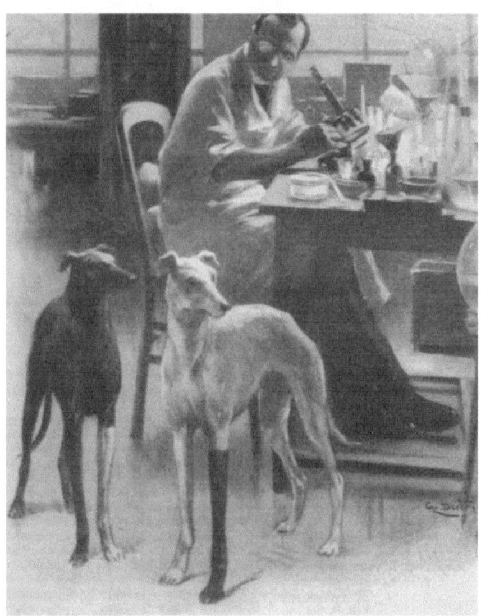

c.

Fig. 3. Alexis Carrel (a) and his surgical technique of vascular sutures (b) exchanging dog legs to prove its efficiency (c). (Küss & Bourget, 1992)[1].

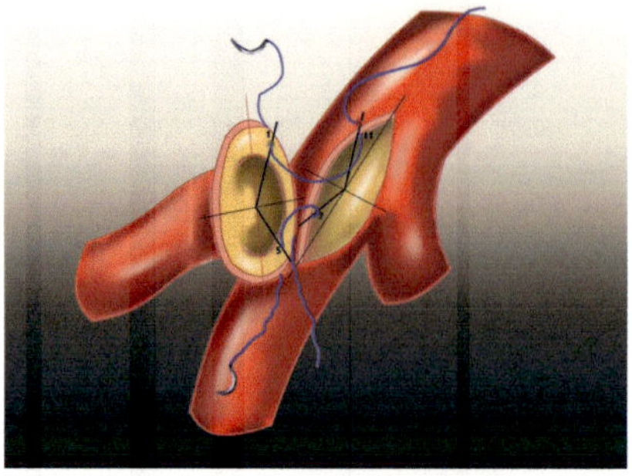

a.

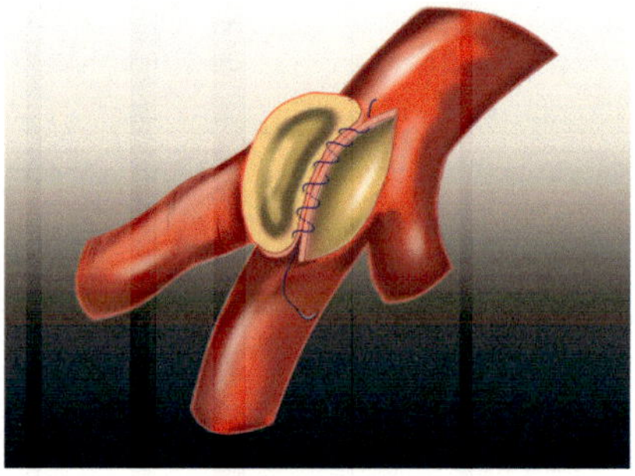

b.

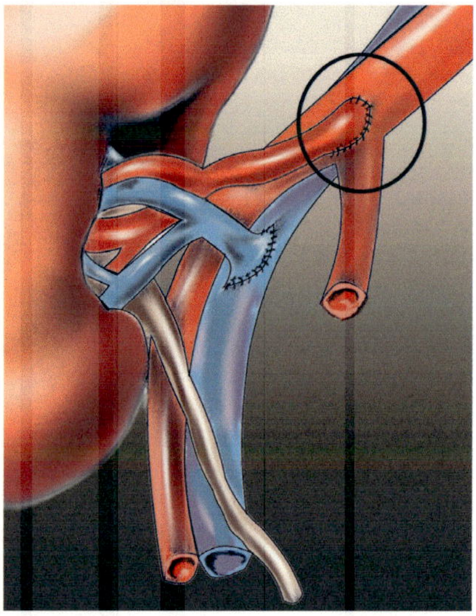

c.

a: two stitches are place on both sides at 1 hour and 11 hour, at 5 hour and 7 hour, in order to correctly tackle the posterior ridge of the vessels, while opening the anterior wall.
b: the posterior running suture is placed from the inside.
c: the anterior running suture.
(Meurisse M., drawings).
Fig. 4. The eccentric biangulation technique for end-to-side vascular anastomosis

homotransplantation in human using a kidney from a deceased-brain trauma, 60-years-old donor (DCD) (Blood group B). The recipient was a 26-years-old woman (Blood group O), who was dying from acute renal failure due to mercury intoxication. The kidney was placed into the groin (Fig. 5). Despite the ABO incompatibility, the urine output remained on 5 ml per hour until PO day 2 while the recipient died on PO day 4 with no vascular thrombosis of graft vessels.

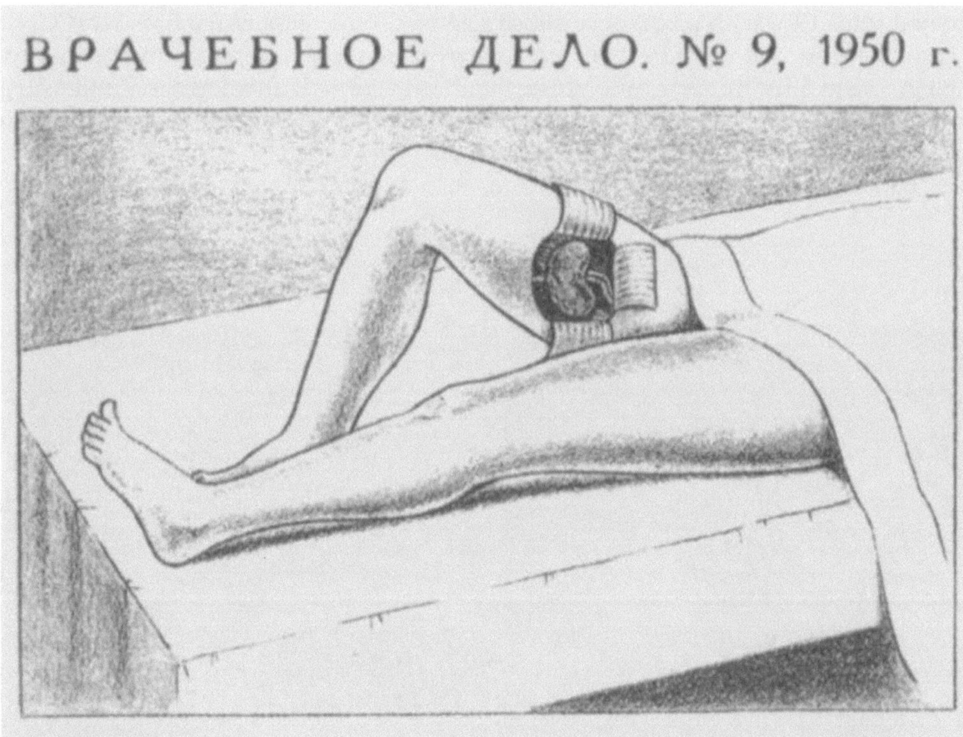

(Küss & Bourget, 1992)[1].

Fig. 5. First renal homotransplantation by Voronoy in 1933. Implantation in the groin of the recipient.

Later on, David Hume in Boston (1947) and Lawler in Chicago (1950), using again DCD kidney did not encounter better success; they used the Voronoy surgical technique for implantation. In 1951, a further and definitive step was taken in the surgical technique of kidney transplantation, by the French School in Paris. Dubost, Œconomos, Servelle and Rougeulle were using kidneys procured in guillotined murderers; Küss, Teinturier and Millez, used also the Matson kidney (nephrectomy of a normal kidney for ventriculo-peritoneal shunt placement to treat hydrocephalia). All kidneys were implanted with the French technique: in the right iliac fossa with vascular anastomosis on the iliac vessels (Fig. 6). That technique was used at the Necker Hospital in Paris on Christmas Eve 1952, to transplant Marius Renard with his mother kidney (Fig. 7). Marius had a single kidney, which had to be removed following a trauma (ladder fall). The mother kidney functioned well without any IS therapy during 3 weeks until rejection occurred, followed by recipient death.

The procedure developed by Küss and the other French surgeons is currently widely used: it inspired Joseph E. Murray, John Merril and their associates at the Peter Bent Brigham Hospital in Boston with their identical monozygotic twin transplantation, which was first attempted two days before Christmas 1954. The US surgeons proved without any IS agents that living renal transplantation could be safely performed for either the recipient who survived eight years, but also, for the donor (Fig. 8) who recently died at the age of 79 years (Murray, 2011)[6]. Following that attempt, other 19 twin transplantations were successfully performed until 1956 with a 30% recurrence rate of chronic glomerulonephritis (CGN). At that time, the principal ingredients of organ transplantation - immunosuppression, tissue matching, organ procurement and preservation - were still unknown or undeveloped. Therefore, the failure of all other types of grafts, usually resulting in the death of the patient, left little room for optimism (Groth & Longmire, 2000)[7].

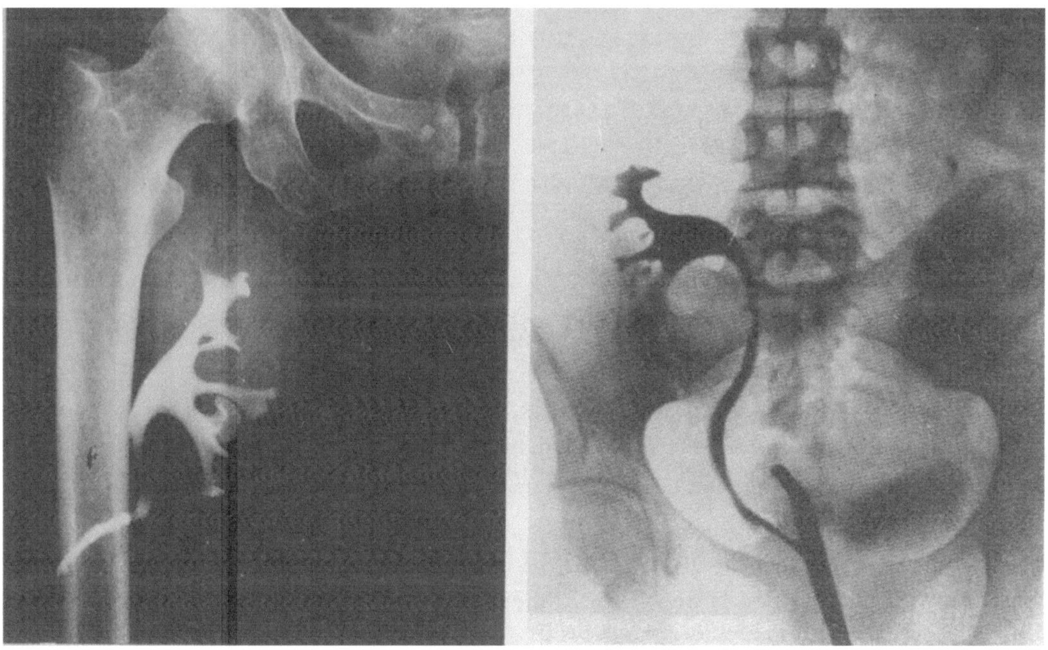

a. b.

(Küss & Bourget, 1992)[1].

Fig. 6. Surgical techniques for kidneys implantation. a. The groin technique (Voronoy). b. The French technique

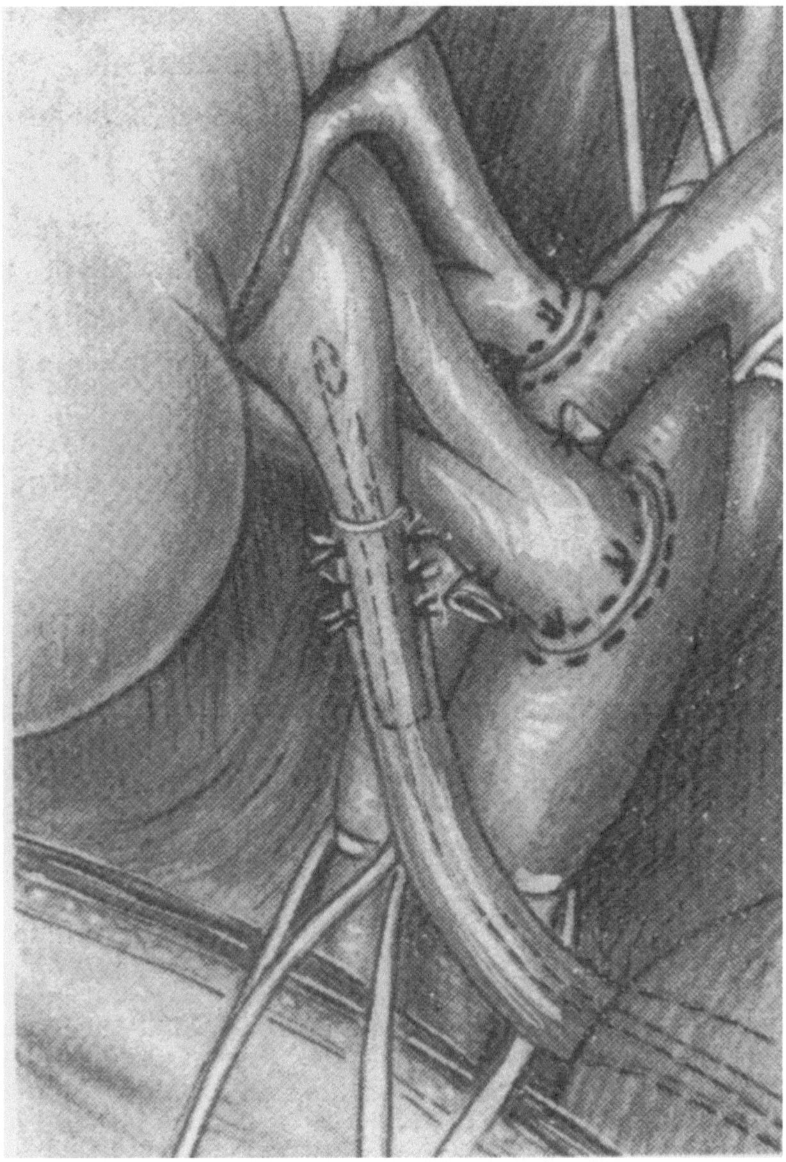

(Küss & Bourget, 1992) [1].
Fig. 7. The French technique used for transplanting Mr. Marius Renard at Necker Hospital (1952).

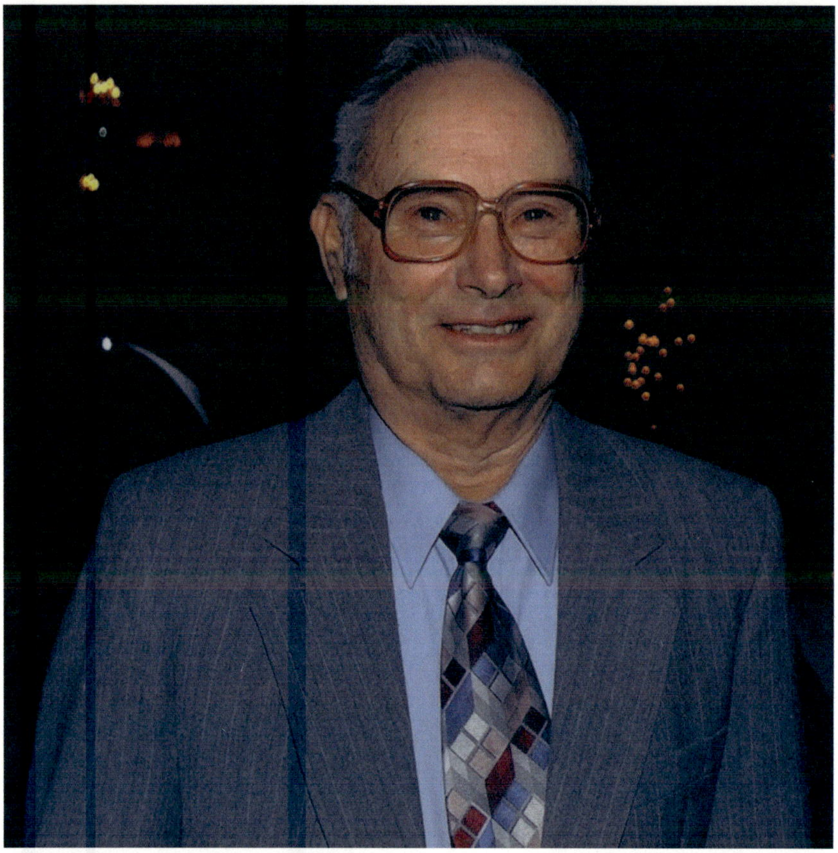

Fig. 8. Ronald Lee Herrick: first living donor for his twin brother, in December 1954 (Murray, 2011) [6].

3. Organ procurement and preservation

The sudden arrival of clinical kidney transplantation during 1962-1963 was so unexpected that little collateral research on the preservation of organs had been done. Kidney transplantation was accomplished at first with total body hypothermia of living volunteer kidney donors using methods developed by cardiac surgeons for open heart operations. In the experimental laboratory, Lillehei et al. simply immersed excised intestine and pancreas in iced saline before its autotransplantation. Thus the principle of hypothermia was understood at an early time, although not efficiently applied (Squifflet et al., 2008)[9].

Today, intravascular cooling is the first step in the preservation of all whole organ grafts. The practice was introduced in 1963 of infusing chilled lactated Ringer's or low-molecular-weight dextran solutions into the renal artery of kidney grafts immediately after their removal. By late 1981, however, it had become obvious that pancreas, liver and thoracic organ transplant procedures were going to be widely used. Methods of multiple organ procurement were required by which the kidneys, pancreas, liver, heart and lungs or various combinations of these organs could be removed without jeopardizing any of the individual organs (Squifflet et al., 1990)[10]. With these methods, all organs to be transplanted are cooled in situ, rapidly removed in a bloodless field, and dissected on a back table (Fig.

9). Fluids of differing osmotic, oncotic, and electrolyte composition are infused into the allografts before placing them in a refrigerated container. The solution described by Collins et al. or modifications of it (Eurocollins®) were used for almost two decades. Renal allograft preservation was feasible for 1 to 2 days, long enough to allow tissue matching and sharing of organs over a wide geographic area (Squifflet et al., 1981)[8]. The introduction of the University of Wisconsin (UW) solution to pancreas, firstly, and then, liver transplantation in 1988 by Belzer, Jamieson and Kalayoglu was the first major development in static preservation since the Collins solution. The superiority of the UW solution for preservation of kidneys and other organs was promptly demonstrated and confirmed in clinical trials.

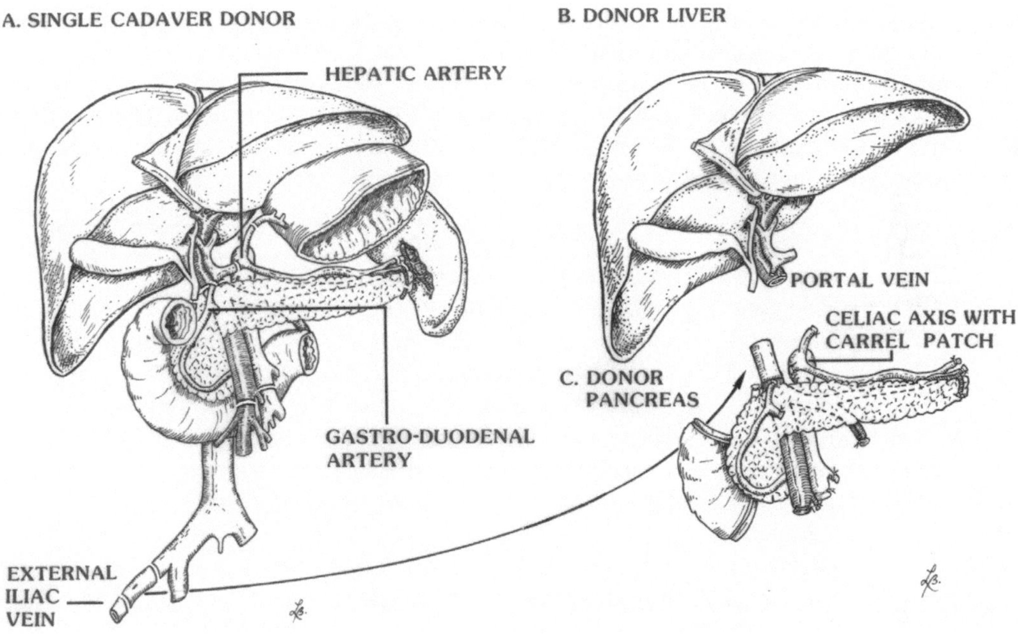

Fig. 9. Maneuvers for en-bloc removal of a whole pancreas and a liver from a cadaver donor with normal vascular anatomy. The gastroduodenal artery must be divided so that the common and proper hepatic arteries can remain in continuity and be retained with the liver. The portal vein is divided just superior to the entrance of the splenic vein. Then, the pancreatic portion is lengthened by an iliac vein graft. The celiac and superior mesenteric arteries can remain with the pancreas with a Carrel aortic patch (Squifflet et al., 1990)[10].

The ex-vivo perfusion technique also permitted good preservation of kidney or liver allografts. However, the complexity of the method precluded its general use. Thus, it was firstly abandoned in most European kidney transplant centers. A renewal of interest in the perfusion technique resulted from the lack of brain-dead cadaveric donors and the search for other sources such as the non-heart beating donors, or extended criteria donors (ECD). In these types of DCD kidneys, agonic ischemic damages are happening. They could be evaluated by a period of re-conditioning on machine perfusion prior to implantation (Moers et al., 2009)[11].

4. The concept of immunosuppression and need for pharmacological agents in transplantation

After Medawar's demonstration in 1944 that rejection was an immunological event, a logical and inevitable question was how to protect the organ allograft by weakening the immune system (Table 2).

Firstly Owen, Medawar and Billingham discovered the phenomena of neonatal tolerance, demonstrating that it was possible to prevent immune responses to allo-antigens. Secondly, works by Dausset and others (Payne, Van Rood, Bodmer, Amos, Ceppellini, Terasaki, Bach and Batchelor) defined what allo-antigens were, namely the major histocompatibility complex (MHC), which in humans is called HLA. Finally, an explosion of information about how the immune system works and further studies on the MHC have led to the concept of tissue typing, histocompatibility and cross-matching. Studies in the early 1960s defined the function of lymphocytes and identified separate roles for T cells (cellular immunity) and B cells (humoral immunity). The T cell receptor and immunoglobulins were discovered, and the role of HLA proteins in presenting antigens to T cells was elucidated (Turka, 2001)[12] (Halloran & Gourishankar, 2001)[13]. Thus, to interfere with that complex reaction, pharmacological agents were introduced for controlling rejection.

Year	Author	Discovery or application
1901	Landsteiner	Discovery of ABO blood groups
1944	Medawar	Rejection as an immunological event
1952	Dausset	Discovered first HLA antigens using antiserum from
1958	Van Rood	transfused patients
1964	Starzl	Demonstrated HLA antibodies in pregnant women
1964	Terasaki	Hyper-acute rejection of ABO-incompatible kidneys
1964	Bach	Description of microcytoxicity test
1966	Terasaki	Described mixed lymphocyte culture test
	Kissmeyer-	
	Nielsen	Hyper-acute kidney rejection with antigraft
1967	Van Rood	lymphocytotoxic antibodies
		First international organ exchange organization (Eurotransplant)

Table 2. A timeline in tissue matching and transplant immunology.

Based upon the demonstration in 1950 that inflammatory diseases could be treated by adrenal steroids, it was natural to apply glucocorticoids to prevent or reserve the severe inflammation of graft rejection.

By the late 1950s, the first attempts to use whole body irradiation to prolong transplant survival were also reported (Halloran & Gourishankar, 2001)[13]. But the real IS options that would allow for successful cadaveric transplantation emerged at the end of the 1950s. During that period, Elion and Hitchings developed 6-mercapto-purine (6-MP) and azathioprine (AZA) (Table 3). By the early 1960s, the practice of using glucocorticoids in conjunction with AZA had been initiated with high-dose steroid used to reverse rejection. The first application of antilymphocyte globulin (ALG) took place in the 1960s. Efforts at immune cell depletion included thoracic duct drainage, irradiation, thymectomy and splenectomy.

In 1963, during a first International Transplantation Congress in Washington, 244 renal allografts were reported. Among them, 28 identical twin transplants. Starlz reported also the first three attempts at orthotopic liver transplantation in humans as well as 25 over 27 successful renal transplantations using 6-MP (Table 1).
With the emerging IS therapy, it was also a period in which attempts of xenografting took place and quickly abandoned.
By the late 1970s, the centers that had access to ALG were reporting improved survival rates in kidney transplantation. However, many patients experienced severe steroid side effects. Graft survival remained poor and only kidney transplants were performed in significant numbers with good success (Squifflet et al. 1981)[8].
The discovery of cyclosporine (CsA) and its first clinical use in 1978 changed transplantation. Results also improved with widespread access to effective ALG - polyclonal antibodies (Ab) therapy and later with the first monoclonal Ab therapy muromonab-CD3 - , which can reduce reliance on high-dose steroids. Many improvements in medical, surgical, anesthetic, and intensive care management improved clinical results. The growth in transplanting hearts, livers, pancreases and lungs, has created the transplantation programs of the present day. CsA, which blocks the transcriptional activation of IL-2 and others cytokines in T cells, made a significant contribution to the basic science of T cell activation.
Tacrolimus (Tac) differed from other drugs in that much that its early development occurred in liver transplants, rather than in kidneys. Acting by the same mechanism as CsA, Tac binds to abundant intracellular protein to create a complex that inhibits the enzyme calcineurin. By the late 1980s, Tac was introduced for use in organ transplants. Today, it is the most common and largely used IS drug.
Mycophenolate mofetil (MMF) is an agent derived from the older drug, mycophenolic acid, which is a potent inhibitor of de novo purine synthesis in lymphocytes and highly effective in combination with CsA and Tac in preventing acute rejection in humans.
Rapamycin (or Sirolimus-Sir) had been discovered in the 1970s as an antifungal, but the potential of its IS properties for commercial development was not recognized until the late 1980s. Large-scale trials have demonstrated its potential and have led to its recent approval for use in kidney transplantation (Table 3).

Year	Immunosuppressive milestones
1950	Glucocorticoid therapy in immune diseases
1959	6-mercaptopurine and azathioprine (AZA)
1968	Polyclonal antilymphocyte globulin (ALG)
1978	First clinical use of cyclosporine (CsA)
1981	Introduction of murine monoclonal anti-CD3 to reverse rejection
1989	First clinical results with tacrolimus (Tac)
1991	First report of clinical use of mycophenolate mofetil (MMF)
1998	First report of clinical use of rapamycin (Sirolimus-Sir)

Table 3. A timeline in transplant immunosuppression.

As the third millennium begins, new humanized or chimeric protein products are becoming available (anti-Il2 receptors; anti-CD2; anti-CTL4 Ig; anti-CD3; anti-CD40 ligand; …). Gene therapy and new classes of agents such as FTY720, FK778, peptides and antisense oligonucleotides are currently being evaluated to determine their potential. The new priority is reduction in toxicity with equivalent efficacy. However, immunosuppression would be tailored by better laboratory measurements of the immunological status, ischemic reperfusion injuries, and stability (Halloran & Gourishankar, 2001)[13].

5. The history of Deceased Donor (DCD) transplantation in Belgium

5.1. The first cadaver – Heart Beating Donor (HBD) – kidney transplant in Belgium

In 1962, Professor G.P.J. Alexandre obtained a fellowship for a year of surgical research to be spent in the laboratory of the Harvard Medical School in Boston, under the direction of Professor Joseph Murray, in the Department of Surgery of the Peter Bent Brigham Hospital directed by Professor Francis D. Moore (Squifflet, 2003)[14]. His initial U.S. contact in Boston was with Professor Roy Calne who was packing to return to England, in whom he put his trust to look at the surviving dogs from his experiments. The dogs were receiving the BW - 57322 - the actual Azathioprine (AZA) - as well as other drug combinations including Azaserine and Actinomycin D. The later drug combination was considered good enough to be used in clinical practice (Fig. 10).

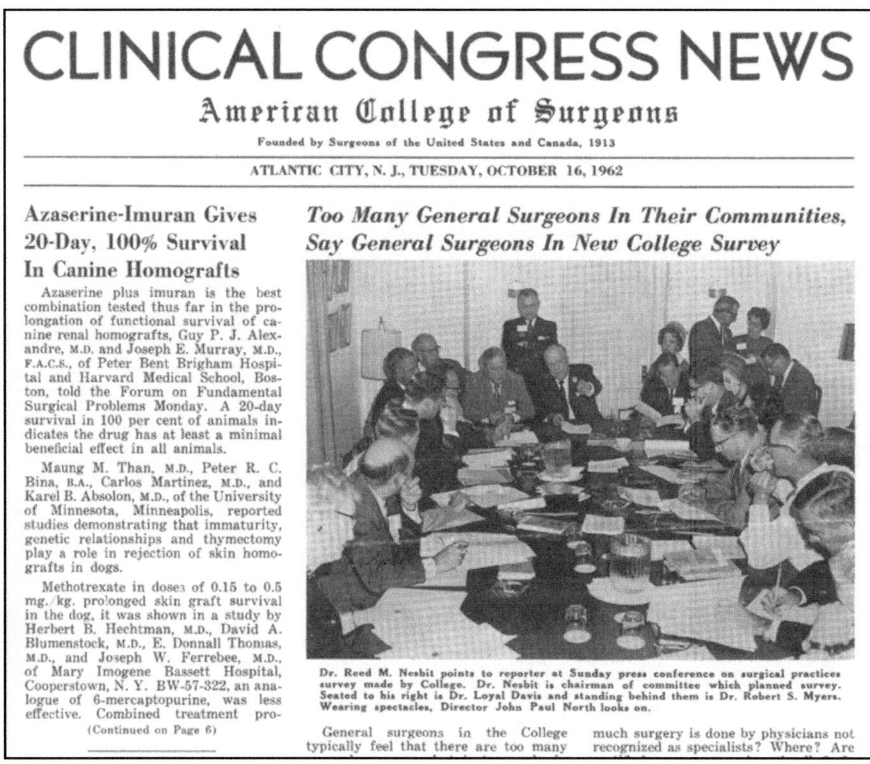

CLINICAL CONGRESS NEWS

American College of Surgeons

Founded by Surgeons of the United States and Canada, 1913

ATLANTIC CITY, N. J., TUESDAY, OCTOBER 16, 1962

Azaserine-Imuran Gives 20-Day, 100% Survival In Canine Homografts

Azaserine plus imuran is the best combination tested thus far in the prolongation of functional survival of canine renal homografts, Guy P. J. Alexandre, M.D. and Joseph E. Murray, M.D., F.A.C.S., of Peter Bent Brigham Hospital and Harvard Medical School, Boston, told the Forum on Fundamental Surgical Problems Monday. A 20-day survival in 100 per cent of animals indicates the drug has at least a minimal beneficial effect in all animals.

Maung M. Than, M.D., Peter R. C. Bina, B.A., Carlos Martinez, M.D., and Karel B. Absolon, M.D., of the University of Minnesota, Minneapolis, reported studies demonstrating that immaturity, genetic relationships and thymectomy play a role in rejection of skin homografts in dogs.

Methotrexate in doses of 0.15 to 0.5 mg./kg. prolonged skin graft survival in the dog, it was shown in a study by Herbert B. Hechtman, M.D., David A. Blumenstock, M.D., E. Donnall Thomas, M.D., and Joseph W. Ferrebee, M.D., of Mary Imogene Bassett Hospital, Cooperstown, N. Y. BW-57-322, an analogue of 6-mercaptopurine, was less effective. Combined treatment pro-

(Continued on Page 6)

Too Many General Surgeons In Their Communities, Say General Surgeons In New College Survey

Dr. Reed M. Nesbit points to reporter at Sunday press conference on surgical practices survey made by College. Dr. Nesbit is chairman of committee which planned survey. Seated to his right is Dr. Loyal Davis and standing behind them is Dr. Robert S. Myers. Wearing spectacles, Director John Paul North looks on.

General surgeons in the College typically feel that there are too many

much surgery is done by physicians not recognized as specialists? Where? Are

Fig. 10. Proceedings of the Meeting of the American College of Surgeons, Atlantic City, October 16, 1962.

Azathioprine plus Imuran is the best combination tested; a 20-day survival in 100% of animals. Therefore, Professor G.P.J. Alexandre returned to Belgium with both drugs in his luggage. Since no chronic dialysis apparatus was available in the Department of Surgery at Saint Pierre Hospital in Louvain where Professor G.P.J. Alexandre was completing his surgical

training, first candidates for renal transplantation were maintained on peritoneal dialysis, performed by medical students on a voluntary basis, in 24-hour rotation.
On June 3, 1963, a patient was brought in the Emergency Department with a head injury and a profound coma. Despite active resuscitation and vasopressive drugs administration, the patient presented all the signs of what Mollaret had previously described and named "coma dépassé" (Mollaret & Goulon)[15]. Professor Jean Morelle, who was the Chief of the Department of Surgery and also experienced in neurosurgery, took the most important decision of his career: to remove a kidney from that patient while the heart was still beating. Moreover, and by contrast to Professor Hamburger's donor management (Legendre & Kreis, 2010)[16], they stopped the mechanical ventilation, immediately after kidney procurement, waiting for the heart beat stop in the OR. No preservation fluid was used; the blood contained in the transplant was not even washed away; the graft functioned immediately without any tubular necrosis (Delayed Graft Function) and the patient's serum creatinine normalized in a few days. The patient died on day 87 from sepsis; at that time of death, three other patients had been transplanted with that effective drug IS regimen. The third patient was transplanted with a living donor kidney (patient's uncle) while the fourth, with a cadaver kidney: both had long term function, more than six years. In this way the kidney transplant program of Professor Alexandre was launched. From then on, the number of transplants performed annually has increased progressively and reached a mean stable number of 100 transplants per year in 1978 when the Department moved to Unit 22 of the Clinic Saint-Luc in Brussels and Professor Jean-Paul Squifflet joined the team. Professor Alexandre left in January 1992 while Professor Squifflet moved to Liege, CHU Sart Tilman in October 2005. From 1963 to 2005, during 42 years, 3.355 renal transplants have been performed (Table 4 and Table 5) (Squifflet J.P., 2007)[17].

Organ	First transplant	Number	
		Total	Live donor
Kidney (Total)	June 3, 1963	3.355	501
Kidney + liver	February 2, 1987	23	
Kidney + heart	February 23, 1986	8	
Pancreas (Total)	November 10, 1982	89	
Pancreas + kidney (SPK)	November 10, 1982	83 (in 82 recipients)	
Pancreas alone (PTA)	February 5, 1983	3	
Pancreas + liver	September 22, 1988	1	
Pancreas after liver	April 4, 1998	1	
Pancreas after failed Kd (SPK)	May 11, 1999	1	
(Islets after kidney)	(October 13, 2002)	(2)	

(Squifflet J.P., 2007)[17].
Table 4. Total number of Organ (Kidney and Pancreas) Transplantations at Saint Pierre Hospital in Louvain (June 3, 1963 to October 30, 1977) and Saint-Luc Hospital in Brussels (November 1, 1977 to September 30, 2005) by G.P.J. Alexandre (June 1963 to October 1991) and J.P. Squifflet (January 1978 to September 30, 2005)

Year	Application
June 3, 1963	First cadaver kidney transplant First heart beating donor First use of AZA and steroids
August 24, 1963	First living related donor renal transplant
January 20, 1965	First haemodialysis
January 20, 1966	First living unrelated donor renal transplant with thoracic duct
June 10, 1966	drainage preparation
1967	First birth of baby from mother kidney recipient
November 8,	Creation of Eurotransplant Foundation
1967	Use of home-made ALG (antilymphocytic globulins) for rejection
March 31, 1971	treatment
September 1976	First pediatric kidney transplantation
November 1977	Use of Eurocollins solution for kidney preservation
January 1978	Move from Saint Pierre Hospital in Louvain to Unit 22 Saint-Luc
	Hospital in Brussels
June 30, 1978	Induction therapy with ALG vs ATGAM
October 1982	AZA and steroids
November 10,	First ABO-incompatible living related donor transplantation
1982	Introduction of cyclosporine A (CsA)
February 5, 1983	First simultaneous kidney and pancreas transplantation in Belgium
March 1985	First pancreas transplant alone in Belgium
March 1985	Introduction of OKT3 for treating acute rejections
February 23,	Honoris Causa: Professor D.E.R. Sutherland, Professor T. Starzl,
1986	Professor J. Van Rood
June 13, 1986	First simultaneous heart and kidney transplantation
February 2, 1987	Belgian law on organ donation and transplantation (presumed
	consent)
July 15, 1987	First simultaneous liver and kidney transplantation
November 7,	Birth of (the 3rd world) baby girl after SPK transplantation
1989	Introduction of bone marrow infusion after kidney transplantation
September 23,	Introduction of deoxyspergualin in kidney transplantation

1992	First use of LoCD2a/BTI-322/MEDI-507 monoclonal Ab in a human
October 12, 1993	kidney recipient
October 18, 1993	Introduction of mycophenolate mofetil (MMF) in kidney
February 17,	transplantation
1997	Introduction of tacrolimus (Tac) in kidney transplantation
March 2, 1997	First video assisted live donor nephrectomy in Belgium
January 1998	Introduction of sirolimus (Sir) in kidney transplantation
December 1998	Start of the EURO-SPK 001 trial
January 31, 2001	Implementation of N.H.B.D. program
June 25, 2001	Introduction of FTY 720 in kidney transplantation
January 2002	Introduction of FK 778 in kidney transplantation
October 13, 2002	Start of the EURO-SPK 002 trial
	First human islet grafting

Table 5. A timeline of the kidney and pancreas transplantation Program at Saint Pierre Hospital in Louvain (June 3, 1963 to October 30, 1977) and Saint-Luc Hospital in Brussels (November 1, 1977 to September 30, 2005) by G.P.J. Alexandre (June 1963 to October 1991) and J.P. Squifflet (January 1978 to September 30, 2005).

5.2 From the brain death concept to the Belgian law on organ donation and transplantation

In November 1957, Pope Pius XII released an important statement for the Catholic Church: he defined death as the "*complete and definitive separation of the soul and the body*" and distinguished "*human life from the mere life of the organs*". He stated also that a Christian "*has to accept the necessary treatments to preserve life and health*" but that "*usually this duty…requires only the use of ordinary means*". The Pope declared furthermore that the treatment of a patient in deep coma without any hope of recovery may be stopped even if this provokes cardiac arrest: "*the interruption of resuscitation attempts is only indirectly the cause of cessation of life*". For deciding when exactly the soul leaves the body, if it is when the brain is destroyed or when the heart stops beating, the Pontiff avoided to answer the question: "*the answer cannot inferred from any religious or moral principle and from that angle is not within the competence of the church*". On the contrary, he charged the clinicians "*to give a clear and precise definition of death and the moment of death of a patient who dies in a state of unconsciousness*" (Kinnaert, 2009)[18]. It was also the period during which Mollaret and Goulon proposed the term "coma dépassé" to describe the absence and complete destruction of cerebral functions in order to stop prolonging futile resuscitation (Mollaret & Goulon, 1959)[15]. Even if the concept was admitted in the transplant community, most of the surgeons were waiting for the heart beat stop before starting the procurement (Legendre & Kreis, 2010)[16]. The further step, taken by Professor Alexandre, in disconnecting the body in the OR after the kidney procurement was eventually more difficult to accept. Indeed, even T. Starzl who had performed the first cadaver liver transplantations in 1963 did not apply it before his participation to the Ciba symposium in London in 1966 on Ethics in Medical Progress (Squifflet 2003)[3] (Kinnaert, 2009)[18], (Ethics in Medical progress, 1966)[19]. The discussions he had with Professor Alexandre illustrate well all doubts that people had during that period.

Alexandre:"*Dr. Gierts spoke about taking organs from a dying person. I would like to make it clear that, in my opinion, there has never been and there never will be any question of taking organs from a dying person who has "non reasonable chance of getting better or resuming consciousness". The question is of taking organs from a dead person, and the point is that I do not accept the cessation of heart beats as the indication of death. We are as much concerned with the preservation of life in a dying person as with the preservation of life in a fœtus: but I think irreversible damage to the central nervous system is an indication of physiological death that permits us to take an organ from a body that is already a cadaver.*"

Starzl: "*Dr. Giertz has drawn a distinction between the Stockholm case and the practice in Belgium which seems to me to be largely quantitative. I assume that when kidneys are removed from "living cadavers" in Louvain, only one organ is removed, so that the patient is not thereby killed. How long did your patients continue to be heart-lung preparations, Dr. Alexandre? Were there any specific differences in the subsequent care of your cases and of the Stockholm patient? The Swedish patient continued to be on the respirator after the kidney was removed. If, in your practice, the respirators is turned off immediately after the kidney is removed this could very easily explain the different survival times of less than one hour in Belgium, and 48 hours in Stockholm.*"

Alexandre: "*In our nine cases we switched off the respirator immediately after the kidneys were removed. The heart beats of all the patients ceased within two or three minutes. In my opinion it is irrelevant whether a heart-lung preparation goes on for two days or even for weeks: it is still a heart-lung preparation and for us it is still a dead person.*"

Starzl: "*The notion of permitting removal of our organs while we still have a circulation is an important one. Personally I would agree to this for myself, but I could not permit this to be done to a member of my family.*"

Nevertheless, that example was followed by other teams in Belgium and in most countries. In 1968, the French Heath Authorities published the "circulaire Jeanneney" following the Ad Hoc Committee of the Harvard School of Medecine (Ad Hoc Communitie, 1968)[20]. It opened the door for the first world pancreas transplantation by Kelley and Lillehei (1966), the first heart transplantation by Christian Barnard (1967) and the first heart transplantation in France by Cabrol (1968).

In Belgium, the first lung transplantation was performed by Fritz Derom (1968), the first adult liver transplantation by P.J. Kestens (1969) and soon later (1970) in children by J.B. Otte, the first heart transplantation by G. Primo (1973) and the first pancreas transplantation by J.P. Squifflet (1982).

Finally, the Belgian Transplantation community had to wait until June 1986 to get a law on Organ Donation and Transplantation. It includes an opting out system. Indeed, the transplant surgeon cannot start any organ procurement if the donor has expressed opposition at the National Registry, or if opposition is communicated in any way to the surgeon. Until 2007, it has been a soft version of the presumed consent principle because a first degree relative could oppose the procurement. A new step was taken in 2007 by suppressing this possibility and therefore turning the presumed consent principle into a strong version. Other important elements of the Belgian Act are that death is not defined – it could be brain death or cardiac death – but must be reported by 3 physicians and violent death must be also reported to the Public prosecutor (Squifflet A.C., 2011)[21]. Like other

European countries with presumed consent laws, Belgium was, in 2007 - and is still - , one of the leading countries for Multiple Organ Donors, with 27.5 cadaver donors by million inhabitants (pmi) and 86.5 cadaver organ transplants pmi (43.0 kidneys; 22.7 livers; 8.7 lungs; 6.7 hearts; 5.3 pancreases/islets). As others, Belgium is also facing challenges such as aging donors, the use of extended criteria donors (ECD) and donors with cerebral bleeding as the main cause of death (Fig. 11) (Roels & Rahmel, 2011) [22]. That's why the Eurotransplant (ET) organization had developed its ET Senior Program (ESP) and the use of non-heart beating donors (NHBD), the so-called deceased after cardiac death donors (DCD) by opposition to the brain death donors (DBD).

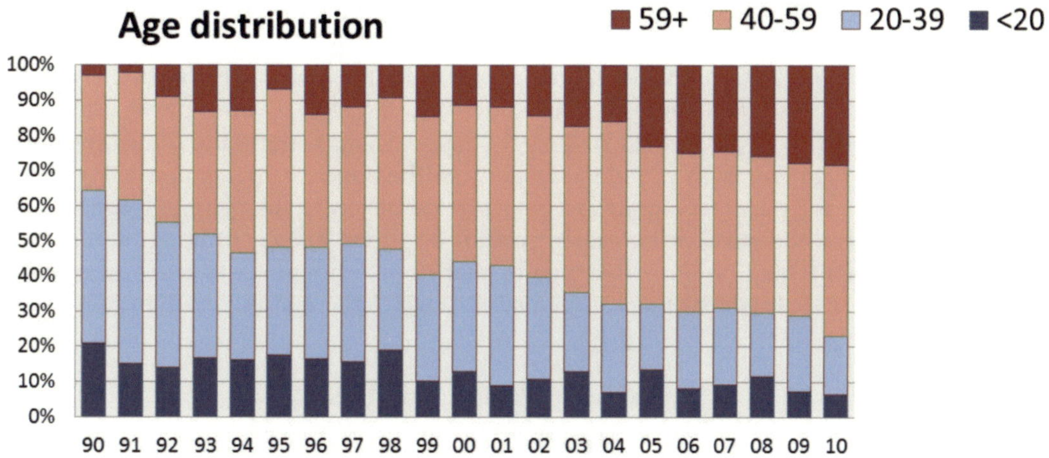

Average age 2010 effective donors: 50 yrs.
Youngest donor: 1 year - Oldest donor: 89 years.
46% women/54% men in 2010.

Fig. 11. Age distribution of (effective) donors between 1990 and 2010 in Belgium.

5.3 The first cadaver pancreas transplant in Belgium

Professor J.P. Squifflet joined Professor G.P.J. Alexandre staff in 1978. After a research fellowship in transplantation at the University of Minnesota in Professor J.S. Najarian department, under Professor D.E.R. Sutherland's supervision, he started a program in pancreatic transplantation in Brussels and performed the first Belgian simultaneous pancreas and kidney transplantation (SPK) in November 10, 1986 (Tables 4 and 5). The women recipient was also one of the first who received cyclosporine A (CsA) as the basic drug in the IS regimen. CsA was used at the dose of 14 mg/kg/day, considered today as a toxic dosage but also in combination with low doses of steroids. The second pancreas transplant was a segmental pancreas transplant alone (PTA). It was performed on a diabetic recipient with pre-end-stage renal failure, in January 1983. Unfortunately, it never functioned due to ischemic damage, pancreatitis and vascular thrombosis. It was promptly removed. By contrast, the first patient rapidly recovered from her double operation; that led to a series of 10 SPK procedures in 10 patients using a segment of pancreas anastomosed to a Roux-en-Y loop. SPK patient number 9 was transplanted in January 86 after chronic rejection of a first cadaver kidney graft. One year later, she delivered a baby girl: she was the third woman ever in the world to enjoy a successful pregnancy after pancreas transplantation. Despite her nephrologist's "disapprobation" she gave birth to a second baby boy in December 1990.

On September 22, 1989, with Professor B. de Hemptinne, J.P. Squifflet performed the first simultaneous liver and pancreas transplant on a 34-years-old man with a type 1 diabetes and a cryptogenic liver cirrhosis. One year later, the patient was back on insulin therapy with a well functioning liver graft. He asked for a second cadaveric pancreas graft that he received on April 4, 1998. Unfortunately, it stopped functioning after several months. A high level of anti-islet antibodies was demonstrated, confirming the recurrence of the type 1 diabetes auto-immune disease (Squifflet, 2007)[17].

The human islet program started in October 2002. The program benefited from the Edmonton experience but it did not succeed in reaching insulin independency with only one pancreatic organ for islet preparation. Therefore that activity remained marginal.

While moving the pancreas transplantation program to the University of Liege, a new surgical technique was implemented (De Roover et al., 2007)[23] and developed with mechanical sutures (De Roover et al., 2008)[24]. It consists in implanting the whole pancreas with a duodenal segment, with portal drainage (into the superior mesenteric vein) of the venous effluent of the pancreatic graft and exocrine diversion to the recipient duodenum. The latero-lateral duodeno-duodenostomy could be done using running sutures or mechanical staplers (Fig. 12). The advantage of that new technique is to allow pancreatic graft monitoring, and duodenal mucosa biopsy through serial endoscopy (Squifflet et al., 2008)[11].

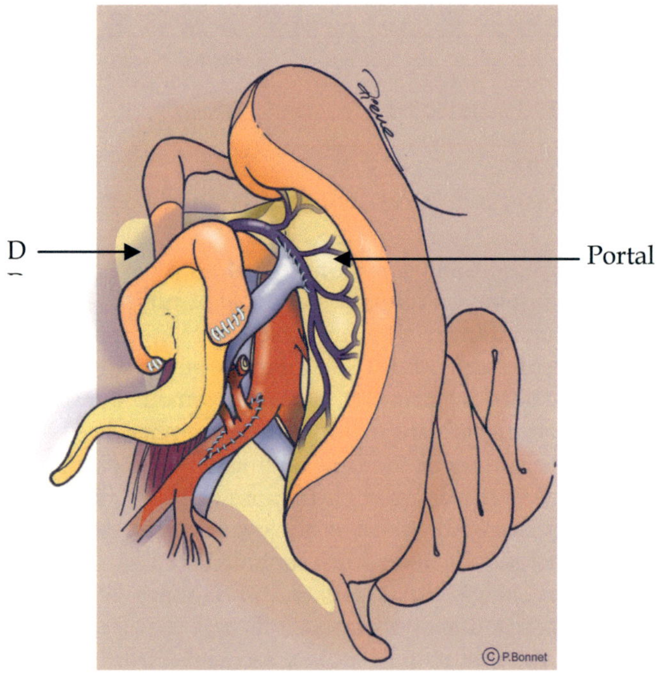

DD: latero-lateral duodeno-duodenal anastomosis.

Portal: portal venous drainage in superior mesenteric vein (De Roover et al., 2007)[23].

Fig. 12. Whole pancreas transplantation technique with enteric drainage and portal drainage.

5.4 Current challenges in Donation after Cardiac Death (DCD)

Like in Austria and Spain which have a huge activity in DBD organ procurement, in Belgium it took almost 40 years to start with DCD organ procurement (Squifflet, 2006)[25]. The main reasons are multiple.

In 1995, the first international workshop on DCD - during that period, one was speaking of Non-Heart-Beating Donors (NHBD) - took place in Maastricht (The Netherlands) where the 4 categories of DCD were defined and published with 12 statements and recommendations (Kootstra et al., 1995)[26]. That was eventually approved by the European Council.

"1. The fact that NHBD organs have to be considered for transplantation is a direct result of the shortage of donor organs in view of the fact that the waiting list continues to increase. The use of NHBD organs can be valuable way to enlarge the number of organs for transplantation.

2. Only sparse data are available on the potential number of NHBDs and the cost of the procedure. More information should be collected to evaluate the efficiency of the procedure.

3. The concept of NHBD is evolving. Therefore, it is important to show that the results are good. Inclusion of NHBD data in registries is necessary.

4. For flush out and preservation methods, one should use solutions that are state of the art. Machine perfusion for kidneys should be considered.

5. No NHBD program should be started without a written protocol approved by the local medical ethical committee.

6. For better understanding and consistency, future reports on analysis concerning procurement and transplantation of NHBD organs should refer to the "Maastricht Categories".

I	*dead on arrival*
II	*unsuccessful resuscitation*
III	*awaiting cardiac arrest*
IV	*cardiac arrest in a brain-dead donor*

7. Category II and III NHBD procedure should only be started 10 minutes after cessation of cardiac massage and artificial ventilation to ensure the "dead-donor rule".

8. Warm ischemia time in NHBDs should be counted from the moment of cardiac arrest until the start of hypothermic flush out, irrespective of the period of cardiopulmonary resuscitation.

9. Better methods for viability testing of NHBD organs should be developed.

10. As in HBD procedures, the diagnosis of death in a NHBD has to me made by (a) physician (s) independent of the procurement team.

11. Public education and openness concerning NHBD are mandatory to keep public trust and to prevent backfiring on the HBD programs.

12. Opting-out or presumed consent systems allow placement of a preservation device before contact with the family. In countries with opting-in legislation, legal approval for placement of such devices should be sought."

Between 1995 and 2003, the Belgian National Council of Physicians established rules for implementing the DCD program according to the local law. Moreover, all 7 transplant centers had to get a formal approval from their own local Ethical Committee.

Finally, it was obvious that such a DCD program could not start without having access to machine perfusion for kidney preservation and re-conditioning. With the help of ET, a large international multicentric study was set up, comparing cold storage and machine perfusion for kidney preservation. In brief, the study demonstrated that 1 year kidney graft survival was 12% higher in recipient of a machine perfused graft which presented a PO delayed graft function (DGF) compared to recipients of a cold storage preserved graft. The length of DGF was also significantly shorter as well as the time for GFR recovery (Moers et al., 2009)[13] (Jochmans et al., 2010)[27]. That study helped the Belgian Centers to implement the use of DCD without jeopardizing the DBD procurement rate (Fig. 13).

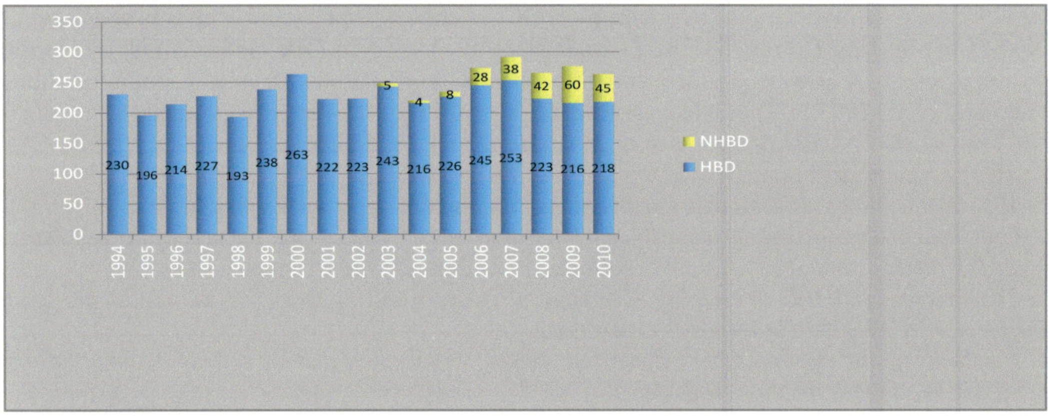

Fig. 13. Effective donor number in Belgium between 1994-2010.
In 2009: 44% University Hospitals - 56% collaborative Hospitals.

At the University of Liege (Le Dinh et al., 2011)[28], the use of DCD had as consequence to double the number of donors (Fig. 14 a), to double the number of kidney transplants (Fig. 14 b), and to 1 ½ time increase the number of liver transplants (Fig. 14 c). But it remains several issues to be solved.

5.4.1 The length of the « no touch » period

The Maastricht statement/recommendation n°7 is proposing a 10 min no-touch period after cessation of cardiac massage for Categories II and III. Indeed Category IV does not need a no-touch period as the cardiac arrest is occurring in a DBD. By contrast, 10 min might be too long if one considers that in categories II and III, the brain has already suffered from irreversible injuries. Then, the Pittsburgh School of Medicine protocol proposes a 2 min waiting time (Institute of Medicine, 1997)[29]. Today, there is a national consensus between all Belgian Centers to declare that a no-touch period of 5 minutes could be enough, but it has not been formally set up yet.

5.4.2 The comfort therapy

Even if intensivists are respecting and protecting all dying patients, they agree to avoid futile sufferances while accompanying the patient in his agonic phase. By contrast, others (Feng S., 2010)[30] think that obstacle against administration of drugs could be the logistics of individual and institutional informed consent for the donor and the potential organ recipients. For the above reason, most intensivists are administering what they call a comfort therapy, while withdrawing the unnecessary support. Therefore improved education of health care professionals and providers on the early recognition and special needs of this DCD population i.e. comfort therapy and implementation of clinical protocol should improve the yield of transplantable organs. Aggressive donor protocols will include early aggressive clinical management of DCD donors including comfort therapy. It requires the help of dedicated health care specialists.

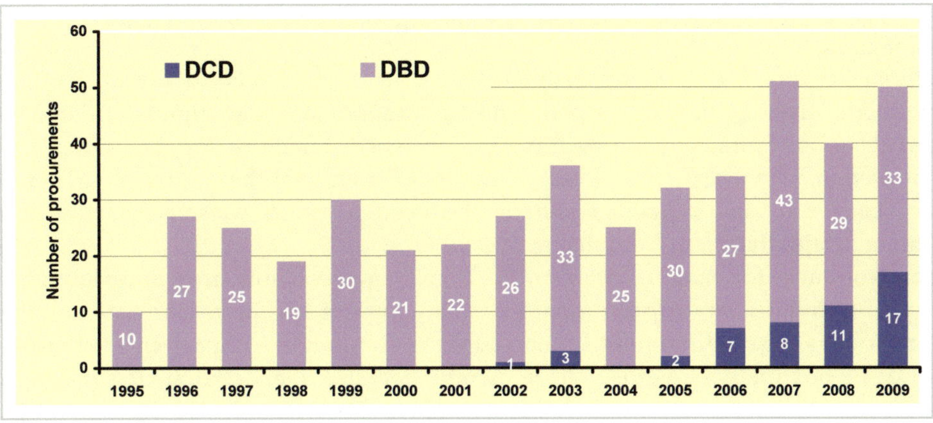

Fig. 14a

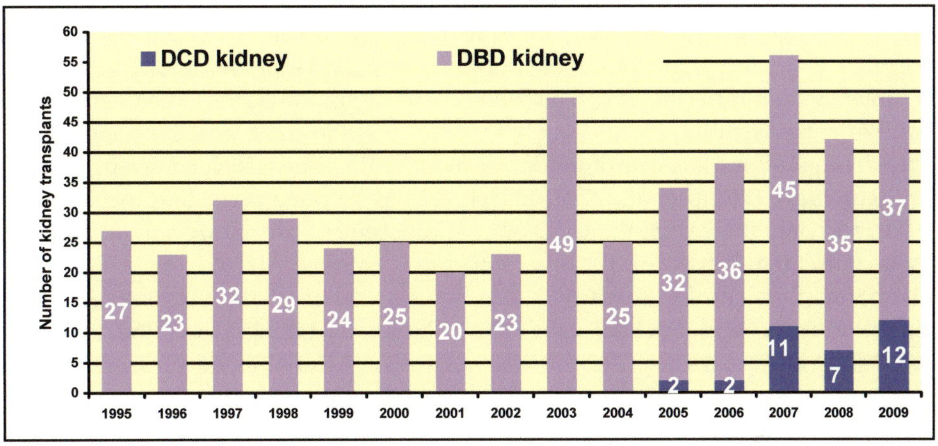

Fig. 14b

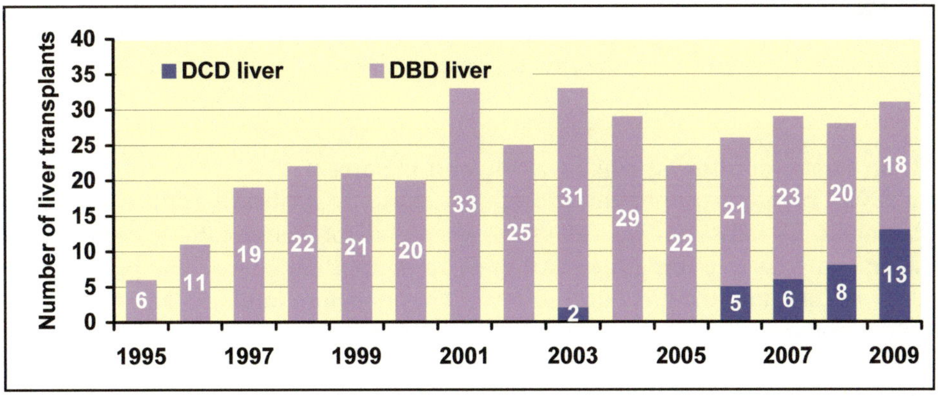

Fig. 14c

Fig. 14. Proportion of DCD/DBD donors (a), kidney (b) and liver (c) transplantations between 1995 and 2009 at the University of Liege (Hieu et al, 2011)[28].

5.4.3 The DCD management: Monitoring awaiting cardiac arrest and drug administration

Unfortunately, today DCD management varies from hospitals to organ procurement organizations, from physicians, nurses, administration and institutional review boards along with donor families (Feng S., 2010)[30]. It is worth remembering that donors are not concentrated in a few hospitals but rather scattered throughout the community. Therefore, a primary barrier to donor management is the need to reach consensus across a broad coalition of parties that stem from distinctive spheres.

A second obstacle for making uniform DCD management and drug intervention is the logistics of individual and institutional informed consent for the donor and the potential organ recipients. The definition of human subjects does not encompass DCD after they are legally dead but there is a grey shade period between the decision of stopping futile reanimation with family consent and the recognition of cardiac death, during which DCD management with drug administration takes an important place. That should require the intervention of independent well trained teams working according to ethical consensus and guidelines. The decision of stopping futile reanimation should be taken by 3 physicians, knowing that a small proportion of patients in a vegetative or minimally conscious state have brain activation reflecting some awareness and cognition. Careful clinical examination will result in reclassification of the state of consciousness in some of these patients, in order to avoid subsequent unuseless prolonged warm ischemic time which contra-indicaties DCD organ procurement (Monti et al., 2010)[31]. That should be done according to family wishes. Thereafter, and only thereafter, the DCD organ procurement procedure should be proposed, discussed with the next-of-skin, and informed consent should be obtained. After administration of the comfort therapy (5.4.2.), mechanical ventilation support is withdrawn with or without the endotracheal tube. If extubation is taking place, the tube must be replaced during organ procurement for lungs recovery. Arterial blood pressure is measured via a femoral - better than radial - artery catheter, along with peripheral oxygen saturation (Spo_2) and Fio_2. Systolic blood pressure should decrease lower than 30 mmHg, the heart rate down to zero, along without any Spo_2 waveform. The patient is pronounced dead by the physical examination 5 minutes after the absence of any systemic anterograde blood flow (through the femoral artery catheter) (DuBose and Salim, 2008)[32]. Drug administration, like heparin, is following Ethics guidelines for research with the recently dead (Pentz et al., 2005)[33].

5.4.4 Brain Death monitoring while waiting cardiac arrest

Current DCD organ procurement procedures make DCD heart graft not suitable for transplantation. Usually, cardiac valves are prepared for homografting. Research is also ongoing and consists in putting the heart graft on normothermic machine perfusion system in order to re-condition the graft during several hours before implantation. Nevertheless, if one could monitor for BD during the DCD procurement procedure, it will allow heart and other organs recovery before waiting for cardiac arrest and the end of the no-touch period, while decreasing the warm ischemic time.

The first attempt to monitor a DCD category III, controlled case for BD was done by J.M. Guerit in 2005, using the somatosensory evoked potentials (Guerit et al., 1999)[34]. By the left median nerve monitoring, he observed the disappearance of the P14 wave, while the dropping blood pressure reached the 51/27 mmHg value (Fig. 15).

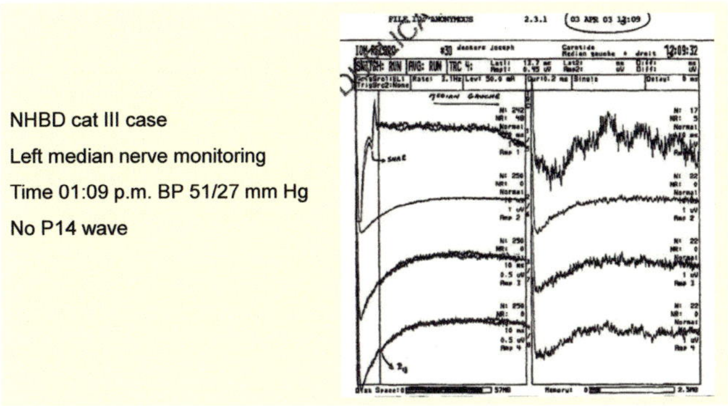

Fig. 15. The brain death (BD) monitoring during the DCD organ procurement procedure (Guerit, 2006)[36]. Disappearance of the P14 wave of somatosensory (left median nerve) evoked potentials with dropping blood pressure.

Another tool, proposed by Auyong et al. is following the bisprectal index (BIS). They presented a case series of increased BIS values during DCD procedure. If these increased BIS values could be a consequence of the catecholamic storm, which could represent a new monitoring tool of BD with the disappearance of BIS. But, limitations of BIS and electroencephelography are well known, the last one being the worst traditionally recommended tool for BD confirmation (Guerit, 2004)[35] (Guerit, 2006)[36]. Nevertheless, if these observed changes were not due to artefact, dosing of hypnotic or anaesthetic drugs might be warranted (Auyong et al., 2010)[37]. Moreover, it will open doors for recovering more DCD organs including hearts for transplantation. But it will need further manipulations to counteract the agonic phase lesions and ischemic injuries, like the intermediate use of machine perfusion for re-conditioning all grafts.

6. The living donor (LD) renal transplantation

The first attempt to LD renal transplantation took place as early as 1962 when no IS drugs were available in Belgium. Indeed, it was a first unrelated LD (LURD) kidney graft which rapidly failed (Kinnaert, 2009)[18]. Soon later, Professor Alexandre was more fortunate in performing living donor renal transplantation (LRD) using the Boston IS regimen. In 1968, he added to the IS armentorium the use of homemade antilymphocyte serum. Horses of the Belgian Police Corps and Army, disqualified for duty, were brought to the Hospital laboratories and injected with thoracic duct lymphocytes. These lymphocytes were being collected from recipients of LD kidneys who, in that period of time, were prepared, during 5 days before the operation, with drainage of the thoracic duct (TDD). After immunization, the horses were bled for extracting the antilymphocyte globulins, for injection into the recipients. Later on, Behringwerke Pharmaceuticals (Germany) took over this preparation known as the Behring horse antihuman ALG (Pressimmum ®) which was still in use until the eighties and from which thousands of patients had benefited. Initially ALG was used to treat steroid resistant acute cellular rejections. Since 1976, it had been used as induction therapy along with Aza and steroids. Moreover in LD recipients, a TDD was added to that protocol along with a per-tranplant splenectomy. In October 1982, CsA was combined to that basic IS regimen: that quadruple drug therapy was the reference treatment for more than 10 years. It allowed using low doses of each IS drug, avoiding toxic side-effects, while hoping an IS synergistic effect (Squifflet et al., 1982)[38]. During the CsA period, for LD transplantation, TDD and splenectomy were abandoned.

6.1 The pediatric renal transplantation

The real advantages of using LD kidneys over DBD during the pre CsA era became obvious with the first results obtained in the pediatric population comparing parental to cadaver donation (Fig. 16) (Squifflet et al., 1981)[39].

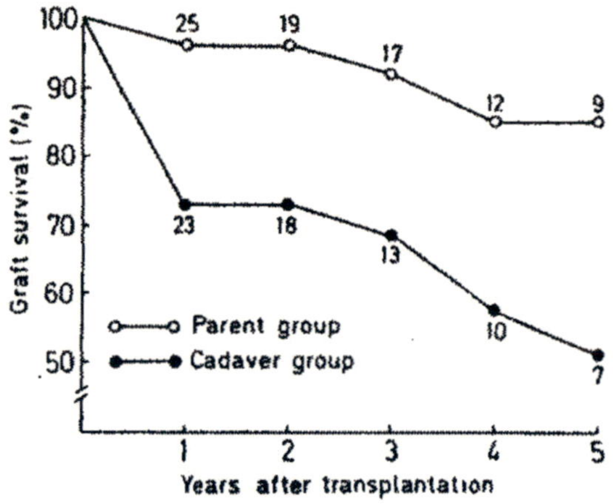

Fig. 16. **Renal Transplantation in Children.**
Graft survival in 32 parental and 35 cadaver graft in pediatric recipients during the pre CsA era (1971-1981). Numbers beside survival curses refer to the number of graft at risk. Difference between the two curses is significant (P < 0.02) and reaches > 30% at 5 years (Squifflet et al., 1981)[39].

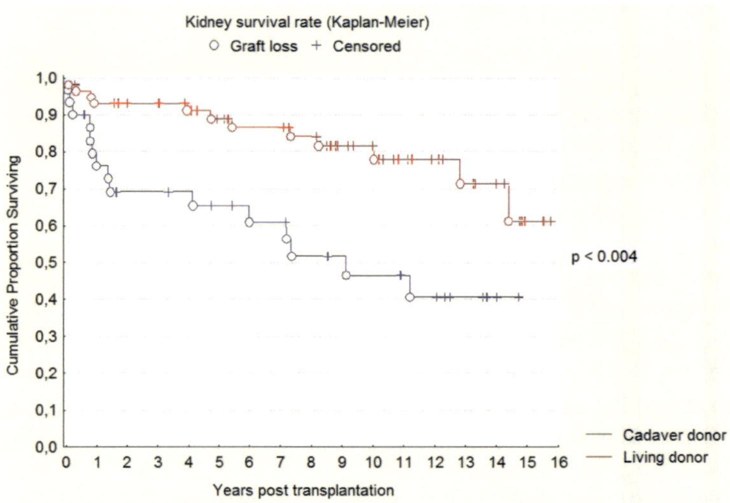

Fig. 17. **Renal Transplantation.** Kidney survival in 56 parental and 26 cadaver graft in pediatric recipients during the CsA era (1983-1994). Difference between the two curves reaches > 30% at 10 years (Malaise et al., 1995)[40].

Twenty years later during the CsA era, that was confirmed in the same pediatric population. Surprisingly, the difference in functional survival rates between the 2 subgroups remained similar but it was more than 30% at 10 years, instead of 5 years (Fig. 17). Even if one year results improved with the CsA use, the slope of the curves were parallel (Malaise et al., 1995)[40].

The children experience underlined the advantages of LD over the DBD renal transplantation. It allows donor selection according to strict medical, serological and anatomical criteria. It insures the quality of the grafts and can help for selection of potential live donors according to the HLA matching (twins, HLA identical siblings, parental...). Moreover the procedure can be programmed without any waiting on dialyse i.e. pre emptive procedure. The recipient can also be prepared by donor specific transfusions and/or pre-transplant IS therapy and/or bone marrow infusion or others. Working in 2 separate operating rooms, it can reduce ischemic injuries with a hemodynamically stable donor. Finally it increases donor self-esteem and the cadaver donor pool.

6.2 The Living Unrelated Renal Transplantation (LURD)

In looking at our LD activity (Table.5 and Fig. 18 a and b) the proportion of LD/DBD was globally 18%, but decreased slowly during the last decade, despite LD promotion.

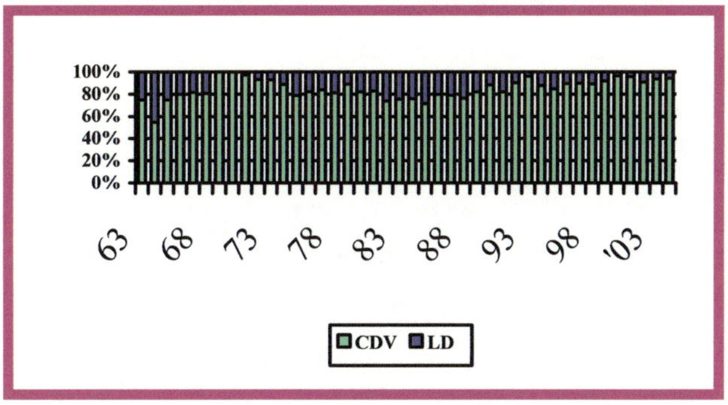

a.

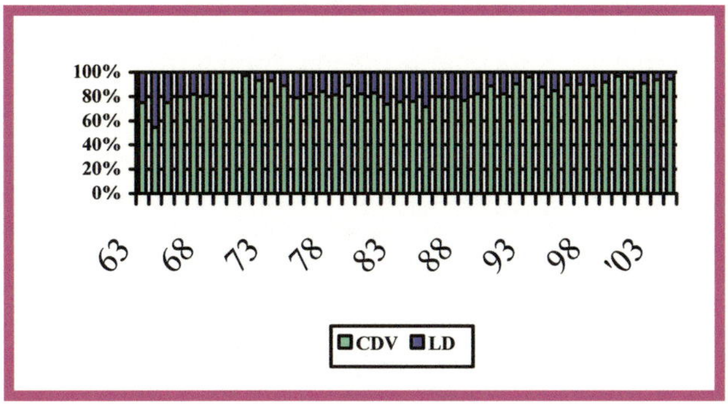

b.

a.: numbers; b.: proportion in %.

Fig. 18. LD/CDV renal transplantation (Prof. G.P.J. Alexandre and J.P. Squifflet activity) from 06/1963 to 12/2004.

The explanation of the phenomena is to be found in looking at mean ages of recipients and donors: for the recipients, it increased from 30 to 50 years and 20 to 40 years for DBD and LD respectively (Fig. 19 a); for the donors, it increased only for DBD from 25 to 40 years but remains stable for LD, around 40 years of age (Fig. 19 b). One can conclude that our selection criteria for the LD did not change over time; for the aging population of recipients, most of their LRD candidates are not fulfilling the donation criteria. Thus, LURD could be another source for renal transplantation; that source in our program, increased slowly over time (Fig. 20).

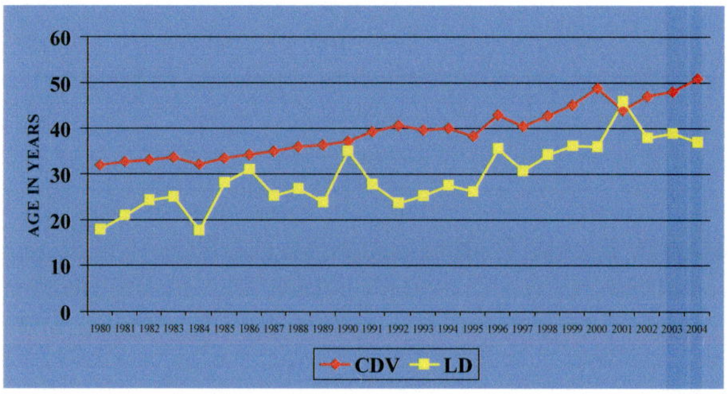

a.

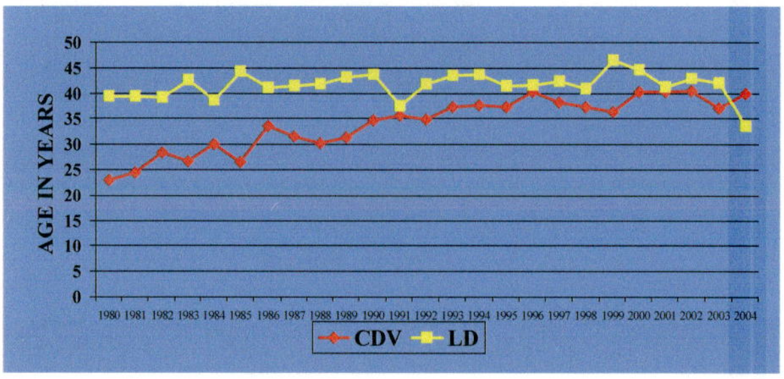

b.

Fig. 19. evolution of mean ages of recipients (a) and donors (b) from 1980 to 2004 according to donor sources: DBD red curves and LD yellow curves.

The LURD program started in 1966. During the pre CsA era, 17 were performed under AZA and Steroids as the basic therapy, plus ALG for induction, TDD and splenectomy (Squifflet et al., 1990)[41]. With the advent of CsA, 41 new LURD were performed between 1983 and 1996, and were compared to paired 82 DBD renal transplantations (Fig. 21) (Malaise et al., 1997)[42].

It is interesting to note that the donor-to-recipient relationship was 22 wife-to-husband, 9 husband-to-wife, 1 aunt-in-law, 1 brother-in-law, 1 wife's niece, 1 mother-in-law, 4 close friends and 2 family's friends. In that series, LURD renal transplantation offered similar results (Fig. 21 a and b) than DBD, despite poorer HLA-A, B and Dr matching and older donor age. The waiting time on dialysis was shorter; early better graft function was encountered in relation to the reduced total ischemia time and better preparation (conditioning) of both donors and recipients. Moreover the video-assisted donor nephrectomy technique introduced for the late cases did not increase the incentive to LD (Berney et al. 2000)[43].

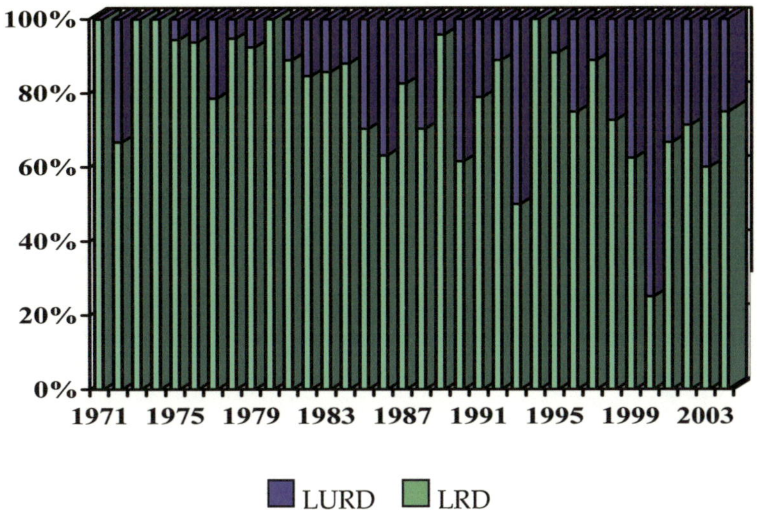

Fig. 20. Proportion LRD/LURD (Squifflet et al., 1990)[41] ; (Malaise et al., 1997)[42].

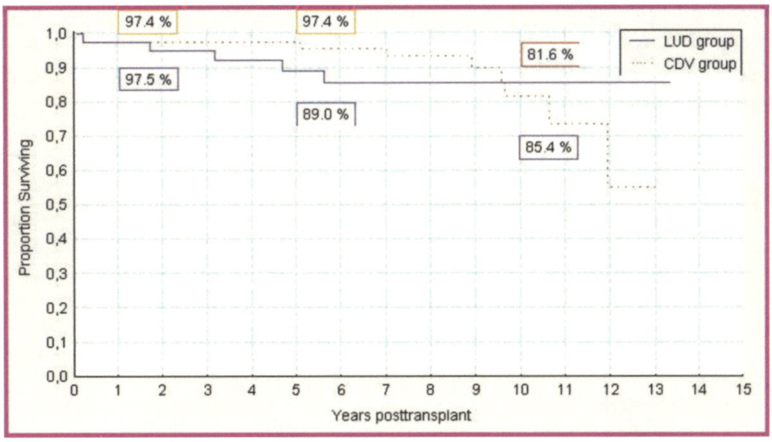

a.

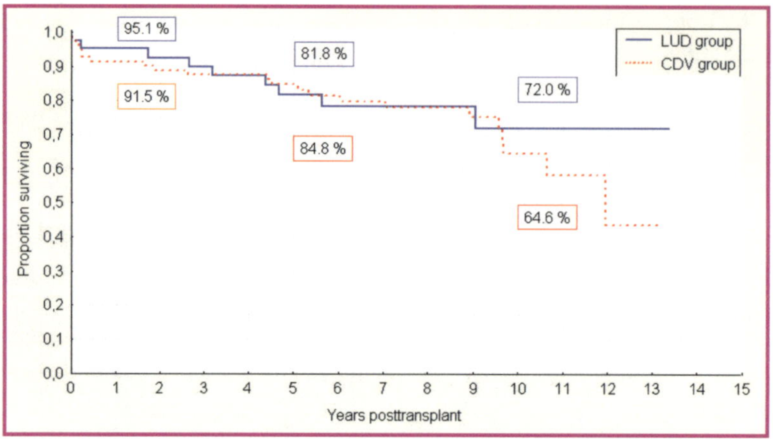

b.

Fig. 21. Comparison of LURD and DBD kidney transplantations under CsA therapy: similar actuarial patient (a.) and renal graft (b.) survival rates (Malaise et al., 1997)[42].

6.3 The ABO-incompatible (ABO-Inc) living donor renal transplantation

Early in 1981, an ABO-Inc cadaver kidney transplant was accidentally performed (blood group A1 into an O recipient). Despite a rejection crisis on the third week with a sharp increase of the anti-A iso-agglutinins, the renal function completely recovered. The patient survived more than 25 years post-transplantation with a functioning kidney graft.

Using a similar approach to that used for achieving ABO-Inc bone marrow transplantation, a series of 39 ABO-Inc live donor kidney transplants (31 related and 8 unrelated donors) was successfully performed (Table 6). The recipients received donor-specific platelet transfusions, 3 to 5 plasmapheresis to get rid of the anti-donor iso-agglutinins and underwent splenectomy at the time of transplantation (Alexandre et al., 1985)[44]. Twenty years graft survival is as high as 76% in the youngest recipients (< 15 years) (Squifflet et al., 2004)[45]. It compares favorably with ABO-compatible LD renal transplantation (Fig. 22 a. and b.).

	N :	Mean age	No RRT Before TP	Death	Graft losses		Functioning graft		
		M ± SD	%		HA Rejection	Chronic Rejection	N :	FU (year) m + sd	Creatinine (mg/dl) m + sd (Median)
Related	**31**	**20 ± 7**	**35**	**0**	**5**	**8**	**18**	**17 ± 3**	**1.9 ± 1.3 (1.5)**
Time to graft loss					11 ± 3 days	9.5 ± 4.8 yrs			
< 15 years	9	11 ± 2	55	0	0	2	7	16 ± 2	1.8 ± 0.6 (1.7)
Time to graft loss						5.5 ± 4.8 yrs			
> 15 years	22	23 ± 6	28	0	5	6	11	18 ± 3	2.0 ± 1.6 (1.4)
Time to graft loss					11 ± 3 days	11 ± 4 yrs			
Unrelated	**8**	**37 ± 9**	**12**	**2**	**4**	**3**	**1**	**20**	**1.0**

Table 6. Outcome of 39 ABO-Inc related and unrelated living donor (LD) kidney transplantations.

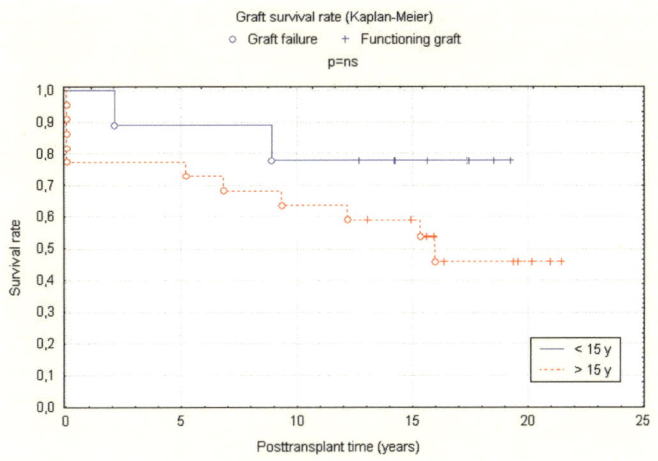

a.

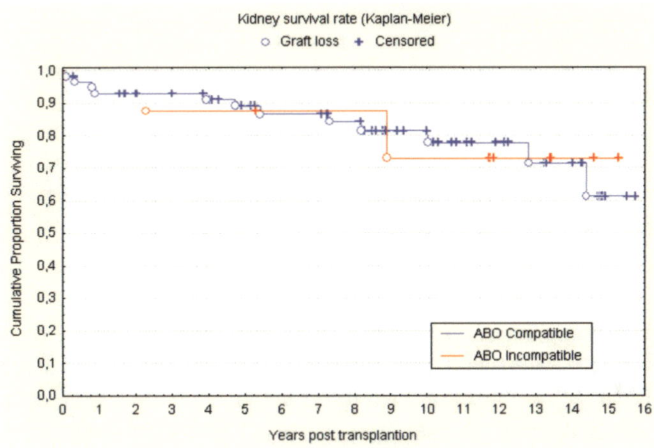

b.

a. Kidney graft survival in recipients < 15 years (n=9) and > 15 years (n=22) of ABO-Inc LRD.
b. Kidney graft survival in recipients < 15 years (n=9) of ABO-Inc LRD compared to a group of recipients < 15 years (n=58) of ABO-Comp LRD (Malaise et al., 1995)[40].
Fig. 22. ABO-Inc LRD: 20 years later (Squifflet et al. 2004)[45].

More surprising is the fact that some patients may carry very high levels of iso-agglutinins with the disappearance of all ABO blood group antigens on the endothelial cells of the transplanted kidney. Later on, Fritz Bach (Bach et al., 1997)[46] proposed the word "accommodation" to name this phenomena; probably there exists a critical period, before the third postoperative week, during which the ABO-Inc transplant is at risk for acute humoral vascular rejection. That is followed by a period of adaptation.
Today, more than 20 years later, each part of the original protocol has been further assessed or modified by different groups. Indeed, plasmapheresis was replaced by immuno adsorption columns. For deleting the last circulating iso-agglutinins, high doses of

intravenous immunoglobulins are communally used. Pre-transplant IS includes Rituximab ®, as well as at the time of transplantation, in order to avoid the splenectomy. In general, the PO IS therapy combines Tacrolimus and Mycophenolate Mofetil with r-ATG induction (Squifflet et al., 2004)[45].

Today, excellent results can be achieved: it is the demonstration that crossing the ABO barrier in LD kidneys transplantation is feasible. The same heavy protocol pertains and can also be applied for hyper immunized recipients with positive crossmatch against potential donors. Others, as well as the Belgian transplant community,

have proposed LD exchange programs (LDEP). Currently, in the Netherlands, that LDEP is very successful in helping numerous pairs of D and R from blood group O, while solving impossibilities (Fig. 23) by incorporating donations from good samaritans.

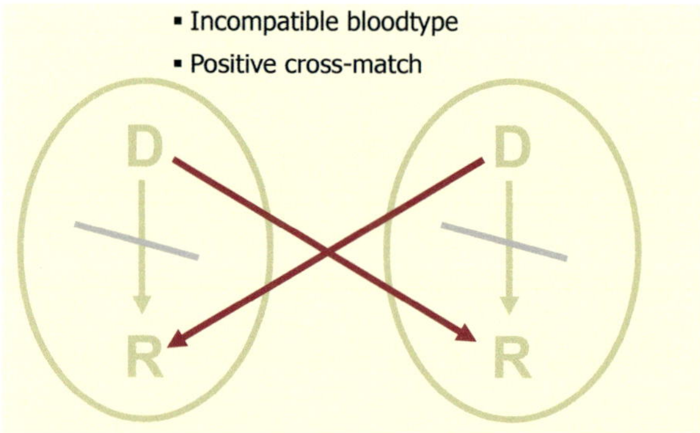

Fig. 23. Solving impossibilities with LDEP.

Based on that human experience and using the same preparation, a dozen pig-to-baboon renal xenografts were achieved in the mid-eighties. Three animal recipients survived 10, 22 and 23 days respectively. The baboon who lived for 10 days died of a pulmonary infection: the renal function was normal at the time of death and histology of the xenograft was remarkably normal. Two baboons, who lived for over three weeks, presented an acute rejection crisis at the end of the first week, vascular in nature for the first animal and cellular in the second one. This demonstrated that, together with an appropriate preparation of the donor animal and the recipient, xenotransplantation could be feasible using new potent immunosuppressive drugs.

7. Present and future perspectives

On May 28, 2002 Belgium adopted the Belgian act on Euthanasia after several months of intensive discussions (Squifflet A.C., 2011)[21]. Euthanasia is described as *'an act on purpose, performed by a third person, in order to end the life of a person who has requested for this act'*. The rules are the following:

The patient must be an adult or an emancipated minor, capable and conscious at the time of his / her request. The request is made voluntarily, is well thought out and reiterated, and is not the result of outside pressure.

The patient is in a hopeless medical condition and complains of constant and unbearable physical or mental pain which cannot be relieved.

If the person is not in the terminal phase of his illness, the 2 doctors must consult with a third doctor, either a psychiatrist or a specialist in the disease concerned.
At least one month must pass between the written request and carrying out the act.
Every euthanasia must be reported to a federal commission that regulate the practice and bring prosecutions when necessary.
Current statistics demonstrate more than 2 acts per day in Belgium and 7 per day in the Netherlands (Fig.24).

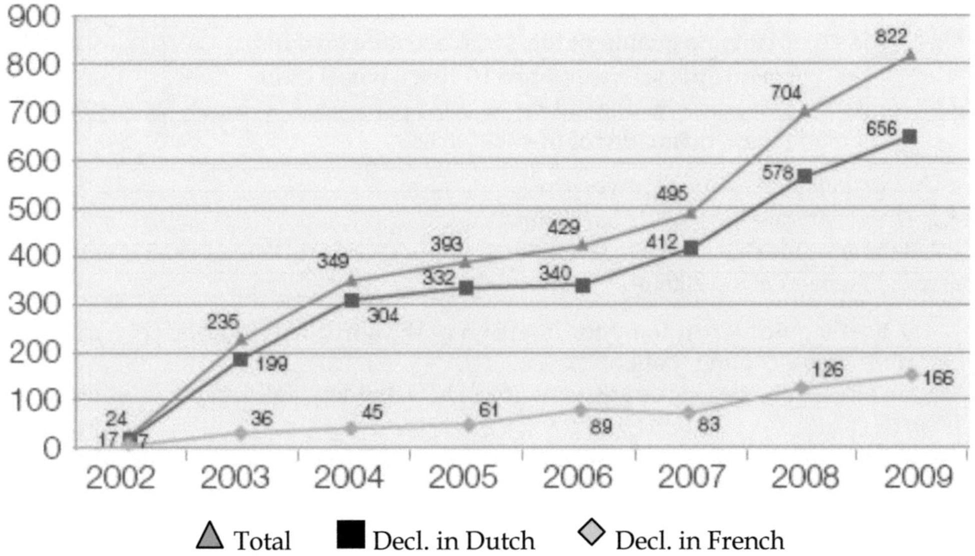

Fig. 24. Annual numbers of legal euthanasia acts in Belgium.

In January 2005, a first woman who was following the procedure of mercy killing asked for organ donation after death (Ysebaert et al., 2009)[47], (Detry et al., 2008)[48]. She was followed by 7 others persons so far. Data concerning the 4 patients are summarised in table 7 and 8 (Ysebaert et al., 2009)[47].
The organ procurement procedure which was adopted after euthanasia was as follow:

- Extensive written informed consent of donor - if possible (see patient 2) - and relatives.
- Strict separation between euthanasia request, euthanasia procedure and organ procurement.
- Euthanasia performed by 2 physicians + neurologist.
- Euthanasia in wheelchair (patients 1, 3, 4) or bed (patient 2), in a special room in the OR, in presence of the family.
- Organ retrieval after clinical diagnosis of cardiac death by 3 physicians.
- Procedures performed by senior staff members and nursing staff on a voluntary basis.
- Euthanasia procedure induced by overdose barbiturates, muscle relaxation and analgesia.
- Heparine given after euthanasia kit.
- The surgical procedure:
  - 3 times femoral vessels cannulation using the DBTL catheter (double balloons triple lumen) followed by a quick laparotomy for topical cooling (patients 1, 3 and 4).

Location	Age	Condition	Date of Euthanasia
1. UZA	44	**CVA** since 6 years, fixed hemliplegia, cortical blindness, special disorientation and dyspraxia.	01/2005
2. U of Lg	43	**CVA** since 4 years, locked-in syndrome, no motor recovery, central hyperthermia episodes, communication only by the eyes.	06/2006
3. UZA	47	**Multiple sclerosis** since 10 years, wheel chair dependent, depending on third parties for personal care, no quality of life, large decubitus wounds.	07/2007
4. UZA	50	**Multiple sclerosis** since 16 years, wheel chair dependent, depending on third parties for personal care, no quality of life.	10/2007

UZA: Universiteit Ziekenhuis Antwerpen
U of Lg: University of Liege, CHU Sart Tilman
Table 7. demographic data of the first 4 Belgian donors who requested organ donation after euthanasia (Ysebaert et al., 2009)[47].

  - 1 time a quick laparotomy for insertion of the aortic and inferior vena cava canule, and topical cooling (patient 2).
- Organ allocation via Eurotransplant (for DCD kidneys, allocation is allowed 4 hrs before).
- Transplant centers informed about the nature of the case and the elements of organ procurement.

Based on that protocol, the first 4 patients donated 8 kidneys, 4 livers, 3 pancreases for islet preparation and 4 lungs. All those organs were successfully transplanted without delayed graft function and need for P.O. dialysis for the kidneys (table 8).

Patient	First warm ischemic times				Outcome			
	Start – Asystoly	Asystoly – Incision	Incision – flush	Total	Kidneys	Liver	Islets	Lungs
1	12′	9′	5′	26′	2	Yes	Yes	No
2	9′	3′	5′	17′	2	Yes	No	No
3	21′	8′	5′	34′	2	Yes	Yes	2
4	6′	5′	3′	14′	2	yes	yes	2

Table 8. First warm ischemic times and outcomes of the organs procured in the first 4 Belgian donors who requested organ donation after euthanasia (Ysebaert et al., 2009)[47].

The potential number of patients asking for euthanasia who fulfilled criteria for organ donation will remain limited and was estimated to be between 5 and 10% (table 9).

That first series demonstrates that organ donation after euthanasia is feasible. It allows respecting strong patient's wish to donate that cannot be denied. The proposed procedure clearly separates euthanasia request, euthanasia procedure and organ procurement. It ensures high quality of DCD organs which might enter in a so-called Fifth Category of Maastricht, of controlled NHBD.

A step further was undertaken by a Pediatric Heart Transplantation team from Denver, Colorado (Boucek et al., 2008)[49] who procured 3 pediatric DCD hearts after a no-touch

	2003	2004	2005	2006	2007	2008	2009
Euthanasia	235	349	393	429	495	704	822
Neuromuscular disorders	22	27	16	33	48	51	58
%	9,5	7,7	4,1	7,6	9,6	7,2	7,0

Table 9. Potential number of patients fulfilling organ donation criteria among Belgian patients requesting euthanasia (Squifflet A.C., 2011)[21].

period of 3, 1.25 and 1.25 minutes. All 3 hearts were successfully transplanted into 3 children. Therefore, the Denver procedure extends the boundaries of organ donation after circulatory death, and perhaps, will require ethical discussions and revisions of the definition of death. Currently the definition of brain death requires the complete absence of all functions of the entire brain (higher-brain definition). The cardiac definition of death requires the irreversible cessation of cardiac function (impossible to reverse). Based on the Denver procedure, the last definition is not valid anymore. It means also, that in DCD organ procurement, with a neuromonitoring of brain death, and adequate analgesic drug management, cessation of cardiac beats could not be waited for, even without any no-touch period. It will also allow heart procurement, reconditioning on artificial device before implantation.

That will necessitate the revision of the dead donor rule and the endorsement of the DCD procedure by separate well trained teams.

The Belgian initiatives in the field of cadaver organ procurement have paid off in terms of number of organs available for allocation. But it remains, like in other countries, that the number of suboptimal organs is increasing for recipients of increasing age and associated morbidities. That will impair the short - and long-term graft and patient outcome.

If there is an urgent need for those centers performing living donor transplantation to turn toward cadaveric organ transplantation, there is also an urgent need for those centers which have DCD programs to turn toward living donor transplantation which offers better results.

Current situation prevails: many persons are willing to offer their organs after death in hoping to help their neighbours. Many patients with end-stage renal disease are turning to live donor kidney transplantation to improve survival and quality of life. Many healthy adults are eager and willing to accept the risk of donor nephrectomy to help their loved ones. Therefore, the responsibility is within the medical community to quantify the risks as best as possible and make the information available to those considering donation. That should be considered and will help for avoiding organ trafficking, tourism and commercialisation in the field of renal transplantation.

8. Acknoledgments

To Professor G.P.J. Alexandre, a pioneer in the field of transplantation
To Professor J. Malaise who initiated most data analysis.
Present address: University of Montreal, Quebec, Canada
Notre Dame Hospital

9. References

[1] Küss R. & Bourget P. (1992). Une histoire illustrée de la greffe d'organes. La grande aventure du siècle. Laboratoires Sandoz, Rueil-Malmaison. ISBN: 2 - 901334 - 05 - 9 France.

[2] Toledo-Pereyra L.H. & Toledo A.H. (2008). History of Living Donor Kidney Transplantation in : Living Donor Organ Transplantation. Gruessner R.W.G. & Benedetti E. (Eds) pp 133-138. The McGraw-Hill Companies. ISBN: 978 - 0 - 07 - 145549 - 7 USA.
[3] Squifflet J.P. (2003). The history of organ transplantation in Belgium 1963-2003. At the honour of the Belgian pioneers in transplantation surgery. Suppl. Acta Chir Belg; 103: 5 - 62.
[4] Squifflet J.P. (2003). From leg transplantation by St Cosmas and St Damian to the Modern Era. Suppl. Acta Chir Belg; 103: 6 - 9.
[5] Squifflet J.P., Sutherland D.E.R., Rynasiewicz J.J., Bentley F.C., Florak G. and Najarian J.S. (1983). Technical aspects of segmental pancreatic grafting in rats. Microsurgery; 4: 61 - 66.
[6] Murray J.E. (2011). Ronald Lee Herrick Memorial: June 15, 1931 - December 27, 2010. Am J of Transplant; 11: 419.
[7] Groth C.G. & Longmir W.P. (2000). Historical landmarks in Clinical Transplantation. World J. Surg; 24: 755 - 843.
[8] Squifflet J.P., Pirson Y., Gianello P., Van Cangh P., and Alexandre G.P.J. (1981). Safe Preservation of human renal cadaver transplants by Euro-Collins Solution up to 50 hours. Transplant Proc; 8: 693 - 696.
[9] Squifflet J.P., Gruessner R.W., and Sutherland D.E.R. (2008). The history of Pancreas Transplantation: Past, Present and Future. Acta Chir Belg; 108: 367 - 378. 10. Squifflet J.P., de Hemptinne B., Gianello P., Balladur P. , Otte J.B., and Alexandre G.P.J. (1990). A new technique for en-bloc liver and pancreas harvesting. Transplant Proc; 22: 2070 - 2071.
[10] Moers C., Smits J., Maathuis M.H., Treckmann J., Van Gelder F., Napieralski B., Van Kasterop M., Van der Heide H.J., Squifflet J.P., Van Heurn E., Kirste G., Rahmel A., Leuvenick H., Paul A., Pirenne J.and Ploeg R. (2009). Machine perfusion or cold storage in deceased donor kidney transplantation. N Engl J Med; 360: 7 - 19.
[11] Turka L.A. (2001). Historical overview of immunobiology and transplantation research. In: Norman and Turka (Eds). Primer on transplantation. American Society of Transplantation National Office. Pages: 1 - 15. ISBN: 0 - 9660150 - 1 - 0
[12] Halloran P.F. & Gourishankar S. (2001). Historical overview of pharmacology immunosuppression. In: Norman and Turka (Eds). Primer on transplantation. American Society of Transplantation National Office. Pages: 73 - 75. ISBN: 0 - 9660150 - 1 - 0
[13] Squifflet J.P. (2003): The History of Transplantation at the Catholic University of Louvain-Belgium. 1963-2003. Suppl Acta Chir Belg; 103: 10 - 20.
[14] Mollaret P. and Goulon M. (1959). Le coma dépassé (Mémoire préliminaire) Rev Neurol ; 101 : 3 - 15
[15] Legendre C. and Kreis H. (2010). A tribute to Jean Hamburger's contribution to organ transplantation. Am J Transplant; 10: 2392 - 2395.
[16] Squifflet J.P. (2007) Pancreas Transplantation at the University of Louvain Saint-Luc Hospital in Brussels (Belgium) and The Euro SPK trial. In: Corry R.J. and Shapiro R. (Eds). Informa Health care USA, Inc - pp 433 - 440. IBSN: 0 - 8247 - 3
[17] Kinnaert P. (2009) Some historical Notes on the diagnosis of death. The Emergence of the Brain Death Concept. Acta Chir Belg; 109: 421 - 428.

[18] Organ transplants: practical possibilities (1966). In: Wolstenholme GEW and O'Connor M. (Eds). Ethics in medical progress: with special reference in transplantation. CIBA foundation Symposium. Boston, Little Brown. pp 65 - 77.
[19] Ad Hoc Committee of the Harvard Medical Scool (1968). A definition of irreversible coma. J Amer Med Ass; 205: 85 - 8.
[20] Squifflet A.C. (2011). Le cadre juridique belge du prélèvement et de la transplantation d'organes: choix éthiques et résultats pratiques. Ethica Clinica: in Press.
[21] Roels L. and Rahmel A. (2011). Strategies to meet organ shortage. The European experience. Transpl Int; 24: 350 - 367.
[22] De Roover A., Coimbra C., Detry O., Van Kemseka C., Squifflet J.P., Honore P., and Meurisse M. (2007). Pancreas graft drainage in recipient duodenum: preliminary experience. Transplantation; 84: 795 - 7.
[23] De Roover A., Detry O., Coimbra C., Squifflet J.P., Honore P., and Meurisse M. (2008). Exocrine pancreas graft drainage in recipient duodenum through side-to-side duodeno-duodenostomy. Transpl Int; 21: 707.
[24] Squifflet J.P. (2006). Why did it take so long to start a NHBD program in Belgium? Acta Chir Belg; 106: 485 - 488.
[25] Kootstra G. and Loveras J., Ploeg R., Squifflet J.P., Van Der Vliet (1995): Statement on Non-Heart-Beating Donor programs. Transplant Proc; 27: 2965.
[26] Jochmans I., Moers C., Smits J.M. et al. (2010) Renal resistance during machine perfusion is a risk factor for delayed graft function and poorer graft survival. Am J. Transplant ; 10 (suppl 4): 107.
[27] Ledinh H., Meurisse N., Delbouille M.H., Monard J., Hans M.F., Bonvoisin C., Weekers L., Joris J., Kaba A., Damas P., Damas F., Lambermont B., Kohnen L., De Roover A., Honore P., Squifflet J.P., Meurisse M., and Detry O. (2010). Contribution of Donors after Cardiac Death to the Deceased Donor Pool: 2002 to 2009. University of Liege Experience. Transplant Proc; 42: 4369 - 4372.
[28] Institute of Medicine (ed) (1997). Non-Heart-Beating Organ Transplantation: Medical and Ethical Issues in Procurement. In: Washington, DC; National Academy Press; 1997.
[29] Feng S. (2010). Donor intervention and organ preservation: where is the science and what are the obstacles? Mini review. Am J Transplant; 10: 1155 - 1162.
[30] Monti M.M., Vanhaudenhuyse A., Coleman M.R., Boly M., Pickard J.D., Tsibanda L., Owen A.M. and Laureys S. (2010). Willful modulation of brain activity in disorders of consciousness. N Engl J Med; 352: 579 - 89.
[31] DuBose J. and Salim A. 2008; Aggressive Organ Donor Management Protocol. Journal of Intensive Care Medicine; 23: 367 - 375.
[32] Pentz R.D., Cohen C.B., Wicclair M., De Vita M.A., Lederman Flam A., Youngner S.J., Hamric A.B., Mc Cabe M.S., Glover J.J., Kittiko W.J., Kinlaw K., Keller J., Asch A., Kavanagh J.J., and Arap W. (2005). Ethics guidelines for research with the recently dead. Nature Medicine; 11: 1145 - 1149.
[33] Guerit J.M., Fischer C., Facco E., Tinuper P., Murri L., Ronne-Engström E., Nuwer M. (1999). Standards of clinical pratice or EEG and EPs in comatose and unresponsive states. Electroencephalogr Clin Neurophysiol; 52: 117 - 131.
[34] Guerit J.M. (2004). The concept of brain death. In: Machado C., Shewmon D.A. (eds). Brain death and disorders of consciousness. Kluwer Academics, New-York, pp 15 - 22.

[35] Guerit J.M. (2007). Electroencephalography: the worst traditionally recommended tool for brain death confirmation. Intensive Care Med; 33: 9 - 10.
[36] Auyong D.B., Klein S.M., Gan T.J., Roche A.M., Olson D. and Habib A.S. (2010). Processed electroencephalogram during donation after cardiac death. Anesth Analg; 110: 1428 - 1432.
[37] Squifflet J.P., Rynasievicz J., Sutherland D.E.R., Field J., Heil J., and Najarian J.S. (1992). Combined immunosuppressive therapy with Cyclosporin A and Azathioprine: a synergistic effect in three or four experimental models. Transplantation; 34: 315 - 318.
[38] Squifflet J.P., Pirson Y., Van Cangh P., Otte J.B., Van Ypersele de Strihou C., and Alexandre G.P.J. (1981). Renal Transplantation in Children. A comparative study between parental and well-matched cadaveric grafts. Transplantation ; 32: 278 - 282.
[39] Malaise J., Baldi A., Setola P., Mourad M., Pirson Y., and Squifflet J.P. (1995). Renal Transplantation in Children : a comparative study between parental and well-matched cadaver grafts. Br. J. Surg 82, suppl: 128 and Eurosurgery; 5: 261 - 264.
[40] Squifflet J.P., Pirson Y., Poncelet A., Gianello P., and Alexandre G.P.J. (1990). Unrelated living donor kidney transplantation. Transplant Int; 3: 32 - 35.
[41] Malaise J., Mourad M., Besse T., Jamar F., Baldi A., Setola P., De Meyer M., Pirson Y., ans Squifflet J.P. (1997). Living Unrelated Kidney Transplantation. Transplantation Proc ; 29 : 2770 - 2772.
[42] Berney T., Malaise J., Mourad M., Morel P. and Squifflet J.P. (2000). Laparoscopic and open live donor nephrectomy: a cost/benefit study. Transplant Int ; 13: 35 - 40.
[43] Alexandre G.P.J., Squifflet J.P., De Bruyere M., Latinne D., Moriau M., Ikabu N. (1985). Splenectomy as a prerequisite for successful human ABO-incompatible renal Transplantation. Transplant Proc ; 17: 138 - 143.
[44] Squifflet J.P., De Meyer M., Malaise J., Latinne D., Pirson Y., and Alexandre G.P.J. (2004). Lessons learned from ABO-incompatible living donor kidney transplantation. Clinical and Experimental Transplantation; 2: 208 - 212.
[45] Bach F.H., Ferrant C., Hechenleitner P., Mark W., Koyamada N., Miyatake T. et al. (1997). Accommodation of vascularised xenografts: host Th2 cytokine environment. Nat Med; 3: 196 - 204.
[46] Ysebaert D., Van Beeumen G., De Greef K., Squifflet J.P., Detry O., De Roover A., Delbouille M.H., Van Donink W., Roeyen G., Chapelle T., Bosmans J.L., Van Raemdonck D., Faymonville M.E., Laurey S., Lamy M. and Cras P. (2009). Organ procurement after euthanasia: Belgian experience. Transplant proc; 41: 585 - 6.
[47] Detry O., Laureys S., Faymonville M.E., De Roover A., Squifflet J.P., Lamy M., Meurisse M. (2008). Transpl Int; 21: 915.
[48] Boucek M.M., Mashburn C., Dunn S.M., Frizell R., Edwards L., Pietra B., and Campbell D. (2008). Pediatric Heart Transplantation after declaration of cardiocirculatory death. N Engl J Med; 359: 669 - 675; 709 - 714.

2

Ethical Controversies in Organ Transplantation

Ehtuish Ehtuish
Surgery Department Tripoli Central Hospital &
National Organ Transplantation Program
Libya

1. Introduction

Since the 1st successful kidney transplant in 1954 done between two identical twins [Merrill etal 1958] organ transplantation has become a life-saving procedure for many disease conditions hitherto considered incurable. Clinical organ transplantation has been recognized as one of the most gripping medical advances of the century as it provides a way of giving the gift of life to patients with terminal failure of vital organs, which requires the participation of other fellow human beings and of society by donating organs from deceased or living individuals [Ehtuish etal 2006 & Hariharan etal 2000]. The gap between the demand for organ transplantation and the supply of donor organs is growing [The economist 2008].The waiting list of the United Network for Organ Sharing has grown from 21,975 names in 2000 to 32,722 in 2008 Fig. (1).

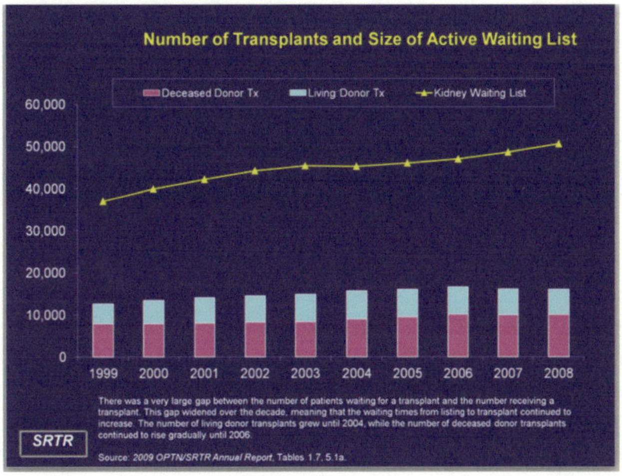

Fig. 1. The gap between the demand for organ transplantation and the supply of donor organs (UNOS) publications

The scarcity of organs has dire consequences. And an average of 19 people dies each day waiting for a transplant that never comes [United Network for Organ Sharing (UNOS) 1999]. The World Health Organization WHO global observatory showed that in 2009 about 100,900 people receive a lifesaving organ transplant, representing only less than 10% of the global needs Fig. (2). the entire issue has raised serious ethical concerns and the debate over

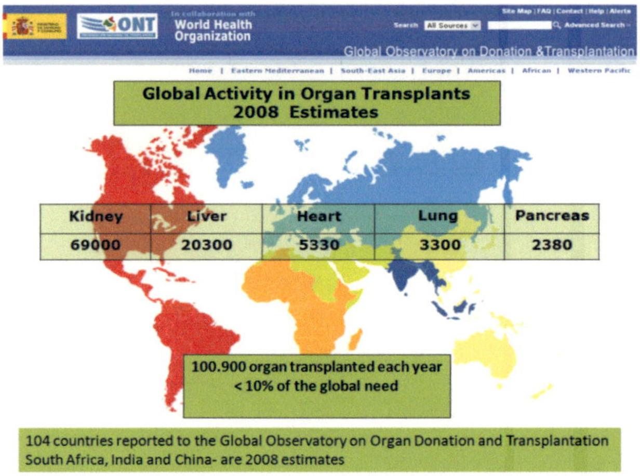

Fig. 2. Number of Transplants done worldwide WHO publication

them rages unabated. As further advances are made in such areas as cloning [Savules etal 1999], the ethical debate should grow more intense. The increasing incidence of vital organ failure and the inadequate supply of organs, especially from cadavers, have created a wide gap between organ supply and organ demand, which has resulted in very long waiting times to receive an organ as well as an increasing number of deaths while waiting. These events have raised many ethical, moral and societal issues regarding supply, the methods of organ allocation, and the use of living donors including minors. It has also led to the practice of organ sale by entrepreneurs for financial gains in some parts of the world through exploitation of the poor, for the benefit of the wealthy the ethical questions are complicated by an outgoing debate over the definitions of certain key terms such as life, death, human, and body. One example is the definition of brain death [Delmonico etal 1973]. People have been confused over the issue because of the highly public cases of people recovering from comas even after many years. The distinction between the idea of brain death and coma becomes a matter that must be clearly defined. A family that is asked to donate body organs from dead relative on the basis of brain death must be confident that there is no hope of recovering. Other ethical issues of organ donation are considered bioethical an important one is the idea of cloning. The technology that would allow the cloning of genetically matched clones for the purpose of body harvesting another issue is known as xenotransplantation which involves the harvesting of certain compatible animal organs for use in humans. A whole new plethora of ethical issues surround this idea due to fear from animals and the diseases might transmitted form them, or to protect them, even animal rights groups have joined in these debates. There is no question that body donation and organ donation will remain a hot topic for many years to come. Organ transplantation in general, and kidney transplants in particular, are fraught with ethical issues and dilemmas worldwide, about which there is ongoing debate, especially because of the shortage of organs The ethical questions associated with transplantation are many [Abouna 2008]. Is the human body a commodity? How should decisions be made about who should receive scarce organs? Who should pay for transplants? Should someone who has received one organ transplant be given a second transplant? Or should people who have not had a transplant be given priority over those who have already had one? Should one person receive several organs or should several people each receive one? Should one person have a

second transplant when the first one fail or should a different person be given a first chance at new organ? Should people who have young children be given an organ transplant over a single person? Should young people be given an organ transplant over an elderly person? Should age and whether or not a person has children even matter? Should organs be given to people who have abused their bodies (smoking and drinking etc,) or only to people whose organs are damaged by disease? Should hands or other appendages, which are not essential to life, be transplanted? Who can "donate" the organs of people who cannot give informed consent to the process? Should money now spent on transplantation be put to other uses? Is it possible to prevent the coercion of some donors? Should suicidal individuals be given an organ transplant? What if they attempted suicide in the past but are not currently contemplating suicide? Should people who can't afford expensive anti-rejection drugs be passed over for a transplant? Should people who don't have Insurance and can't pay for a transplant be allowed to go on the National waiting list? Should condemned prisoners receive organ transplants? What if they are serving a life sentence without parole? Should country lawmakers be involved in transplantation? When should courts be involved in these questions?
The questions go on and on; the answers are never simple. Knowing that there are more people who need organs than there are organs available, how would you answer these questions? Are your answers based on a belief of equal access or maximum benefit distribution?

2. What is organ transplantation?

An organ transplant is a surgical operation involves removing of an organ from one person (donor) and transferring it to another (recipient), keeping the native organs like Kidneys or removing them like Livers and Hearts. The need to obtain informed consent from both persons (and their surrogate decision-makers) is compulsory. This is in keeping with the ethical principle of respect for persons and is expressed in many ethical guidelines today.

3. Important milestones in the history of organ transplantation

- 1950 – 1954 The first successful kidney transplant. A kidney is taken from one identical brother and transplanted in another, where it worked for 8 years.
- 1960 - 1962 The first successful cadaveric transplant used deceased donor kidney. The kidney worked for almost 2 years.
- 1966 First successful liver transplant. The liver worked for over one year.
- 1967 First successful heart transplant. The heart worked for 2 1/2 weeks.
- 1980 – 1981 First successful heart-lung transplant. The organs worked for 5 years.
- 1982 First artificial heart transplant.
- 1983 Cyclosporine, an immunosuppressant drug, was approved by the FDA.
- 1986 A baboon heart was transplanted into Baby Faye and worked for 20days.
- 1989 The first successful living-related liver transplant.
- 1990 – 1996 The first "split liver" transplant was performed where one cadaveric liver was split into several pieces to transplant into more than one person.
- 2000 First culture of human embryonic stem cells.

4. Types of organ donors

The sources of organs for transplantation, i.e., living donor (related and nonrelated), cadaveric donor, and brain-dead patients. In countries where transplantation is well established, organs are sourced from living and cadaveric donors using different strategies, i.e., an opt-in (explicit consent), opt-out (presumed consent), and donation after brain death, donation after controlled cardiac death, and extended criteria for deceased donors.

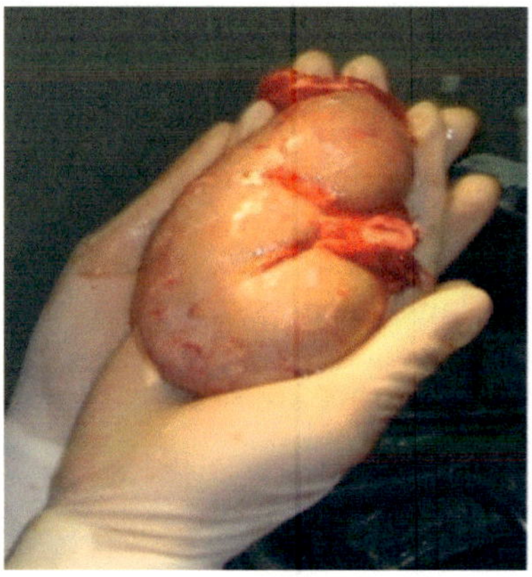

Gift of Life

4.1 Living organ donation

Four categories of donation by living persons can be distinguished: **Living Related Organ Donation "blood or emotional"**: directed donation to a loved one; **Altruistic Organ Donation:** non-directed donation, in which the donor gives an organ to the general pool to be transplanted into the recipient at the top of the waiting list; **Living Non-Related Organ Donation:** directed donation to a stranger, whereby donors choose to give to a specific person with whom they have no prior emotional connection; and **Cross donation** where a living donor wants to donate to his blood or emotional relative an organ but blood groups does not match, there is a complete mismatch or cross matching is positive. Two families or more can cross donate if matches exist. Each type of donation prompts distinct ethical concerns. Living Related Organ Donation is presumed to be the most ethical form of organ donation [Spittal A 1997]. One can argue that the psychological and non-specific benefits to the donor are real, particularly when a close relative is returned to normal health. There can, however, be no doubt that the physical consequences of living donation are entirely detrimental to the donor. Motives behind the 1st degree living renal donation are understandable and one may assume that the living donation between relatives carries the same altruistic motives. In related organ donation, the donor saves the life and attains the wellbeing of its immediate relative by accepting a physical injury and debilitation to itself. While many related donors fall neatly into this altruistic categorization, unfortunately, there are many examples where the related donors have attained physical, emotional or financial toll from the recipient. With directed donation to loved ones or friends, worries arise about the intense pressure that can be put on people to donate, leading those who are reluctant to do so to feel coerced. In these cases, transplantation programs are typically willing to identify a plausible medical excuse, so that the person can bow out gracefully. Equally important, however, are situations in which people feel compelled to donate regardless of the consequences to themselves. In cases like these, simply obtaining the informed consent of the relative is insufficient; physicians are obligated to prevent people from making potentially life-threatening sacrifices unless the chance of success is proportionately large. Non directed donation raises different ethical concerns. The radical altruism that motivates a person to make a potentially life threatening sacrifice for a stranger calls for careful scrutiny [Garwood etal 2007].

Transplantation teams have an obligation to assess potential donors in all these dimensions and prohibit donations that arouse serious concern. Directed donation to stranger raises similar ethical questions with a few additional wrinkles. This type of donation usually occurs when a patient advertises for an organ publicly, on television or billboards or over the Internet. Such advertising is not illegal, but it has been strongly discouraged by the transplantation community. Two central objections are that the practice is unfair and that it threatens the view that an organ is a "gift of life," not a commodity to be bought and sold. Some argue that just as we have a right to donate to the charities of our choice, so should we be able to choose to whom to give our organs. In practice, however, this means that those who have the most compelling stories and the means to advertise their plight tend to be the ones who get the organs — rather than those most in need. This strikes some ethicists as unfair. Unlike monetary gifts, they argue, organ transplantation requires the involvement of social structures and institutions, such as transplantation teams and hospitals. Hence, the argument goes, these donations are legitimately subject to societal requirements of fairness, and transplantation centers should refuse to permit the allocation of organs on the basis of anything but morally relevant criteria [Hull etal 1997].

The most ethically problematic cases are those in which the recipient is chosen on the basis of race, religion, or ethnic group [Epstein 2007]. A person with organ damage or organ failure may look for a living donor to donate an organ, allowing the patient to bypass the national waiting pool to receive a cadaveric organ.

4.1.1 Directed versus anonymous donation

Currently there is some debate whether altruistic donation should be anonymous or the donor should choose the recipient that he wishes to donate the organ to [Epstein etal 2009]. Donation could be criticized ethically that it unfairly favors some potential recipients by allowing them to jump to the top of the waiting list; however, many transplant surgeons and ethicists believe that this is a very special kind of advantage when a good Samaritan donates one of his organs to a friend or colleague who is on the waiting list. For this not only helps the recipient, but actually also helps those who are on the waiting list who will move up the ladder and will have a better chance of having a cadaveric organ.

4.1.2 Benefits to living donation [Abouna 1998]

- The operation can be pre-arranged so, the hot and cold ischemia will be minimized which will have a good impact on the transplantation outcome.
- There are often better matches between donors and recipients with living donation, because many donors are genetically related to the recipient.
- Psychological benefits for both the donors and recipients.

Not everyone encourages the practice of living donation for all people.

4.1.3 Drawbacks of living donation [Landolt etal 2001]

- Health consequences: Pain, discomfort, infection, bleeding and potential future health complications.
- Psychological consequences: Family pressure, guilt or resentment.
- Pressure: Family members may feel pressured to donate when they have a sick family member or loved one.
- No donor advocate: While the patients have advocates, like the transplant surgeon or medical team (who are there to advise the patient and work in favor of his or her best interests) donors do not have such an advocate and can be faced with an overwhelming and complicated process with no one to turn to for guidance or advice.

A few medical and ethical professionals argue that living donation is inappropriate under any circumstances and should not only be discouraged but abandoned all together because of the risk and dangers associated with donating organs.

WHO publications

Other critics seek to discourage living donation because they think extending life through costly and physically taxing medical procedures is not the purpose of health systems. Although there are some who object to the practice of living donation, this potential source of organs is currently a major focus as a way to reduce the shortage of organs. Increasing the number of living donors could occur through a variety of strategies from education and civic duty promotion to the sale and purchase of organs Fig. (3).

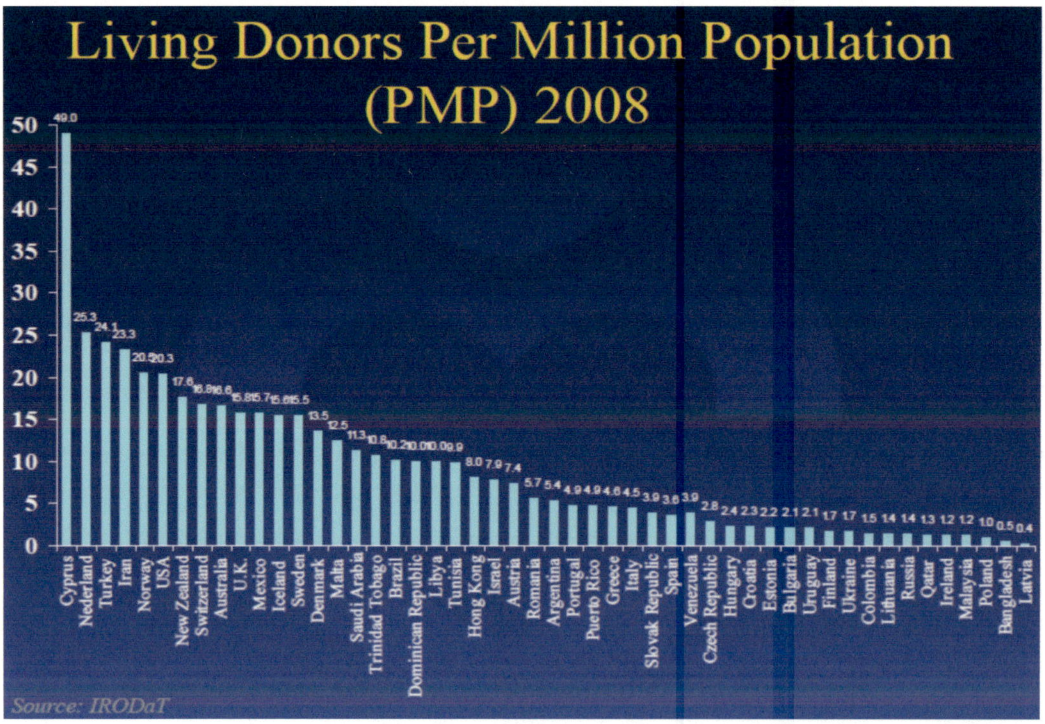

Fig. 3. International Registry of Organ Donation

4.1.4 Justification of transplantation from living donors

Living related donation, emotional related or altruistic are very justifiable on humanistic grounds and they are ethically and medically acceptable, providing that donor evaluation both medical and psychological is carried out in accordance with accepted protocols and that a fully informed consent is given by the donor. Also, the rate of donor complications after kidney donation is extremely small. The reported mortality rate after kidney donation is 1 in 10,000 [Delmonico etal2007].

On the side of the donor, there are many psychological and spiritual benefits, and most donors express an increased sense of pride and satisfaction and the joy of giving a gift of life to a relative, a friend or to another fellow human being. Another justification is that the success rate of living donor kidney transplantation is considerably higher than that of cadavers [Hunsicker 1999]. The expected patient survival rate and graft function at 5 years in 2007 is 99 and 96%, respectively, with living donors and 96 and 91% with cadaver donors, which is much better than 1998 statistics and that is most probably due to the recent introduction of more effective immunosuppression medications Fig. (4a&b).

In living donor transplantation it must be shown that the benefits to both donor and recipient outweigh the risks associated with donation and transplantation.

Unadjusted 1-Year Graft and Patient Survival by Organ (1998 and 2007)

Graft Survival	Year of Transplant			
	1998	2007	% Change	P-Value
Kidney: deceased donor graft survival	89%	91%	3%	<0.0001
Kidney: living donor graft survival	95%	97%	2%	<0.0001
Pancreas transplant alone	78%	76%	-1%	0.8341
Pancreas after kidney	72%	82%	10%	0.0302
Kidney-pancreas: kidney	91%	93%	2%	0.1355
Kidney-pancreas: pancreas	83%	86%	4%	0.0392
Liver: deceased donor graft survival	80%	86%	6%	<0.0001
Liver: living donor graft survival	70%	87%	16%	0.0022
Intestine	50%	75%	25%	0.0004
Heart	85%	88%	3%	0.0006
Lung	75%	80%	5%	0.0115
Heart-lung	54%	90%	36%	0.0001

Patient Survival	Year of Transplant			
	1998	2007	% Change	P-Value
Kidney: deceased donor patient survival	95%	96%	1%	0.0055
Kidney: living donor patient survival	98%	99%	1%	0.0015
Pancreas transplant alone	98%	98%	0%	0.9320
Pancreas after kidney	94%	97%	3%	0.2472
Kidney-pancreas	94%	97%	3%	0.0093
Liver: deceased donor patient survival	86%	89%	3%	<0.0001
Liver: living donor patient survival	80%	91%	11%	0.0173
Intestine	67%	78%	11%	0.0995
Heart	86%	89%	3%	0.0006
Lung	77%	82%	6%	0.0016
Heart-lung	57%	90%	34%	0.0003

SRTR

Source: *2009 OPTN/SRTR Annual Report*, Table 1.11b, 1.12b.

Fig. 4a. Patient & Graft survival (UNOS Published Reports)

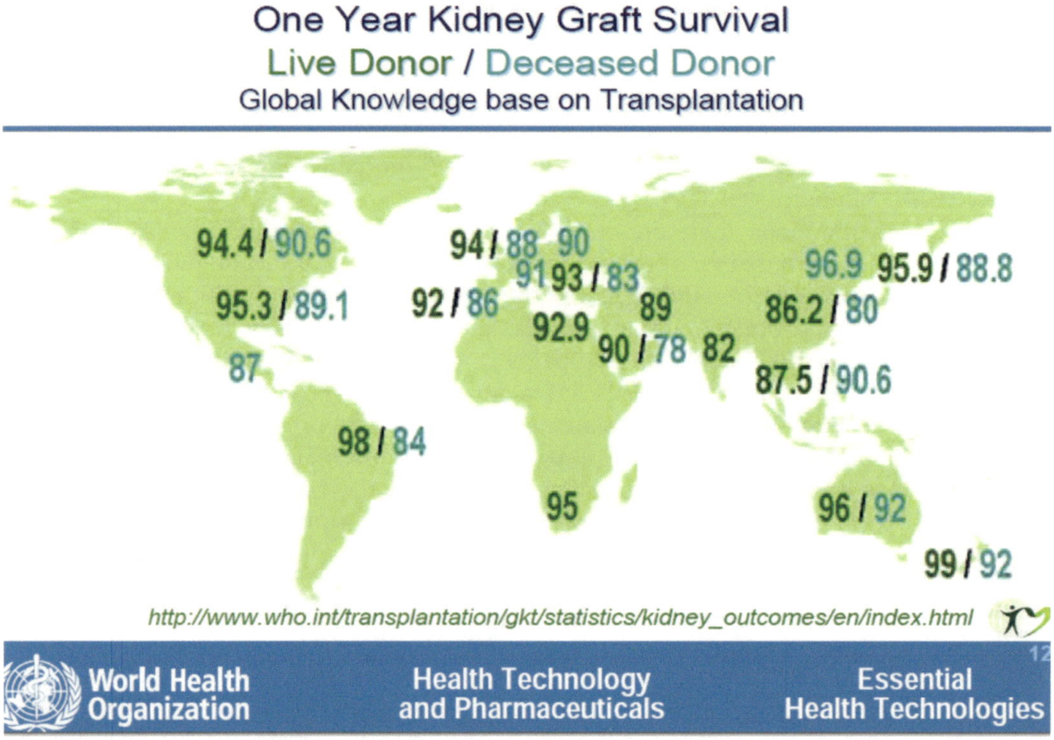

Fig. 4b. Patient & Graft survival (WHO Published Reports)

4.1.5 The decision to donate organs within the family

Many decisions to be living donors will be made within a family context - whether blood relations or less commonly, spouses, or in-laws - and involve the needs of specific members of that family. Very often, in living donation, there will be a host of pressures and family complexities to take into account. These may affect the extent to which a decision to donate or not to donate is genuinely free. Understanding some of these complexities and family dynamics can assist greatly in reaching a decision that is genuinely voluntary. It is important to distinguish between different kinds of pressure that a person faced with the decision about living donation may feel Avoidable pressures or Unavoidable pressures [Spital A 1996]. The decision to be a living donor should be based on adequate information and understanding, an informed decision is one based on information relevant to the making of that decision. Of course, in assisting a potential donor to make his or her decision about donation, doctors have an ethical and legal duty to warn about material risks in a treatment [Danovitch 2007]. Material risks are those that most people would want to know and also those that would be significant for a particular individual. It follows that a donor, before deciding about donation, should ask the appropriate medical practitioner to disclose the risks of the intended procedure and of its short and long term effects.

4.1.6 Psychological issues in live donation

This includes information and understanding about possible emotional and psychological consequences of making a decision one way or the other, for the potential recipient, the potential donor, the relationship between these two people, and for other family members. These questions can only be answered within the context of understanding a particular family and/or the particular individuals involved whatever the outcome, certain issues may take some time to resolve.

Tissue typing and other medical checks may identify only one suitable donor in a family, which can lead to great pressure being put on that person. There may be more than one suitable donor and in these cases there can be complex pressures again as a choice is made between these people. As examples of such pressures, focus may fall on one of the suitable people for various reasons, perhaps without sufficient thought. In other cases there may be one person who is extremely eager to donate and so perhaps too willing to overlook possible difficulties that may be encountered. Often, such very willing people may need even more careful counseling to ensure that their decision is sound.

Living donation offers the recipient immediate hope. Because the results are generally favorable, the mood of the recipient, family and donor are usually optimistic. Against this background, other issues need to be considered [Jarvis 1995]:

Chances of survival of recipient:

It is argued by some that it is preferable to donate to recipients who are not critically ill, because choosing recipients with higher chances of survival better balances the risk to the donor. In addition, when such recipients are chosen, there is less need to make a decision under pressure and the additional time allows thorough medical and psychological evaluation of the proposed donor.

Changes in donor/recipient relationship:

The exceptional nature of what has happened and what both the donor and recipient have shared may be mutually enhancing. After a donation, there is often increased contact between a donor and the recipient where they are known to each other. Our experience suggests that reaction to being identified as a donor is very positive [Mathieson 1999].

Feeling if the transplant fails:

If the donation does fail, the donor may have feelings of guilt or inadequacy or feelings of anger, sadness, or that the donated organs or tissues have been wasted, and that the discomforts he or she has suffered have been made for nothing.

Feelings of 'ownership' towards the recipient:

Living donors can feel closer to recipients and have expressed attitudes of ownership about the state of health and activities of the recipient. They may feel that they have a right to ensure that the recipient is taking good care of his or her health and therefore of the donated organ or tissue. Conversely, the recipient may identify with the donor and feel that part of the donor is living in them. Ultimately such feelings may not be in the best interest of either party.

Recipient feelings of guilt if the donation has harmful effects on the donor:

A recipient may feel guilty and responsible if the donor suffers from his or her donation.

Consequences of not donating:

A decision not to donate can have a major impact on relationships within a family. The recipient's illness is often life-threatening and death may occur before or after transplantation. It is therefore important that the family, including prospective donors, do not have unrealistic expectations for the recipient nor underestimate the difficulties for the donor. A decision not to donate might be entirely appropriate for the individual, but still have profound effects on family relationships if the proposed recipient dies. It is very important to consider whether such factors amount to undue pressure on a potential donor

4.2 Deceased organ donation

Organs for transplantation which obtained from living donors unfortunately, have so far been unable to keep up with demand. As a result, there are a large and steadily increasing number of potential recipients awaiting transplantation, some of whom will die before an organ can be found. This scarcity of organs for transplantation can only be met from the cadavers Fig. (5). Cadaveric source is beneficial in another way that it provides multi-organ donation. To utilize cadaveric organs effectively, it needs legal formalities and most of the countries have passed cadaveric law [Alashek, Ehtuish etal 2009].

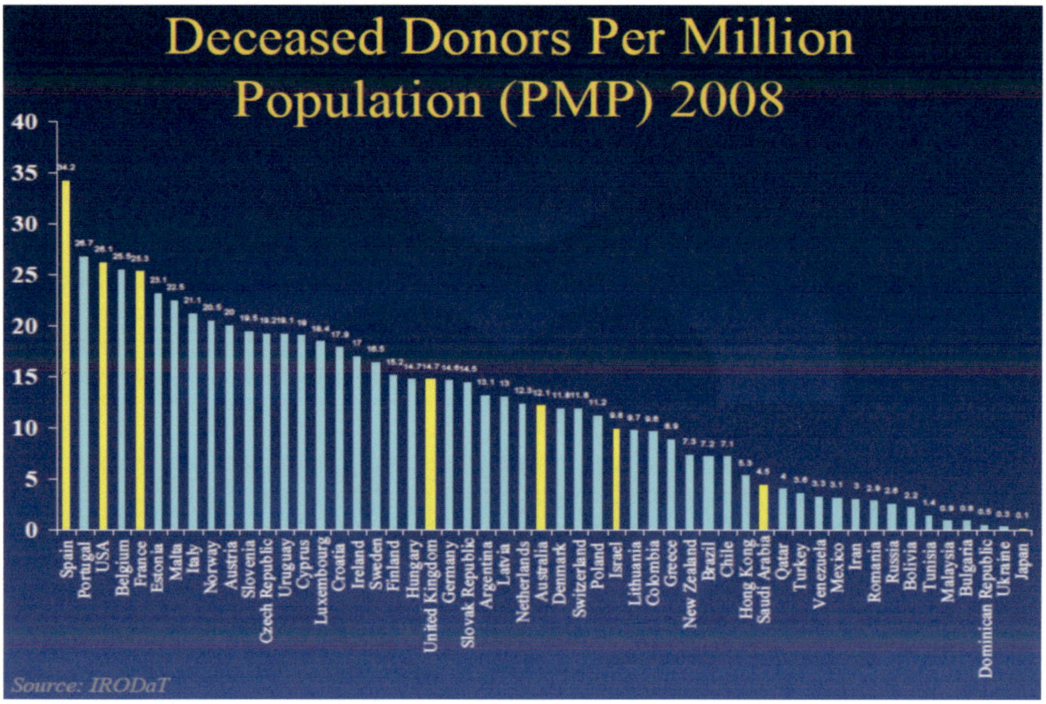

Fig. 5. International Registry of Organ Donation WHO Publications

4.2.1 Strategies to promote cadaveric organ donations and self sufficiency

a. Education

Educational efforts focus on increasing the number of people who consent to be an organ donor before they die. And educating families when they are considering giving consent for their deceased loved one's organs. Social responsibility and the idea of "the gift of life" should be popularized

b. Mandated choice

Under this strategy, every individual would have to indicate his wishes regarding organ transplantation, perhaps on driver's licenses. When a person dies, the hospital must comply with their written wishes regardless of what their family may want. The positive aspect of this strategy is that it strongly enforces the concept of individual autonomy of the organ donor. A mandated choice policy would require an enormous level of trust in the medical system. People must be able to trust their health care providers to care for them no matter what their organ donation wishes

c. Presumed consent

This method of procuring organs is in fact the policy of many European nations. In countries with presumed consent, their citizens' organs are taken after they die, unless a person specifically requests to not donate while still living. Advocates of a presumed consent approach might say that it is every person's civic duty to donate their organs once they no longer need them (i.e. after death) to those who do. People against presumed consent would argue that to implement this policy, the general public would have to be educated and well-informed about organ donation, which would be difficult to adequately achieve. Doubters of the presumed consent approach might also argue that requiring people to opt out of donating their organs requires them to take action and this might unfairly burden some people. The countries having presumed consent principles like Spain and Canada shows higher donation rate 40-50 per million population [Miranda etal 1998 & Rithalia etal 2009].

d. Incentives

Incentives take many forms [Beier etal 2008]. Some of the most frequently debated incentive strategies are:

1. Give assistance to families of a donor with funeral costs
2. Donate to a charity in the deceased person's name if organs are donated
3. Offer recognition and gratitude incentives like a plaque or memorial
4. Provide financial or payment incentives

One of the most highly debated incentives would give donating families assistance with burial or funeral costs for their loved one this could be an attractive incentive for many families.

Proponents say that since the person will be dead and unable to receive the recognition, that this would not be a coercive action. Some ethicists believe that many of the incentives above, while not attached directly to cash money, are still coercive and unfair. They believe that some people will be swayed to donate, in spite of their better judgment, if an incentive is attractive enough. They further argue that a gesture may seem small and a mere token to one person, but others might interpret it quite differently. A final anti-incentives argument offered by some ethicists discourages the practice of incentivizing organ donation [Jasper etal 1999]. They believe that society should instead re-culture its thinking to embrace a communitarian spirit of giving and altruism where people actively want to donate their organs

4.2.2 Maximizing donation form deceased donors

In order to maximize the donation from deceased donors it is important to consider the following:

- Legal and organizational framework

- Coordinating authority over health system
- Citizen's understanding: donation in school curriculum
- Ongoing reality and momentum in media
- Adaptation of relevant models (Spain) in emerging countries

4.3 Minors and children as donors

It is another issue that needs considerate discussion. Living donors provide the best outcome for children undergoing renal transplantation. Most of these donors are parents. When parents are unable to donate, siblings are often considered. But what if the siblings are also children? Should they be permitted to donate? They are below 18 years of age and not able to consent and they might be pushed or convinced to donate. And what about those who are mentally subnormal and their families wants to use them as donors?

Sometimes there are reports that children have been kidnapped, only to re- appear later lacking one kidney, or that they simply disappear and are subsequently killed to have all their transplantable organs removed for profit. However, the issue is covered in a broader sense by more general provisions. There are endless rumors surrounding this area. Members of various organizations who travel in the suspected countries say that the trafficking in children who are sold for transplantation is well known, but it is too difficult and very dangerous to catch the people involved [Spital A 1997],

4.4 Executed prisoners as donors

Several authors and ethicists have recently commented on the current practice in some countries of the use of organs from executed prisoners. While all societies strongly condemn the arbitrary use of taking organs from executed prisoners, which is a common practice in some countries, where organs are taken and given to various institutions for transplantation or even sold to other countries. It is suggested that it will be ethically permissible to allow a prisoner on death row to donate an organ to a relative or a friend. [Miller 1999].

One argument in favor of taking organs from prisoners, who are put to death, is that it is the execution that is ethically unsound and not the organ removal. Indeed, in light of the severe organ shortage, some ethicists could make the argument that to not use the organs for transplantation is wasteful. Some ethicist, put forth the argument that obtaining organs from condemned prisoners is allowable if the prisoner or their next of kin consents to donation, as long as organ donation is not the means by which the prisoner is killed because that violates the principle that a cadaveric donor be dead prior to donation. Some could argue that organ retrieval from executed prisoners is morally justifiable only if a "presumed consent" donation practice was in place. Many, if not most, bioethicists consider taking organs from condemned prisoners a morally objectionable practice. And immoral [Cameron etal 1999].

4.5 Alternative organ sources

Some potential non-traditional sources of organs are:

4.5.1 Animal organs – "xenotransplantation"

Animals are a potential source of donated organs. Experiments with baboon hearts and pig liver transplants have received extensive media attention in the past. One cautionary argument in opposition to the use of animal organs concerns the possibility of transferring animal bacteria and viruses to humans. Some argue that xenotransplantation is the only potential way of addressing this shortage. As immunological barriers to xenotransplantation are better understood, those hurdles are being addressed through genetic engineering of donor animals and the development of new drugs therapies [Starzl etal 1964 & Grant etal 2001]. The focus of ethical attention has changed from the moral correctness of using animals for research/therapy to an increasingly appreciated danger of the establishment and spread of xenozoonses in recipients, their contacts and the general public. There are a number of reasons for not using subhuman primates for xenotransplantation, including their closeness to humans, the likelihood of passing on infections, their availability (gorillas, chimpanzees), their slow breeding and the expense of breeding them under specified pathogen free conditions. The pig, although domesticated and familiar, is too distant to evoke the same feeling as we have for primates, has the correct size organs, is probably less likely to pass infections, breeds rapidly and is not endangered; moreover, millions of them are eaten every year. Although drawing ethical conclusions is difficult at the stage of knowledge and debate, it seems acceptable to manipulate pigs genetically and to proceed to using their organs for xenotransplantation trials when infection control measures and the scientific base justify it [Bukler etal 1999 & Sim etal 1999]. The use of pigs in Muslim countries would be more controversial and disruptive although it is acceptable by Islamic religion in case of a real need and when there is no alternative [Rahman 1998]. In this case the question of informed consent is likely to be ambiguous and awkward. It might end up more of a binding legal contract than consent, as we understand it now. Xenotransplantation is also unlikely to cost less than or significantly alleviate the shortage of cadaveric organs in the short term. The international dimension of the risk of infection is becoming obvious, but there has so far been no effort to convene an international forum to agree on universally acceptable guidelines However, before xenotransplantation can be fully implemented, both the scientific/medical communities and the general public must seriously consider and attempt to resolve many complex ethical, social and economic issues that it presents [Platt 1999].

4.5.2 Artificial organs

Artificial organs are yet another potential option.

The ethical issues involved in artificial organs often revert to questions about the cost and effectiveness of artificial organs. People who receive artificial organ transplants might require further transplanting if there is a problem with the device.

4.5.3 Organs from fetuses

The ethics of using tissues and organs from fetuses have been a matter of enormous discussion. Aborted fetuses are a proposed source of organs. Debates address whether it is morally appropriate to use organs from a fetus aborted late in a pregnancy for transplantation that could save the life of another infant. Many people believe that this practice would encourage late-term abortions, which some individuals and groups find morally objectionable. Another objection comes from people who fear that encouraging the use of aborted fetal organs would encourage "organ farming," or the practice of conceiving a child with the intention of aborting it for its organs[Golmakani etal 2005]., but the use of spontaneously aborted fetus or anencephalic newborn could be encouraged. Although there is ethical debate concerning the possible use of organs of anencephalic babies for transplant. Some have argued that because of the absence of neocortex these are 'nonpersons 'and are 'brain-dead' and thus, such infants should be available for organ donation if this is the wish of the parents. However, as brain stem function is present in these infants, the 'whole of the brain' or 'brain stem' requirement for certification of brain death precludes removal of organs until cardiorespiratory death occurs.

4.5.4 Stem cells –"The future"

Stem cells are cells that can specialize into many different cells found in the human body. Researchers have great hopes that stem cells can one day be used to grow entire organs, or at least groups of specialized cells [Bartholomew etal 2001 & Eradini 2002]. Some of the very recent developments in transplantation over the past decade have been the use of stem cells from bone marrow, cord blood, and from fetal and adult tissue, including somatic cells and neural cells. These cells have the great potential for differentiation and proliferation into other types of body cells including neuronal, hepatic, hemopoietic and muscular and thus help many patients with organ failure after their transplantation into the patients. These stem cells have also been shown to induce immunological tolerance and chimerism when they are transplanted into recipients of vital organ grafts and their rejection of a transplanted organ such as bone marrow, kidney, heart, liver, is prevented [Fandrich 2002]. A new hope is emerging now with the possibility of preserving the architecture of an organ i.e. preserving capsule, vascular structures and draining system and removing the destroyed or fibrosed cells and replace them with new cell mass produced by stem cells like removing all non-functioning Hepatocytes and replacing them with a new Hepatocyte cell mass, The ethical objections concerning stem cells have focused primarily on their source. While stem cells can be found in the adult human body, the seemingly most potent stem cells come from the first few cells of a human embryo. When the stem cells are removed, the embryo is destroyed. Some people find this practice morally objectionable and would like to put a stop to research and medical procedures that destroy human embryos in the process.

5. Life & death

With the development of mechanical ventilators, new drugs, and other forms of treatment, it became possible to artificially maintain circulatory and respiratory functions, even after the brain had stopped functioning. In the past four decades many countries amended their death statutes to include a definition of death by the complete and irreversible cessation of all brain functions. Since that time almost all cadaveric organs have been recovered from patients who have been declared "brain dead." Veatch has never been comfortable with the term "brain death," preferring instead "brain-oriented definition of death." Since the 1970s he has argued that the entire brain does not have to be dead for the individual as a whole to be dead. Instead, he advocates a "'higher-brain-oriented definition' of death—in other words, one is dead when there is irreversible loss of all 'higher' brain functions" he further proposes creating a new definition of death law that incorporates the notion that one need only have an irreversible loss of consciousness as opposed to an irreversible loss of all brain functions [Veatch 2008]. Veatch's proposal is clearly controversial. It suggests a violation of an ethical boundary most clinicians are currently unwilling to cross. Perhaps he is correct that such a change is inevitable and that the "definition of death at the conceptual level is a religious/philosophical/social policy choice rather than a question of medical science" .There was clear leadership from individuals such as pioneering transplant surgeon, Dr. David Hume; Dr. Hume wrote "there is only one definition of death, irreversible brain damage. Cessation of heart beat does not constitute death unless it has caused irreversible brain damage there must be no spontaneous respirations" [Delmonico 2010]. These observations were later corroborated by Dr. William Sweet published in the New England of Medicine when he wrote "it is clear that a person is not dead unless his brain is dead [Sweet 1978]. The time-honored criteria of stoppage of heart beat in circulation are long enough for the brain to die". Dr. Sam Shemie has clarified the paradigm for donation and death by emphasizing on the "required absence of circulation" and by underscoring the vital functions of the brain as an essential criterion of life [Shemie 2007]. "Where the extracorporeal machines of transplantation can support or replace the function of organs such as the heart, lung, liver or kidney, the brain is the only organ that cannot be supported by medical technology". On the other hand Byrne and others have rejected brain death as constituting death of the person contending the "cessation of the entire brain function, whether irreversible or not, is not necessarily linked to total destruction of the brain or the death of the person". Byrne, apparently, bases his opinion regarding death as philosophically constituting a separation of the soul from the body [Byrne 1979]. However, applying that personal philosophy to the diagnosis of death defies a legal and medical standard, and an ethical and practical sensibility. No one knows when the soul may separate from the body at the time of death. However, the legal and medical definition of death is clear in terms of neurological and circulatory function. It becomes unethical to impose futile clinical treatments to a comatose individual, if the function of the entire brain is irreversibly lost. What would opponents of the brain death determination do with a patient on a ventilator with such a clinical condition have them maintained indefinitely in such a state? To propose the brain death criteria as constituting death was the central issue that confronted the Harvard Committee in 1967 [Ad Hoc 1968]. No one knows when the soul separates from the body, but a precise time of death must be specified for obvious legal, medical and social reasons, so that futile treatment can be concluded (without further obligation or responsibility to provide resuscitative or supportive technologies) and proper disposition of the body with burial and estate and property transfer, etc can be exercised. For many years, Truog has also objected to the determination of death by neurologic evaluation and by circulatory function. He wrote in the New England Journal of Medicine that "arguments about why these patients should be considered dead have never been fully convincing [Truog 1997]. The definition of brain death requires a complete absence of all functions of the entire brain yet many of these patients retaining essential neurologic function, such as regulated secretion of hypothalamic hormones". The rebuttal to this assertion has been given by Shemie [Shemie etal 2006] who claimed that "the release of antidiuretic hormone (ADH) from the hypothalamus is not considered to be essential neurologic function. Brain death is determined by an absence of consciousness, receptivity and responsiveness, spontaneous movement, spontaneous breathing and absence of brainstem reflexes". Brain death does not require every brain cell to be nonviable but the criteria require an irreversible loss of neurologic function of a patient interminably supported by a mechanical respirator. For Truog and others however, these patients are not considered dead because they indeed can be supported indefinitely beyond the acute phase of their illness. It is well known however that despite the irreversible loss of brain function the remainder of the body can be maintained by mechanical support; for example, even by patients who become brain-dead during pregnancy yet successfully have their fetuses brought to term. The clinical condition still constitutes the death of the mother and a viable fetus buys continued mechanical support until birth. Again in the New England Journal of

Medicine. Truog and Veatch [Veatch 2008 &Truog etal 2008 & Life 9 November 1962] have asserted the donation after cardiac death (DCD) is not acceptable; that is, the recovery of organs after the determination of death by circulatory and respiratory criteria. Troug suggests that recovery of the heart following DCD is "paradoxical" because the hearts of patients who have been declared dead on the basis of the irreversible loss of cardiac function have in fact been transplanted and successfully functioned in the chest of another". Veatch is similarly not convinced that the donor is dead and stated that "if someone is pronounced dead on the basis of irreversible loss of heart function, after all. It would not be possible for heart function to be restored in another body. Both Veatch and Truog misinterpret the uniform declaration of death act UDDA which precisely stated that it applies to an individual who had sustained irreversible cessation of circulatory and respiratory functions. It is not a matter of the cessation of heartbeat or cardiac function per se but an irreversible cessation of circulation in the donor. The consequence of the absence of circulation is upon the function of the brain results in an irreversible loss or neurologic function - the UDDA definition of death [Ad Hoc committee 1968 & President Commission 1981 & Delmonico etal 1999].

Bernat has written that circulation - not heartbeat - is the critical function that must be lost using circulatory-respiratory tests to determine death [Bernat 2008]. For example, we do not declare patients dead who are on heart lung machines during cardiac surgery, on ECMO awaiting heart transplantation (even if they never receive a heart), or carrying artificial hearts because, despite absence of heartbeat, their circulation remains continuously maintained. That is why the death standard requires absence of circulation. "Whether the asystolic heart is subsequently left alone, removed and not restarted or removed and restarted in another patient is irrelevant to the circulatory status of the just-declared dead patient [Norton 1992]. Removing and restarting the heart elsewhere simply has no impact on the previous death determination because that patient remains permanently without circulation in exactly the same way as if the non-beating had been left in place". And as an everyday example after slaughtering the rooster it jumps higher and stronger as never than done in its life, this movement doesn't indicate that he is still alive and it continues bleeding strongly indicating that the heart is still functioning, and on the opposite side the heart beating may stop spontaneously, known as cardiac arrest and attempts of rescue continue, in many cases the restitution succeed. The heart start beating again and life gets back to its normal state, moreover doctors can stop the heart for hours during the operation of the open heart, however the blood circulation does not stop, not even for seconds, therefore the heart beating does not mean life and the stoppage of heart beating does not necessarily mean death. Irreversible loss of consciousness may be due to partial or total brain injury [Shewmon 1998]. For the determination of brain death, irreversible coma must be due to injury to the brain so severe as to cause loss of brain functions

Death is when blood stop reaching the brain causing a permanent harm to the brain and leading to a permanent loss of all its functions including the brainstem functions and to diagnose death it is necessary to prove the cessation of the functions of the brain, and then brain commences disintegration and its known that many cells from a dead person remain alive after the declaration of his death. Therefore we find that the muscular cells responds to electrical stimulations and some cells within the liver continue transforming the glucose to glycogen, so cells do not die all at once, however they differ in their timing of death and perish after death of the person. We can extend the life of these cells if they are put in saline solution, especially with the flow by means of a pump hence allowing the use of organs and cell of the dead person for another patient needing them, the death is a process and not an event.

Brain death can be defined as follows: When the brain is damaged, and its activities completely cease, brain death is present, even if it is possible for the patient to be kept breathing and his heart is beating with artificial respiration and medications; even if the heart and liver are functioning that is not live it is just artificial. The consideration of legality of brain death as "true death" was first considered in the early 1960's; with the 1968 Harvard report becoming the "standard" definition of brain death. the majority of countries and international professional associations have accepted it.

5.1 Islamic opinion

The majority of Muslim jurisprudents consider organ transplantation to be permissible on the basis of principles that needs of the living outweigh those of the dead. Saving a life is of paramount value in Islam as the following verse from the Quran illustrates "And if any one sustains life, it would be as if he sustained the life of all mankind" [Ebrahim 1995 & Ebrahim 1998 & Van Bommel 1999 & Al Faqih 1991]. The Islamic jurisprudence Assembly Council in its meeting in Saudi Arabia on Feb 6-11, 1988 ratified resolution number 26.1.41 declared the following fatwa the permissibility of proxy consent: "Transplantation of an organ of the dead to a living human being whose life or essential function of the body would rely on the donated organ is allowed, provided that the dead (before his death) or his heirs permit it. Shiite scholars have made similar rulings. The majority of Shiite jurisprudents confirm organ transplantation especially when human life is at stake.[Moqaddam 2000 & Ghods etal 2006 & Zargooshi 2008].

Ordinarily, the dead have a right in Islam to the sanctity and wholeness of their body, but as we have already noted, the need to save a life overrides this injunction as it has a prima facie importance in the mundane affairs of mankind. While saving a life is of paramount importance in Islam, the family of the deceased must consent and there are in no way obliged to consent to organ donation even if it involves the death of another person who is alive but gravely ill. It has been reasoned that the "ownership" of organs, like that of property, is relative and subjective because God is the ultimate "owner" of the universe having created it. Therefore, it would be permissible to donate them because God had placed great value on saving a life.

5.2 Church opinion

In the address of pope John Paul II to the Transplantation Congress in Rome in 2000, regarding the determination of death, he said ..."it is helpful to recall that the death of the person is a single event, consisting in the total disintegration of the unitary and integrated whole that is the personal self". And that "it is a well-known fact that for some time certain scientific approaches to ascertaining death have shifted the emphasis from the traditional cardio respiratory signs to the so-called neurological criterion. Specifically, this consists in establishing, according to clearly determined parameters commonly held by the international scientific community, the complete and irreversible cessation of all brain activity (in the cerebrum, cerebellum and brain stem). This is then considered the sign that the individual organism has lost its integrative capacity" [Abouna 1984 & Pope John Paul II 2000].

6. Brain death is death

6.1 Misuse of terminology

Patients who fulfill the brain function criterion for death are commonly said to be 'brain dead'. This term, unfortunately, suggests that there are two ways of being dead, being 'brain dead' and being 'really dead'. The term 'brain death' is also used, incorrectly, in other contexts to describe much lesser degrees of neurological dysfunction than it strictly implies. This misuse of the term is to be found in the medical and related professions as much as in the general public. It has lead to confusion surrounding the idea of a brain function criterion and its relation to 'brain death'. It may be that it is too late to reclaim the term for its legitimate use. Whenever it is used, it is important that it is sufficiently qualified to ensure that its meaning is clear, and professional medical bodies may have a role to play in encouraging correct application of the term.

6.2 Explaining brain function criterion to the family of the deceased donors

Even apart from confusion over the use of the term 'brain death' it can be very difficult for families to fully understand the reality of death based on a brain function criterion. To casual observation, patients fulfilling the brain function criterion for death appear to be sleeping rather than dead. The skin is warm. The chest rises and falls with mechanical ventilation. The heart and the kidneys continue to function. There are even reports that pregnancy may be maintained in patients fulfilling the brain function criterion for death. This ambiguity is reflected in the way medical and paramedical staff relates to the beating-heart cadaver in the period before organ donation. Nurses will often talk to such a cadaver as they carry out their nursing care as if the body retained the ability to hear. Acceptance of death by the brain function criterion in the context of organ donation asks much more of a family than does the same diagnosis with a view to cessation of treatment. Community education programs might go part way in helping families understand the issues involved. Detailed explanations with appropriate written material should be provided. Practitioners dealing with families should be trained in the process of explaining the brain function criterion and in grief counseling in general. Families should be provided with the opportunity to ask relevant questions and to have their questions answered in a genuinely sympathetic environment. Sufficient time should be provided to ensure that families really understand the brain function criterion before the issue of organ donation is broached. Families should then be allowed whatever time and assistance are necessary to make a decision concerning organ donation and then to deal with the particular grieving problems over the ensuing days and weeks. They should be offered the opportunity to view the body after the retrieval process has occurred when it has the appearance of being dead [Shemie etal 2006 & Delmonico etal 1999 & Norton 1992].

6.3 Deciding to donate or not to donate organs after death

The main reason why people may consider donating organs is because of the very great benefit that this can bring to others. Organ transplantation may be a lifesaving treatment for patients with liver or heart disease, and it may be the only hope of treatment there is. For kidney patients, having a transplant can mean being able to cease, and this can bring a great improvement in health and lifestyle. For instance, it may enable a kidney patient to return to the workforce, or to work longer hours, and it can even mean that a woman can now have a baby. The transplantation of a cornea can give someone back his or her sight [Ehtuish etal 2006 & Abouna 1998 & Hunsicker 1999 & Alashek etal 2009 & Cohen etal 1995].

Transplantation is generally a very successful procedure. The success rates of transplantations vary, but in all cases these have increased considerably since transplantation first began (Fig. 4b). It can be difficult in medical science to predict which procedures will become more successful and eventually routine. However, kidney transplantation is now considered to be accepted medical treatment and this is likely to happen in other areas of transplantation. Some people decide not to donate organs because they are not confident that donation would be in accordance with their dead relative's wishes. Some people think that transplantation is a very costly procedure from which relatively few people benefit. If you believe that your family may gain some comfort from donation, this may be a reason to consider it for yourself. On the other hand, if you feel that your family may be upset about donation, you may decide against it. This shows the importance of discussing donation with your family. You need also to bear in mind that the people who donate organs are mostly those who have died suddenly and unexpectedly and they are often quite young. For the families of these patients, death may be especially traumatic. When deciding about donation for yourself before death, you may begin by thinking of how you would feel if you were in the position of needing lifesaving organ or tissue transplantation. In making your decision, you also may feel, for instance, that you no longer need your body, and would like to feel that you had done something to help others. Or you may feel that it is important that your body remains intact for burial or cremation. If you belong to a religious faith, you may want to consider how organ donation and transplantation is understood from that religious point of view. Indeed you may wish to consult a religious advisor on the appropriateness of organ donation in your particular circumstances.

6.4 Making a decision when a relative has died

Deciding about organ donation on behalf of a loved relative who has just died may be a very difficult decision to make. Often the relative's death will have been the result of a traumatic event such as a car accident or a head injury. This makes the death an especially sad one for family and friends, means that people are asked to make a serious decision at a difficult, stressful and emotional time. You may feel shocked, bewildered, angry, and numb [Norton 1992]. But, for practical reasons, if organ donation is to occur, it must take place within a certain time period: so there will be only a limited time in which to make this decision. The difficult circumstances in which the decision has to be made make it all the more important that you are well-informed and that you feel confident that you have considered the matter as fully as you wish. Families are greatly assisted in their decision-making at a time of crisis if they have previously discussed organ and tissue donation and the wishes of individuals are known. There are three scenarios that need to be considered: (1) Your relative dies having made known his or her wish to donate organs after death: in this case the family is consulted in order to clarify what the person's wishes were in relation to organ donation and to see whether the family has any objections to the deceased's wishes being acted on. Donation will not proceed in the face of objection from families. If you know that your relative wished to donate his or her organs and/or tissues, this may provide you with a substantial reason for you to consent to the request for donation. Islamic religion respect the intestate and wishes of the person before he died and the relatives are obliged to implement the intestate that is clear in many verses in Quran. (2) Your relative dies having made known to you his or her wish not to donate organs: in this case, made this known to hospital staff and organ donation will not be discussed further. (3) Your relative dies and either had no views about organ donation (as in the case of a young child) or had not made his or her views known to you: in this case the hospital authorities will consult the family to find out whether anything is known about the deceased person's wishes and/or to find out whether the family will consent to donation on behalf of their deceased relative. One thing that you may like to do in this situation is to make a judgment based on your knowledge of that person. What was his or her attitude to transplantation: had he or she ever shown any sign of being in favor or against it? What were his or her beliefs and feelings about the body and about how it should be treated after death? Was he or she the kind of person who would want to help others? Would he or she have been likely to have discussed organ donation with someone outside the family? It is professional practice not to pressure people in any way. The decision that you have to make is not a purely rational or 'head' decision but also an emotional or 'heart' decision. You may need time to come to terms a little more with the emotional significance of events, may be to accept that your relative really is dead. You may wish for time to imagine how you may feel afterwards, whatever decision you make; and how others in your family may feel. You may feel you need time alone, or time with just your family [Evans 1993 & Courtney etal 2009].

6.5 Some key questions you might consider in case of organ donation

Do I think that donating organs and/or tissues for transplantation (or other purposes) is a worthwhile cause? How would I feel if I needed a transplanted organ? How does organ donation fit with my religious, spiritual and moral beliefs? How would I feel if a friend or relative needed an organ? What do my other family members think about organ donation? Have I made my wishes about organ donation known to my family? If I decide I want to donate organs, how will this affect my family? Am I satisfied that I understand the concept of 'brain death' as a way of determining death? Do I feel that I could trust the medical staff involved if I were ever in a situation to be a potential organ donor? How do I think of my body after death? Are there some organs I would like to donate, and not others? Will my family try to carry out my wishes? Will counseling be available for my family if they need it? Am I satisfied that respect will be shown to my body? Are there other people I would like to consult? [Miranda etal 1998 & Jasper etal 1999 & Cameron etal 1999 & Cohen etal 1995]

7. Entry of patients to transplantation programs

Decision-making becomes necessary at two stages of the process of organ and tissue allocation. The first stage deals with those considerations which should be taken into account in deciding on the identity of the individual patients to whom offers of transplants are to be made. Decisions of this type, by reason of the technical details involved, will remain a responsibility of medical personnel. Entry to, and exclusion from, a transplantation program both raise ethical issues.

Entry to a program is offered following assessment of patients by the program personnel. Exclusion criteria include age restrictions, abnormalities in other organ systems, previous history of malignant disease and other medical considerations. In making decisions about which patients are to be admitted to a program, there is merit in more than one medical practitioner being involved.

The second stage of decision-making relates to whether an individual chooses to become a transplant recipient. This is a decision to be made by the patients in the light of advice received from their medical attendants and consultation with their families. Acceptance of the offer requires an informed decision on the part of a patient and/or their family. Prior to this decision, a patient should receive a full description of what is entailed in being in the program, what procedures can be expected and their possible risks and benefits. On the other hand, if a patient is excluded from a transplantation program, he or she is entitled to know why? [Turcotte etal 1989].

In an attempt to ensure that transplanted kidneys have the best outcome possible for individual patients, concurrent medical conditions that introduce a potential risk following transplantation should be managed before acceptance on to the waiting list, If a pre-existing condition is likely to be affected adversely by the ongoing immunosuppression required after transplantation (for example, immunosuppression increases the risk of recurrence of cancer and of persistence of chronic infection) a patient may be excluded from transplantation in his or her own interest. Though some may think it is unfair to deny a patient the opportunity to receive a transplanted kidney because of renal disease which could recur in the graft, others might consider it unreasonable to inflict repeated transplantation when there is a high risk of rejection. In rare circumstances, the kidney allocation system may be suspended to provide an organ for transplantation to a critically ill patient. To ensure fairness in allocation, the selection criteria and weighting of different criteria are subject to repeated review by personnel from all institutions involved in renal transplantation.

7.1 Factors influencing entry to, and ranking in, a transplantation program

a. The patient sickness.
b. The patient most likely to benefit based on medical or other criteria.
c. The length of the patient on the waiting list.
d. All patients on the waiting list should have an equal chance.
e. The patient's importance for the well-being of others, for example previous organ donors.
f. The patients who have previously had one or more transplants.
g. Capacity of the patient to pay.

8. Allocation of kidneys

The allocation of kidneys occurs under circumstances not paralleled in the case of other organs because candidates for transplantation are drawn exclusively from patients already within a dialysis program. This introduces the difficulty that, whereas selection to receive a kidney is determined by clearly defined and promulgated criteria that are uniformly applicable nationally, selection to enter dialysis programs is affected by a variety of sets of guidelines. In some cases uniform criteria for entry to dialysis are being formulated. However, in other instances, individual clinics have their own guidelines, not all of which are readily available. This lack of transparency precludes ethical assessment of the procedures employed and this should occasion concern: it is an ethical issue in itself. As kidneys can be preserved safely by simple cold storage for at least twenty-four hours, the results of a blood T-cell cross match and tissue matching can be available before transplantation is undertaken. Because of the length of waiting lists, several potential recipients are commonly equally well matched with each presenting donor. Allocation of kidneys should be organized on a national basis so that recipients with the closest tissue matching with the donor are selected to receive the organs. This provides the best chance of success. Currently, kidneys are raised by allocation of transplant resources allocated to potential recipients according to the best available tissue match. If there are no suitably matched potential recipients on the national waiting list, the length of time on dialysis usually determines the recipient. Factors such as recipient age, period on dialysis, pre-sensitization to tissue antigens, presence of diabetes mellitus and the previous receipt of a transplant are likely to be taken into account.

The concept of distributive justice - how to fairly divide resources - arises around organ transplantation. Distributive justice theory states that there is not one "right" way to distribute organs, but rather many ways a person could justify giving an organ to one Particular individual over someone else. Equal access criteria include [UNOS 2001]:

- Length of time waiting (i.e. first come, first served)
- Age (i.e. younger to younger, older to older or youngest to oldest)
- Organ type, blood type and organ size
- Distance from the donor to the patient
- Level of medical urgency

Equal access supporters believe that organ transplantation is a valuable medical procedure and worth offering to those who need it. They also argue that because the procedure is worthy, everyone should be able to access it equally.

Successful transplants are measured by the number of life years gained. Life years are the number of years that a person will live with a successful organ transplant that they would not have lived otherwise. This philosophy allows organ procurement organizations to take into account several things when distributing organs that the equal access philosophy does not - like giving a second organ transplant to someone who's already had one or factoring in the probability of a successful medical outcome.

Three primary arguments oppose using the maximum benefit distribution criteria. First, predicting medical success is difficult because a successful outcome can vary. Is success the number of years a patient lives after a transplant? Or is success the number of years a transplanted organ functions? Is success the level of rehabilitation and quality of life the patient experiences afterward? These questions pose challenges to those attempting to allocate organs using medical success prediction criteria. The second argument against maximum benefit distribution is that distributing organs in this way could leave the door open for bias, lying, favoritism and other unfair practices more so than other forms of distribution due to the subjective nature of these criteria. Third, some ethicists argue against using age and maximizing life years as criteria for distributing organs because it devalues the remaining life of an older person awaiting a transplant. Regardless of how old someone is, if that person does not receive a transplant they will still be losing "the rest of his or her life," which is valuable to everyone.

9. Organ trafficking

Organs trading

The transfer, traveling, hosting, receiving living or deceased persons, or their organs, through threat, by force or any other forms of oppression or kidnapping or fraud, or deceit, or misuse of power or position, mis-receipt by a third party of money or subsidies submitted to oppress the contingent donor and use him as an organ donor.

Commercialization of organs

It is the policy or conduct by which the organ is dealt with as if it is a trade goods, including their purchase, sale or use for material gain.

Travel for organs transplantation

It is the travel of organs, donors, recipients or professionals of organs transplantation over the international borders for purpose of organs transplantation.

9.1 Methods and means used for organ trafficking and transplant tourism

The donor, recipient and surgeon may be of the same country. The agreement may be done before they get to the surgeon. The donor and recipient may travel to the country of the surgeon. The patient may travel to the donor country and vice-versa. The donor may be from one country, the patient from another country and the surgeon from third country, and all may travel to a fourth country to perform the transplantation
[Bramstedt 2007] Fig (6a&b). This needs organizers and coordinators, until the matter arrived to the existence of organized gangs aiming for benefit and do not care of the donor or the patient. They are standing on extortion principle and earning profits on the account of poor people and those in need. The matter arrived to even stealing organs, yet to kidnap children and women and even men in order to get their organs for selling them to whom pays more [Fasting etal 1998].

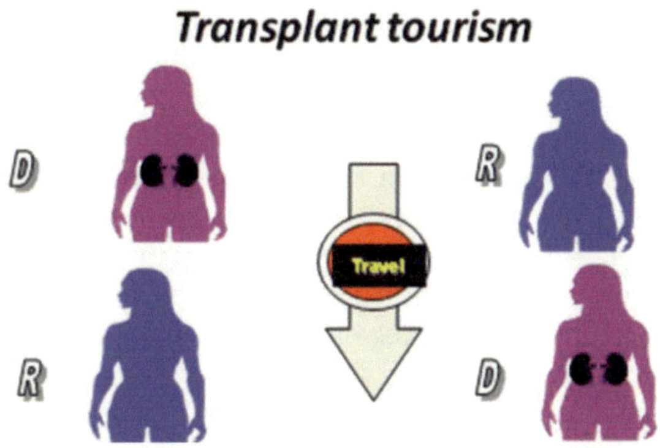

Fig. 6a. The patient may travel to the donor country and vice-versa

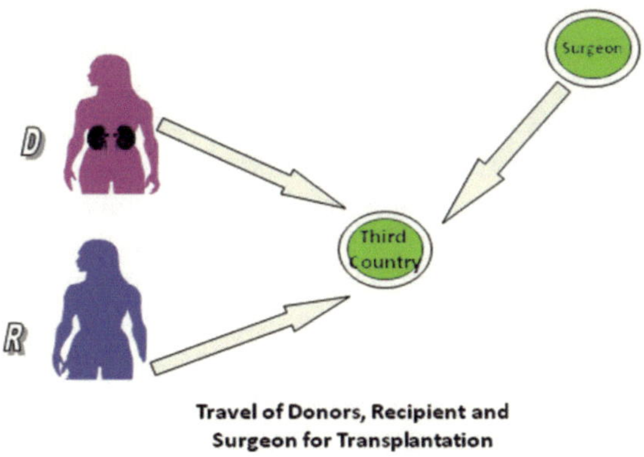

Fig. 6b. The travel of donors, recipients and surgeons for Transplantation

9.2 Organ sale

Paying people to donate their kidneys is one of the most contentious ethical issues being debated at the moment. The most common arguments against this practice include:

- Donor safety
- Unfair appeal of financial incentives to the economically disadvantaged
- Turning the body into a money-making tool "commodity'
- Wealthy people would be able to access more readily

The idea of nonfinancial incentives may be rising in popularity as a way to entice people to donate their organs. Financial incentives aimed at encouraging living donation have received much attention from bioethicists lately. Most experts argue that buying and selling human organs is an immoral and disrespectful practice [Daar 1998]. The moral objection raised most is that selling organs will appeal to the socioeconomically disadvantaged (poor, uneducated people) and these groups will be unfairly pressured to sell their organs by the promise of money. This pressure could also cause people to overlook the possible drawbacks in favor of cash incentives. On the other hand, wealthy people would have unfair access to organs due to their financial situations. It has been noticed that almost all of the people sold their kidneys to pay off debts and those will still had debt some time later but they will have a deterioration in their health status after donation and most of them would not recommend to others that they sell kidneys. Arguments that favor the buying and selling of human organs are scarce, but a few do exist. One of them is that payments aren't necessarily a bad idea if they work to increase the number of donated organs. The position contends that donating an organ is a relatively small burden compared to the enormous benefit reaped by recipients. Some argues that buying and selling organs is not morally objectionable, but that the system as it exists is inadequate to provide appropriate safeguards. This critique extends not only to the medical system, but also to legal and religious safeguarding organizations as well. It is an important ethical issue in organ transplantation. Whatever the perceptions of this practice in developed countries, it is widespread across the world. There are regional variations in its acceptance and practice. In France it is crime to get involved in paid organ donation. Most of the international organizations and forums have called fora moratorium against the sale of organs [Budiani-Saberi etal 2008] but the debate is not yet over. Recently the existing arguments against paid organ donation have been re-examined and found to be unconvincing. It is argued that the real reason why organ sale is generally thought to be wrong is that (a) bodily integrity is highly valued and (b) the removal of healthy organs constitutes a violation of this integrity [Wilkinson etal 1996]. Both sale and (free) donation involve a violation of bodily integrity. In case of free donation the violation of bodily integrity is typically outweighed by the presence of other goods: mainly, the extreme altruism involved in free donation. There is usually no such outweighing feature in the case of paid donation. Given this, the idea that we value bodily integrity can help to account for the perceived moral difference between sale and free donation. International trade in human organs, particularly in the developing countries of the world where cadaveric organs are not easily available and where there is marked disparity in wealth. As a consequence, a deplorable type of medical practice has emerged, where human kidneys are bought from the poor for transplantation into the wealthy clientele with soaring profits for brokers, private hospitals and physicians [Danovitch 2008]. It is estimated that since 1980, over 2,000 kidneys are sold annually in India, Iraq, Philippines, Iran and elsewhere. to wealthy recipients from the Middle East, the Far East and Europe. Human organ ("Kidneys") trade which has shifted from India to

Pakistan [Noorani 2008 & Naqvi etal 2007 &Delmonico 2007]. Media, in particular had gone to the extent of labeling it as shifting of "Kidney Bazar", "Bombay Bazar" from India to Karachi, Lahore and Islamabad [Naqvi etal 2008 & Sajjad etal 2008 & Beasley etal 2000 & Amerling 2001]. Fig (7).

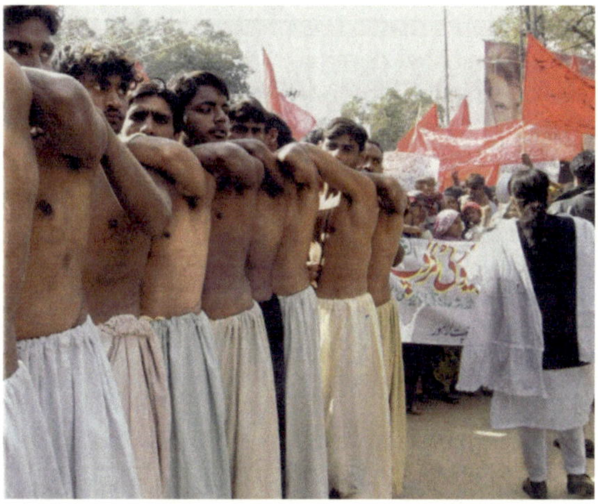

Fig. 7. Kidney bazar

The drawback is that physical harm comes to one person for the benefit of another. However, this is considered an acceptable side effect because of the rule of choosing between the lesser of two maladies, i.e. one person dies and one lives, or, two people live, both with physical deformities. It is not surprising, therefore, that this practice of trading in human organs has alarmed the medical profession, the public and many governments and it has rightly been condemned by all major religions, and by most transplant societies. Organ sale has serious negative impact on all aspects and on everyone involved in the process of transplantation, including the donor, the recipient, the local transplant program, the medical profession and the moral and ethical values of the society. Most ethicists believe that organ sale is an affront not only to altruism, but also to basic human dignity as opposed to a utilitarian approach to the important issue of transplantation for the following main reasons: (a) Organ sale promotes coercion and exploitation of the poor. (b) It promotes poor quality of care to the donor and particularly to the recipient as a result of poor standards of donor selection and inadequate screening for transmissible disease. (c) It benefits ruthless entrepreneurs, greedy doctors who care for their egos and financial gain. It is also against the patient's right for autonomy. It is contrary to accepted moral and ethical beliefs of most societies, including the major religions of Islam, Christianity, and Judaism. It diminishes the current benefit of altruistic donation by living donors and the families of cadaveric donors. It makes human organs a commodity for profit and sale thus inviting corruption and an unjust and unfair system of organ access and distribution and it predisposes to criminal tendencies of selling, kidnapping or killing children and women for organ sale, which has been reported [Spital 1997 & Danovitch etal 2006]. Some proponents of organ sale claim that well-controlled organ purchase does have several major advantages: by making more organs available it can reduce the waiting time for organs, reduce the number of deaths among waiting list patients as well as reduce the overall cost of treatment of patients with end-stage kidney disease. Some professionals in the transplant community believe that it will be much more productive as well as protective from sale of organs by vendors, at least in the developing countries where cadaver organs are not available, if the practice of organ sale is regulated by an independent organization. They argue that the feeling of repugnance of organ sale for the rich and the healthy should not justify removing the only hope for the destitute and dying. Cameron and Hoffenberg [Cameron etal 1999 & Ghods etal 2006 & Friedman 2006 & Laurance 2008] have recommended that organs be paid for through nationally established organ sharing networks to ensure the quality of care received by donors and to promote the equity of distribution which will involve the ethical and medical problems that exist with organ sale. Radcliffe-Richards et al. [Radcliffe etal 1998] have emphasized that current exploitation of donors and lack of informed consent through organ purchase are due to poverty and lack of education, which do not justify banning organ sale. They suggest that a national organization be established to regulate the sale of organs or provide educational and appropriate consultation to patients to enable them to have informed consent and even a 'guardian' for the donor. Also this organization will regulate and control organ vending, proper selection, payment of fees and provision of necessary care which will prevent the current exploitation, the risk of removing organs, both for the donor and the recipient, and provide screening and counseling, together with reliable payment and financial incentives [Friedman E 2006 & Friedman Al 2006 & Surman etal 2008]. They believe that this will not affect cadaveric donation, since payment can also be made to the family of the deceased. Some have proposed a market for organ donation or sale. The proponents of this model propose a legitimate governmental or nonprofit nongovernmental organization to take charge for the responsibility of compensating the donor, without any direct contact between donors and recipients. This would eliminate profit-seeking middlemen and organ brokers. While in certain instances, this practice has led to elimination of the waiting list [Matas 2008], evidence for negative impact of kidney donation for the donors have been reported. The best is to avoid people and their organs of being a commodity in the market weather it is an open black market or an organized and controlled market. In addition to direct payment, various other forms of compensation such as life and health insurance, medal of honor, reimbursement for travel expenses, compensation for time out of work, or a tax credit have been proposed. The potential problem with this model is that if it is not well organized, it will open the door to an organ market, where the organs are sold to the highest bidder, benefiting the rich and disadvantaging the poor [Chapman 2008 & Godlee 2008 & Thomas 2000]. Concern has also been raised that this will reduce altruistic kidney donation and discourage deceased multi-organ donation. However, some believe that it does not preclude increased donation, and others have shown that it has not inhibited the establishment of deceased donor transplantation programs. Opponents to any form of compensation and an organ market cite the concern that the poor will be viewed as mere providers of spare parts and will live with fewer organs, adding to this their list of disadvantages. According to this viewpoint, the market will be driven by poverty and the poor will be a disadvantage compared to the ealthier, feeling a disproportionately higher pressure to sell their organs Fig (8). On a global scale this could translate into people from rich nations travelling to poor countries to buy organs. There is the concern that the market could potentially lead to demeaning bodies to "articles of trade". Degrading human relationships, and particularly damaging the altruistic bond. There is also the concern about the occasional coercion of a spouse by an addicted spouse into selling an organ to pay for the addiction.

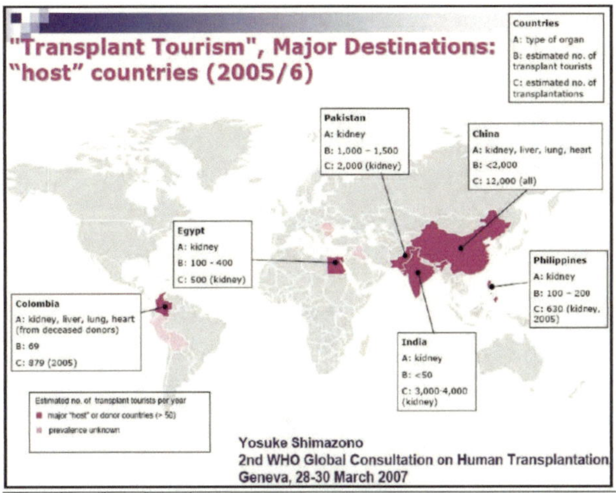

Fig. 8. Major destination host countries WHO publications

With related donor transplantation, altruism is the expected driving force; however, regarding unrelated donors, several valid question have been raised. Why should the unrelated donors not be at least partially rewarded for their donation? Why should they be expected to undergo the surgery and live with one less organ for the rest of their lives? Are the other parties involved (physicians, surgeons, nurses, etc,) providing their services only altruistically? Why should the only individuals sacrificing their bodies not be appropriately acknowledged? Although current laws in most countries and guidelines by WHO and professional societies prohibit the sales of organs, it has been debated that provision of financial incentive seems not only fair, but may also encourage donation and subsequently benefit the patients on the waiting list [Novelli etal 2007 & Satel etal 2008 & Kranenburg etal 2008]. The main opponents of providing financial incentives have voiced concern over "devaluing" the body to a mere commodity and the potential for commercialization. Some would argue that the body is a property and, in fact, the most valuable commodity that an individual possesses. They would contend that the owner of this property has a right to sell part of it for his/her better good.

There is little doubt that commercialization of organ donation is fraught with drawbacks, dangers and potential immoral consequences. On the other hand, it is clear that efforts to increase the rate of organ donation through education have failed and sole moral incentives have not worked [Delmonico etal 2008 & Colakgin etal 1998 & Prasad etal 2006]. Organs are currently limited by supply, and in the hope of expanding the available organs, it seems prudent to provide incentives not only to encourage donation, but also in order to express appreciation. In the process, we should be cognizant of the fact that we might be sacrificing some good for the sake of other potentially more meritorious goods, weighing the ethical and morals risks of one against the other. The obligation of society is to establish safeguards to protect all parties involved, as well as the humane inter-relationship between donor and recipient. In this regard, the method of acknowledging the good deeds of donors is of paramount importance.

It is clear that we need to look for feasible, ethical alternatives to the current model. This is not limited to whether or not donors should be compensated. Now that living unrelated transplant (LURT) has become an ever increasing reality Fig (9). Society and the transplant community should devise safeguards to scrutinize the process [Matas 2007 & Chapman 2008 & Godlee 2008 & Novelli etal 2007 & Satel etal 2008 &Kranenburg etal 2008 & Leung 2006].

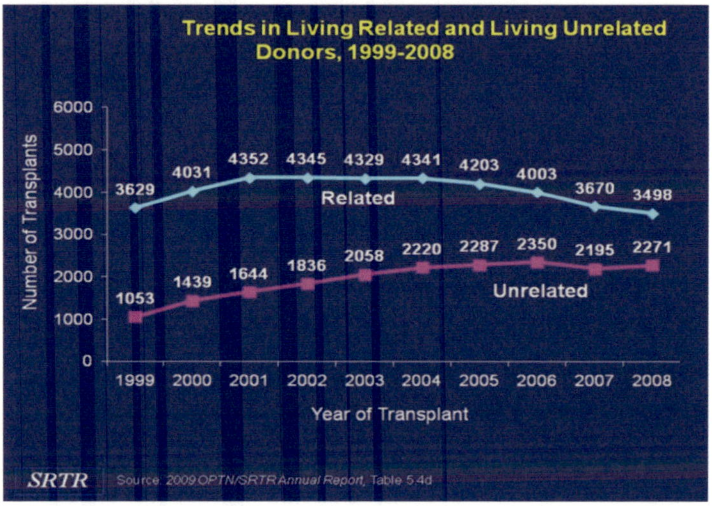

Fig. 9. Trends in living related and living unrelated donors UNOS publications

10. The struggle against international organ trafficking

The antimarket campaign could change things. To be able to do so, however, it needs to embrace a strategy combining new discursive and practical elements.

The campaign against transplant commercialism could be coherent and possibly successful only if it explained that the suffering-preventing capacity of a kidney disease-free and poverty-free world is considerably greater than that of any regulated market in organs [Danovitch etal 2008 & Turner 2008].

10.1 WHO guiding principles for cell, tissue and organ transplantation

WHO has condemned the commercialization of organs in several occasions, starting from the decision of the General assembly No. 40.13 in year 1987 and No. 42.5 in year 1989, and requested the countries to consolidate efforts to implement the decision, then the decision No. 44.25 for the year 1991 which has adopted the first draft of the WHO guiding principles regarding the human cells, tissues and organs transplantation, and which has contoured the methodological and ethical standard framework.

Among the most important recommendations issued by the general assembly, are those issued in its fifty-seventh session (decision 57.18) in may 2004, where the organization has required from the member countries the necessity of existence of an actual supervision on the organ transplantation, and promotion of both living and deceased donation, and to take the necessary measures to protect the poorest and exposed to the organs transplantation tourism. In year 2008, the guiding principles of the WHO have been updated regarding the human cells, tissues and organs transplantation [WHO 2008]. They were adopted by the executive council in its session held in November 2008 these guidelines are.

- Consent for deceased donation
- No conflict between physicians determining death

- Deceased but also live consenting donors
- Minors and incompetent persons be protected
- No sale or purchase
- Promotion of donation no advertising nor brokering
- Physician responsibility on origin of transplant
- Justifiable professional fees
- Allocation rules
- Quality safety efficacy of procedures and transplants
- Transparency and anonymity

10.2 International consultation for the organization of organ transplantation

A group of meetings were held by the WHO joined number of scientists and international and national organizations in order study the challenges facing human cells, tissues and organ transplantation. Open consultations were done in Karachi, Geneva and Madrid, different experts were invited The purpose of all such consultations is to determine the problem about such a matter and also to extract preparatory ideas in order to make them implemented and to encourage countries to have national or regional strategies for self sufficiency by promoting both living and deceased donation and to cooperate towards organ trafficking free world. They urge the need for an international binding treaty to regulate transplantation and to combat organ trafficking [Carmi 1996]. Fig (10)

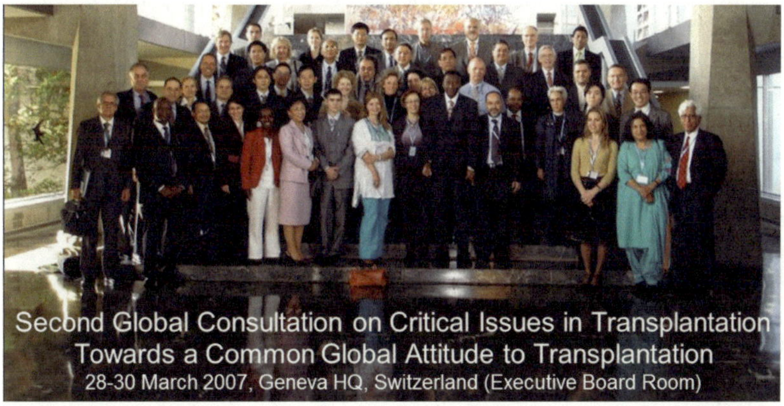
Second Global Consultation on Critical Issues in Transplantation
Towards a Common Global Attitude to Transplantation
28-30 March 2007, Geneva HQ, Switzerland (Executive Board Room)

Fig. 10.

10.3 Amsterdam forum on the care of the kidney donor: Data and medical Guidelines

Kidney and transplant surgeons met in Amsterdam. The Netherland, from April 1-4, 2004 for the international forum on the care of the live kidney donor. Forum participants included over 100 experts and leaders in Transplantation representing more than 40 countries from around the world. The Forum analyzed the sentinel events associated with live kidney donation; the data emphasized the extremely low Operative mortality rates and the long-term safety of this procedure. Forum participants affirmed the necessity for live donors to receive complete medical and psychosocial evaluation prior to donation. A great detail of discussion focused on prevention of transmissible infectious diseases through live kidney transplantation [Delmonico etal 2007].

10.4 Lisbon conference for the care of kidney transplantation recipients in February 2006

An international conference about the care of the kidney transplantation recipients, held in Lisbon, Portugal, February 2nd-4th 2006, with the cooperation between the WHO and different international and national societies of organs transplantation. The conference has joined more than 100 experts and leaders in organ transplantation. It represents more than 40 countries from all over the world. The conference aimed to determine the main issues and to set recommendations to improve the outcome of kidney transplantation all over the world [The Consensus Statement of the Amsterdam Forum 2004].

10.5 Asian campaign against organs commercialization

A meeting was held in Taipei - January 2008, About the immoral and unfair practices related to the organs transplantation in Asia by local citizens and by others from other areas. The recommendation of the Asian campaign stressed the importance of collective measures against organ trafficking [Bagheri 2005].

10.6 Istanbul declaration

An international summit was held in Istanbul on May 2nd 2008, joining more than 150 representatives for medical professional, governmental and non governmental organizations, and transplant societies from 78 countries and 20 international organizations, The meeting was organized by The Transplantation Society (TTS) and the International Society of Nephrology (ISN). The recommendations of Istanbul Declaration have added very important dimensions to the international standards of organ transplantation and emphasized the encouragement of living and deceased donation and stressed on the living donors care and to view their act as a championship as they are sharing in the Gift of life and the necessity to evaluate the donors medically and psychologically before and after donation [Steering Committee of the Istanbul Summit 2008]. The declaration was centered on Organ commercialism, which targets vulnerable populations (such as illiterate and impoverished persons, undocumented immigrants, prisoners, and political or economic refugees) in resource-poor countries, has been condemned by international bodies such as the World Health Organization for decades. Yet in recent years, as a consequence of the increasing ease of Internet communication and the willingness of patients in rich countries to travel and purchase organs, organ trafficking and transplant tourism have grown into global problems.

The Istanbul Declaration proclaims that the poor who sell their organs are being exploited, whether by richer people within their own countries or by transplant tourists from abroad. Moreover, transplant tourists risk physical harm by unregulated and illegal transplantation. Participants in the Istanbul Summit concluded that transplant commercialism, which targets the vulnerable, transplant tourism, and organ trafficking should be prohibited. And they also urged their fellow transplant professionals, individually and through their organizations, to put an end to these unethical activities and foster safe, accountable practices that meet the needs of transplant recipients while protecting donors.

Countries from which transplant tourists originate, as well as those to which they travel to obtain transplants, are just beginning to address their respective responsibilities to protect their people from exploitation and to develop national self-sufficiency in organ donation. The Declaration should reinforce the resolve of governments and international organizations to develop laws and guidelines to bring an end to wrongful practices. "The legacy of transplantation is threatened by organ trafficking and transplant tourism. The Declaration of Istanbul aims to combat these activities and to preserve the nobility of organ donation. The success of transplantation as a life-saving treatment does not require—nor justify—victimizing the world's poor as the source of organs for the rich" [Epstein 2008]

10.7 Madrid conference March 23th-25th, 2010

A conference was held in Madrid. It has concentrated about the self-sufficiency of organs for each country or region. The conference has recommended the necessity to set national plans and strategies to promote the donation of organs from deceased and living persons, arriving to the self-sufficiency and to fight, struggle and limit organ trafficking and transplant tourism.

10.8 Global leadership symposium on organs donation

During the period May 10th-13th, 2010, the global leadership symposium on organs donation was held in California. It was attended by a lot of workers in the promotion of organs donation and a number of the international experts in the organs donation and transplantation and ethicists from several countries to more support the organs donation and fight organ trafficking.

11. References

Abouna GM: Recent Pronouncements by Two Major Religions on Organ Transplantation: Current Status of Clinical Organ Transplantation. The Hague, Nijhoff, 1984, pp XI–XII.

Abouna GM: Kidney transplantation from live donors: Benefits, possible risks and dilemmas. *J Kuwait Med Assoc* 1998; 30:89–92

Abouna GM. Organ shortage crisis: problems and possible solutions. *Transplant* Proc 2008; 40:34-38

Ad Hoc Committee. A definition of irreversible coma: report of the Ad Hoc. Committee of the Harvard Medical School to Examine the Definition of Brain death. *JAMA* 1968; 205: 337-40

Alashek WA, Ehtuish EF, Elhabashi A, Emberish W, Mishra A: Reasons for Unwillingness of Libyans to Donate Organs after Death. *LIBYANJOURNAL OF MEDICINE,* VOL 4, NO 3 2009

Al-Faqih SR: The influence of Islamic views on public attitudes towards kidney transplant donation in a Saudi Arabian community. Public Health, 1991; 105(2): 161-65.

Amerling R: A market for living organs revisited. Transplant News Issues 2001; 2:S16–S17.

Bagheri A. "Organ Transplantation Laws in Asian Countries: A Comparative Study," Transplantation Proceedings 37, no. 10 (December 2005): 4159-4162

Bartholomew A, Sher D, Sosler S, Stock W, Lazda V, Koshy M, Devine S, van Besien K:Stem cell transplantation eliminates allo-antibody in a highly sensitized patient. *Transplantation* 2001;72:1653–1655.

Beasley Cl, Cherry MJ: Body parts and the market place: insights from Thomistic philosophy. Christ Bioethics, 2000; 6(2): 17193.

Beier UH, Hidalgo G, John E. Financial incentives to promote prolonged renal graft survival: potential for patients and public health. Med Hypotheses 2008; 70:218-220.

Bernat JL. The Boundaries of organ donation after circulatory death. N Engl J Med 2008:359" 669-71

Bramstedt KA, Xu J. Checklist: passport, plane ticket, organ transplant. Am J Transplant 2007; 7:1698-1701.

Budiani-Saberi DA, Delmonico FL. Organ trafficking and transplant tourism: a commentary on the global realities. Am J Transplant 2008; 8:925-92

Bukler L, Cooper DK: Xenotransplant: *State of the art. Front Biosci* 1999;4:416.

Byrne PA, O'Reilly S. Quay PM. Brain Death an opposing viewpoint. *JAMA* 1979; 242:1985-90

Cameron JS, Hoffenberg R: Ethics of organ transplantation reconsidered: Paid organ donation and the use of executed prisoners as donors. Kidney Int 1999; 55:724–732.

Carmi A: Organ transplantation in the mirror of the recent world- wide legislation. Med Law, 1996; 15: 341-9

Chapman J. Should we pay donors to increase the supply of organs for transplantation? No.BMJ 2008; 336:1343.

Cohen B, D'Amaro J: Some contemporary ethical consideration related to organ transplantation. Transpl Int 1995;8:238–243.

Colakgin M, Yenicesu M, Akpolat T, et al: Nonrelated living donor kidney transplantation: Medical & ethical aspects. Nephron, 1998; 79: 447-51

Courtney AE, Maxwell AP. The challenge of doing what is right in renal transplantation: Balancing equity and utility. *Nephron Clin Pract.* 2009;111:62–6778.

Daar AS: Paid organ donation-the grey basket concept. J Med Ethics, 1998; 24: 365-8

Danovitch GM, Leichtman AB. Kidney vending: the 'Trojan horse' of organ transplantation. Clin J Am Soc. Nephrol 2006 1: 1133-1135

Danovitch GM. The doctor/patient relationship in living donor kidney transplantation. Curr Opin Nephrol Hypertens 2007; 16:503-505.

Danovitch GM. Who cares? A lesson from Pakistan on the health of living donors. Am J Transplant 2008; 8:1-2.

Danovitch GM, Delmonico FL. The prohibition of kidney sales and organ markets should remain. Curr Opin Organ Transplant 2008;.

Delmonico FL, Radolph JG. Death: a concept in transition. *Pediatrics* 1973;51:234-9

Delmonico FL, Murray JE.A medical defense of brain death.Ethics & Medics1999;224:1-268.

Delmonico FL, Dew MA Living donor kidney transplantation in a global environment. Kidney Int. 2007 Apr;71(7):608-14. Epub 2007 Feb 7

Delmonico FL. The Pakistani revelation. Transplant Int 2007; 20:924-925.

Delmonico FL, Danovitch GM. Regulated market for organs is unattainable. Minn Med 2008; 91:6.2

Delmonico FL. The concept of Death and Deceased organ donation. *Int J OrgTransplantation Med.*, 2010; 1(1): 15-20.

Ebrahim AF: Organ transplantation: contemporary Sunni Muslim, legal and ethical perspectives. Bioethics, 1995; 9(3-4): 291-302.

Ebrahim AF: Islamic jurisprudence and the end of human life. Med Law, 1998; 17(2): 189-

Ehtuish EF, Abouna GM, Shebani AH, Abdulmola TS, Shawesh TZ. Kidney transplantation in Libya: a North African and Middle Eastern perspective Exp Clin Transplant. 2006 Jun;4(1):425-8

Epstein M. The ethics of poverty and the poverty of ethics: the case of Palestinian prisoners in Israel seeking to sell their kidneys in order to feed their children. *J Med Ethics* 2007; 33:473-474.

Epstein M. The Declaration of Istanbul on Organ Trafficking and Transplant Tourism: an important international achievement with one disturbing loophole. BMJ 2008.

Epstein M, Danovitch G. Is altruistic-directed living unrelated organ donation a legal fiction? Nephrol Dial Transplant 2009; 24:357-360.

Eradini S:Stem cells for all seasons ? Experimental and clinical issues. *JR Soc Med* 2002;95:5–8.

Evans RW: Organ transplantation and the inevitable debate as to what constitutes basic health care benefit. Clin Transpl 1993:359- 391.

Fandrich F: Pre-implantation stage stem cells induce allogeneic graft acceptance with host conditioning. *Nat Med* 2002;8:171.46.

Fasting U, Christensen J and Glending S: Children sold for transplant: Medical & legal aspects. Amnesty International-Danish Working Group for children. Nurs Ethics, 1998; 5: 518-

Friedman AL. Payment for living organ donation should be legalized. BMJ 2006; 333:746-748.

Friedman E, Friedman AL. Payment for donor kidneys: pros and cons. Kidney Int 2006; 69:960-2.

Garwood P. Dilemma over live-donor transplantation. Bull World Health Organ 2007; 85:1

Ghods AJ, Savaj S. Iranian model of paid and regulated living-unrelated kidney donation. *Clin J Am Soc Nephrol*. 2006;1:1136–1145.

Godlee F. Is it time to pilot paying for organs? BMJ 2008; 336.

Golmakani MM, Niknam MH, Hedayat KM. Transplantation ethics from the Islamic point of view. *Med Sci Monit*. 2005;11:105–109.

Grant D, Mendicino M, Levy G: Xenotransplantation: Just around the corner? Surgery 2001;129:243–247

Hariharan S, Johnson CP, Bresnahan BA, Taranto SE, McIntosh MJ, Stablein D. Improved graft survival after renal transplantation in the United States, 1988 to 1996. *N Engl J Med*. 2000;342:605–612.

Hull AR & Rosenthal JT: Living kidney donation: A survey of professional attitudes & practices. *Am J Kidney Dis*, 1997; 30: 549-57

Hunsicker LG: Survival advantage for renal transplantation. N Engl J Med 1999; 341:1762–1763.

Jarvis R: Join the club: A modest proposal to increase availability of donor organs. J Med Ethics 1995;21:199–204

Jasper JD, Nickerson CA, Hershey JC Asch DA: The public's attitudes toward incentives for organ donation. Transplant Proc, 1999; 31(5): 2181-84.

Kranenburg L, Schram A, Zuidema W, *et al*. Public survey of financial incentives for kidney donation. Nephrol Dial Transplant 2008; 23:1039-1042.

Landolt MA, Henderson SJ, Barrable WM, Greenwood SD, McDonald MF, Soos JG, Landsberg DN: Living anonymous kidney donation: What does the public think? *Transplantation* 2001; 71:1690–169

Laurance J. Surgeon: organ trade should be legalized. The Independent 13 June 2008.

Leung G. Fun, sun, get a surgery done! The growing trend of transplant tourism. Issues Berkeley Med J 2006; 13:7-8.. BMJ 2008; 336:1377.

Life, They decide who lives, who dies: Medical miracle puts a moral burden on a small committee." Life, 9 November 1962,102

Matas AJ. A gift of life deserves compensation: how to increase living kidney donation with realistic incentives. Cato Institute Policy Analysis 2007; 604:15.

Matas AJ. Should we pay donors to increase the supply of organs for transplantation? Yes. BMJ 2008; 336:1342.

Mathieson PW, Jolliffe D, Jolliffe R, Dudley CR, Hamilton K & Lear PA: The spouse as a kidney donor: Ethically sound. Nephrol Dial Transplant, 1999; 14: 46-8

Merrill JP, Murray JE, Harrison JH, Guild WR: Successful homotransplantations of human kidneys between identical twins. *Am J Surg* 1958; 148:343

Miller DB: Ethics of paid organ donation and the use of executed prisoners as donors. Kidney Int 1999; 55:733–737.

Miranda B and Matesanz R: International issues in transplantation. Setting the scene & flagging the most urgent & controversial issues. Ann N Y Acad Sci, 1998; 862: 129-43

Moqaddam A: Organ transplant not a non-religious act in Iran any more. Tehran Times, 2000 27 September.

Naqvi SAA, Ali B, Mazhar F, *et al*. A socioeconomic survey of kidney vendors in Pakistan. Transplant Int 2007; 20:934-939.

Naqvi SAA, Rizvi SAH, Zafar MN, *et al*. Health status and renal function evaluation of kidney vendors: a report from Pakistan. Am J Transplant 2008; 8:1444-1450.

Noorani MA. Commercial transplantation in Pakistan. BMJ 2008; 336:1378.

Norton DL: Clinical application of brain death protocol. J Neurosci Nurs 1992;24:354–35883.

Novelli G, Rossi M, Poli L, *et al*. Is legalizing the organ market possible? Transplant Proc 2007; 39:1743-1745.

Platt JL: Genetic engineering for xenotransplantation. Transplant Proc 1999;3:1488.

Pope John Paul II. Address to International Congress on Transplants. August 29,2000. (available from http://www.cin.org/pope/organ- transplant-cloning.html)

Prasad GV, Shukla A, Huang M, *et al*. Outcomes of commercial renal transplantation: a Canadian experience. Transplantation 2006; 82:1130-1135

President's Commission for the Study of Ethical Problems in Medicine and Biomedical and Behavioral Research. *Defining Death: A report on medical legal, and ethical issues in the determination of death*. Washington, DC: The Commission; 1981.

Radcliffe-Richards J, Daar AS, Guttmann RD, Hoffenberg R, Kennedy I, Lock M, Sells RA, Tilney N: The case for allowing kidney sales. Lancet 1998;351:1950 –1952.

Rahman F: Haealth and medicine in the Islamic tradition: change and identity. Chicago, IL: ABC International Group, 1998.

Rithalia A, McDaid C, Suekarran S, Norman G, Myers L, Sowden A. A systematic review of presumed consent systems for deceased organ donation. *Health Technol Assess.* 2009;13:1–95.

Sajjad I, Baines LS, Patel P, *et al*. Commercialization of kidney transplants: a systematic review of outcomes in recipients and donors. Am J Nephrol 2008; 28:744-754.23.

Satel S, Hakim N. 'What's wrong with selling kidneys?' International Herald Tribune 20 June 2008

Savules J: Should we clone human beings? Cloning as a source of tissue for transplantation. *J Med Ethics*, 1999; 25: 87-956

Shemie SD, Baker AJ, Knoll G, et al. National recommendations for donation after cardiocirculatory death in Canada: Donation after cardiocirculatory death in Canada. *Can Med Assoc J*. 2006;175:S1..

Shemie SD. Clarifying the paradigm for the ethics of donation and transplantation: was "dead" really so clear before organ donation? *Philos Ethics Humanit Med* 2007;2:18

Shewmon DA. Chronic "brain death": meta-analysis and conceptual consequences. Neurology 1998;51:1538-45.

Sim KH, Marinov A & Levy GA: Xenotransplantation: A potential solution to the critical organ donor shortage. Can J Gastroentrol, 1999; 13: 311-8

Spital A: Do US transplant centers encourage emotionally related kidney donation? Transplantation, 1996; 61: 374-7

Spital A: Should children ever donate kidneys? *Views of US transplant centers. Transplantation*, 1997; 64: 232-6

Spital A: Ethical & policy issues in altruistic living & cadaveric organ donation. *Clin Transplant*, 1997; 11: 77-78.

Starzl T, et al: Renal transplantation from baboon to man: Experience with six cases. Transplantation 1964;2:752.

Steering Committee of the Istanbul Summit. Organ trafficking and transplant tourism and commercialism: the Declaration of Istanbul. Lancet 2008; 372:5-

Surman OS, Saidi R, Purtilo R, *et al*. The market of human organs: a window into a poorly understood global business. Transplant Proc 2008; 40:491-493.

Sweet WH. Brain death. *N Engl J Med* 1978;299:410-2

The Consensus Statement of the Amsterdam Forum on the care of the live kidney donor. Transplantation 2004; 78: 491-492.

The Definition of Irreversible Coma: Report of ad hoc Committee of Harvard Medical School of Definition of Brain Death. JAMA 1968;205: 337

The Economist The gap between supply and demand. 11-17 October 2008:85- 87

Thomas C: Living donor receives leave benefits. Transplant Chronicle 2000;7:4.

Truog RD. Is it time to abandon brain death? Hastings Cent Rep 1997;27:29-37

Truog RD Miller FG. The dead donor rule and organ transplantation. *N Engl J Med* 2008;359:674-5

Turcotte JT, Benjamin M, Caplan AL: Patient selection criteria in organ transplantation: The critical questions. Transplant Proc 1989;21: 3377–3445.

Turner L. Let's wave goodbye to ' transplant tourism' BMJ 2008; 36:1377

United Network for Organ Sharing (UNOS): Annual Report,1999.

United Network for Organ Sharing (UNOS): Policy of Organ Distribution. June 2001

Van Bommel A: Medical ethics from the Muslim perspective. Acta Neurochir Suppl (Wien), 1999; 74: 17-277.

Veatch RM. Donating hearts after cardiac death – reversing the irreversible. N *Engl J Med* 2008;359:672-3

WHO. WHO guiding principles on human cell, tissue and organ transplantation. EB123/5 2008:1-8. Another document that reaffirms the principles of the international campaign against transplant commercialism and global transplant commercialism in particular.

Wilkinson S & Garrad E; Bodily integrity & the sale of human organs. J Med Ethics, Lancet, 1996; 22: 334-9

Zargooshi J. Iran's commercial renal transplantation program: results and complications. In: Weimar W, Boss MA, Busschbach JJ, editors. Organ transplantation: ethical, legal and psychosocial aspects. Lengerich: Pabst Science Publishers; 2008. pp. 80-94

3

Preemptive Kidney Transplantation

Burak Sayin
Baskent University Faculty of Medicine, Ankara
Turkey

1. Introduction

End-stage renal disease (ESRD) is a severe health problem with high mortality and morbidity rates and growing incidence worldwide. Recently, two main renal replacement therapy modalities have been used for ESRD patients: Dialysis and kidney transplantation. It is undoubtedly clear that transplantation is the best choise for long term survival and every transplantation candidate is also a preemptive transplantation candidate.

Preemptive kidney transplantation(PKT) may be summarized as transplantation before the commencement of dialysis in ESRD patients. Preemptive transplantation confers a significant benefit in terms of both patient and allograft survival. The benefit thought to be the result of avoidence of cardiovascular adverse effects of long term dialysis. Current opinion allows ESRD patients to receive PKT when their GFR is 20 mL per minute or less and preparation for transplantation should be started at the time of the diagnosing chronic renal disease.

Kidney transplantation should be the choise of therapy in ESRD patients not only because of improving graft and patient survival and also preventing dialysis related comorbidities and lower cost in the long term(1,2,3). New and more effective immunsupressive drugs, growing experience in transplantation surgery are making kidney transplantation a more common and safe option.

Although there are studies showing nephrologists have the same opinion that preemptive transplantation is the best treatment modality for eligible ESRD patients, that has been convincingly shown to improve posttransplant graft and patient survival. Unfortunately, while PKT is much more beneficial over transplantation, preemptive kidney transplantation seems to be underutilized specially as a result of late referral of the patients to a nephrologist and transplantation center. Only 2% of ESRD patients receive PKT while one forth of transplantation procedures are preemptive in children in the USA. Of course, there are other difficulties for PKT such as poor health status, lack of compliance, comorbidities, older patients, longer waiting time for deceased kidney donors and lack of social insurance.

Ideally, preparation for transplantation should be initiated as soon as progressive chronic kidney disease (CKD) is recognized because cardiovascular morbidity and mortality rates increases while CKD progresses. Early referral to a nephrologist has a vital importance in this situation. Unfortunately, just about 50% of CKD patients come upon a nephrologist in end stage of chronic renal disease. Early referral not only allows careful preparation for PKT and also evaluation of potential living donor candidates and selecting the exact time for transplantation. Because the course of CKD varies according to the primary disease, earliest referral is synonymous to early preparation and beter outcome for transplantation.

GFR 20 mL per minute or less is widely accepted to be the time for preemptive kidney transplantation regardless of the etiology of the kidney disease. Diabetic CKD patients should also be evaluated for pancreatic islet cell transplantation. Kidney biopsy may be helpful for potentially recurring primary kidney diseases after transplantation. A living kidney donor enhances the chance for PKT but deceased kidney donor may be an alternative that should not be failed to remember and all patients should be added to waiting list when GFR decreases under 20 mL per minute. Previously transplantated patients may also be candidates for another PKT.

Recent studies show that preemptive transplantation has better outcomes than non-preemptive transplantation. Lower infection, lower hypertension and less acute rejection episode rates in preemptive transplant patients may be the main reasons for these results. PKT allows preventing from complications during hemodialysis, higher hemoglobin levels before transplantation, lower cardiovascular disease and coronary artery calcification rates, better consistency to immunsuppressive therapy and beter life-quality. Long term graft and patient survival are two major motivators for PKT.

Although kidney transplantation has many advantages against other therapeutic approaches, has its own problems. While kidney transplantation becomes more prevalent, post transplant problems growing as well and transplant recipients becomes a "special patient group". Minimazing the problems of this "special patient group" is a significant target and may only be achieved by proper choise of recipients, appropriate preparation and finally exact timing of transplantation.

Is preemptive kidney transplantation exact time of transplantation? Until mid 80's preemptive transplantation has been thought to have worse results than non preemptive (4,5). But after 90's more recent studies referred just the opposite (6,7). Currently, the question stil remains controversial for nephrologists.

Both in Turkey and in the world, widening of transplantation centers and experienced surgeons and nephrologists PKT has become a more common option. Specially in stage 3 and stage 4 CKD patients early referral to a transplantation center carries a high importance for long term survival.

In USA, PKT constitude 25% of living donor transplantations and 10% of deceased donor transplantations, while the rates are 34% and 14% for chidren recipients respectively(8,9). PKT in children has beter percentages because of family relationships, easier to find a donor for children and probably more doubt of adult nephrologist for PKT (10).

PKT offers preventing dialysis related co-morbidities. Approximately 20% of hemodialysis patients have been hospitalized for vascular access problems and 50% has cateter infections per year. In addition prolonging of hemodialysis process results irreversible cardiovascular problem even after transplantation (7,11). PKT has beter outcomes for both post transplant graft and patient survival and also co-morbidities happening during a dialysis period (10,11).

Mange et al showed improved graft survival of PKT in 8481 living donor transplantation with 52% decrease for graft loss for PKT over non preemptive (12). Kasiske et al found similar results for both living and deceased donor transplantation(13). Chronic allograft nephropathy rates are lower for PKT (14). Some investigators suggest that improved graft survival in PKT patients is a natural result of beter patient survival of selected patients for PKT. Besides other factors for graft survival are similar (15).

It is clear that prolongation of dialysis period in non-preemptive transplantation may result irreversible complications such as cardiovascular disease, renal allograft vascular disease, malnutrition, chronic inlammation,impaired immunologic functions and inadequate clearence in ESRD patients (16,17). Immun system impairment may cause unavoidable infections during dialysis period (18,19,20). Non-preemptive transplantation patients expose to dialysis membranes that may cause activations in immun system which may even cause acute rejection (21,22,23). Hypertensionand left ventricular hypertrophy are more common in nonpreemptive group because of the interdialytic weight gain.

Kidney transplantation should be the first choise in ESRD patients. PKT may be termed as *créme de la créme* and should never be underestimated. Preparation for transplantation should be initiated at the time CKD has been diagnosed and every CKD patient should be accepted as a candidate for PKT for better survival and life-quality.

2. Results and offers

Every CRD patient is a candidate for PKT.

PKT is an important alternative to avoid from dialysis related co-morbidities and complications.

PKT has improved graft and patient survival rates over non preemptive KT.

Early referral to a transplantation center allows proper choise of recipients, appropriate preparation and finally exact timing of transplantation.

PKT offers lower infection rates, lower cardiovascular disease and better life quality.

Every transplantation candidate is also a preemptive transplantation candidate.

3. References

[1] Meier-Kriesche HU, Kaplan B. Waiting time on dialysis as the strongest modifiable renal transplant outcomes: a paired donor kidney analysis. Transplantation 74: 1377–1381, 2002.

[2] Wolfe RA, Ashby VB, Milford EL. Comparison of mortality in all patients on dialysis, patients on dialysis awaiting transplantation, and recipientss of a first cadaveric transplant. N Engl J Med 341: 1725, 1999.

[3] Evans R. Cost effectiveness analysis of transplantation. Sug Clin North Am 66: 603-608, 1986.

[4] Jacobs C, Brunner FP, Chantler C. Combined report on regular dialysis and transplantation in Europe. Proc Eur Dial Transplant Assoc 14: 3-9, 1977.

[5] Kramer P, Broyer M, Brunner FP. Combined report of regular dialysis in Europe. Proc Dial Transplant Assoc 19: 4-8, 1981.

[6] Migliori RJ, Simmons RL, Payne WD. Renal transplantation done safely without prior chronic dialysis therapy. Transplantation 43: 51-56, 1987.

[7] Katz SM, Kerman RH, Golden D. Preemptive transplantation. An analysis of benefits and hazards in 85 patients. Transplantation 51: 351-355, 1991.

[8] John AG, Rao M, Jacob CK. Pre-emptive live-related renal transplantation. Transplantation 66:204-209, 1998.

[9] Papalois VE, Moss A, Gillingham KJ. Preemptive transplant for patients with renal failure. Arguments against waiting until dialysis. Transplantation 70(4): 625-631, 2000.

[10] Mange K, Joffe MM, Feldman HI. Effect of the use or nonuse of long term dialysis on the subsequent survival of renal transplants on living donors. N Eng J Med 8: 726-731, 2001.
[11] Vats A, Donaldson L, Fine R. Pretransplant dialysis status and outcome of renal transplantation in north american children: a NAPRTCS study. Transplantation 69: 1414-1419, 2000.
[12] Mange K, Weir M. Preemptive renal transplantation: Why not? Am J Transplant 3: 1336-1340, 2003.
[13] Wali RKGW, Bellimokunda L, Blahut S. What happens to patients with CHF due to left ventricular sistolic dysfunction defined as left ventricular ejection fraction (LVEF) of less than 40% (congestive cardiomyopathy in uremia) in dialysis dependent patients after successful renal transplantation? Am J Transplant 3(S5): 313, 2003.
[14] Kasiske BL, SJ.Matas AJ, Ellison MD. Preemptive kidney transplantation: the advantage and the advantaged. J Am Soc Nephrol 13: 1358-1364, 2002.
[15] Innocenti GR, Wadei HM, Prieto M. Preemptive living donor kidney transplantation: Do benefits extend to all recipients? Transplantation 83: 144-149, 2007.
[16] Gill JS, Tonello M, Johnson N. Why do preemptive kidney transplant recipients have an allograft survival advantage? Transplantation 78: 873-879, 2004.
[17] Wolfe RA, Ashby VB, Daugirdas JT. Body size, dose of hemodialysis, and mortality. Am J Kidney Dis 35: 80-88, 2000.
[18] Drukker A, Schlesinger M. The Immune system in uremia. Child Nephrol Urol 10: 61-64, 1990.
[19] Meier-Kriesche HU, Port FK, Ojo A. Effect of waiting time on renal transplant outcome. Kidney Int 58: 1311-1317, 2000.
[20] Nishimoto A, Matsumoto Y. Increase of periferal natural killer T cells in hemodialysis patients. Clin Nephrol 55: 121, 2001.
[21] Kaul H, Girndt M, Sester U. Initiation of hemodialysis treatment leads to improvement of T-cell activation in patients with end stage renal disease. Am J Kidney Dis 35: 611, 2000.
[22] Cooper AC, Mikhail A, Lethbridge MW. Increased expression of erytropoiesis inhibiting cytokines (IFN-gamma, TNF-alpha, IL-10, IL-13) by T cells in patients excibiting poor responce to erytropoietin therapy. J Am Soc Nephrol 14: 1776, 2003.
[23] Joo KW, Shin SJ, Lee JW. Preemptive transplantation and long term outcome in living donor kidney transplantation, single center experience. Trans Proceed 39: 3061-3064, 2007.

4

Proactive Management Approach in Prevention of Kidney Transplantation

Levent B. Kıdak
Izmir Bozyaka Training and Research Hospital
Hospital and Health Care Institutions Management
Deputy of Head Physician, Izmir,
Turkey

1. Introduction

Chronic kidney disease (CKD) is a serious health problem that increases both in terms of prevalence and importance all around the world. However, while the number of patients is steadily increasing, not enough organs are available for transplantation and the gap between the patients who need transplantation and the number of existing donors has widened considerably. In order to address the problem of the increased demand for kidneys, we need to review the real issues underlying the existing situation. Is the problem related to the insufficient number of donors? Or are there too many diseased kidneys? If we can accurately define the problem referred to as the "organ shortage", a major step towards the solution can be achieved. The goal of this chapter is to discuss an applicable strategy that aims to reduce or prevent kidney transplantations using a proactive management approach that includes medical as well as managerial strategies.

2. Proactive management approach

Proactive management is based on preventing a mistake before it happens being one step ahead of that mistake. The concept of proactive means taking action before an event happens; and proactive management is an approach based on designing the desired future and the managerial environment in the said future. Proactive management approach is frequently used in management field to change the course of existing conditions deliberately or create new conditions. The essence in this approach which requires developing new paths and strategies to shape the future for organisations and services is long term gains. (Charles, 2008; Kocel, 2005).

Above all, proactive management represents a philosophy, understanding and a belief. This philosophy and belief do not follow after the events but instead shape events by predicting and having an impact on the future. Proactive management or mainly proactive planning approach is to review and explore strategies that enable us to foresee future events (Teixidor, 2006). The beginning of proactive management, i.e. planning is to understand that we have to to look into the future. Planning stage requires to understand that there are opportunities to be used or certain events which may interfere with the structure are about to happen. Planning is the main tool of proactive behaviour. Especially to achieve such an understanding in long term strategic planning, it should be clearly defined as to with what goals the organisation is established, what the organisation plans to do and where the organisation wants to see itself (Kocel, 2005).

Whereas reactive management is defined as a working and management style to look for solutions for the problems already encountered. Reactive management approach means to react to the conditions already encountered, to search to find what needs to be done to adapt to the conditions encountered. Most of the reactive approaches or reactive actions are based on the practices of reactive planning algorithm after the problem happens. The major disadvantage of these processes is that they also include the flexibility which may change the processes assuring the quality of the services. Reactive approach is generally used in situations where the degree of uncertainty is high or there is no information regarding the uncertainty (Teixidor, 2006)

Proactive approach is beyond being dull and over analytical. It is a starting point for change and creativeness. As a result of reactive approach managers become too busy running from crisis to crisis and give a wrong impression that they are constantly working. In reality this situation should be seen as an indication that the management has lost the control. Proactive management includes tools, methods and applications which enable the replacement of reactive managerial habits with a dynamic management style that can actually respond to needs. Proactive approach is related with critical work behaviours for success; it is to develop assertive goals, to frequently review these goals, to develop open policies, to focus on preventing problems, to inquire why work is done in a certain way instead of defending blindly the way in that the work is done (Procen, 2010).

Proactive approach is always more preferred than reactive approach. In proactive approach, it is necessary to monitor the conditions closely to foresee possible developments and to make changes within the organisation. Proactive managerial approach enables organisations to make necessary arrangements so that they could be the least affected by the conditions that they may face in the future. In that sense, developing an early warning system for individuals and organisations is an effective method (Toland, 2007). Early warning system increases the awareness of individuals and at the same time creates a database contributing to the decision making process of organisations while defining paths and strategies.

Although this approach corresponds to preventive medicine approach, this is also a managerial approach which includes calculating risks and challenges in advance, making predictions and developing strategies accordingly. Due to the above qualities, it is used in certain fields of healthcare services such as monitoring and preventing some chronic diseases such as diabetics, cardiac failures and obesity (MacStravic, 2008; Daleiden-Burns & Stiles, 2007). This approach has started to be used also in activating databases in healthcare services and reducing health expenditures of social security organisations (Overhage, 2008; Richardson, 1997).

3. Kidney transplantation and proactive management approach

3.1 Definition

Chronic kidney disease (CKD) is a nephrological syndrome characterised by chronic, progressive and irreversible nephron loss resulting from multiple etiologies. Chronic kidney disease is one of the most important public health issues in Turkey and in the world. Nowadays, the number of people suffering from chronic kidney disease is increasing (Levey, 2007; Obrador & Pereira, 2010).

3.2 Importance

As of the end of 2008, there were 60,592 patients with chronic kidney disease in Turkey. Of these patients 13,346 were added to the total figure within the same year (TSN, 2009). These patients need dialysis treatment or kidney transplantation. 54,700 chronic kidney disease patients were on dialysis treatment and at the same time hoping for kidney transplantation. According to the data of the Ministry of Health, only 2502 of these patients received kidney transplants in 2010. Every year, 110 of 1000 End Stage Renal Disease (ESRD) patients lose their lives waiting for kidney transplantation; and 4506 patients lost their lives in 2008 (TSN, 2009; MHT, 2011). As of the end of 2007, there were 527,283 ESRD patients in the USA. Of these patients 111,000 were included in the ESRD programme in 2007 (Obrador & Pereira, 2010). According to the yearly report of the U.S. Organ Procurement and Transplantation Network and the Scientific Registry of Transplant Recipients, in 2007 16,120 patients and in 2008 16,067 patients of the above received kidney transplantation. In the USA 87,812 ESRD patients lost their lives in 2007. One, two and five year life expectancy of dialysis patients is 81, 65 and 34 percent respectively (Obrador & Pereira, 2010).

CKD is a condition which in addition to causing loss of lives, creates serious social problems for patients especially for paediatric patients, patients' families and the society as with many chronic diseases (Richardson, 1997; Şirin et al., 1995). For adult patients, in addition to economical, social and psychological problems, an important loss of working time is assigned. Children with CKD have growth failure, and their education is hampered and severe psychological problems emerge in their families (Karakavak, 2006; Falkenstein, 2004). CKD does not only cause loss of lives and social losses but also with a yearly expenditure of USD 25,000 per patient, and although relatively less, a yearly expenditure of USD 10,000 for patients who have undergone kidney transplantation, it also causes major economic losses (Kapuagası, 2010). In the USA the total of the costs of ESRD treatment programmes is estimated to be USD 28 billion based on the number of patients in 2010 (Obrador & Pereira, 2010). Such economic consequences of ESRD cause problems in appropriation and use of the resources allocated for healthcare service (El Nahas & Bello, 2005).

3.3 Etiology and reasons

There are certain risk factors leading to the occurrence of CKD. Generally, history of diabetes mellitus, cardiovascular disease, hypertension, hyperlipidemia, obesity, metabolic syndrome, smoking, HIV or hepatitis C virus infection, and malignancy are among risk factors for CKD. In addition to those, family history of CKD, advanced age and treatment with potentially nephrotoxic drugs are other risk factors. Among these risk factors diabetes mellitus, high blood pressure and cardiovascular diseases are the ones which require the most attention to prevent the occurrence of CKD (Obrador & Pereira, 2010).

In the report prepared by The Turkish Society of Nephrology (TSN, 2009) in Turkey, in haemodialysis patients, diabetes mellitus and high blood pressure ranked in the top two among the risk factors of CKD. In addition to these, glomerulonephritis, polycystic kidney diseases, pyelonephritis, amyloidosis and other diseases are also among the risk factors. The frequency and ratios of these risk factors are shown in Table 1.

When the etiology of chronic renal failure in children is examined, the chief ethiologies are found to be vesico ureteral reflux (VUR) and recurrent urinary tract infection (25.9%), then primary glomerulonephritis (18.4%), other known causes (15.1%) and congenital urologic anomalies (excluding VUR) (13.4%) (TSN, 2009). Urinary tract infection (UTI) known to be the most common cause of CKD is usually a preventable disease coming second after respiratory tract infections among childhood infections. According to the studies, UTI is currently an important etiology of CKD even in the developed countries (Warady & Chadha, 2007). Except some congenital diseases, early diagnosis and suitable treatment of almost all anomalies and of UTI and monitoring results can prevent permanent and dangerous results. Additionally children are especially susceptible to permanent kidney damage (ISM, 2005).

Diseases	N	%
Diabetes mellitus	10762	27.9
Type 1 DM	*1761*	*4.6*
Type 2 DM	*9001*	*23.3*
Hypertension	10177	26.4
Glomerulonephritis	3343	8.7
Polycystic kidney diseases	1707	4.4
Pyelonephritis	1616	4.2
Amyloidosis	793	2.1
Renal vascular disease	477	1.2
Other	3005	7.8
Unknown etiology	6210	16.1
Missing data	514	1.3
Total	38604	100.0

Table 1. Distribution of chronic HD patients followed, according to etiology.
National Hemodialysis, Transplantation and Nephrology Registry Report of Turkey (TSN, 2009).

Today it is known that every year, an average of 60 per million people are diagnosed with CKD in Turkey and we know that these patients consult a physician at a very late stage (Kocak, 1993). In the study, the urinary tract disease found in 543 (3.2 %) children coming to clinics for regular vaccinations without any complaints indicates that this is a disease progressing without any symptoms (Kıdak, 2010). In other studies, it is expressed that urinary tract disease constitutes a major health problem due to the reasons that its clinical symptoms can sometimes be very inconspicuous, that it is difficult to obtain valid urine samples and reach to a definitive diagnosis, has a high recurrence rate, is frequently coinciding with urogenital system anomalies, and that it leads to permanent kidney failure in the long term (El Nahas & Bello 2005; Ardissino et al. 2003; Prodjosudjadi, 2006; ISM, 2005).

Consequently, CKD is generally an insidious disease. Most patients are diagnosed with a kidney disease during routine examinations performed without any symptom or sign. Some of the etiologies of CKD are treatable diseases if they are diagnosed at early stages; thus CKD can be prevented or delayed. The most frequently seen and easily detected indicator of kidney damage is proteinuira (ISM, 2005).

3.4 Treatment

There are currently two main strategies to be followed for the treatment of CKD patients diagnosed with ESRD (El Nahas & Bello, 2005; Warady, 2007). These are;

- Dialysis and
- Kidney transplantation.

A good and regular dialysis treatment process is the first strategy to follow. Dialysis treatment which is the treatment method of ESRD is performed to improve the general condition of a patient, to restore water-electrolyte balance and to remove uremic toxins accumulated in the body. When we consider the 10 % possibility for CKD patients to undergo organ transplantation, the importance of dialysis in treatment of patients becomes apparent. Under good circumstances, the life expectancy of the patient can be 10 years in average and sometimes, though seldom, this can go up to 25 years (Kocak, 1993).

Kidney transplantation is the second strategy serving to far less number of patients and with which patients continue to hope for kidney transplantation waiting in the organ waiting lists. Advances in medical technology, improvements in surgical techniques and developments in post operative medications have made organ transplantation an effective and powerful treatment (Fuzzati, 2005). After successful kidney transplantations there remains no need for dialysis treatment and patients become independent. Therefore interest, on reasonable grounds, on human tissue and organ transplantations is continuously increasing.

The goal of these two strategies is to improve quality of life of patients and provide more permanent solutions to patients with transplantation of organs obtained through organ donation. However both strategies serving effectively to the ESRD patients are reactive approaches based on providing solutions after the problem has occurred. In other words, as in most reactive behaviour, actions are carried out after the problem has occurred based on a reactive planning algorithm.

3.5 Problem

Although the number of donors has been constantly increasing in all European countries, this said number is still not sufficient to meet existing donor kidney needs (Fuzzati, 2005). There has been a growing gap between the frequency ESRD in Turkey and in the world and organ donation (Fuzzati, 2005; Ateş, 1998). New alternative solutions are needed for "shortage of donor organs" problem which is still growing in the world. To solve this problem, scientists have been working on both epidemiology of the disease in terms of frequency and diagnosis and treatment management (Ardissino et al., 2003; El Nahas & Bello, 2005; Prodjosudjadi 2006; Warady & Chadha, 2007). In these studies, there is strong evidence that CKD can be screened and treated using simple laboratory tests. It is also indicated that with the same tests, cardiovascular risks causing CKD are lowered, the progression of renal diseases is slowed down, complications are delayed or eliminated (Kıdak, 2010; Levey, 2007). Therefore, in addition to the existing two strategies, new strategies to solve organ shortage problem are needed.

In order to make real and true assessment about CKD incidence and prevalence, epidemiologists and clinicians have been working on different population groups management (Ardissino et al., 2003; El Nahas & Bello, 2005; Warady & Chadha, 2007). Within this scope, protective medicine has been approached with a different understanding all around the world since it has been understood that only a medical perspective is not sufficient for healthcare issues which are increasing in numbers and becoming more complex and contribution of healthcare management sciences is also needed. Donor organ need, besides being a medical problem to be solved, is also a healthcare management problem and managerial solution options should also be considered. Here at this point proactive management approach comes to the scene (MacStravic, 2008; Overhage, 2008).

In some relevant studies conducted, efforts to slow down the progress of CKD and improve clinical results were evaluated and costs of such services were assessed. It is indicated that early diagnosis of CKD and early treatment of patients reduce the costs of the disease and improve clinical results (Jabs & Warady, 1999). At the same time, it is also concluded that early diagnosis diminishes the need for organ transplantation. The proactive management approach may lower the incidence rate of the disease, slow progress of the disease, and therefore improve clinical results and economic aspects of the disease (Khan & Amedia, 2008). In Pereira's study about renal anaemia management period, the importance of early diagnosis and aggressive treatment of anaemia which causes a serious mortality and morbidity in CKD is emphasized (Pereira, 2001). These studies demonstrate that proactive management approach is highly considered for the early diagnosis and treatment of kidney diseases.

3.6 Solution proposal - Proactive management approach in prevention of kidney transplantation

This chapter aims to contribute to the prevention of ESRD and hence decrease the number of kidney transplantations with proactive management approach. In proactive management approach, problems or uncertainties present in the development of ESRD must be defined. It will be advisable to identify what level of performance weaknesses or risks cause uncertainties or problems.

It is known that 10 % of ESRD patients have the chance of organ transplantation, that the disease develops and progress insidiously and most patients consult to a physician at later stages of the disease. When some diseases causing ESRD are detected at an earlier stage, they can be treated thus kidney disease can be prevented or delayed. In light of this information, the importance of the proactive approach becomes apparent. Since proactive approach means taking actions before the event, it is clearly understood that it is of vital importance to detect the signs of the insidious disease before it becomes apparent and monitor the cases. Proactive management of the disease represents an approach based on a desire for a future which will prevent the increase of the number of ESRD patients and on designing the future environment. The goal here is to establish the management structure which identifies risks not after but before patients become sick and takes necessary precautions.

What needs to be done is strategic analysis and this analysis is the starting point of proactive management. It is the stage where problems are defined again, strategies are developed and proactive planning is made (Dincer, 2005). Some basic questions are needed to be asked to make the analysis necessary at this stage (Teixidor, 2006). The first question to be asked in this regard is "what should we do to understand this uncertainty or problem?" This question is the basic question to identify and analyze characteristics of the origins of the problems causing ESRD. The second question is "how can we examine the uncertainty or the problem with proactive approach?" Proactive and reactive approaches address essentially the most prominent and the biggest problems. Identifying and defining problems in a healthy and accurate way will act as a guide not only for implementation but also for controlling activities. Some problems such as determining the implementation time can be solved very easily. Third question is "how can we understand whether the model is suitable and healthy?" The aim of this question is to prevent differences between goals and objectives although they are defined in a suitable and healthy manner and the implementation. Fourth question is "can the problem be identified and solved scientifically?" This question can help us to make progress with solving the problem and also contribute to defining the limits and boundaries of activities. And fifth question is "what are the benefits of the approach and how can it be improved?" This final question is directly related with the basics of research and development activities (Teixidor, 2006).

In this respect, the existing problem should be redefined, the right question should be found and asked. With reactive approach, donor organ need is accepted as the main problem and organ donation is encouraged to be increased thus corrective actions can be taken. However, unless we address the real problems which render organs dysfunctional, donor organ need will grow despite increasing organ transplantations. Is the existing organ need a problem or a consequence of another problem? We need to identify what the problem is and for what we should look for solutions.

According to proactive management approach, the main question here is why there are so many organ failures. When we look into the problem with this approach one of the important options to improve the existing situation of organ transplantation is to lower the need for donor organs. Therefore, it is understood that there are critical processes in this field, which should be managed with proactive management approach; and the first of these processes is to determine the factors causing organ failure and to look for solutions. In other words, the purpose here is to minimise organ failures or to prevent organs from becoming dysfunctional.

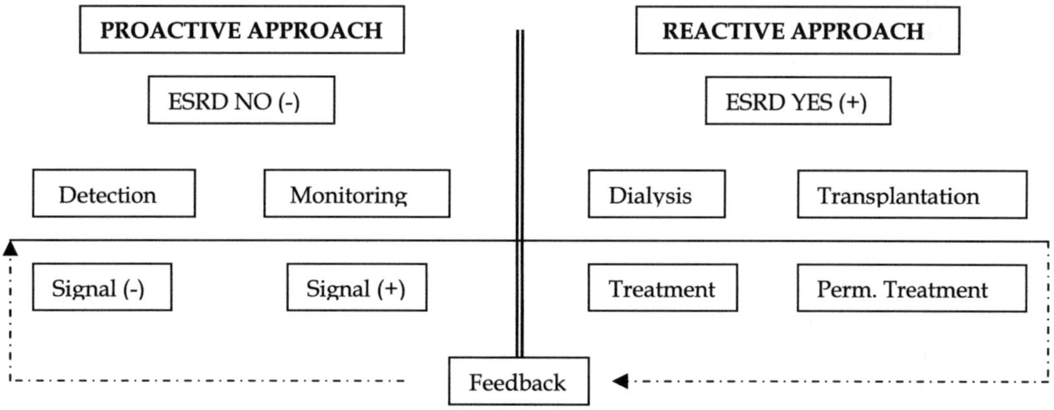

Fig. 1. ESRD in proactive and reactive approach processes

Proactive management approach, as seen in the above Figure 1 focuses on the stage before the disease develops. "Modern medicine" which includes preventive medicine can be considered as the common point between the approach and healthcare services. Accordingly, three main strategic plans; namely primary, secondary and tertiary prevention, can be made in relation to the proactive management of ESRD. These are (Irgil, 2006);

- Primary prevention level is to define risk factors for ESRD, control and monitor signals, and to prevent the disease before it starts and develops. Activities can be oriented to individuals or to the society. Special preventive measures for the diseases are included in this group.
- Secondary prevention level is early detection and treatment of symptoms and diseases causing ESRD and to reduce the number of severe cases. With this method, serious progression of the disease can be monitored, minimised or slowed down. It is a strategy applicable to the diseases which can be diagnosed at early stages and against which there are effective treatments.

- Tertiary prevention level is to prevent the progression of already developed diseases and its complications. It is to mitigate the problems caused by the disease. It enables to improve the life quality by preventing the progression of especially chronic diseases.

The main strategy of proactive management is to systematically investigate signals of the disease in otherwise healthy people before ESRD occurs and to monitor cases giving positive signs more closely taking risk factors into consideration. CKD gives out some signals before reaching to the disease stage. If these signals are detected early, evaluated correctly and necessary measures are taken, it is believed that the existing situation which could be described as the "organ shortage" can be improved and be more problem free. It is assumed that proactive management approach with early diagnosis of insidious kidney diseases, investigation of reasons, slowing progression and prevention of complications has a major effect on the prevention of future negative consequences. With the implementation of this approach, a third strategy could be added to the existing two strategies to solve the problem. Then, these three strategies are; to increase organ donation for more organ supply, to improve the life quality of existing patients by treating them and to work with proactive management approach to lower the need for donor organs.

4. Proactive management algorithm in prevention of kidney transplantation

Healthcare institutions are compelled to deal with diseases which develop as a result of common health risks that, for various reasons, are not evaluated correctly. Proactive methods and strategies are developed to prevent before it becomes a disease. Therefore, the importance of immediate implementation of such methods and strategies which can make the provision of healthcare services effective is clear. Otherwise, or if no new strategy is developed, more resources will be allocated for these services; organ shortage and this vicious circle will become increasingly problematic. In other words, since available structures and resources are not used effectively and efficiently, people who may be prevented from developing ESRD or who should not die of ESRD will continue to die.

In order to the healthcare services to be effective in a social sense i.e. to make the desired changes in the health status of the society, the healthcare services should have certain qualities. It would be useful to take such qualities into consideration when micro and macro planning, organising and delivering the healthcare services. Management in organisations are shaped according to the different structures in the organisation hierarchy. As seen in the Figure 2, there are 3 main management levels in an organisation. These are called senior management level, middle management level and lower management level. Each management level carries out different managerial activities. Accordingly, senior level managers are responsible for strategic management, middle level managers are responsible for functional and tactical management and lower level managers are responsible for operational and program management. There is a close relation among the plans made at these three management levels. Senior level plans are binding decisions for lower level plans. Plans of senior level management should provide guidance for lower level plans whereas lower management level plans should support senior level plans (Dincer, 2004). Plans made at these three levels should constitute a whole connected in terms of the goals and the activities of all units. Plan implementations should not conflict with each other. Realisation of strategic plans is possible only with the realisation of lower level plans. As the management level rises, scope of planning widens.

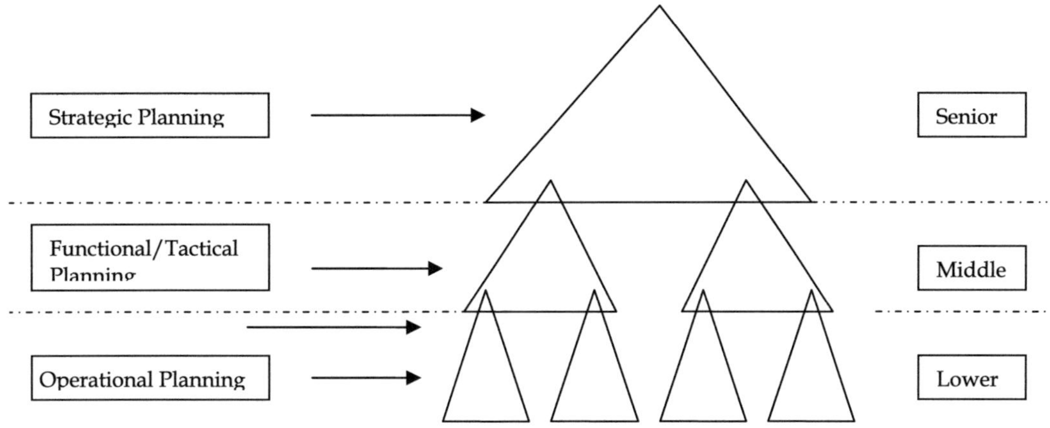

Fig. 2. Types of planning and organisation levels in proactive management (Kocel, 2005)

In line with the above information, ESRD prevention planning and implementation organisation is required through proactive management approach according to the management levels of the healthcare services. Healthy design of this stage plays an important role in the efficiency and success of implementation. Converting strategies into action plans requires suitable organisational structure. Organisation structure refers to differentiating of activities and work as vertical, horizontal and spatial to prevent and reduce ESRD. At the end of this differentiation, activities need to be coordinated. Differentiation is the process in which activities are described for each to management level and for each healthcare institution. These descriptions should be compatible with the characteristics of the work, people and institutions and goals of the organisation (Kocel, 2005). Therefore, to organise the implementation of reduction and prevention plan of ESRD using proactive management;

- Work to be carried out,
- Authorities and responsibilities of the individuals and organisations which carry out the work,
- Knowledge and skills necessary for the individuals and organisations which carry out the work should be defined.

To structure this implementation organisation; exogen factors such as goals, departments, necessary equipment, and endogen factors such as qualifications of employees and environmental factors are used. Senior management should link these factors with each other and define the structure. The structure achieved as a result of this process should be described with an organisation chart. At the same time main responsibilities, duties and authorisation relations which constitute this structure should be explained in a written document called the handbook (Kocel, 2005).

4.1 Proactive management algorithm in the health care organisation for prevention of ESRD

The management levels in the healthcare services organisation are respectively; senior management level is the Ministry of Health, middle management level is Local Health Directorates and lower level management is the management of local healthcare institutions. Each of these three main management levels should carry out different managerial activities within proactive management of ESRD. Therefore in the organisation of healthcare services to prevent and mitigate ESRD activities, authorities and responsibilities, duties of individuals and organisations together with necessary information and competencies should be defined for all management levels. According to the above explained information, decision and planning types of the healthcare management regarding this implementation should be as following:

1. **Senior of Health Management - Ministry of Health:** Strategic planning and new politics
2. **Local Health Directorate**: Functional planning and tactics
3. **Primary Secondary and Tertiary Health Care Facilities - Family Physicians and Hospitals:** Detection and monitoring of ESRD candidates, treatments of patients for prevention of ESRD.

The first step in the algorithm is the integrated strategy of the senior management (Ministry of Health) which manages various institutions and various services. The senior management should develop new policies to prevent ESRD. The Local Health Directorates coordinating and organising activities of healthcare institutions in provinces should determine tactics to implement strategies. Lower management levels which are the management units to carry out activities for individuals and patients should develop implementation plans. Healthcare institutions in all three levels should carry out the activities assigned to them. At first, due to the reasons such as possible lack of information in the primary level healthcare institutions, terminology confusion, difficulties in the recording system, a coordinated work should be planned together with primary, secondary and tertiary health care levels. These activities which will be explained in detail later are shown collectively in Table 2. The study of Teixidor (2006) was referred to while preparing this table.

Ministry of Health Strategic Plannings	**Local Health Directorate Functional and Tactical Plannings**	**Health Care Institutions Operational Plannings**
• Strategic goals and objectives • Vision and mission • Population data (General) • Social and environmental conditions • Medical and technologic developments • Disease information and data • Regional/specific qualities • International aspect • Government regulations • Laws and legal factors • Financial issues • Clinical experiences	• Information flow • Personnel training • Population information (Local) • Capacities of institutions *-Primary* *-Secondary and Tertiary level* • Material supply • Demands of patients and patient relatives • Budgeting	• Business processes • Time plans • Continuity of resources • Quality of resources • Recording system • Collecting of data • Control systems

Table 2. Contents of plan types according to the management levels

4.2 Senior of health management – the Ministry of Health: Strategic planning and new politics

The first stage of proactive management is to identify long term goals which are a part of the strategic planning. This is done by the senior management of the organisation. The most important feature of strategic planning is the time period set forth and the operational activities covered. A strategic plan maintains its qualities to the extent that the time period is prolonged and the plan deals with the organisation in its entirety (Kocel, 2005). The strategic planning under the responsibility of the senior management involves mainly identifying and solving problems in the external environment. Answering the questions about where the organisation will be in the long run, strategic planning is the process in which activities to determine the direction are defined.

"New" ways and strategies should be developed using proactive management approach to shape the future for ESRD on behalf of the healthcare services. Such "new" ways and strategies should be developed by the senior management. Therefore the main activity that the senior management (Ministry of Health) should carry out is strategic analysis which is the starting point of proactive management. At this point, the problem of kidney failure should be redefined, strategies should be developed and proactive plans including new policies should be prepared.

The main duties of the Ministry of Health are to protect individuals' and the society's health and to make, implement and enforce plans and programs covering the entire country for this purpose; to take all kinds of measures, establish necessary organisations or oversee that such organisations are established (Eren, 1985). Goals and objectives should be defined under the scope of prevention of ESRD; the defined vision and mission should be explained to all relevant units and institutions. Information about the present condition of the disease should be monitored and evaluated together with the epidemiologic result of the disease. Future path of the disease should be foreseen using suitable techniques and alternative plans should be prepared. Financial resources should be reviewed to make necessary allocations for the implementation. Medical technology that can prevent the disease should be explored, appropriate techniques should be identified. Characteristics and structure of the population should be studied to ascertain whether there are any local differences. Structural arrangements required for the success of the implementation should be made, legal and statutory requirements should be complied with. These are explained below (Teixidor, 2006; Kocel, 2005; Dincer, 2004);

- Vision and mission: This could be summarised as the way the senior management expresses its opinions about ESRD. What the basic services to prevent ESRD are, which patient groups are offered which services in which institutions, what the main technologies to be used in these institutions are, what the opinions are about the incidence and prevalence of the disease and what kind of image is desired should be identified. All these should be kept in writing and distributed to relevant people, mainly health care providers and institutions. Thus, health care providers will understand why they do what they do, use initiative and decide better about how they can contribute to this service. To achieve these, the senior management should combine existing realities with anticipated conditions to design a future hoped for ESRD. The senior management should visualise its vision regarding this disease, and express its dreams about the future outlook of the disease. The senior management should also define the "game plan" to prevent ESRD and to reduce the number of kidney transplantations.
- Strategic goals and objectives: Goals and objectives of the management play a central role both in decision making and planning. "New" methods should be developed using proactive management approach to shape the future of ESRD on behalf of the

healthcare services. The goals and objectives involving these new methods and strategies can be defined as the strategy to change the conditions. Change in ESRD can be achieved not through better treating patients but through changing the conditions of the existing situation. At this stage, the organisation should decide, in a given period of time, what and how much they want to achieve or where they want to be with regard to ESRD. The number of people screened for ESRD, the number of patients treated, the number of ESRD cases prevented, the desired incidence and prevalence rates, the number of personnel to be employed in a given time, for example 5 years later and the number of training programmes in this period of time should be determined. The most important principle of setting goals and objectives is that the goals are measurable, that they indicate necessary actions and have a time dimension.

- Population data (General): Is to analyse the structure of the population constituting the society. These analyses cover the age, sex, education, economic condition, place of residence etc and other characteristics of the population. Data obtained from these analyses enable managers to make accurate projections, to take proactive actions. This data allows them to identify the risks related with the changes that will happen to the structure of the population, and allows them to take necessary measures in advance. On the other hand, a population structure which can be defined, calculated and estimated will mitigate the risks included in the decision of the senior management. Thus, data about the structure of the population stands out as a secure way for resource planning of the future (Drucker, 2003).
- Social and environmental conditions: Changes and developments in social and environmental conditions are one of the most important determining factors in strategic planning decisions and implementation. Continuous changing of the environment and long time horizon of strategic planning further increases the uncertainty in the environment and emphasises its importance for the organisation. Threats and opportunities introduced by ESRD are evaluated in this context forming the decision focus of the senior management.
- Medical and technologic developments: Medical and technological developments are the fastest changing factors in the healthcare services. What is meant here by technology is the tools and equipment-devices together with the information and processes which are used in the operations. Medical materials, methods and processes used in screening, treatment and monitoring of ESRD, changes and improvements in the devices used should be followed closely. The existing structure and development potential of the technology both in the country and abroad should be identified. In order to do this, in which areas of activities the research and development funds are focused should be established.
- Disease information and data: People with ESRD risk nationwide should be identified, common characteristics of the patients diagnosed with ESRD should be established, results of medical treatments should be monitored, costs of the disease should be calculated, mortality rates and incidence and prevalence rates should be estimated. By investigating the epidemiology of the disease it will be easier to find the reasons of the problem, and parameters to be monitored in controlling activities will be identified. Researches regarding the etiology of the disease which is explained in this chapter and in other studies should be followed; parameters applied to the model should be established.
- Regional/specific characteristics: Tracking regional distribution of ESRD disease, related factors and characteristics is useful in mapping population with risk factors of

this disease and layering risk factors. The prevalence of the disease in certain regions, whether the distribution in cities and towns is clustered in certain areas should be investigated. Demographic characteristics of ESRD patients according to regions should be identified and reported to the concerned local health directorates (Varol, 2009). Infrastructures of the health care services in the regions should be examined, and compared with the regional characteristics of the disease.

- International aspect: Social and economic problems occurred due to ESRD and organ shortage problem should be monitored together in the international arena. The dimensions of the relevant social and economic problems experienced in the developed and developing countries at certain times should be explained. Perhaps if this problem continues to increase, ESRD approaches of all countries will have to be redesigned. Developments and changes with regard to the diagnosis, treatment and monitoring of the disease at the international level are of particular concern to senior managements.
- Government regulations: Governments and ministries are executive authorities. They are responsible for implementing the budget and the programme. Government regulations have strategic influence on defining working conditions about the strategic planning of the implementation, provision of materials and resources, deciding about motivational elements such as rewards, incentives. Furthermore, to increase the efficiency of the implementation, individuals and organisations which will be affected by the model should be informed, suggestions coming from these individuals and institutions should be received and evaluated, a structure to include suitable ones into the regulations should be created.
- Political and legal factors: Political tendencies and legal regulations at both national and international levels may change in time. Such regulations have effects on the success of the implementation of the government and local authorities. With political and legal regulations, in addition to the efforts to further the implementation, development strategies should continue to be created. Furthermore, strategic, political and legal developments in different platforms should be explored. It is advisable to build cooperation between different institutions such as education and social services and create separate mechanisms and structures for these institutions.
- Financial issues: Success of the implementation requires the provision of financial resources reserved for the planned services. And this depends on the balances in the financial structure. The important element here is that the activities planned to prevent ESRD and reduce the number of kidney transplantations should above all achieve the desired results. The beginning, development and maturation stages of the implementation should be defined. Implementation activities are affected by the changes in these stages. Changes in the financial requirements deemed necessary for these stages should be identified and met. Furthermore, the amount saved from the existing expenditures as a result of the implementation should be established and monitored; the possibility of these savings returning to other investment areas in the healthcare services should be investigated.
- Clinical experiences: Clinical studies both national and international should be followed; the applicability of the innovations achieved through research and development activities, their suitability to the country's conditions, financial effectiveness should be monitored comparing long term results. Hence, existing associations (e.g. TSN) should be actively effective; they should support and improve

clinical studies not only about organ transplantation and dialysis but also to prevent ESRD nationwide. Or new structures for which clinical studies have been completed at all three stages to prevent and monitor this disease can be created.

4.3 Local health directorate: Functional plannings and tactics

Local health directorates are responsible for planning and delivering functional and tactical planning services, making human resources and finance related decisions. A directorate makes the connection between strategic plans and operational plans. It is focused more on increasing the efficiency of the resources. At this level, plans are closer to implementation stage and the directorate provides coordination of activities. At this stage, cooperation between organisations, collaboration and mutual support become prominent. The effect of existing organisation on the success of the planned new strategies and new activities should be evaluated. These plans about the synergy of inter-organisational harmony and skills allow to build a connection between the strengths and weaknesses of the organisation and the desired objectives (Dincer, 2005).

- Information flow: Information flow should be addressed in two main groups. The first is the information flow among the levels of the healthcare services, and the second is the information flow among the healthcare management levels. Thus an information flow effectively established between healthcare institutions will enable individuals and organisations to easily reach to information. Cooperation and sharing that ensure an information flow via the internet among the primary, secondary and tertiary level healthcare services will also increase the value of the present infrastructure of the organisation. This structure will allow the problems and opportunities which could not previously be noticed to be seen. With the strengthening of the information flow both between organisations and between organisations and individuals more synergy will be created and the information flow between the levels of healthcare services will become healthier.

  The local health directorates play an effective role in providing information flow between the healthcare management levels. The key role of the Directorates stems from the fact that there is a continuous information and data flow coming from healthcare institutions and they are the local authorities to evaluate such information. Relevant branches of the directorates should monitor and control the results of the implementation comparing them with the plans and goals. The implementation status of the plans and early detection and correcting possible deviations from the plans are vital for the success of the implementation. The local health directorates should periodically report data and information they receive in a predefined format to the senior management (Ministry of Health). This reporting may allow the senior management to follow the implementation. Therefore strategic plans can be controlled and updated.

  Provision of information flow will enable the information flow between primary healthcare institutions which are one of the most important bases of the implementation and hospitals. In order to achieve this there should be a computer network ready to be used. An effective computer network is as vital as the blood circulation in a body in terms of sharing information and generating new information; it will strengthen the connection between the local healthcare directorates and the senior management in addition to the above institutions.

- Personnel training: In this category, teams consisting of doctors and nurses working in the primary level institutions should receive training. Training materials should be prepared by nephrologists, urologists, other clinicians and relevant healthcare services managers. The training materials should consist of intelligible work flow algorithms and be of standard quality nationwide. Trainings of personnel in groups of predefined numbers in a province should be given, if applicable, by expert teams working in the same province. Here the training activities should include operational activities as well as the information about the importance of clinical substructure, registration system, provision of communication and information flow.
- Population information (Local): With the demographic information about the local population, data providing a basis for the planning of the implementation can be prepared. Population and its characteristics registered with primary healthcare institutions or family physicians in that region should be identified. Risk groups in male, female, infant, children and senior population over 60 years of age registered with the primary healthcare institutions which represent the basis for ESRD screening should be identified. To contribute to the ESRD screening activities, information about changes of residence and household density should be obtained.
- Institution capacity: In this category, primary, secondary and tertiary healthcare services for reducing kidney transplantation and preventing ESRD in line with proactive approach should be explained; capacities and roles of these healthcare institutions should be defined.
  - Primary healthcare institutions: The number of primary health care institutions and family physicians in the province should be reviewed. Those who execute the programme at the primary level are family physicians. Therefore, first the quality of accuracy and content of the data of population registered with family physicians should be controlled; problems, if any, should be solved. Additionally, physical structure, number of rooms, laboratory infrastructure, availability, number of employees and their qualifications, consumables and the condition of equipment of institutions, daily, monthly and yearly number of patients in a routine schedule should be reviewed. The number of people to be screened in a given period of time within the capacity of each family practice should be specified. Computer network providing information flow and data processing programme to be used, connections with other people and institutions should be checked.
  - Second and tertiary health care institutions: The purpose of determining hospital capacities is to define their limits in terms of providing treatment to all diagnosed patients. Hospital personnel medically and administratively responsible for the programme should be identified. Number of specialist physicians in the relevant specialty, number of nurses, the quality of laboratory and specific tests, necessary equipment and devices, number of beds and yearly number of patients and number of operations of secondary healthcare institutions in a province should be reviewed. Furthermore, localisations of hospitals should be reviewed to determine with which primary healthcare institutions they are connected. Tertiary health care training and research hospitals should be designated for the patients who require further research and treatment. Yet, the number of nephrologists, paediatric nephrologists and other specialists and other assets of these institutions should be

established. In order to implement strategic plans, number of estimated patients and capacity targets should be identified to provide treatment to all diagnosed patients. It should to determine compatibility with the functional plans. At the same time a structure to provide information flow should be established.

- Provision of materials: Infrastructure of the institutions at all three levels should be examined. Human force, materials, devices, equipment and information flow infrastructure should be reviewed. Personnel shortage, if any, should be solved, and employees should be equipped with necessary information through trainings. Consumables for all institutions, especially urine testing strips, urine collection containers etc should be supplied continuously for primary health care providers.
- Demands of patients and patient relatives: The main goal of the implementation is ESRD patients thus their demands are important. Increase of patients' awareness, their opinions about the medical and support services provided changes of the preferences of patients along the process and factors affecting those have an influence on the understanding and sensitivity of the managers towards patients' demands. Demands and wishes of patients which may be expressed during diagnosis, examination or treatment stages are vital to uncover and solve existing problems. Identifying the problems experienced by patients and their relatives and by those who were treated in the past play an important role for the success of the implementation. Demands and expectations of patients have an impact on the screening monitoring and treatment plans of ESRD and creating algorithms. Identifying medical and social needs of patients will improve patient satisfaction and contribute to faster and lower cost treatment and recovery of patients.
- Budgeting: is to express the plans and the anticipated results in numbers. This activity involves measuring and calculating in numbers and expressing in monetary terms all the activities such as human force, working hours, devices and equipments used etc. Budgeting shows the outcome of the model, what kind of earnings there will be and what level of resources is needed. Obtaining and using the resources economically, effectively and efficiently is necessary to evaluate the performance of the implementation model. It also enables the implementation to be transparent, its accountability to be maintained. Budgeting enables that the results of the applied strategy can be reviewed with different perspectives and the reasons behind can be studied.

4.4 Primary secondary and tertiary health care facilities-family physicians and hospitals: Operational planning, detection and monitoring of ESRD candidates, treatments of patients for ESRD

Multi-level health care services model is used to provide health care services. Multi level health care services refer to providing services which are complementary to each other. This classification involves primary health care services, secondary health care services and tertiary health care services (Hayran, 1998; Kartal, 2004). The main purpose of having multi-level health care services is to enable people to have the right kind of services at the right place. This multi-level structure of health care services ensures that the services provided are efficient and effective and prevents unnecessary utilisation of resources (Belek, 2001). There should be an integrity between the levels of health care services and these services should be provided in coordination. The one which is the most available one to the public and the most frequently used among health care services is the primary health care service. In an effective health care system there should be a relation between the levels. In most of the countries, people are first required to use primary health care services. Provided that primary health care providers find it suitable and necessary, other levels, namely secondary and tertiary can be utilised (Kavuncubası, 2000).

Operational planning is to plan implementation activities. This is the stage which comes after the plans are prepared in line with the objectives, approved according to the operational conditions, and the alternatives to be implemented are identified. Implementation plans should be prepared in a more detailed manner; how and by whom, where and when each activity to reach the goal will be carried out should be explained. At the same time, implementation plans should describe the structure of the organisation and should also include coordination activities (Gözlükaya, 2007).

The purpose of operational planning is to screen patients with ESRD risk, to treat and monitor ESRD patients. Therefore, provision of health care services requires an effort which involves and coordinates all three levels. At this stage, primary, secondary and tertiary prevention principles explained in the proactive management of ESRD are appropriately coordinated between the three levels of health care services.

The success of the implementation depends on the power of the infrastructure of the health care services organisation. Suitability of the organisation's structure, accessibility level of the services, effectiveness of the communication and correspondence systems, technologic advantages of the organisation, cooperation and coordination, qualifications and motivation of human resources, the quality of the materials, devices and equipment used, and maintenance of continuity are the main elements defining the strength of the infrastructure. Success will be achieved within the existing activities of the health care institutions, with the help of the compatibility of the existing resources and structures with the resources necessary for the implementation aimed with proactive approach.

4.4.1 Primary health care facilities: (Family physicians, health centres)

Primary health care services involve the services which combine and provide preventive health care services together with home care and outpatient health care services. These are the health care services which are designed in a way that people can easily access to and use. Healthcare institutions providing these services are the basic and important service facilities which people refer to first. These services are provided in facilities which are positioned and designed to be in locations where people in that area can easily reach to. Primary health care services are considered to be the main starting point in defining health plans and policies of countries, and achieving health care goals (Rico, 2003). These services, depending on the individual country, are provided either in family practices or in clinics.

Primary health care institutions constitute the basis of proactive management implementation with regard to prevention of ESRD due to their availability throughout the country, accessibility and personal data infrastructure. Special preventive measures for diseases are planned in these institutions. The purpose here is to screen and control predefined signals of the risk factors of ESRD, to prevent the disease before it develops. Planned activities should be designed, in addition to addressing individuals and the society, to detect otherwise healthy people who have underlying risk factors without showing any signs or symptoms. Screening and monitoring the symptoms and the diseases defined in the algorithm should be made in these institutions which have an integrated service approach.

- Business processes: Processes and work flows regarding the activities carried out in primary health care. Certain norms should be created for these. Designing business processes allows the distribution of strategic and tactical plans to lower level units and people. In addition to business processes, short term programme objectives or personal success goals should be defined.
- Time planning: Time planning helps to steer the strength of the organisation towards goals and objectives. Time planning is one of the critical processes determining the contribution of the activities for the efficiency. In order to do this, the plan should be kept under control and necessary monitoring should be made to detect any problem. With the help of a schedule, each responsible person can both create his/her own plan and define and track cooperative work activities with other people With time planning; activities for ESRD which are important and not urgent can be identified; those that are vital and have the priority can be emphasised and prioritised.
- Continuity of resources: The final objective of screening and monitoring activities of ESRD is to continue their existence. Availability and continuity of the model depends on the success of the results. Existence and continuity of the resources is also closely related with the success and improvement of the model.
- Quality of resources: Quality of the resources used in ESRD screening has an important role in the implementation of the model. Improving the quality and the features of the resources consisting of materials, equipment and devices is important for successful results and to lower the costs.
- Recording system: Developments in patient recording system contribute significantly to the improvement of the health care services provided during ESRD screening and monitoring activities. The recording system combines physician's records, laboratory records and health care providers' records in all three levels. Here, it should be stressed that the hidden quality of the primary health care services is the recording system.
- Collecting data: Since ESRD is one of the most important public health problems, healthcare data systems are the biggest data sources for this kind of screening monitoring activities. Today, owing to the developments in information systems and communication technologies a lot of medical and health care data can be stored in digital media and are easily accessible. Information systems created with the purpose of collecting, processing and sharing data contain demographic information, disease and treatment condition, tests made, invoicing and administrative information about patients (Yıldırım, 2007).
- Control systems: Control systems are used to control the conformity of the results achieved through the implementation model with the planned outcomes and whether the anticipated success has been achieved. Control process is closely related with the other functions of the model, notably planning. This process which determines the conformity of the strategic plans and plans of implementation with the current situation should be conducted in a very delicate manner and control techniques suitable for the plans should be used.

Urine samples of those coming to primary health care institutions should be tested for leucocytes, nitrite, albumin, protein, blood and glucose parameters using simple analysis techniques (strip); in the event that any of the parameters is found positive, these findings should be subjected to further testing (Kıdak, 2010; Levey, 2007). Since primary health care institutions are the first to accept people, they act as gate keepers, filters for secondary health care institutions (Willems, 2001). Therefore, screening should first be carried out in primary health care institutions; positive cases diagnosed by health care personnel working in these institutions should be referred to secondary and tertiary health care institutions. Gate keeping means that primary health care physicians have the authority to control the access of patients to other levels of the health care system and that patients could access to secondary and tertiary health care services only by referrals of primary health care physicians (Guy, 2001). Therefore, patients with values outside the normal ranges should be planned to be referred to nephrology clinics of consultant hospitals (centres) of the model for further tests and treatment. Screenings can be made during check-ups of healthy people or when they come to health care institutions for other reasons. Positive cases found during these checks should be referred to higher level institutions and results and feedback should be tracked again by primary health care institutions.

The important point to be emphasized in this chapter is the effective role primary health care institutions play in reducing the number of kidney transplantations. This role is basically the result of the integrated/holistic perspective already present in primary health care services. The efficiency level of the role is directly linked to the strength of the primary health care services infrastructure. The stronger this infrastructure is the more efficient the model will work and ease the workload of secondary and tertiary health care institutions.

4.4.2 Secondary and tertiary health care facilities (hospitals)

Secondary health care services consist of inpatient and outpatient health care services including examination, diagnosis, treatment and rehabilitation. They are hospital-based services. They are also referred to as secondary level or therapeutic health care services. The main function of a hospital should be to provide inpatient treatments; outpatient clinic services are not their main services. Secondary health care services in which more advanced technologies are used are evaluated in two groups; outpatient and inpatient therapeutic health care services (DPT, 1989). Tertiary health care institutions, in addition to secondary health care services, are the places where high end medical technologies are used, diseases requiring research to diagnose and treat are intended to be treated. These hospitals are advanced treatment centres where cutting edge medical technologies are used. These mostly include university hospitals, training and research hospitals and specialty hospitals. Therapeutic health care services provided in secondary and tertiary levels involve situations where diseases are treated. These services consist of medical and complementary medical services.

In secondary and tertiary health care institutions early diagnosis and treatment of signs and symptoms leading to ESRD and mitigating severe conditions should be aimed. Monitoring, minimising and delaying the progress of the diseases which can be diagnosed at early stages and be treated effectively should be aimed. Thus, positive cases diagnosed in primary health care institutions should be referred to secondary and tertiary health care institutions (hospitals). Here, people with CKD risk should be identified and monitored for CKD and progression of ESRD in patients diagnosed with CKD should be halted or retarded. Especially patients with diabetes, cardiovascular diseases, high blood pressure, hyperlipidemia, malignancy etc should be closely monitored (Obrador & Pereira, 2010). Urine samples received by health care centres should be tested again with urine test strips and urine microscopy for pyuria and/or nitrite positive. Urine cultures should be taken directly from asymptomatic patients; and from symptomatic patients and patients in whose urine culture samples growth is detected, urine cultures should be taken with catheters.

In hospitals, patients who have developed the disease earlier should be treated to prevent progression and complications. The goal here is to prevent problems caused by the disease and to improve the quality of life by preventing especially the progression of chronic diseases.

4.4.3 Evaluation and sharing of data

One of the most important stages of proactive management implementation is the stage of data collection, evaluation and converting into information. The main purpose of this stage is to develop an early warning and monitoring system. The information obtained will support control activities (measuring the level of goal achievement). The information should be used in updating organisational goals and developing new strategies.

Some of the important elements of the proactive management approach are to develop proactive monitoring tools, activate recording system and improve data flow process (Daleiden-Burns & Stiles, 2007). For this purpose in order to collect necessary information from all three levels, tracking forms which include and detail all data should be created and distributed to the institutions. Clinical examination and laboratory test results on these forms together with monthly activity reports of the institutions should be sent to the Local Health Directorates (relevant department) in electronic format and data should be systematically evaluated. The database created will assist decision makers to make more accurate decisions when defining strategies and goals. On one side, organisational information is produced and shared and on the other side this will contribute to transforming the entire organisation into a **learning organisation**.

In light of this information, despite the negative situation described above, it is observed that most of the present problems can be solved even with the available resources. The existing health care service infrastructure allows developments and improvements to be effected on health care services without necessitating large scale changes. The efficiency and effectiveness of health care services regarding screening and monitoring of ESRD should be improved. With such new strategies existing resources can be utilised more effectively, and with the prevention of ESRD without increasing the resources an improvement in efficiency will be achieved.

5. Application of proactive management model and its results

Up to that part of chapter, theoretical frame work of proactive management approach to prevent ESRD was explained. A summary of the study wchich described the implemented proactive management model is given in last part of the Chapter. This study was published with the title "Decreasing the need for kidney transplantation through proactive management" in Journal of Nobel Medicus in 2010.

In order to prevent ESRD, a program has been started in 2005 in the city of Izmir, Turkey. The aim of this program was to determine the incidence of UTIs in children and diagnose kidney anomalies at an early stage. Also the objective of this program was to start treating the affected children immediately and prevent the occurence of permanent kidney damage. This program, under the leadership of Healt Authority in Izmir city, academicians and specialists in pediatric nephrology that working in two training and research hospitals were included in this study. This study includes all the primary care facilities within the boundaries of the city of Izmir with 239 (91%) health centers and 25 (9%) maternity and child health and family planning centers. The program has been planned and realized for a period of one year between 2005 and 2006. The target grup of the study consisted of all the children within the city limits who applied to these healthcare facilities for inoculation. The most appropriate and efficacious period to reach the target age group has been chosen as the rubella vaccination scheduled at the 9th month, and the diphtheria, pertussis and tetanus boosters together with the polio booster at the 16th month. The population of Izmir is 3.5 million people and the population at the age of 0 is around 45 thousand.

In this study, teams from each facility consisting of a physician and a nurse or midwife (responsible of the laboratuar) have been given a training. The training material has been prepared by the teams serving at the children's nephrology clinics of the related hospitals and the same team also completed the training of the 528 employees in groups of 50. The urine samples of the children applying to primary care facilities have been tested for leukocytes, nitrites, proteins, blood and glucose parameters using a strip. If one of these parameters were positive, the cases have been taken under further examination. The cases outside the normal values are planned to be referred to the pediatric nephrology clinics of the advising (central) hospitals of the project for further analysis and treatment. The urine samples of the cases referred to the centers have been re-analysed using strips and urine microscopy, and bag and urine cultures have been taken from the asymptomatic patients positive for pyuria and/or nitrites. The symptomatic patients and those whose bag and urine cultures showed evidence of multiplication have been taken catheterized culture specimens for the final diagnosis of the UTI. Data collection forms have been designed, printed and distributed for the documentation of the project. Every month, all the urine test results documented with these forms have been sent digitally to the ACSAP Department of the Local Health Authority and assessed using frequency analysis.

Within the one year period when the study was conducted, 16908 children in Izmir aged 0-30 months have been assessed for urinary tract infections. Of these 9080 (53.7%) were male and 7828 (46.3%) were female. Their mean age was 15.6±13.4 months with a median value of 12 months; and the age distribution was 0 to 30 months. During the first evaluations made in the primary care facilities using a urine strip, the samples taken from 14098 (83.4%) children were assessed as normal, whereas 2810 (14.8%) samples tested positive for findings. The 302 (1.8%) children who tested positive have been treated in the primary health facilities, 2508 (14.8%) children have been referred to screening centers for further analysis. Among these children referred to the centers, 1096 (44%) reached the screening centers, whereas 1412 (56%) did not. 490 (44.7%) of the 1096 cases evaluated further in the screening centers have been assessed as normal while 543 (49.5%) of them were classified as pathological. 483 (44.1%) of these cases had UTI, 32 (2.9%) proteinuria, 28 (2.6%) hematuria and 27 (2.5%) urogenital anomalies. 27 (2.5%) patients having UTI together with a urogenital anomaly have been detected. Among the patients in this last group, 63 (5.8%) have discontinued investigations after the first examination (Table 3).

Evaluated Children	Number	Ratio (%)	Further Evaluation	Number	Ratio (%)
Total	16908	100.0	Total	1096	100
Normal	14098	83.4	Normal	490	44.7
Abnormal (Positive finding)	2810	16.6	Pathological	543	49.5
-Treated	*302*	*1.8*	*-UTI*	*483*	*44.1*
-Referred to hospital	*2508*	*14.8*	*-Proteinuria*	*32*	*2.9*
			-Hematuria	*28*	*2.6*
			Discontinued	63	5.8

Table 3. Results of the evaluated cases and the cases after further evaluation

The most important result of this study is the revelation of the fact that the urinary tract disease detected in 543 children (3.2%) who had no complaints at all and had applied to the local healthcare facility only for vaccination, has been demonstrated to be a disease progressing insidiously without giving any evidence. The main issue here is that most of these cases are preventable cases of UTI (483). This number is 2.8% of all the children screened. According to the study findings, there have been a significant number of cases without any complaints or clinical evidence. Of course not all of the detected cases shall develop CKD; but still, unless they are treated appropriately, all of them are candidates for CKD.

This study constitutes an important example for the training, solidification and application of the infrastructure, and the collection and evaluation of the data throughout the three steps in healthcare services. Evaluation of the targeted number of children and complete training supports this view. As in this study, the primary, secondary and tertiary health services may be supplementary and complementary for each other even in a highly technical subject like organ transplantation. The study has also shown that the health system must be managed with a multidisciplinary approach for a more effective and productive use of the sources allocated to healthcare services.

Another finding of the study, that only 1069 of all the cases that tested positive in primary care facilities applied to screening centers and that some of the cases discontinued tests and treatment after the initial application to the centers indicates the shortcomings of this cooperative effort that must be worked on. In additionally, this study pointed out that proactive monitoring systems as a vital part of this proactive management approach must therefore be formed with the registration system activated and the data flow process improved.

6. Conclusion

Evidently, the application of screening and prevention programs in order to reduce the need for kidney transplants arises as a basic necessity. Therefore, through the proactive management approach involving early diagnosis and screening programs, preventable etiologies of ESRD such as UTIs, diabetes mellitus, hypertension, etc beneath the visible part of the iceberg can be diagnosed and treated at an early stage and the number of the ESRD cases may be reduced. The early diagnosis and screening techniques must be in a way applicable in primary care facilities. This screening test must be integrated into the routine healthcare. This method will help reduce the number of the patients undergoing dialysis and waiting for an organ transplant, making comprehensive social and economic improvement possible.

7. Acknowledgments

I would like to thank Dr. Nese Nohutcu, Chief of ACSAP Department; Ass. Prof. Mustafa Bak, Chief of Pediatric Nephrology; Ass. Prof. Nejat Aksu, Pediatric Nephrology Specialist; and their teams and the primary healthcare staff in the city of Izmir for their contributions to the screening program of UTIs in children. Also, I would like to thank Ass. Prof. Nazif Erkan General Surgery for his contribution.

8. References

Ardissino, G.; Daccò, V. Testa, S. Bonaudo, R. Appiani, A. C. Taioli, E. Marra, G. Edefonti, A. & Sereni, F. (2003). Epidemiology of Chronic Renal Failure in Children: Data From the ItalKid Project, *Official Journal of the American Academy of Pediatrics*, Pediatrics; 111; pp. 382-387. ISSN: Print, 0031-4005; Online, 1098-4275

Ates, E.; Erkasap, S. Ihtiyar, E. Yılmaz, S. & Kiper, H. (1998). Böbrek Transplantasyonu Için Donör Havuzunun Genişletilmesinde Bir Kavram: Non-Heart Beatıng Donor Bir Yıllık Retrospektif Inceleme, *Türk Nefroloji Dializ ve Transplantasyon Dergisi* ; 1: pp. 32-34. ISSN 1300-7718

Belek, I. (2001), *Sosyal Devletin Çöküşü ve Sağlığın Ekonomi Politiği*, Sorun Yayınları, Istanbul. ISBN: 975-431-039-4

Charles, S. (2011). Proaktif Yönetim: Yenilik & Strateji, Sabancı Universty, Executive Development Unit, Penn State University, ABD, 17.02.2011, Available from www.su-edu.com.

Daleiden-Burns, A. & Stiles, P. (2007). Proactive Monitoring: Implications Of Implantable Devices For Future Heart Failure Management. *Critical Care Nursing Q*. Oct-Dec;30(4): pp.321-8. ISSN: 08879303 EISSN: 15505111

Dincer, Ö. (2004). *Stratejik Yönetim ve Işletme Politikası*, Beta Basım Dağıtım, Istanbul. ISBN: 9789754865547

DPT, (1989), Türkiye Sağlık Sektörü Masterplan Etüdü Mevcut Durum Raporu, Price Waterhouse, Ankara.

Drucker, P. (2003). *On the profession of management*. The Harvard Business Review Book Series, Boston. ISBN 1-59139-322-1

El Nahas, A. M. & Bello, A. K. (2005). Chronic Kidney Disease: The Global Challenge, *Lancet*, 365: pp. 331-40.

Varol, E. Varol, S. & Tokgözlü, A. (2009). Isparta Ilinde Koroner Arter Ektazisinin Demografik Özellikleri ve Hastalığın Bölgesel Dağılımının Coğrafi Bilgi Sistemleri Ile Gösterilmesi, *S.D.Ü. Tıp Fak. Derg*, 16(1)/ pp. 11-15. ISSN 1300-7416

Falkenstein, K. (2004). Proactive Psychosocial Management Of Children And Their Families With Chronic Liver Disease Awaiting Transplant, *Pediatric Transplantation,* Jun;8(3): pp. 205-7. Print ISSN: 1397-3142 Online ISSN: 1399-3046

Fuzzati, R. Faltings, B. & Calisti M. (2005). Organ Transplantation Management, Swiss Federal Institute of Technology Lausanne, EPFL Technical Report IC/2005/022, Switzerland.

Obrador, G. T. & Pereira, B.J.G. (2010). Epidemiology Of Chronic Kidney Disease And Screening Recommendations, UpToDate Available from: http://www.uptodate.com

Gözlükaya, T. (2007). Yerel Yönetimler Ve Stratejik Planlama: Modeller Ve Uygulama Örnekleri, Pamukkale Üniversitesi, Y. Lisans Tezi.

Guy, M.H.J. (2001). How Do Primary Health Care Systems Compare Across Western Europe, *The Pharmaceutical Journal;* 267; pp. 269-73.

Hayran, O. & Sur H. (1998). *Sağlık Hizmetleri El Kitabı Örgütlenme Finansman Yönetim Mevzuat,* Çevik Matbaası, Istanbul.

Irgil, E. (2006). Sağlığı Koruma, Uludağ Üniversitesi Halk Sağlığı ABD, 2005-2006 Eğitim Programı ve Ders Notları, 11.02.2011, Available from: http://halk-sagligi.uludag.edu.tr/EGITIM.HTM

ISM, Izmir Il Sağlık Müdürlüğü (2005). Izmir Ili 5 Yaş Altı Çocuklarda Idrar Yolu Enfeksiyonlarının Kontrolü Programı, AÇSAP Departman.

Jabs, K. & Warady, B.A. (1999). The Impact Of The Dialysis Outcomes Quality Initiative Guidelines On The Care Of The Pediatric End-Stage Renal Disease Patient, *Advances in Renal Replacement Theraphy,* Jan;6(1): pp. 97-106.

Kapuağası, A. (2010). Sağlık Bakanlığı Tedavi Hizmetleri Genel Müdürlüğü, 27. Ulusal Nefroloji, Hipertansiyon, Diyaliz ve Transplantasyon Kongresi, *Sağlık Dergisi,* 10/22/2010. Available from: http://www.aymedilac.com/tr_haber/haberdetay.asp?hid=5

Karakavak, G. & Çırak, Y. (2006). Kronik Hastalıklı Çocuğu Olan Annelerin Yaşadığı Duygular, *İnönü Üniversitesi Eğitim Fakültesi Dergisi* Cilt: 7 Sayı:12 Güz, pp. 95-112. ISSN: 1300 - 2899

Kartal, M. & Mollahaliloğlu, S. (2004). OECD Sağlık Hesapları Sistemine Göre Türkiye Ulusal Sağlık Hesapları 1999 - 2000, T.C. Sağlık Bakanlığı Refik Saydam Hıfzıssıhha Merkezi Başkanlığı, Ankara.

Kavuncubaşı, Ş. (2000), *Hastane ve Sağlık Yönetimi,* Siyasal Kitabevi, Ankara. ISBN: 975735151-2

Khan, S. & Amedia, C.A. Jr. (2008). Economic Burden Of Chronic Kidney Disease. *Journal of Evaluation in Clinical Practice,* Mar 24, Epub ahead of print ISSN 1356-1294

Kıdak, L.B. (2010). Decreasing The Need For Kidney Transplantation Through Proactive Management, Journal of Nobel Medicus, 16, 6(1): pp. 61-67. ISSN 1305-2381

Kocak, H. (1993). *Doku ve Organ Transplantasyonları,* Haberal M.A., (ed). Haberal Eğitim Vakfı, Ankara.

Kocel T. (2005). *İşletme Yöneticiliği, Yönetim ve Organizasyonlarda Davranış Klasik-Modern-Çağdaş ve Güncel Yaklaşımlar,* Arıkan Bas. Yay. Dağ. Ltd. Şti, 2005 Istanbul. ISBN 9756145447

Levey, A.S.; Atkins, R. Coresh, J. Cohen, E.P. Collins, A.J. Eckardt, K.U. Nahas, M.E. Jaber, B.L, Jadoul, M. Levin, A. Powe, N.R. Rossert, J. Wheeler, D.C. Lameire, N. & Eknoyan, G. (2007). Chronic Kidney Disease As A Global Public Health Problem: Approaches and Initiatives–A Position Statement From Kidney Disease Improving Global Outcomes. *SO Kidney Int.* 72(3): pp. 247-59.

Levin, A. (2001). Identification Of Patients And Risk Factors In Chronic Kidney Disease--Evaluating Risk Factors And Therapeutic Strategies, Nephrology Dialysis Transplantation. *Oxford Journals, Medicine*, 16 Suppl 7: pp. 57-60.

MacStravic, S. (2008). The Real Potential In Proactive Health Management, *Marketing Health Services*, Spring; 28(1): pp. 44. ISSN: 1094-1304

MHT (The Ministry Of Health Of Turkey) (2011). Health Statistics Yearbook 2010, Refik Saydam Hygiene Center Presidency, School of Public Health, Ankara.

Overhage, J.M. (2008). Proactive Medicine. The Benefits Of An EMR In Locations Without One, *Modern Healthcare*, Feb 4;38(5): pp. 24.

Pelczarski, K.M. (2007). Take A Proactive Approach To Bariatric Patient Needs, *Material Management in Health Care*, Jun;16(6): pp. 24-6. ISSN: 1059-4531

Pereira, B.J. (2001). Management Of Chronic Renal Insufficiency: A Call For A Proactive Approach, *Nephrology News and Issues*, Feb;15(3):32, pp. 35-39. ISSN: 0896-1263

Yıldırım, P.; Uludağ, M. & Görür, A. (2008). Hastane Bilgi Sistemlerinde Veri Madenciliği, *X. Akademik Bilişim Konferansı*, Çanakkale Onsekiz Mart Üniversitesi, Çanakkale, 30 Ocak - 01 Şubat 2007

Procen. (2010). Egitim ve Danısmanlık Hizmetleri, 18.02.2011, Available from: http://www.procen.com.tr/altisigma5.htm

Prodjosudjadi, W. (2006). Incidence, Prevalence, Treatment and Cost of End-Stage Renal Disease in Indonesia, *Ethn Dis.* Spring;16(2 Suppl 2):S2- pp. 14-6. pISSN = 1049-510X

TSN (Turkish Society of Nephrology) (2009). 2008 Registry of The Nephrology, Dialysis and Transplantation in Turkey, Istanbul.

Richardson, R.C. (1997). Discipline And Children With Chronic Illnesses: Strategies To Promote Positive Patient Outcomes, *ANNA J.* 1997 Feb;24(1): pp. 35-40. ISSN:8750-0779

Rico, A.; Saltman, R. & Boerma, W. (2003). Organizational Restructuring in European Health Systems: The Role of Primary Care, *Social Policy and Administration;* 37 (6): pp. 592-608. Online ISSN 1467-9515

Süleymanlar, G. (2007). Kronik Böbrek Hastalığı ve Yetmezliği: Tanımı, Evreleri ve Epidemiyolojisi, *Turkiye Klinikleri J Int Med Sci*, 3(38): pp. 1-7. ISSN: 1300-0292

Şirin, A.; Emre, S. Alpay, H. Nayır, A. Bilge, I. & Tanman, F. (1995). Etiology of Chronic Renal Failure in Turkish Children, *Pediatric Nephrology*, Volume, 9, No:5, pp. 549-552. pISSN 0931-041X online ISSN 1432-198X

Teixidor, A.B. (2006). Proactive Management Of Uncertainty To Improve Scheduling Robustness In Process Industries, A thesis submitted for the degree of Doctor Universitat Politμecnica de Catalunya Barcelona.

The U.S. Organ Procurement and Transplantation Network and the Scientific Registry of Transplant Recipients the 2009 OPTN/SRTR Annual Report: Transplant Data 1999-2008.

Toland, C. Meenan, C. Warnock, M. & Nagy, P. (2007). Proactively Monitoring Departmental Clinical IT Systems With An Open Source Availability System. *J Digit Imaging*. Nov; 20 Suppl 1: pp.119-24. ISSN 0897-1889

Warady, B. A. & Chadha, V. (2007). Chronic Kidney Disease In Children: The Global Perspective, *Pediatric Nephrology* 22: 1999–2009. ISSN 0931-041X

Willems, D. L. (2001). Balancing Rationalities: Gatekeeping In Health Care. *Journal of Medical Ethics*; 27: pp. 25-9. ISSN 0306-6800

5

Transplantation in Diabetics with End-Stage Renal Disease

Elijah Ablorsu
Department of Nephrology and Transplant Services
University Hospital of Wales, Cardiff,
United Kindgdom

1. Introduction

Pancreas transplantation is well recognised and established treatment for selected patients with type-1 diabetes. Furthermore, this treatment remains the only therapeutic modality to offer excellent and reliable glycemia control, without the administration of insulin in type-1 diabetics.

It is well documented that combination of pancreas and kidney transplant (i.e. Simultaneous Pancreas and Kidney Transplantation or Pancreas After Kidney Transplantation) gives to patients who suffer from type-1 diabetes and End-Stage Renal Failure superior outcomes, improved patients' survival and better quality of life compared to other therapeutic modalities.

In this chapter will be reviewed current status of pancreas transplantation with focus on recipient selection, management and outcomes.

2. Diabetic Nephropathy

2.1 Definition

Diabetic nephropathy (DN) has been acknowledged as the most common disorder leading to End-Stage Renal Failure (ESRF) in adults (Fig. 1). Renal disease is associated with higher morbidity and mortality in diabetics compared to patients who do not suffer from diabetes. Approximately 0.5% of the population in developed countries (United States and Europe, i.e. Western societies) is thought to have diabetes (ADA, 1999). It is well known that DN is the most common diabetic complication. Patients with type-1 diabetes have the highest risk of developing nephropathy, but those with type-2 have significant risk, too. This condition develops in 50% of type-1 diabetics progressively over a period of 10 to 15 years. In contrast, people suffering from type-2 diabetes can undergo a more variable course and approximately 30% of them will develop DN at some point.

2.2 Etiology

The patho-physiologic mechanisms of diabetic nephropathy are not completely understood yet, but they include hyperglycemia (causing hyperfiltration and renal injury), glycosylation of circulating and intrarenal proteins, hypertension, and abnormal intrarenal hemodynamics.

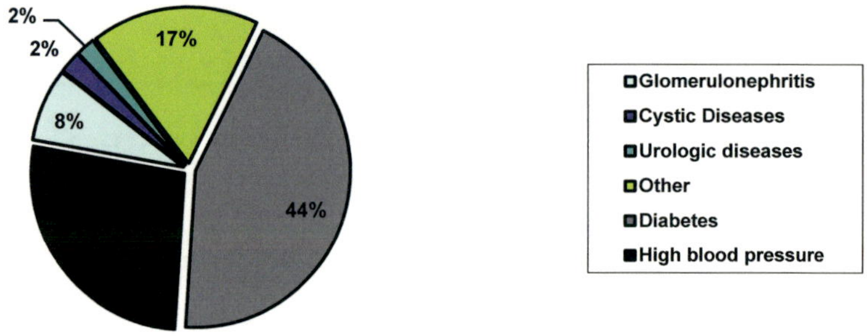

Fig. 1. Primary Causes of Kidney failure (Collins et al., 2008).

For DN are typically three major histological changes that seem to have a similar prognostic impact. Mesangial expansion is induced by hyperglycaemia, causing matrix production or glycosylation of matrix proteins. Another common feature is glomerular sclerosis caused by intraglomerular hypertension; induced by renal vasodilatation or from ischemic injury induced by the hyaline narrowing of the vessels supplying glomeruli. Glomerular basement membran thickening is another common feature, too.

2.3 Secondary complication of diabetes

Among patients with DN we see an increased prevalence of other secondary diabetic complications. Hypertension significantly increases diabetes-related morbidity and is the second most common cause of morbidity in diabetics. It has been documented that hypertension increases mortality in diabetics with renal failure by 37 folders (MacLeod & McLay, 1998). Hypertension also contributes to the developing of DN, microvascular and macrovascular complications.

Diabetic micro and macroangiopatic complications develop simultaneously and have a widespread effect on many organs as well as participating on the development of various diseases (diabetic nephropathy, retinopathy, coronary artery disease, peripheral vascular disease, cerebrovascular disease, etc).

Diabetic retinopathy is the leading cause of visual loss in diabetics due to retinal damage. This condition affects up to 80% of patients who have suffered from diabetes for more than 10 years (Kertes & Johnson, 2007). The main mechanism of diabetes induced retinal damage is a combination of cytotoxic effect of high blood glucose levels and hypertension. Characteristic retinal lesions include the formation of retinal capillary microaneurysms, extensive vascular permeability, vascular occlusion, angio proliferation and basement membrane thickening (Matthew et al., 1997). Some studies have demonstrated (Wong et al., 2008) that the prevalence of retinopathy rises with the increasing duration and severity of the diabetes. However, good glycaemia control reduces retinopathy development by more than 40% (TDCCTG, 1993).

In some diabetics, mainly in patients with long standing or poorly controlled diabetes, symptoms of hypoglycaemia (e.g. palpitation, sweating, tremor, headache, etc.) do not occur. The absence of these symptoms during hypoglycaemia is called hypoglycaemic unawareness. Patients suffering from this condition have a lack of warning signals and cannot actively correct their hypoglycaemia before plasma glucose falls to extremely low levels. The main factor responsible for the development of hypoglycaemic unawareness is autonomic diabetic neuropathy and brain desensitization to hypoglycaemia.

Absence of glucose homeostasis in diabetes also causes pathological damage and functional disturbance of the peripheral (motor and sensor) and autonomic nerves. Frequently, patients suffer from motor neuropathy: pain, paresthesia and anesthesia. Autonomic neuropathy (arrhythmia, postural hypotension, diabetic diarrhoea, gastroparesis, neurogenic bladder, impotence, etc) is less common than peripheral neuropathy, but is a more symptomatic and has limited therapeutic effect (Watkins & Edmonds, 1997).

The development of complications is related to the severity and length of diabetes, and its management involves glucose control and symptomatic treatment which seems to have a positive effect (Ward, 1997).

2.4 Management

In recent years, there has been significant progress in the management and treatment of diabetics. We have seen not only a reduced morbidity but also increased patients' survival and improved patients' quality of life. Median patient survival in recent years amongst this population has increased from 6 to 15 years (Wiesbauer et al., 2010).

It is well known that poor diabetic control is responsible for developing various diabetic complications; mainly DN. The risk of developing nephropathy is significantly reduced if HbA1c stays below 7.5-8.0% (Deferrari et al., 1998; Di Landro et al, 1998). For that reason the American Diabetes Association highlights in their "Guidelines for Glycemic Control" to target HBA1c level below 7% to achieve a normal or near normal glycemia (ADA, 2005).

It was documented in two large studies on a cohort of 1349 patients, the DCCT (Diabetes Controlled and Complication Trial) and EDIC (Epidemiology of Diabetes Intervention and Complications) that tight glycemic control decreases the risk of development of microvascular disease (retinopathy, nephropathy, and neuropathy) and even slows down established DN (TDCCTRG, 1993), (DCCT, 2003).

In brittle type-1 diabetes serum glucose levels can rapidly swing between extremely low and high levels. This can lead to the development of acute and life threatening conditions: keto-acidosis, coma or even death. Often patients have absent warning symptoms. In some diabetics it is difficult, and even impossible, to achieve a good glycemic control with conventional management.

Nowadays, varieties of insulin preparations are available. The type, the dose and the frequency of insulin doses depends on patient's individual factors. For type-1 diabetics "Basal-bolus insulin regiment" (a combination of high frequency boluses of short-acting insulin with long-acting insulin) is often used. Some people benefit from "Mixed insulin regiment". This includes a mixture of short and long-acting insulin delivered two to three times a day. Regardless of meticulous blood glucose monitoring and accurate insulin dosage, some patients may still have problems achieving an appropriate blood glucose level. These patients may be considered for an insulin pump. The disadvantage of this method is increased frequency of hypo/hyper glycemia episodes and also the fact that it requires a cannula implantation (Collins et al., 2007).

The innovations in insulin formulation and delivery have had a significant impact on the management of type-1 diabetes and they have improved glycaemic control. Despite this

progress, many patients cannot achieve a good degree of serum glucose control and keep suffering from frequent sudden hypoglycaemia episodes. These circumstances have a negative impact on patients' quality of life and can even be life threatening.
In addition, sufficient management of DN also includes rigorous treatment of hypertension in combination with conventional management of renal failure, hyperlipidemia, anaemia, etc.

3. Pancreas transplantation

The first pancreas transplant was performed at the University of Minnesota, in Minneapolis, on 17 December 1966 by the team led by Dr William Kelly and Dr Richard Lillehei (Kelly et all., 1967). A pancreas, together with a kidney, was implanted to a 28-year old woman. Immediately after the transplantation the patient became euglycemic, but unfortunately she died three months later from a pulmonary embolism with functioning grafts. The same team in Minneapolis, on 3 June 1969, performed the first successful pancreas transplant and the pancreas graft functioned for more than one year (Lillehei & et al., 1970). Early experiences with pancreas transplantation were disappointing, as they were associated with a high incidence of rejection, infectious complications and early graft failure. Progressively in the late 70's and early 80's the results of pancreas transplantation improved. First of all, the original Lillehei surgical technique was modified and refined. In 1988 Starz published a technique of anastomozing graft duodenum to the recipient jejunum for draining a pancreas graft exocrine secretion (Fig 2) (Starzl et al., 1988). Subsequently, his technique was adopted by other big pancreas transplant institutions; by Dr Hans Sollinger at the University of

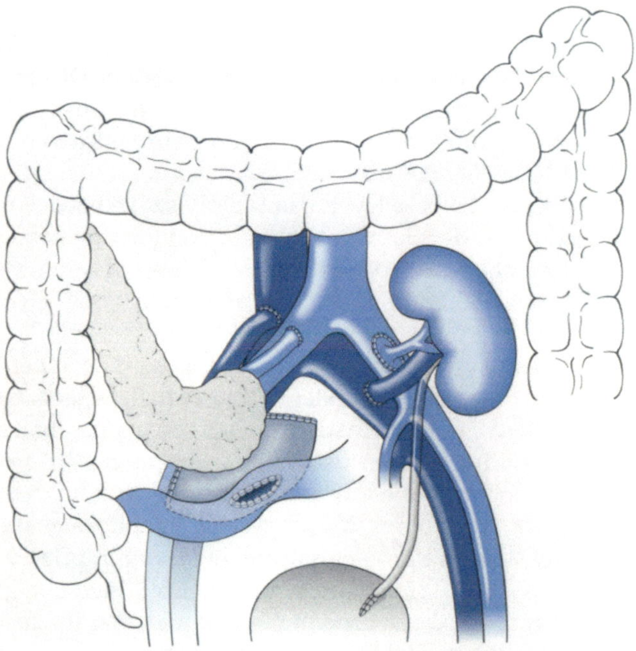

Fig. 2. The Enteric drainage technique in simultaneous pancreas and kidney transplantation. Pancreas graft duodenum is anastomosed side-to-side to the jejunum of a recipient.

Wisconsin and Dr Robert Corry at the University of Iowa. Later, all three centres employed to their routine practice the technique of draining graft duodenum to the bladder (Fig 3) (Sutherland et al., 1988; Sollinger & Belzer, 1988; Corry, 1988). Both techniques, with minimal modifications are still used these days. A number of studies compared the outcomes between bladder and enteric drained pancreas transplants. Most of them showed similar complication rates (Lo et al., 2001; Stratta et al., 2000), graft and patient survival (Sugitani et al., 1998).

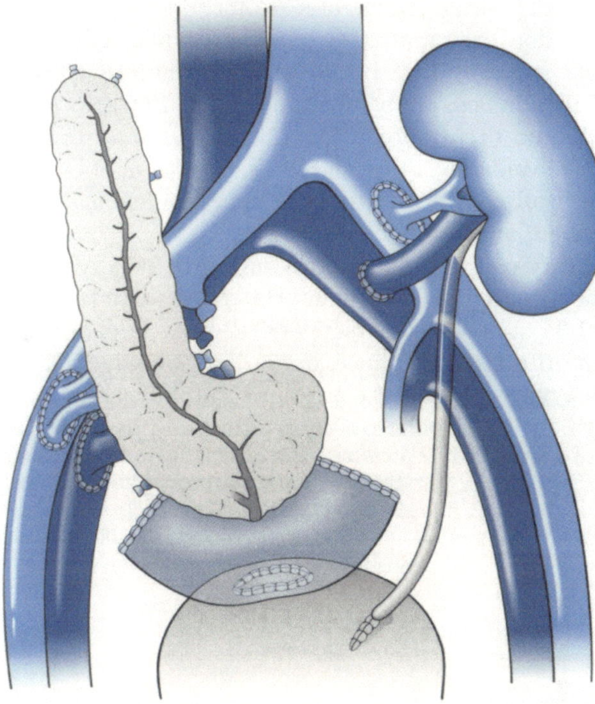

Fig. 3. The Bladder drainage technique in simultaneous pancreas and kidney transplantation. Pancreas graft duodenum is anastomosed side-to-side to the bladder of a recipient.

The Enteric Drainage pancreas technique compared (ED) to the Bladder Drainage pancreas technique (BD) is a more physiological option because it drains pancreatic enzymes into intestinal track. However, this technique is associated with a higher rate of surgical complications (anastomotic leak, chemical and infectious peritonitis, ileus, intra-abdominal abscess formation, etc.). A typical complication of bladder drainage technique is the recurrence of urinary track infections, haematuria, urethral strictures, prostatitis, pyeloneophritis, reflux pancreatitis, etc. Additionally to these complications, the urinary diversion of exocrine pancreas graft secretion potentiates excessive loss of bicarbonates, sodium and fluid. This results in acid-base and electrolytes disturbance (metabolic acidosis) and fluid depletion. Metabolic acidosis is even more exacerbated by renal dysfunction. For those reasons, serum electrolytes must be closely monitored in patients with bladder drained pancreas, patients must be well hydrated and receive bicarbonate supplements.

Enteric conversion is a surgical alternative to manage sever complications related to the bladder drainage of pancreas graft (Stephanian et al., 1992). The United Network for Organ Sharing (UNOS) and the International Pancreas Transplant Registry (IPTR) data from 2005 reports the overall conversion rate from BD to ED of 9% at 1 year and 17% at 3 years after transplant (Gruessner & Sutherland, 2005). The major indications for conversion were recurrent episodes of haematuria, graft pancreatitis, chronic urinary track infections, dehydration and bladder calculi (Jimenez-Romero, et al., 2009).

In terms of pancreas venous drainage there are two available variations: portal venous and systemic venous drainage. Portal drainage is a more physiological alternative, but with regards to the complication rate; graft and patient survival there are not any significant differences. Some data suggests that portal venous drainage is an important factor to determine peripheral insulin sensitivity (Radziuk et al., 1993). In portal venous drainage, serum glucose and insulin concentration recover to normal in contrast with systemic venous drainage, where plasma insulin levels are increased, as a result of bypassing liver circulation (Gu et al., 2002). Hyperinsulinemia contributes to hyperlipidemia, hypercholesterolemia and accelerate the development of atherosclerosis.

A milestone in the history of transplantation occurred in 1976, when Calne published the first clinical experiences with Cyclosporin-A. He reported improved graft and patients' survival in a cohort of 34 transplant recipients (32 kidneys, 2 pancreases and 2 livers) who received only Cyclosporin-A maintenance immunosuppressive regiment (Lillehei et al., 1979). A Cyclosporin-A helped to achieve a better control of rejection and minimise steroid dependence. Although, the introduction of new immunosuppressive drugs (tacrolimus,

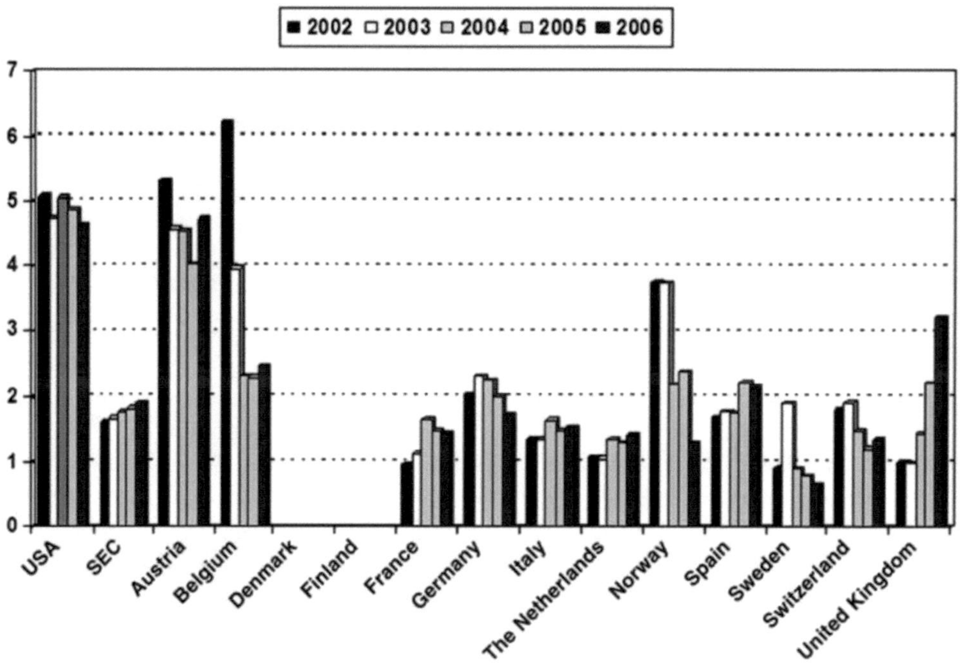

Fig. 4. Pancreas transplant activity rate (incidence per million population) in USA and 13 European countries considered together (SEC) and individually during the period 2002–06 (Gonzales-Posada et al. 2010).

	USA	Europe[a]	Austria	Belgium	Denmark	Finland	France	Germany	Italy	Netherlands	Norway	Spain	Sweden	Switzerland	UK
Population[b]															
2002	287.67	366.73	8.07	10.31	5.37	5.19	61.40	82.44	56.99	16.10	4.52	40.96	8.91	7.25	59.22
2003	290.34	368.82	8.10	10.36	5.38	5.21	61.83	82.54	57.32	16.19	4.55	41.66	8.94	7.31	59.44
2004	293.03	371.05	8.14	10.40	5.40	5.22	62.25	82.53	57.89	16.26	4.58	42.34	8.98	7.36	59.70
2005	295.73	373.34	8.21	10.45	5.41	5.24	62.64	82.50	58.46	16.30	4.61	43.04	9.01	7.41	60.06
2006	298.44	375.29	8.27	10.51	5.43	5.26	63.00	82.44	58.75	16.33	4.64	43.76	9.05	7.46	60.39
Pancreas Tx[c]															
2002	1460	591	43	64	0	0	59	161	77	17	17	69	8	13	59
2003	1373	614	37	41	0	0	70	191	77	17	17	74	17	14	59
2004	1483	657	37	24	0	0	103	187	95	22	10	74	8	11	86
2005	1444	678	33	24	0	0	92	165	87	21	11	96	7	9	133
2006	1386	718	39	26	0	0	90	141	90	23	6	94	6	10	193
Pancreas WL[d]															
2002	2835	897	38	56	0	0	189	180	245	15	11	47	20	6	90
2003	2747	877	42	56	0	0	199	145	213	14	11	75	19	5	98
2004	2388	918	36	53	0	0	178	158	216	34	13	79	14	8	132
2005	2071	920	38	34	0	0	169	169	197	40	10	87	15	16	145
2006	1984	1009	32	30	0	0	169	190	222	40	10	73	15	21	207
DD[e]															
2002	6190	6422	195	223	73	89	1198	1001	1020	202	62	1409	98	75	777
2003	6457	6598	187	248	75	85	1119	1110	1042	223	87	1443	114	95	770
2004	7150	6898	181	220	64	109	1291	1052	1203	228	90	1495	123	91	751
2005	7593	7159	200	237	63	85	1371	1185	1197	217	76	1546	128	90	764
2006	8024	7340	201	273	62	109	1442	1227	1231	200	76	1509	137	80	793

[a] All 13 countries.
[b] Million inhabitants.
[c] Tx = transplants.
[d] WL = waiting list.
[e] DD = deceased donors.

Table 1. Population, total number of pancreas transplants, pancreas waiting list and DD in USA and 13 European countries (Gonzales-Posada et al. 2010).

MMF, sirolimus, antibody based agents) contributed to further improved graft survival, reduction of rejection rate and the overall expansion of transplantation.

These days, pancreas transplantation has become a worldwide popular therapeutic alternative for type-1 diabetics. According to data from the United Network for Organ Sharing (UNOS) and the International Pancreas Transplant Registry (IPTR), more than 30,000 pancreas transplants have been performed worldwide (>22,000 reported from the United States and >8,000 from rest of the world) between December 1966 and 31 December 2008 (UNOS & IPTR, 2008). The majority pancreas transplants have been performed in North America and Western Europe (Fig 4), (Tab. 1) (Gonzales-Posada et al. 2010).

4. Indication of pancreas transplantation

At the present, Pancreas Transplantation is the only therapeutic modality that can achieve full insulin independence and euglycemic state in type-1 diabetic patients. It is well known that normoglycemia has a positive impact on preventing secondary diabetic complications. Therefore, this modality does not only improve patients' quality of life but also it has a positive impact on patients' medical conditions. Nevertheless, this therapeutic alternative is recommended only to a selected group of diabetics.

For a pancreas transplantation should be considered patients with brittle type-1 diabetes who suffer from secondary diabetic complications (diabetic nephropathy, diabetic retinopathy, diabetic neuropathy, diabetic gastro-enetopathy, etc); frequent hypoglycaemic episodes or hypoglycaemic unawareness and failure to achieve eu-glycemia even on intensive insulin treatment (insulin pump, etc.).

A detailed assessment of potential candidates for pancreas transplantation is mandatory because many of these patients have pre-existing cardiac diseases or other medical problems related to diabetes, and these may significantly increase per-operative morbidity, mortality and early graft failure.

4.1 Diabetes assessment

The first part of the evaluation is to determine the type of diabetes. It is generally accepted that pancreas transplantation should be reserved for type-1 diabetics. However, there are published data repording successes of pancreas transplantation also in type-2 diabetic patients. Nevertheless, a more strict patients' selection is required (Orlando et al., 2010). For diagnosis type-1 diabetes it is satisfactory to detect an absence or very low levels of C-peptide together with raised HbA1c (>7.5%). However, the patient's considered for pancreas transplantation cannot exceed insulin requirements beyond 1.5mg/kg/day; as this is the marker of peripheral insulin resistance. These patients do not achieve full insulin independence even with successful pancreas transplantation. Patients who are failing to achieve a reasonable serum-glucose control with conventional insulin treatment should be also considered for pancreas transplantation. Usually, they suffer from frequent hypo and hyper-glycemic episodes. Sever hypoglycaemia is the most common casualty in diabetics on insulin treatment. These complications are potentially life-threatening, associated with high morbidity and mortality rate.

4.2 Cardiac evaluation

Diabetes doubles the risk of developing cardio-vascular disease; coronary-artery disease, cerebro-vascular disease and peripheral vascular disease (Grundy et al., 1999). Over 50% of diabetics have some degree of coronary artery disease. Also, it is well known that diabetics suffer from accelerated atherosclerosis and a high incident of silent ischemia and cardio-myopathy compared to the non-diabetic population. Furthermore, cardio-vascular disease is the leading cause of death in the general population (35%) but diabetic patients are two times (67%) more likely to die due to this cause (Watkins, 2003).

The key purpose of the pre-transplant cardiac assessment is to identify risk factors (reversible ischemia, impaired left ventricular function, coronary artery disease, etc.) that may increase per-operative morbidity and mortality; and minimize them with the appropriate management and treatment. For cardiac evaluation standard echocardiography, Dobutamine stress echocardiography (DSE), exercise tolerance testing, nuclear (thalium) myocardial perfusion scan and formal coronary angiogram are routinely used. Because each of these tests has some limitations, there is not a consensus yet regarding which method has the highest predicting value.

Dobutamine stress echocardiography (DSE) is a non-invasive imaging modality which combines two-dimensional echocardiography with cardiovascular stress induced by dobutamine infusion. This test is sensitive to detect coronary artery disease in asymptomatic, high risk (diabetic, patients with peripheral vascular disease, etc.) patients.

The nuclear myocardial perfusion study (MPI) is a sensitive, non-invasive test for the assessment of myocardial perfusion, ejection fraction, wall motion and wall thickness. Stress radionuclide myocardial perfusion imaging, on the other hand, displays the downstream functional consequences of epicardial coronary artery disease in the myocardium. It also may visualize the regional effects of micro vascular endothelial dysfunction and impairment of regional coronary flow reserve.

DSE and MPI methods are generally accepted as standard and non-invasive screening studies useful to identify patients (diabetics with ESRF) with significantly increased risk of myocardial infarction or cardiac death (Rabbat et al., 2003; Cai et al., 2010). Nevertheless, they have low sensitivity and specificity to define coronary artery disease in patients with ESRD (Letine et al., 2010).

On the other hand, the coronary-angiogram (CA) offers high sensitivity to detect coronary-artery disease but it is limited in regards to predicting survival. This is mainly because myocardial infarction is more likely to be caused by plague instability rather than angiographic stenosis. Additionally, the contrast used for this test is nephro-toxic and it can have a catastrophic impact on impaired kidney function (Letine et al., 2010).

There is only one published study which directly compares doputamine stress echocardiography to coronary angiogram in renal transplant candidates (Herzog et al., 1999). Fifty potential transplant candidates underwent DSE followed by CA. Twenty of fifty DSE were positive for inducible ischemia. Sensitivity and specificity of DSE were 52% and 74%, respectively, for stenosis ≥50%; 75% and 71% for stenosis greater than 70%; 75% and 57% for stenosis greater than 75%. At the end the authors concluded that DSE is a good screening method, in spite of low sensitivity to detect coronary artery disease. For that reason, CA is reserved for high risk groups of patient with a previous history of cardiac problems (cardiac event, ishemic heart desease etc) or for patients with positive stress echocardiography or MPI scan.

4.3 Dietitian management

4.3.1 Pre-transplant assessment

A well balanced nutrition in transplant recipients plays a vital role in a pre and pos-transplant period to ensure the best possible outcomes. The role of a dietician is to evaluate the patient's nutrition status and design a nutrition plan for a pos-transplant period. For that reason it is important we ensure pre-operatively the following parameters:

a. *Good glucose control:* It is well documented (Kuo et al., 2010) that diabetes mellitus is a major predictor of cardiovascular morbidity and mortality in kidney transplant recipients. A recent study (Sato et al., 2010) analysed the outcomes of patients undergoing cardiac surgery and revealed that increased of HbA1c levels (>6.5%) predicts insulin sensitivity and increases the incidence of major complications. In addition, a well controlled diabetes improves gastroparesis and delays gastric empting (Reddy, 2010) as well as preventing other gastro intestinal symptoms including nausea, vomiting, bloating, early satiety and abdominal pain (Kashyap & Farrugia, 2010).

b. *Weight maintenance:* A Body Mass Index (BMI) ≥25kgs/m^2 is a strong predictive factor with significantly negative impact on long term renal graft outcomes (Cheung et al., 2010). So, in these patients weight loss is strongly recommended.

c. *Balanced nutrition status*: Prior to transplantation it is also crucial to optimize good nutrition status in patients with low BMI. According to some data (Meier-Kriesche et al, 2002) poor nutrition is associated with significantly worse patient and graft survival.
d. *Adequate electrolyte balance:* Patients with chronic renal failure may be on a low potassium, phosphate and low salt diets and fluid restrictions. Raised levels of potassium and phosphate are associated with increased mortality in these patients (Noori et al 2010; Ganesh et al., 2001).

4.3.2 Immediate pos-transplant management

The transplant recipient must receive adequate nutrition support (25-30 kcal/kg ideal body weight per day) during the first seven pos-operative days to avoid starvation and to enhance postoperative recovery (Braga et al., 2009). We should aim to identify the patient's post-transplant nutrition requirements prior to a surgery and in advance to design an individual sufficient nutrition plan.
The European Society for Clinical Nutrition and Metabolism (ESPEN) developed guidelines on enteral nutrition management after surgery (Weiman et al., 2006). These guidelines suggest that oral diet and supplements should be initiated early after surgery, where possible. Furthermore, enteral nutrition should be considered in patients with obvious under-nutrition and those whose oral intake will be inadequate (<60% of requirements) for 10 days after surgery. These patients should ideally have a naso-jejunal tube placed during surgery and feeding commenced on the first pos-operative day. According to these guidelines, parenteral nutrition is reserved for those patients who are unable to tolerate enteral feeding; due to complication including interstinal obstruction, ileus and sever shock (Braga et al., 2009).

4.3.3 Pos-transplant surveillance

In the long term, it is important to maintain a healthy weight and maintain good nutrition status. A team from the Netherlands (Hoogeveen et al., 2011) reports that 1-year post-transplant BMI is more strongly related to death and graft failure than pre-transplant BMI. According these data, patients who reached pos-transplant BMI>30 kg/m^2 have a 20-40% higher risk of death and graft failure compared to patients with lower BMI.

4.4 Other tests

A routine part of the pre-transplant assessment includes blood tests:
a. *Haematology Blood Tests:* Blood group identifying, antibody screen, full blood count, Thrombophilia screen, APTT, PT, and INR.
b. *Biochemistry Test:* Urea & electrolytes, creatinine, uric acid, calcium, phosphate, 24-hour urine collection (tested for protein/micro albuminuria and creatinine clearance), eGFR (radioisotope glomerular filtration rate if needed), liver function tests, amylase, thyroid function, fasting blood glucose, fasting and stimulated C-peptide levels if needed, fasting blood lipids.
   Additional studies may include oral or intravenous glucose challenge, anti-insulin and islet cell antibodies, proinsulin level and lipoprotein.
c. *Viral screen:* Hepatitis B and C, HIV, HTLV, BK virus, Polioma virus, Syphilis, Rubella, Epstein Barr Virus, Toxoplasma, Varicella-Zoster, Herpes , simplex, Cytomegalovirus.
d. *Immunology Blood Tests:* HLA typing and antibody screening.

5. Contraindications

Overall, contraindications to pancreas transplantation are the same as for kidney transplantation, and they are often determined by patient co-morbidity.

5.1 Absolute contraindications

a. Insufficient cardiovascular reserve:
   - Ejection fraction below 50%
   - Myocardial infarction within 6 months
   - Non-correctable coronary artery disease or refractory congestive heart failure

b. Non curable malignancy (excluding localised skin malignancy)

c. Active sepsis

d. Active peptic ulcer

e. Major psychiatric history likely to result in non-compliance

f. Inability to withstand surgery and immunosuppression

(UKT, 2003)

Some contraindications are relative and must be individually assessed and discussed with the responsible specialist on multidisciplinary bases and with the patient, too.

5.2 Relative contraindications

a. Cerebrovascular accident with long term impairment.

b. HIV (subject to discussion).

c. Chronic liver disease: Candidates with Hepatitis B/C need recent viral screen, LFT and assessment by hepatologist prior activating on a WL. The aim is to exclude active viral disease as well as advanced irreversible liver disease.

d. Body Mass Index greater than 30.

e. Malignancy: In patients with a history of cancer a cancer free interval from three to five years according the type of cancer, stage and cancer therapy are required. This issue must be discussed in detail with an oncologist. A valuable source of information is "Israel Penn International Transplant Tumor Registry" (www.ipittr.org).

f. Type-2 diabetes was originally an absolute contraindication to pancreas transplantation. However, a recently published review reports that selected group type-2 diabetics benefit from whole organ pancreas transplantation, too. Transplant outcomes (after SPK) are comparable between type 1 and 2 diabetics. But a strict patient selection is required; BMI less than 30 kg/m^2, insulin requirements <1.0 units/kg/day, C-peptide level less than 10 ng/ml, etc. (Orlando et al., 2010).

g. Extensive aorta/iliac and/or peripheral vascular disease.

h. Continued abuse of alcohol, smoking or other drugs.

(UKT, 2003)

6. Transplant alternatives for diabetic patients

For diabetic patients with ESRF three transplant alternatives are currently available: kidney transplantation (including cadaver and living donor kidney transplantation); Simultaneous Pancreas-Kidney Transplantation (SPK) and Pancreas After Kidney Transplantation (PAK). Each of them has some recognised advantages and disadvantages (Tab. 2).

	Advantages	Disadvantages
CKT	Provides better survival than dialysis options	Inferior to other transplant options with respect to kidney graft survival and patient survival
LRD	Minimizes waiting time, time spent on dialysis Very low early morbidity and mortality	Absence to normalize of blood glucose Inferior patient survival over time when compared with SPK recipients with functioning grafts
SPK	Glycemic control, with recent median pancreas graft survival of >10 years High-quality, deceased donor kidney graft	Higher morbidity and mortality due to larger operation If pancreas fails within the first year, outcomes are worse than LRD
PAK	Glycemic control If living donor kidney transplant, comparable/better patient and kidney graft survival than LRD	Two separate surgical procedures, increased mortality early postoperatively following pancreas transplant Historically inferior pancreas graft survival (35% at 10 years) than SPK

Table 2. Summary of advantages and disadvantages of transplant options for diabetic kidney disease (Wiseman, 2010).

6.1 Kidney transplantation

Kidney transplantation is a widely used and well accepted transplant option for patient with ESRF secondary to DN. It is indisputable that this alternative gives survival advantages to these patients over chronic dialysis. The estimated survival of a diabetic on dialysis is only 30-40% at five years, while kidney transplantation increases their 5 year survival to up to 70% for Cadaver Kidney Transplantation (CKT), and to up to 80% for Living Donor Kidney Transplantation (LRD) (Reddy et al., 2003; USRDS 1998; Cecka et al. 1997). As we know, LRD is associated with better outcomes due to a superior quality of kidney graft and reduced cold ischemia time. This type of transplantation has relatively low risk of post-transplant complications (10-12%) and compared to pancreas transplantation it is less traumatic, too. For that reason, a greater population of diabetic patients with ESRF is eligible for renal transplantation rather pancreas transplantation. A successfully treated ESRF with renal transplantation does not only improve overall patients' medical conditions (anaemia, hypertension, etc) but in many cases it also stabilises brittle diabetes.

6.2 Simultaneous pancreas and kidney transplantation

During recent years, Simultaneous Pancreas and Kidney Transplantation (SPK) has become the most popular transplant alternative and golden standard for type-1 diabetic with ESRF. Additionally to renal transplantation in these patients pancreas transplantation helps to achieve euglycemia, insulin independence and enhances patients' quality of life (Sureshkumar et al., 2006). Also, the tight glycaemic control prevents the recurrence of diabetic nephropathy and improves secondary diabetic complications; mainly diabetic retinopathy, cardiovascular disease, diabetic neuropathy, etc.

Overall, it has been proven that SPK gives some survival benefits to these patients. In one of the largest studies (Ojo et al., 2001) SPK was associated with a 10-year patient survival of 67% compared to 46% in a CKT recipient group. However, in comparison with the LRD benefit of SPK, in terms of patient and graft survival, it does diminish. Wisconsin experiences (Tab. 3) (Rayhill et al., 2000) have shown that patient and renal graft survival was not different between the LRD and the SPK groups, but it was significantly lower in the CKT group (Fig 5,6) (Young et al., 2009).

The main advantage of LRD is the low immunological risk and good quality kidney graft that participates on excellent kidney function and prolongs graft survival. However, only an additional pancreas transplant gives a protective role to prevent the recurrence of DN, maintain a good kidney function, improve the quality of life and eliminate secondary diabetic complications. On the other hand, we cannot forget that SPK is associated with a double level of morbidity (20-40%) and mortality (2-5%) compared to kidney transplantion. For that reason, younger patients with better medical conditions (Rayhill et al., 2000) should be considered for SPK.

	1y patient survival	5-y patient survival
LRDi	100%	94%
LRDh	99%	85%
SPK	96%	88%
CKT	94%	72%

	1y graft survival	5-y graft survival
LRDi	96%	85%
LRDh	94%	72%
SPK	87%	78%
CKT	86%	64%

LRDi - HLA-identical living related donor, LRDh - haplotype-identical living related donor

Table 3. The 1-year and 5-year pos-transplant outcomes (Rayhill et al., 2000).

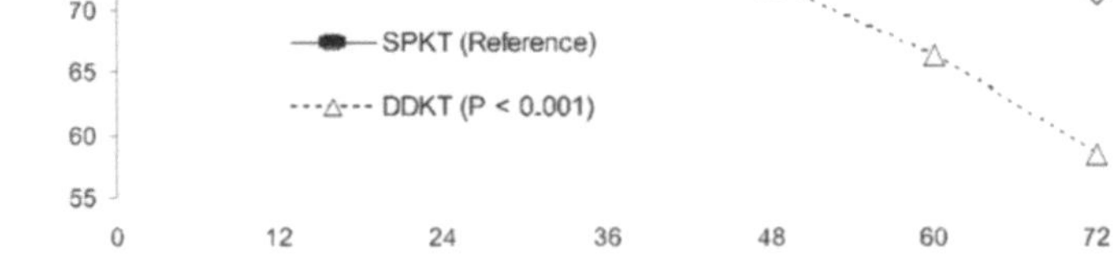

(LDKT - living donor kidney transplant; SPKT - simultaneous pancreas kidney transplant; DDKT - deceased donor kidney transplant).

Fig. 5. Unadjusted kidney graft survival by transplant type (Young et al., 2009).

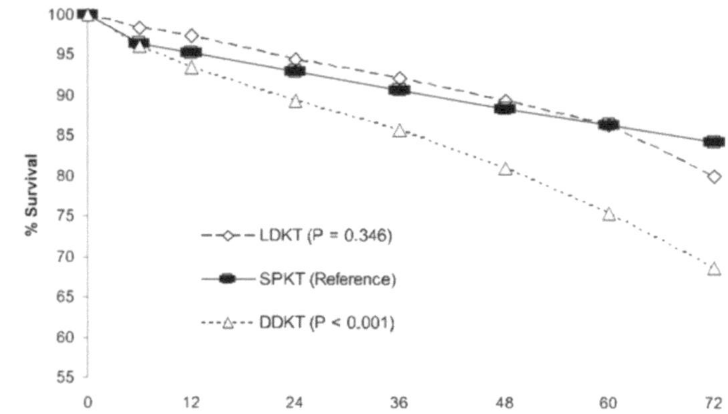

(LDKT - living donor kidney transplant; SPKT - simultaneous pancreas kidney transplant; DDKT - deceased donor kidney transplant).

Fig. 6. Unadjusted patient survival by transplant type (Young et al., 2009).

6.3 Pancreas after kidney transplantation

Historically, Pancreas After Kidney Transplantation (PAK) was not a very popular pancreas transplant alternative due to the inferior pancreas graft survival compared to SPK. The impact of pancreas graft on patients with kidney graft from two different donors was associated with high immunological graft failure. However, the development of new immunosuppressive regiments based on depleting antibody induction and Tacrolimus and MMF maintenance reduced the risk of immunological graft loss and improved graft survival outcomes. For those reasons, this alternative has become more popular (Larson et al., 2004).

Diabetic patients who have undergone kidney transplant or who underwent SPK and have lost pancreas graft might be today considered for PAK. With increased frequency, this two-stage procedure involves a living donor kidney transplantation followed by a cadaver pancreas transplant (PALK). This alternative has the advantage of a short waiting time and of a superior quality kidney graft (Kleinclauss et al., 2009). The second great advantage of PAK is performing major pancreas transplant surgery on a non-uremic patient. This minimizes the risk of per-operative morbidity and mortality related to renal failure.

Pominipanin analysed data of the Organ Procurement Transplant Network/United Network of Organ Sharing (OPTN/UNOS) database and compared outcomes of SPK with CKT and PALK. He reports that renal graft outcomes were superior in PALK compared to SPK. The 1-year pancreas graft survival was marginally higher for the SPK cohort (86%) vs. 80% for PALK. The overall patient survival was better in PALK compared to SPK (Fig 7 a,b). Even this study showed that PAK is an alternative with competitive results to SPK.

6.4 Simultaneous cadaver pancreas and living donor kidney transplantation

At present, SPK and PAK are the most common options for uremic type-1 diabetics. SPK is a one-stage procedure and this is its main advantage over PAK. On the other hand, PAK has the advantage of involving living donor with superior quality of kidney graft function and subsequently of performing pancreas transplantation on a non-uremic patient. Simultaneous Cadaver Pancreas and Living Donor Kidney Transplantation (SPLK) is an innovative approach that merges some benefits of both alternatives; superior quality of living donor kidney and s single procedure with shorter waiting time for cadaver pancreas graft.

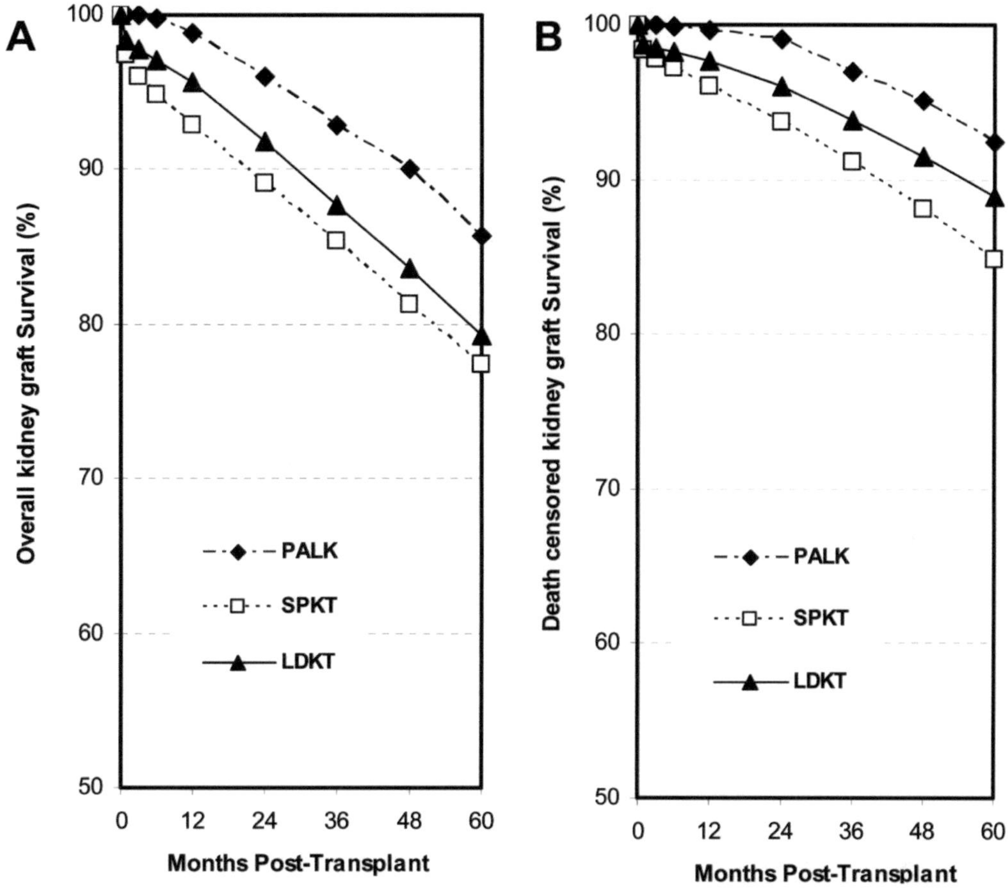

No at risk

	A						B					
PALK	807	755	669	547	403	283	807	755	669	547	403	283
SPKT	5580	4457	3527	2737	2057	1453	5580	4457	3527	2737	2057	1453
LDKT	3461	2888	2340	1799	1326	937	3461	2888	2340	1799	1326	937

a/ Overall kidney graft survival (%)
b/ Death censored kidney graft Survival (%)
PALK - pancreas after living kidney transplant,
SPKT - simultaneous pancreas kidney transplant,
LDKT - living donor kidney transplant.

Fig. 7. Kidney graft survival (Poommipanit et al., 2010).

Despite increased immunological risk, SPLK showed comparable results with SPK and PAK (Boggi et al., 2004). In a study from Maryland (Farney et al., 2000), it was reported that 1-year pancreas graft survival in the SPLK group was not significantly higher than in SPK and PAK (88% vs. 84% vs. 71%) Fig. 8,9,10 (Farney et al., 2000). The 1-year patient survivals were 95% (SPLK), 94% (SPK) and 100% (PAK). The SPLK group showed lower incidence of delay graft function and better kidney function.

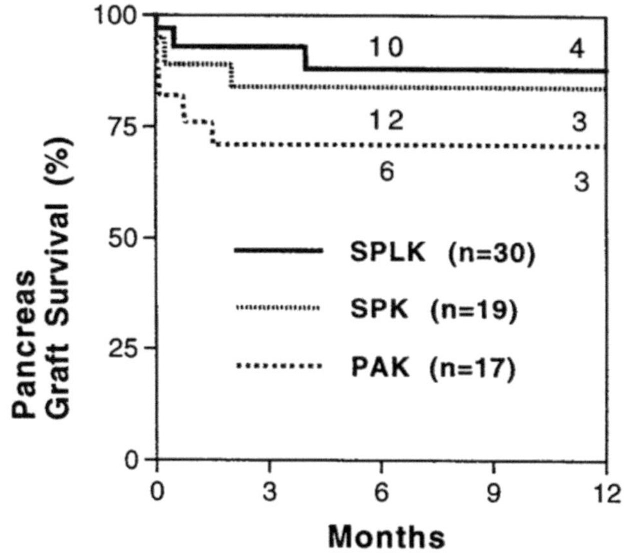

One-year pancreas graft survival rates were 88%, 84%, and 71%, respectively, for simultaneous cadaver-donor pancreas and living-donor kidney transplantation (SPLK), simultaneous cadaver kidney and pancreas transplantation (SPK) and living-donor kidney transplantation alone followed by a solitary cadaver-donor pancreas transplant (PAK)

Fig. 8. Pancreas graft survival rates (Farney et al., 2000).

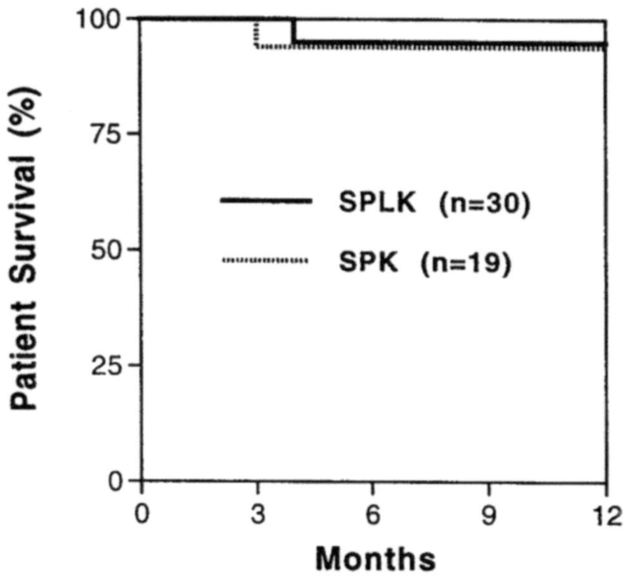

One-year patient survival rates were 95% and 94% for simultaneous cadaver-donor pancreas and living-donor kidney transplant (SPLK) and simultaneous cadaver kidney and pancreas transplant (SPK) recipients. The patient survival rate was 100% in living-donor kidney transplantation alone followed by a solitary cadaver-donor pancreas transplant (PAK) recipients (not shown).

Fig. 9. Patient survival rates (Farney et al., 2000).

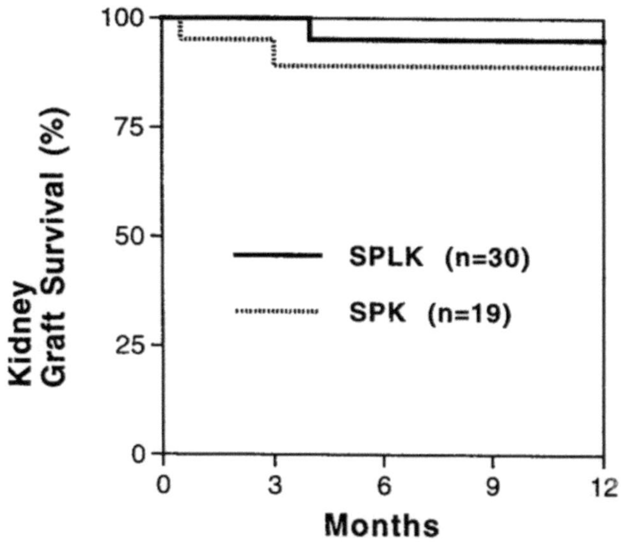

One-year kidney graft survival rates were 95% and 89% for simultaneous cadaver-donor pancreas and living-donor kidney transplant (SPLK) and simultaneous cadaver kidney and pancreas transplant (SPK) recipients. The only SPLK loss was death with function. No living-donor kidney transplantation alone followed by a solitary cadaver-donor pancreas transplant (PAK) kidney grafts were lost (not shown).

Fig. 10. Kidney graft survival rates (Farney et al., 2000).

7. Surgical complications

Despite worldwide growing experience with pancreas transplantation, this procedure is still associated with high incidence of pos-transplant complications; and compared with other solid organ transplants; it has the highest incidence of serious intrabdominal complications and reoperations. We know that up to 50% of pancreas recipients develop pos-transplant complication and around 32% of patients require further surgery to deal with these problems (Troppmann et al., 1998). According the United Network for Organ Sharing report, from 11% to 21% of all pancreas grafts are lost because of surgical complication (Gruessner & Sutherland, 2005).

There are recognised several factors that participate in development of postransplan complications. Diabetes was found to be the strongest independent risk factor. It is well documented that diabetics have significantly higher complication rate compared with non-diabetic population. Also, these patients receive strong immunosuppressive regiment, compared to other solid organ recipients. This makes patients more immunocompromised and vulnerable to infection. Open bowel or bladder, during pancreas implantation is other possible source of abdominal contamination and infection. Furthermore, SPK recipients are compromised by uraemia and PAK recipients are chronically immunosuppressed at the time of transplant. Additional risk factors include: older donors and recipients, long cold ischemia time and high BMI (UNOS & IPTR, 2008).

The most common surgical complication after pancreas transplantation is abdominal infection and graft pancreatitis (38%), followed by pancreas graft thrombosis (27%) and anastomotic leak (9%) (Troppmann et al., 1998).

7.1 Thrombosis

Vascular thrombosis is the second leading cause of pancreas graft failure after rejection. Incidence is reported between 2-20% and it can be either arterial or venous (Gruessner & Sutherland, 2000).

It is well known that pancreas is more susceptible to thrombosis than other organs. Pancreas has naturally low microvascular flow. Removing the spleen from pancreatic graft as a part of the pancreas bench-work, venous flow does reduce even more. The pancreas also requires vascular reconstruction because blood supply to the pancreas is divided during explantation. The donor iliac artery extension "Y" graft is joined to the superior mesenteric artery and the splenic artery to create a single arterial conduit (Fig. 11). The venous extension graft is an additional risk factor causing venous thrombosis. Furthermore, hyper-coagulable status in renal failure patients and endothelial damage are recognised as other negative factors in developing venous thrombosis (Muthusamy et al., 2010).

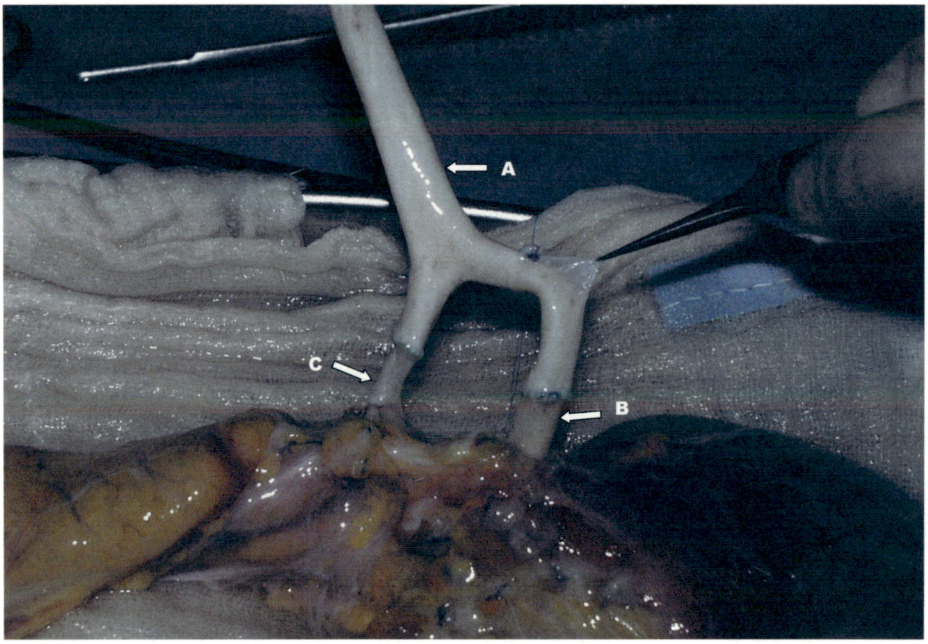

An end-to-end anastomosis between limb of internal iliac artery of the "Y" graft and stump of the splenic artery of the pancreas graft; and limb of external iliac artery and stump of the superior mesenteric artery.

A - "Y"graft, B- superior mesenteric artery, C – splenic artery

Fig. 11. Vascular reconstruction

If venous thrombosis occurs, often a patient develops abdominal pain due to organ swelling with an acute drop of haemoglobin levels. Raising levels of serum glucose are usually late sings of thrombosis. Arterial thrombosis is much less common with a less dramatic clinical picture. In the majority of cases, the pancreas graft is non-salvageable and requires urgent graftectomy. Some data report that in an early stage urgent radiological intervention with thrombectomy or thrombolysis can salvage a pancreas allograft (Stockland et al., 2009) (Fig. 12).

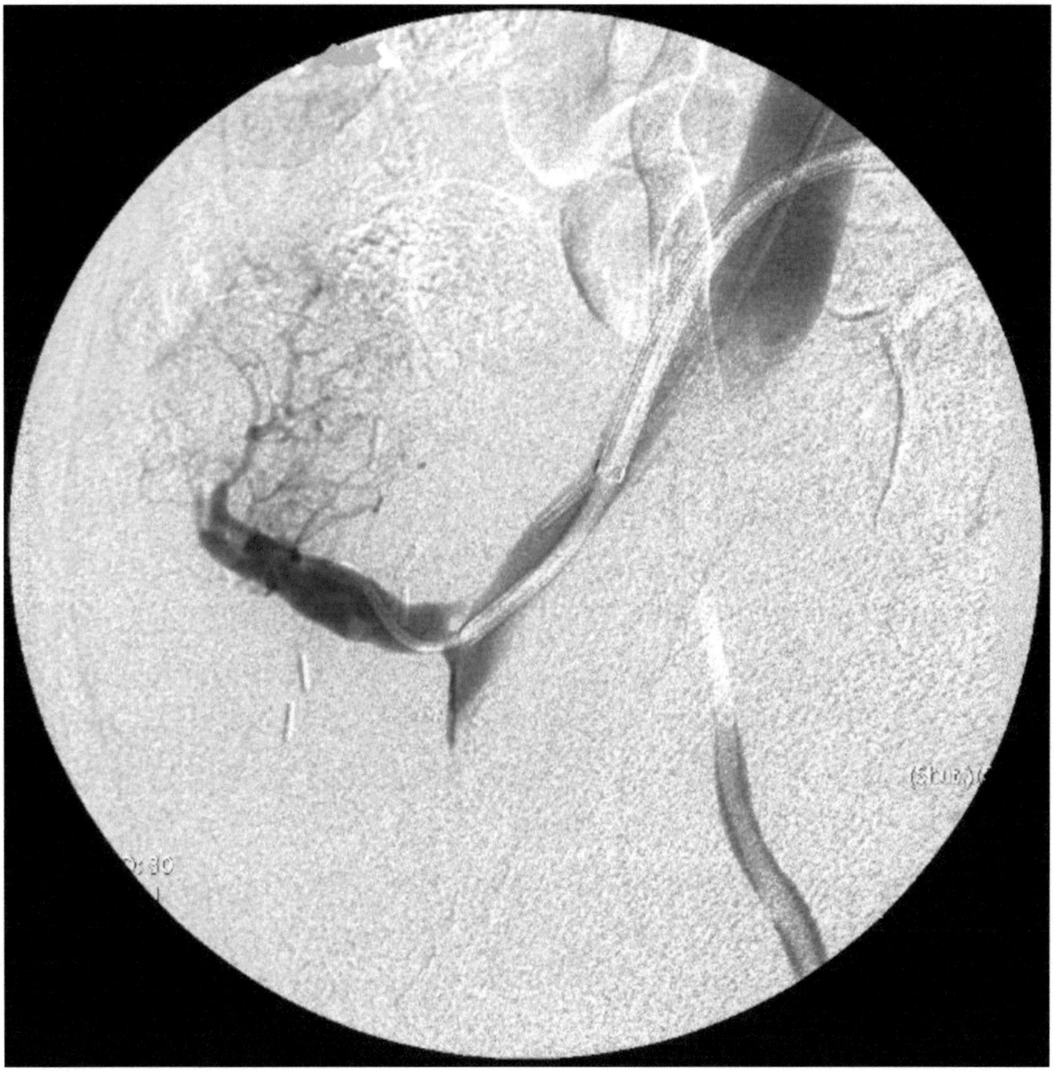

Fig. 12a

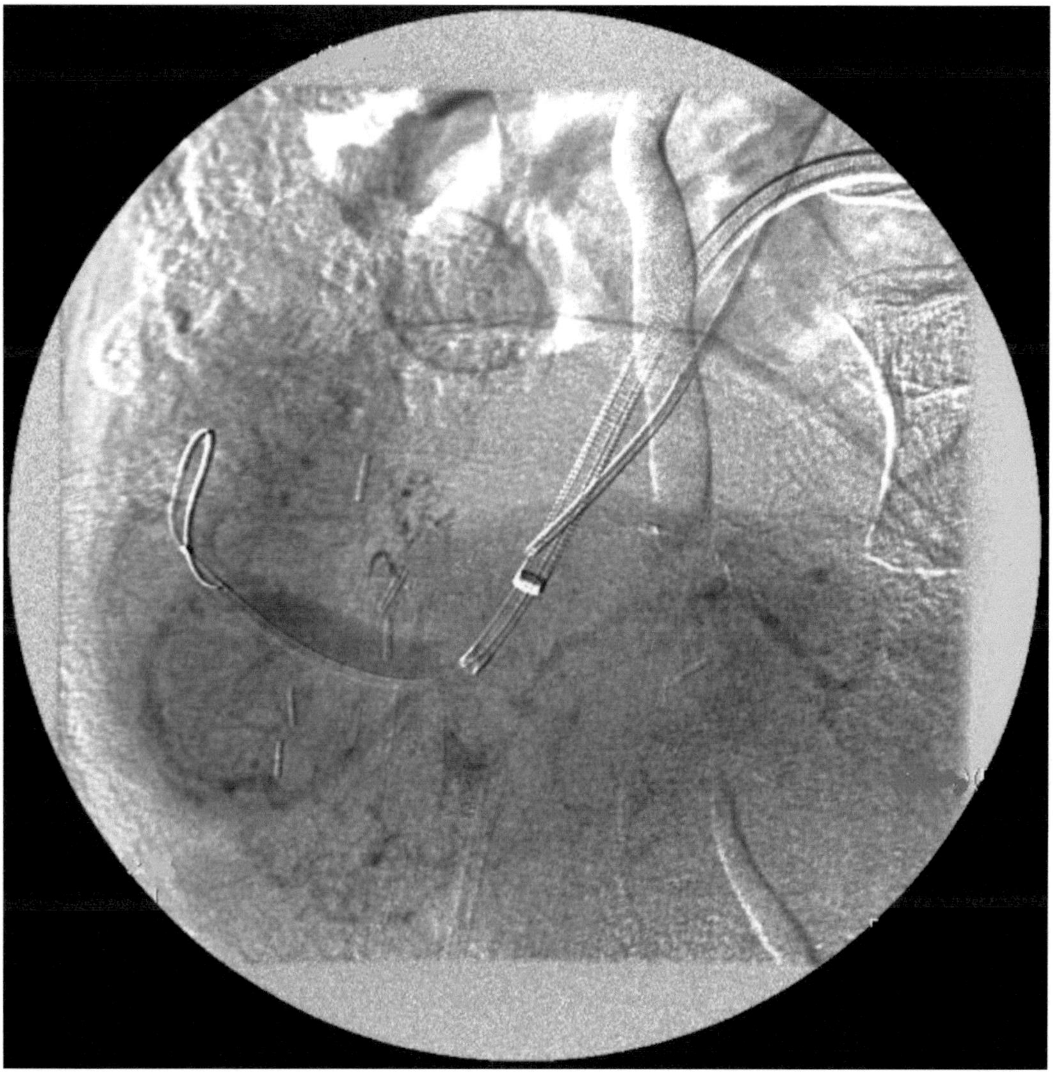

Fig. 12 b

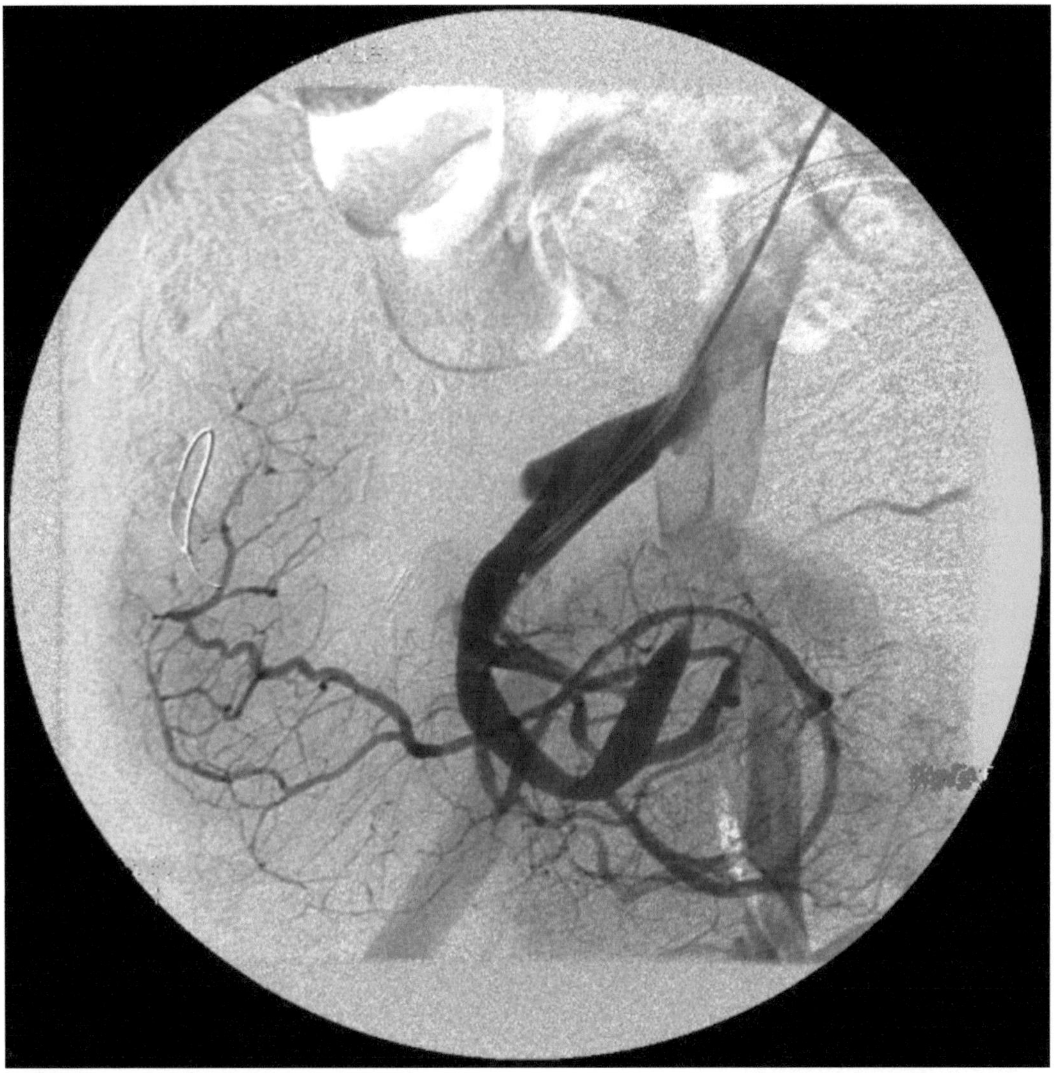

Fig. 12 c

a/ Thrombus in the portal vein of pancreas graft (black arrow points on filling defect, thrombus, in portal vein). A thrombectomy catheter is in the graft's portal vein via right external iliac vein by cannulation right femoral vein.
b/ Status after thrombectomy. Improvement in venous flow and full patency of portal vein without a thrombus.
c/ Normal angiogram of pancreas graft.

Fig. 12. Conventional angiography of pancreas graft.

A key part of the post-operative thrombosis management is prevention, close monitoring, early diagnosis and early intervention, but mainly meticulous vascular reconstruction, bench-work and refine implantation technique. Patients after transplantation receive a high dose of fractionated/continued infusion heparin to develop hypo-coagulable status to reduce clot formation. Sensitive markers for careful coagulation monitoring are APTT ratio (INR) and Thromboelastogram (TEG) (Burke et al., 2004). Several diagnostic methods are recommended for graft monitoring and diagnosis vascular complications: duplex ultrasound, CT-angiography or MR-angiography and formal angiography.

7.2 Bleeding

This vascular complication does mainly occur in combination with intra-abdominal infection or during sever hypo-coagulable status secondary to heparin treatment. Heparin induced bleeding usually has a slow progress and it is often managed conservatively; with antibiotics and blood transfusions. Bleeding secondary to infection is a serious event and it can be life-threatening. Clinical presentation is rapid, sudden hypotension, significant fall of haemoglobin levels and pulsative intra-abdominal mass. In that case urgent laparotomy is vital to control bleeding and abdominal sepsis. At presence of advanced abdominal sepsis or infection involving pancreas graft it is recommended to perform graftectomy to prevent fatal bleeding.

7.3 Pancreatitis

Graft pancreatitis usually occurs instantly after transplant as a result of excessive handling of an organ during retrieval, storage, bench-work and transplantation, as well as a consequence of ischemic-reperfusion injury. Most episodes of pancreatitis resolve uneventfully, however some may lead to secondary complications (fistula, pseudocyst, etc.). Also, Octreotide (synthetic somatostatin analog that inhibits exocrine pancreatic secretion) has been used to prevent and treat some pos-transplant complications (i.e. graft pancreatitis, pancreatic fistula). But data from published studies are controversial with no statistical difference in complication rate between recipients who received octreotide and patient treated by placebo (Stratta et al., 1993).

7.4 Miscellaneous

Other common early surgical complications involve anastomotic leak, pancreatic fistula, intra-abdominal sepsis, ileus, wound infection, etc. They may cause graft lost and recipients' mortality so it is important to actively search for them, to detect them early and to treat them.

8. Immunosuppression

The key role of immunosuppression in transplantation is to minimize graft lost due to rejection. Despite this major benefit, all immunosuppressive medication has some side effects. For that reason, a good immunosuppressive regiment should balance both aspects to deliver the best possible outcomes. The pancreas is a more immunogenic organ than the kidney, and precisely for that reason the majority of immunosuppressive regiments for pancreas transplantation are mainly based on quadruple drug therapy; including antibody agents for induction in combination with calcineurin inhibitors (CNI) and mycophenolate mofetil (MMF) or sirolimus and steroids (Singh & Stratta, 2008).

Initially, the IL-2 receptor antagonists (basiliximab, daclizumab) have been used as induction agents in pancreas transplantation for long period. In the PIVOT Study daclizumab induction was compared to no antibody induction in pancreas transplantation. The results showed that daclizumab significantly reduced the incidence of acute rejection. The 1-year rejection free interval in the daclizumab group was 68% compared to 51% in the non antibody induction group (Stratta et al., 2003). T-cells depleting antibody agents, such as antithymocyte globulin (ATG) and alemtuzumab (Campath), have gained great popularity these days. According to the United Network of Organ Sharing data, this type of induction significantly decreases incidence of immunologically related pancreas graft failure (Gruessner & Sutherland, 2003).

According to a review published in 1999 (Stratta, 1999), a combination of MMF and tacrolimus in primary immunosuppressive regiment resulted in an improved 2-years patient, kidney and pancreas survivals; 97.7%, 93.3% and 90%, respectively.

Lymphocyte-depleting antibody agents in combination with tacrolimus, and MMF or sirolimus, are effective in preventing acute rejection and allow corticosteroids elimination or even full avoidance (Heilman et al., 2010). The principle of the steroid sparing regiment is to avoid steroids related side effects (increased risk of hypertension, glucose intolerance, cholesterol, infection, cardiovascular events, anaemia, osteoporosis, etc.) in pancreas transplant recipients. There is strong evidence that steroid sparing/avoidance regiments are safe and effective with a positive impact on patient and graft survival. Also, we have seen significantly improved the short-term outcomes whereas the long-term outcomes are still insufficient (Mineo et al., 2009).

9. Monitoring pancreas function

The development of surgical techniques and immunosuppressive drugs has significantly improved short-term outcomes of pancreas transplantation (Fig. 13). So these days the main target is to improve long-term results and minimize late graft dysfunction.

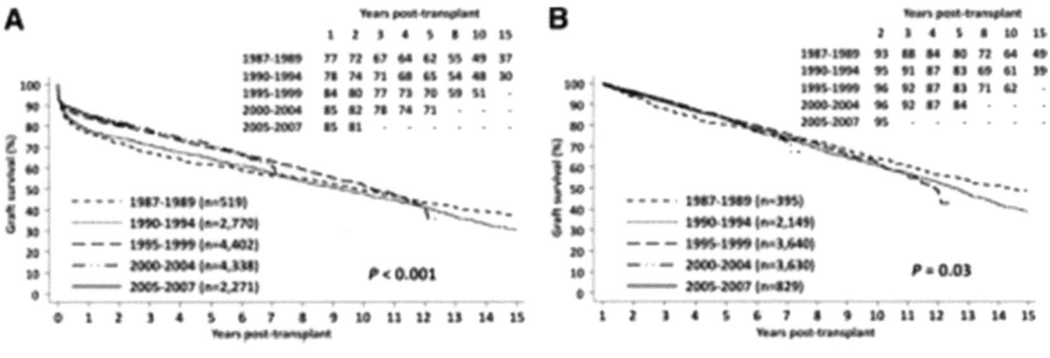

Fig. 13. Pancreas graft survival by era for all transplants, 1987–2007: UNOS registry analysis. *B*: Pancreas graft survival by era for transplants surviving more than 1 year, 1987–2007: UNOS registry analysis (UNOS, 2010).

Immunological graft loss still remains the main cause of graft failure; its rate in 1-year is significantly lower in SPK groups (2%) compared to solitary pancreas transplants (6% for PAK and PTA) (Fig 14) (Gruessner et al., 2008).

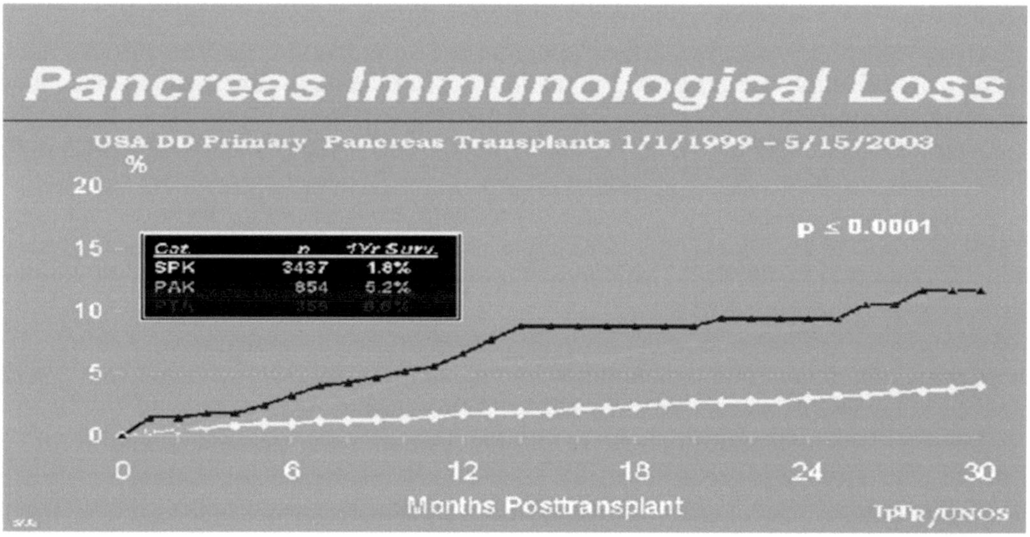

Fig. 14. Pancreas Immunological loss (Waiki et al., 2010).

The incidence of acute rejection is at its highest early after the transplantation. Induction regiments based on antibody depleting agents (i.e. ATG, Campath) delay the repopulation of lymphocytes; so the peak of rejection rate is around six to nine months after transplantation instead of three months as we see in regiments based on IL-2 receptor antagonists induction. A clinical picture of acute rejection is non-characteristic (fever, abdominal pain, ileus, tenderness, diarrhea, haematuria in bladder drained pancreas) or in the majority of cases absent.

Close monitoring of the pancreatic graft is a crucial part of pos-transplant surveillance. Unfortunately, there are not any biomarkers that can sensitively predict rejection yet. For that reason routinely are monitored the levels of fasting blood glucose, fasting C-peptide, HbA1c, serum amylase, serum lipase, oGTT and CRP; but with limited sensitivity and specificity. In SPK patients we do monitor serum creatinine as an indirect marker, too. Also, we know that islet function is resistant to pancreas damage so serum glucose elevation is a late manifestation of pancreas graft dysfunction and predicts poor prognosis; i.e. acute or chronic rejection, pancreatitis, thrombosis, etc.

The bladder-drained pancreas technique gives easy and convenient access to monitor pancreas graft function by measuring urine amylase. A low amylase level is a marker of graft dysfunction (rejection, pancreatitis, etc). Also, cystoscopy enables to perform repeated pancreas graft biopsies with a relatively low risk of complication rate.

The only objective way to diagnose rejection is a histological evaluation of the pancreas graft. Precise diagnoses help to tailor management and subsequently improve graft function. Despite a higher incidence of biopsy related complications pancreas graft biopsy is now widely employed (Gaber, 2007). SPK cases have a high incidence of synchronous pancreas and kidney rejection rate, around 62.5%. Kidney graft biopsy has lower risks of complications compared to pancreas biopsy. Also for that reason, kidney biopsy is routinely employed to diagnose pancreas graft rejection. On the other hand, there is a 25% occurrence of kidney only rejection; that usually correlates with elevation of serum creatinine. In 12.5% cases rejection involves only pancreas without involvement of renal graft (Kitada et al., 2009).

A successful Banff scheme of grading rejection in kidney (Solez et al., 2007) and liver (ICD, 1997) transplantation was subsequently applied in pancreas transplantation, too. On the 9th Banff conference on Allograft Pathology in 2007 (La Coruña, Spain) a final version (Tab. 4,5) of Banff Schema for Grading Pancreas Allograft Rejection was agreed (Drachenberg et al., 2008).

10. Benefits of pancreas transplantation

The main purpose of pancreas transplantation is to achieve eu-glycemia, insulin independence and improve the quality of life in diabetics. A number of studies examined the impact of successful pancreas transplantation also on secondary diabetic complications (nephropathy, retinopathy, neuropathy, etc).

Nephropathy: Diabetic nephropathy has a high recurrence rate, effects almost all kidney grafts and can lead to graft failure. Development of histological sings of diabetic nephropathy is seen within two years after transplantation (Bohman et al., 1984). It has been well documented that functioning pancreatic grafts have a protective role on kidney graft function. Achieving permanent normo-glycemia not only prevents the development of DN but it can also reverse histological lesions characteristic for DN (Fioretto et al., 1998).

Retinopathy: There is good evidence that pancreas transplantation and subsequent normoglycemia stabilizes and even improves retinopathy. However, patients with a high grade of retinal damage before a transplant may get a progression of retinopathy (Königsrainer et al., 1991).

1. Normal. Absent inflammation **or** inactive septal, mononuclear inflammation not involving ducts, veins, arteries or acini. There is no graft sclerosis. The fibrous component is limited to normal septa and its amount is proportional to the size of the enclosed structures (ducts and vessels). The acinar parenchyma shows no signs of atrophy or injury.
2. Indeterminate. Septal inflammation that appears active but the overall features do not fulfill the criteria for mild cell-mediated acute rejection.
3. Cell-mediated rejection
Acute cell-mediated rejection
- Grade I/Mild acute cell-mediated rejection
Active septal inflammation (activated, blastic lymphocytes, ± eosinophils) involving septal structures: venulitis (sub-endothelial accumulation of inflammatory cells and endothelial damage in septal veins, ductitis (epithelial inflammation and damage of ducts).
Neural/peri-neural inflammation.
and/or
Focal acinar inflammation. No more than two inflammatory foci^per lobule with absent or minimal acinar cell injury.
- Grade II/Moderate acute cell-mediated rejection
Multi-focal (but not confluent or diffuse) acinar inflammation (≥3 foci^per lobule) with spotty (individual) acinar cell injury and drop-out.
and/or
Minimal intimal arteritis

- Grade III/Severe acute cell-mediated rejection
Diffuse, (widespread, extensive) acinar inflammation with focal or diffuse multi-cellular /confluent acinar cell necrosis.
and/or
Moderate- or severe-intimal arteritis
and/or
Transmural inflammation-Necrotizing arteritis
Chronic active cell-mediated rejection. Chronic allograft arteriopathy (arterial intimal fibrosis with mononuclear cell infiltration in fibrosis, formation of neo-intima)
4. Antibody-mediated rejection = C4d positivity[∞∞] + confirmed donor specific antibodies + graft dysfunction
Hyperacute rejection. Immediate graft necrosis (≤1 h) due to preformed antibodies in recipient's blood
Accelerated antibody-mediated rejection. Severe, fulminant form of antibody-mediated rejection with morphological similarities to hyperacute rejection but occurring later (within hours or days of transplantation).
Acute antibody-mediated rejection. Specify percentage of biopsy surface (focal or diffuse). Associated histological findings: ranging from none to neutrophilic or mononuclear cell margination (capillaritis), thrombosis, vasculitis, parenchymal necrosis.
Chronic active antibody-mediated rejection. Features of categories 4 and 5.
5. Chronic allograft rejection/graft sclerosis
- Stage I (mild graft sclerosis)
Expansion of fibrous septa; the fibrosis occupies less than 30% of the core surface but the acinar lobules have eroded, irregular contours. The central lobular areas are normal.
- Stage II (moderate graft sclerosis)
The fibrosis occupies 30–60% of the core surface. The exocrine atrophy affects the majority of the lobules in their periphery (irregular contours) and in their central areas (thin fibrous strands criss-cross between individual acin).
- Stage III (severe graft sclerosis)
The fibrotic areas predominate and occupy more than 60% of the core surface with only isolated areas of residual acinar tissue and/or islets present.
6. Other histological diagnosis. Pathological changes not considered to be due acute and/or chronic rejection. e.g. CMV pancreatitis, PTLD, etc.

[a] Categories from 2 to 6 may be diagnosed concurrently and should be listed in the diagnosis in the order of their clinico-pathological significance.
[o] See Table 2 for morphological definition of lesions.
[∞∞] If there are no donor-specific antibodies or these data are unknown, identification of histological features of antibody-mediated rejection may be diagnosed as 'suspicious for acute antibody- mediated rejection', particularly if there is graft dysfunction

Table 4. Diagnostic categories Banff working grading schema[a/o] (Drachenberg et al., 2008).

Diagnosis	Main histological findings	Clinical presentation
Posttransplant ischemic pancreatitis	Inflammation: neutrophils, foamy macrophages. Location: septal if mild or diffuse if severe Other features: fat necrosis, edema and interstitial hemorrhage. Patchy coagulation necrosis of clusters of acinar cells may be present. No fibrosis, the septa may be expanded due to edema/fat necrosis.	Increase in amylase and lipase in serum. Decrease in urinary amylase.* Hyperglycemia if there is extensive necrosis.
Peripancreatitis/peri - pancreatic fluid collection	Inflammation: mixed (lymphocytes, plasma cells, eosinophils, neutrophils). Location: septa and periphery of lobules Other features: dissecting bundles of active fibroblastic proliferation with obliteration of septal structures, relative preservation of the center of lobules ('cirrhotic appearance')	Local or systemic infectious symptoms, abdominal pain, peri-tonitis. Peripancreatic fluid accumulation.Increase in amylase and lipase in serum.
Cytomegalovirus pancreatitis	Inflammation: mostly mononuclear. Location: septal and acinar, patchy. Other features: cytomegalovirus cytopathic changes in acinar, endothelial or stromal cells.	Increase in serum amylase and lipase. Decrease in urinary amylase.* Systemic symptoms if generalized disease. Other: Duodenal cuff perforation.
Posttransplant lymphoproliferative disorder	Inflammation: ranging from polymorphic with lymphoblasts, plasma cells, eosinophils in low-grade disease, to monomorphic, predominantly lymphoid in high-grade disease (lymphoma). Other features: lymphoid proliferation is nodular, expansive. Necrosis may be present.	Asymptomatic, or increase in serum amylase and lipase. Lymphadenopathy. Tumor mass. May coexist with acute rejection.
Bacterial or fungal infection	Inflammation: variable; acute, chronic, purulent, necrotizing (abscess), granulomatous. Location: random. Other features: same as bacterial and fungal infections in other organs.	Systemic and/or localized infectious symptoms. Peritonitis, duodenal cuff perforation. Increase in serum amylase and lipase.
Recurrent autoimmune disease/diabetes mellitus	Inflammation: islet-centered lymphocytic inflammation (isletitis). No inflammation in late stages after disappearance of beta cells. Other features: immuno-histochemical stains for insulin and glucagon demonstrate absence of insulin producing beta cells in some or all islets depending if early or late disease.	Acute or chronic deterioration in glucose metabolism with increasing need for insulin. Although not pathognomonic, islet cell auto-antibodies typically present (i.e. GAD 65, IA-2, etc.).
Acute calcineurin inhibitor toxicity	Absence of inflammation. Variable degrees of islet cell injury (cytoplasmic swelling, vacuolization, islet cell drop-out. formation of empty spaces (lacunae), apoptotic fragments). Immuno-peroxidase stains: markedly diminished staining for insulin in comparison to controls and to glucagon stain. Electron microscopy: loss of insulin dense core granules with preservation of glucagon dense core granules.	Acute hyperglycemia. High levels of cyclosporine or tacrolimus with return to normoglycemia with adjustment of drug dose or discontinuation.

* In bladder-drained grafts.

Table 5. Pathological changes "other" than rejection in pancreas needle biopsies (Drachenberg et al., 2008).

Neuropathy: Initially after transplantation (SPK) neuropathy improves with correction of uraemia. Several studies reported improvement in motor and sensory nerve functions; confirmed by improved nerve conduction velocity. Less clear is the impact on autonomic function (arrhythmia, postural hypotension, diabetic diarrhoea, gastroparesis, neurogenic bladder, impotence, etc). Some data suggest that patients improve even with these symptoms but it is difficult to quantify (Nusser et al., 1991).
Cardio-vascular disease: Also, the positive impact of functioning pancreas graft on micro-vascular disease and cardiac function is well documented. This involve improvement in ventricular ejection function, reversal of diastolic function, and improved endothelial function.
Quality of Life: The main benefit of pancreas transplantation is the improved patients' quality of life. Sureshkumar, in his study (Sureshkumar et al., 2006), used three quality of life questionnaires (Diabetes Quality of Life Questionnaire, Medical Outcomes Questionnaire and Quality of Well-being Questionnaire) to compare outcomes of diabetics after SPK with patients on the Waiting List. He reports that SPK groups showed better diabetes-related quality of life.
Patient Survival: Results of SPK suggests that this group of patients do better over diabetics receiving cadaveric kidney transplants but there are no survival benefits compared to LRD recipients. The same study concludes that pancreas transplantation is not only life enhancing but also a life saving procedure (Reddy et al., 2003).

Algorithm of transplant alternatives in diabetics

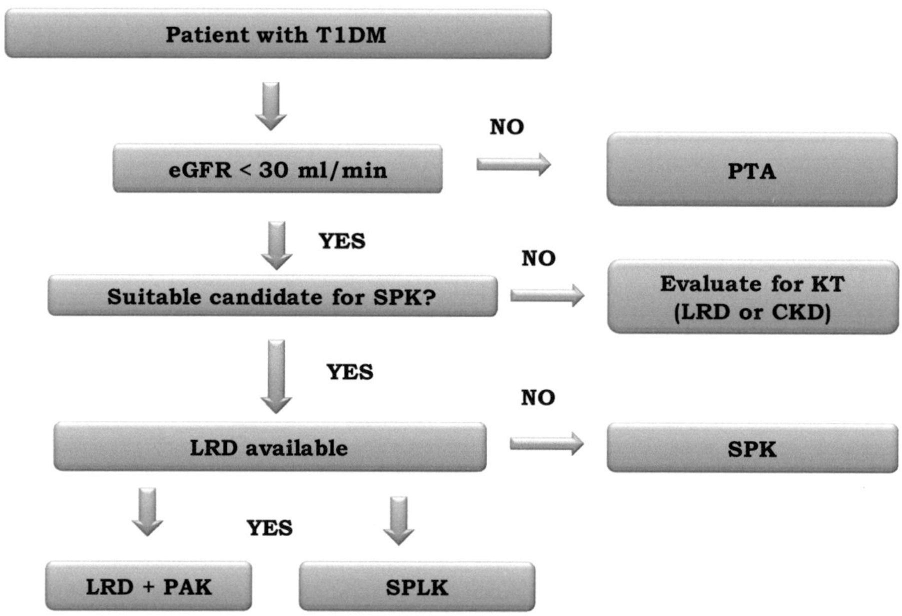

T1DM - type-1 diabetes mellitus, KT - kidney transplant, LRD - living related donor, CKD - cadaver kidney donor

Fig. 15. Algorithm to choose the best transplant alternatives for diabetics.

11. Summary

The outcomes following pancreas transplantation have significantly improved in the last decade. Careful patient selection, better organ procurement, refinements in surgical technique, new immunosuppressive drug regiments and better graft monitoring have all contributed to excellent outcomes. The available data provides strong evidence that pancreas transplantation not only improves diabetics' quality of life but also improves their medical conditions and prolongs their life expectancy.

Pancreas transplantation has become the option of choice to treat patients with type-1 diabetes. Currently several alternatives for these patients are available. The best option should be selected after careful patient assessment and individually weight pros and cons of each alternative (Fig. 15).

12. References

American Diabetes Association. (1999) Position statement: Diabetic nephropathy. *Diabetes Care*. Vol. 22, Suppl 1, pp. 66-69, ISSN 1935-5548

American Diabetes Association. Diabetes management in correctional institutions. *Diabetes Care*. Vol. 28, Suppl 1, (January 2005), pp. 53-60. ISSN 1935-5548

Bode BW. (2010) Comparison of pharmacokinetic properties, physiochemical stability and pump compatibility of three rapid-acting insulin analogs: aspart, lispro and glulisine. *Endocr Pract*. Vol. 6, (December 2010), pp. 1-36, ISSN 1530-891X

Boggi, U.; Pietrabissa, A.; Vistoli, F.; Del Chiaro, M.; Signori, S.; Coletti, L.; Morelli, L.; Moretto, C.; Barsotti, M.; Marchetti, P.; Del Prato, S.; Rizzo, G.; Mosca, F. Simultaneous pancreas-kidney transplantation is improved by living kidney donation program. *Transplant Proc*. Vol. 36, No. 4, (May 2004), pp. 1061-3, ISSN: 0041-1345

Bohman, S.O.; Wilczezck, H.; Jaremko, G.; Lundreg, G. (1984) Recurerance of diabetic nephropathy in human renal allografts: Preliminary report of a biopsy study. *Transplant proc*. Vol. 16, No. 3, (Jun 1984), pp. 649-53, ISSN 0041-1345

Braga, M.; Ljungqvist, O.; Soeters, P.; Fearon, K.; Weimann, A.; Bozzetti, F.; ESPEN. (2009) ESPEN Guidelines on Parenteral Nutrition: surgery. *Clin Nutr*. Vol. 28, No. 4, (August 2009), pp. 378-86, ISSN 1938-3207

Weimann, A.; Braga, M.; Harsanyi, L.; Laviano, A.; Ljungqvist, O.; Soeters, P.; DGEM (German Society for Nutritional Medicine); Jauch, K.W.; Kemen, M.; Hiesmayr, J.M.; Horbach, T.; Kuse, E.R.; Vestweber, K.H.; ESPEN (European Society for Parenteral and Enteral Nutrition). (2006) ESPEN Guidelines on Enteral Nutrition: Surgery including organ transplantation. *Clin Nutr*. Vol. 25, No. 2, (April 2006), pp. 224-44. ISSN 1938-3207

Burke, G.W. 3rd; Ciancio, G.; Figueiro, J.; Buigas, R.; Olson, L.; Roth, D.; Kupin, W.; Miller, J. Hypercoagulable state associated with kidney-pancreas transplantation. Thromboelastogram-directed anti-coagulation and implications for future therapy. *Clin Transplant*. Vol. 18, No. 4, (August 2004), pp. 423-8, ISSN 1399-0012

Cai, Q.; Serrano. R.; Kalyanasundaram, A.; Shirani. (2010) A preoperative echocardiographic predictive model for assessment of cardiovascular outcome after renal transplantation. *J Am Soc Echocardiogr*. Vol. 23, No. 5, (May 2010), pp. 560-6), ISSN 1532-2114

Calne, R.Y.; Rolles, K.; White, D.J.; et al. (1979) Cyclosporin A initially as the only immunosuppressant in 34 recipients of cadaveric organs: 32 kidneys, 2 pancreases, and 2 livers. *Lancet*. Vol. 314, No. 8151, (November 1979), pp. 1033-1036, ISSN 0140-6736.

Cecka, J.M. (1996) The UNOS Scientific Renal Transplant Registry. In: Clinical Transplants. Cecka, M.J.; Terasaki, P.I. eds. 1-14, UCLA Tissue Typing Laboratory, ISBN 0-7216-0409-9., Los Angeles, US

Cheung, CY., Cha, YH, Chan, HW., Chau, KF., Li CS. (2010) Optimal body mass index that can predict long term graft outcome in Asian renal transplant patients. *Nephrology*. Vol. 15, No. 2, (March 2010), pp. 359-65, ISSN 1533-3450

Collins, A.J.; Foley, R.; Herzog, C.; Chavers, B.; Gilbertson, D.; Ishani, A.; Kasiske, B.; Liu, J.; Mau, L.W.; McBean, M.; Murray, A.; St Peter, W.; Xue, J.; Fan, Q.; Guo, H.; Li, Q.; Li, S.; Li, S.; Peng, Y.; Qiu, Y.; Roberts, T.; Skeans, M.; Snyder, J.; Solid, C.; Wang, C.; Weinhandl, E.; Zaun, D.; Zhang, R.; Arko, C.; Chen, S.C.; Dalleska, F.; Daniels, F.; Dunning, S.; Ebben, J.; Frazier, E.; Hanzlik, C.; Johnson, R.; Sheets, D.; Wang, X.; Forrest, B.; Constantini, E.; Everson, S.; Eggers, P.; Agodoa, L.. Excerpts from the United States Renal Data System 2007 annual data report. Am J Kidney Dis. Vol. 51, Supplement 1, (January 2008), pp. 1-320

Corry RJ. Pancreatico-duodenal transplantation with urinary tract drainage. (1988) In: Groth, C.G., ed. Pancreatic Transplantation. 131-146, WB Saunders Company, ISBN 0. 7216 1614 3, Philadelphia, PA

Deferrari, G.; Repetto, M.; Calvi, C.; Ciabattoni, M.; Rossi, C.; Robaudo, C. (1998) Diabetic nephropathy: from micro- to macroalbuminuria. *Nephrol Dial Transplant*. Vol. 13, Suppl 8, (December 1998), pp. 11-15, ISSN 0931-0509

DiLandro, D.; Catalano, C.; Lambertini, D.; Bordin, V.; Fabbian, F.; Naso, A.; Romagnoli, G. (1998) The effect of metabolic control on development and progression of diabetic nephropathy. *Nephrol Dial Transplant*. Vol. 13, Suppl. 8, (1998), pp.35-43, ISSN 1460-2385

Document. (1997) Banff schema for grading liver allograft rejection. An international consensus document. *Hepatology*. Vol. 25, No. 3, (March 1997), pp. 658–663, ISSN 1527-3350

Drachenberg, C.B.; Odorico, J.; Demetris, A.J.; Arend, L.; Bajema, I.M.; Bruijn, J.A.; Cantarovich, D.; Cathro, H.P.; Chapman, J.; Dimosthenous, K.; Fyfe-Kirschner, B.; Gaber, L.; Gaber, O.; Goldberg, J.; Honsová, E.; Iskandar, S.S.; Klassen, D.K.; Nankivell, B.; Papadimitriou, J.C.; Racusen, L.C.; Randhawa, P.; Reinholt, F.P.; Renaudin, K.; Revelo, P.P.; Ruiz, P.; Torrealba, J.R.; Vazquez-Martul, E.; Voska, L.; Stratta, R.; Bartlett, S.T.; Sutherland, D.E. (2008) Banff schema for grading pancreas allograft rejection: working proposal by a multi-disciplinary international consensus panel. *Am J Transplant*. Vol. 8, No. 6, (April 2008), pp. 1237-49, ISSN 1600-6143

Farney, A.C.; Cho, E.; Schweitzer, E.J.; Dunkin, B.; Philosophe, B.; Colonna, J.; Jacobs, S.; Jarrell, B.; Flowers, J.L.; Bartlett, S.T. (2000) Simultaneous cadaver pancreas living-donor kidney transplantation: a new approach for the type 1 diabetic uremic patient Ann Surg. Vol. 232, No. 5, (November 2000), pp. 696-703, ISSN 1528-1140

Fioretto, P.; Steffes, M.W.; Sutherland, D.E.; Goetz, F.C.; Mauer, M. (1998) Reversal of lesions of diabetic nephropathy after pancreas transplantation. *N Engl J Med.* Vol. 339, No. 2, (Jul 1998), pp. 69-75. ISSN 1533-4406

Gaber, L.W. (2007) Pancreas allograft biopsies in the management of pancreas transplant recipients: histopathologic review and clinical correlations. Vol. 131, No. 8, (August 2007), pp. 1192-9, ISSN 1543-2165

Ganesh, SK., Stack, AG., Levin, N., Hulbert-Shearon, T., Part, F. (2001) Association of elevated serum phosphate, calcium x phosphate product and parathyroid hormone with cardiac mortality risk in chronic haemodialysis patients. *Journal of American society of nephrology.* Vol. 12, No. 10, (October 2001), pp. 2131-2138, ISSN 1533-3450

González-Posada, J.M.; Marrero, D.; Hernández, D.; Coll, E.; Tamajón, L.P.; Gutiérrez, P.; Martín, E.; Bravo, A.; Alarcó, A.; Matesanz, R. (2009) Pancreas transplantation: differences in activity between Europe and the United States. Nephrol *Dial Transplant.* Vol. 25, No. 3, (March 2010), pp. 952-9, ISSN 1460-2385

Gruessner, A.C.; Sutherland, D.E.R. Pancreas transplant outcomes from United States (US) cases reported to the United Network for Organ Sharing (UNOS) and non-US cases reported to the International Pancreas Transplant Registry (IPTR) as of October, 2000. In: Cecka JM, Terasaki PI, eds. Clinical Transplants. 45-72, UCLA Immunogenetics Center, ISBN 0965952207 Los Angeles, US

Gruessner, A.C.; Sutherland, D.E. (2005) Pancreas transplant outcomes for United States (US) and non-US cases as reported to the United Network for Organ Sharing (UNOS) and the International Pancreas Transplant Registry (IPTR) as of June 2004. *Clin Transplant.* . 19, No. 4, (August 2005), pp. 433-55, ISSN 1399-0012

Gruessner, A.C.; Sutherland, D.E. (2008) Pancreas transplant outcomes for United States (US) cases as reported to the United Network for Organ Sharing (UNOS) and the International Pancreas Transplant Registry (IPTR). *Clin Transpl.* Vol. 22, No.1, (January-February 2008), pp. 45-56, ISSN 0902-0063.

Grundy, S.M.; Benjamin, T.J.; Burke, G.L. et al. (1999) Diabetes and cardiovascular disease: a statement for healthcare professionals from the American Heart Association. *Circulation.* Vol. 100, No. 10, (September 1999), pp 1134-46, ISSN 0009-7322

Gu, Y.; Li, J.; Li, N. Insulin sensitivity after pancreaticoduodenal transplantation with systemic and portal venous drainage in inbred rats. *Chin Med J.* Vol. 115, No. 4, (April 2002), pp. 549-51, ISSN 0021-9738

Heilman, R.L.; Mazur, M.J.; Reddy, K.S. (2010) Immunosuppression in simultaneous pancreas-kidney transplantation: progress to date. *Drugs.* Vol. 70, No. 7, (May 2010), pp. 793-804, ISSN 0012-6667.

Herzog, C.A.; Marwick, T.H.; Pheley, A.M.; White, C.W.; Rao, V.K., Dick. C.D. Dobutamine stress echocardiography for the detection of significant coronary artery disease in renal transplant candidates. *Am J Kidney Dis.* Vol. 33, No. 6, (Jun 1999), pp. 1080-90, ISSN 0272-6386

Hoogeveen, E.K.; Aalten, J.; Rothman, K.; Roodnat, J.; Mallet, M.; Borm, G.; Weimer, W.; Haitsman, A.; de Fijter, J. (2011) Effect of obesity on the outcome of kidney transplant: A 20 year follow up. *Transplantation.* Published ahead of print, ISSN 1534-0608

Jiménez-Romero, C.; Manrique, A.; Morales, J.M.; López, R.M.; Morales, E.; Cambra, F.; Calvo, J.; García-Sesma, A.; Praga, M.; Moreno, E. (2009) Conversion from bladder to enteric drainage for complications after pancreas transplantation. *Transplant Proc.* Jul-Aug;Vol. 41, No. 6, (Jul-August 2009), pp. 2469-71, ISSN 0041-1345

Kashyap, P., Farrugia, G. (2010) Diabetic gastroperesis: what we have learned and had to unlearn in the past 5 years. *Gut.* Vol. 59, No. 12, (December 2010), pp. 1716-26, ISSN 1468-3288

Kelly, W.D.; Lillehei, R.C.; Merkel, F.K.; Idezuki, Y.; Goetz, F.C. (1967). Allotransplantation of the pancreas and duodenum along with the kidney in diabetic nephropathy. *Surgery.* Vol. 61, No. 6, (Jun 1967), pp. 827–37, ISSN 0002-9610

Kertes, PJ.; Johnson, TM. (Eds.) (2007). *Evidence Based Eye Care.*, Lippincott Williams & Wilkins. ISBN 0-7817-6964-7. Philadelphia, Ph

Kitada, H.; Sugitani, A.; Okabe, Y.; Doi, A.; Nishiki, T.; Miura, Y.; Kurihara, K.; Tanaka, M. (2009) Availability of pancreatic allograft biopsies via a laparotomy. *Transplant Proc.* Vol. 41, No. 10, (December 2009), pp. 4274-6, ISSN 0041-1345

Kleinclauss, F.; Fauda, M.; Sutherland, D.E.; Kleinclauss, C.; Gruessner, R.W.; Matas, A.J.; Kasiske, B.L.; Humar, A.; Kandaswamy, R.; Kaul, S.; Gruessner, A.C. (2009) Pancreas after living donor kidney transplants in diabetic patients: impact on long-term kidney graft function. *Clin Transplant.* Vol. 23, No. 4, (August-September 2009), pp. 437-46, ISSN 1399-0012

Königsrainer, A; Miller, K.; Steurer, W.; Kieselbach, G.; Aichberger, C.; Ofner, D.; Margreiter, R. (1991) Does pancreas transplantation influence the course of diabetic retinopathy? Diabetologia. Vol. 34, Suppl. 1, (Augusta 191), pp. 86-88, ISSN 1432-0428

Kuo, HT., Sampaio, MS., Vincenti, F., Bunnapradist, S. (2010) Association of post transplant diabetes mellitus, new onset diabetes after transplantation and acute rejection with transplant outcomes: an analysis of the organ procurement and transplant network/united network for organ sharing (OPTN/UNOS) database. *American Journal of Kidney Disease.* Vol. 56, No. 6, (December 2010), pp. 1127-39, ISSN 0272-6386

Larson, T.S.; Bohorquez, H.; Rea, D.J.; Nyberg, S.L.; Prieto, M.; Sterioff, S.; Textor, S.C.; Schwab, T.R.; Griffin, M.D.; Gloor, J.M.; Kudva, Y.C.; Kremers, W.K.; Stegall, M.D. (2004) Pancreas-after-kidney transplantation: an increasingly attractive alternative to simultaneous pancreas-kidney transplantation. *Transplantation.* Vol. 77, No. 6, (March 2004) pp. 838-43. ISSN 1534-0608

Lentine, K.L.; Hurst, F.P.; Jindal, R.M.; Villines, T.C.; Kunz, J.S.; Yuan, C.M.; Hauptman, P.J.; Abbott, K.C. (2010) Cardiovascular risk assessment among potential kidney transplant candidates: approaches and controversies. *Am J Kidney Dis.* Vol. 55, No. 1, (January 2010), pp. 152-67, ISSN 1523-6838

Lillehei, R.C.; Simmons, R.L.; Najarian, J.S.; Weil, R.; Uchida, H; Ruiz, J.O.; Kjellstrand, C.M.; Goetz, F.C. Pancreatico-duodenal allotransplantation: experimental and clinical experience. *Ann Surg.* Vol. 172, No. 3, (September 1970) , pp. 405-36, ISSN 1528-1140

Lo, A.; Stratta, R.J.; Hathaway, D.K.; Egidi, M.F.; Shokouh-Amiri, M.H.; Grewal, H.P., Winsett, R.; Trofe, J.; Alloway, R.R.; Gaber, A.O. (2001)Long-term outcomes in simultaneous kidney-pancreas transplant recipients with portal-enteric versus systemic-bladder drainage. *Transplant Proc.* Vol.33, No. 1-2, (February-March 2001), pp. 1684-6, ISSN 0041-1345

MacLeod, M.; McLay, J. Drug treatment of hypertension complicating diabetes mellitus. *Drugs*. Vol. 56, No. 2, (1998), pp. 189-202, ISSN 0012-6667

Matthew, D.D.; Thymothy, S.K.; Lawrence, I.R. (1997) Diabetic Retinopathy, In: Alberti, K.G.M.M.; Zimmet, P.; DeFronzo, R.A.; Keen, H. *International Textbook of Diabetes mellitus*, second edition, vol2, 1441-1446, John Wiley and Son, ISBN 0471939307, Canada

Meier-Kriesche, H.U., Arndarfer, J.A., Kaplan, B. (2002) The impact of BMI on renal transplant outcomes: A significant rick factor for graft failure and patient death. *Transplantation*. Vol. 73, No. 1, (January 2002), pp. 70-4, ISSN 1534-0608

Mineo, D.; Sageshima, J.; Burke, G.W.; Ricordi, C. (2008) Minimization and withdrawal of steroids in pancreas and islet transplantation. *Transpl Int*. Vol. 22, No. 1, (January 2009), pp. 20-37. ISSN 1432-2277.

Muthusamy, A.S.R.; Giangrande, P.L.F.; Friend, P.J. (2010) Pancreas Allograft Thrombosis. *Transplantation*. Vol. 90, No. 7, (October 2010), pp. 705-707, ISSN 1534-0608.

National Institutes of Health, National Institute of Diabetes, Digestive, and Kidney Diseases. United States Renal Data Systems. Digestive and Kidney Diseases. (April 1998), ISSN 1533-3450

http://www.usrds.org/download/1998/ch07.pdf

Noori, N., Kalantar-Zadeh, K., Kavesdy, CP., Murali, SB., Bross, R., Nissenson, AR., Kapple, JD. (2010) Dietary potassium intake and mortality in long term haemodialysis patients. *American Journal of Kidney Disease*. Vol. 56, No. 2, (August 2010), pp. 338-47, ISSN 0272-6386

Nusser, J.; Scheuer, R.; Abendroth, D.; Illner, W.D.; Land, W.; Landgraf, R. (1991) Effect of pancreatic and/or renal transplantation on diabetic autonomic neuropathy. *Diabetologia*. Vol. 34, Suppl. 1, (August 1991), pp. 118-20, ISSN 1432-0428.

Ojo, A.O.; Meier-Kriesche, H.U.; Hanson, J.A.; Leichtman, A.; Magee, J.C.; Cibrikm, D.; Wolfe, R.A.; Port, F.K.; Agodoa, L.; Kaufman, D.B.; Kaplan, B. (2001) The impact of simultaneous pancreas-kidney transplantation on long-term patient survival. *Transplantation*. Vol. 71, No. 1, (January 2001), pp. 82-90, ISSN 1534-0608

Orlando, G.; Stratta, R.J.; Light, J. (2010) Pancreas transplantation for type 2 diabetes mellitus. *Curr Opin Organ Tranplsnt*. Vol. No. , (December 2010), pp. ISSN 1531-7013

Pommipanit, N.; Sampaio, M.S.; Cho, Y.; Young, B.; Shah, T.; Pham, P.T.; Wilkinson, A.; Danovitch, G.; Bunnapradist, S. (2010) Pancreas after living donor kidney versus simultaneous pancreas-kidney transplant: an analysis of the organ procurement transplant network/united network of organ sharing database. *Transplantation*. Vol. 89, No. 12, (Jun 2010), pp. 1496-503, ISSN 1534-0608.

Rabbat, C.G.; Treleaven, D.J.; Russell, J.D.; Ludwin, D. Cook, D.J. (2003) Prognostic value of myocardial perfusion studies in patients with end-stage renal disease assessed for kidney or kidney-pancreas transplantation: a meta-analysis. J Am Soc Nephrol. Vol. 14, No. 2, (February 2003), pp. 431-9, ISSN 1533-3450

Radziuk, J.; Barron, P.; Najm, H.; Davies, K. (1993) The effect of systemic venous drainage of the pancreas on insulin sensitivity in dogs. *J Clin Invest*. Vol. 92, No. 4, (October 1993), pp. 1713-21, ISSN 0021-9738

Rayhill, S.C.; D'Alessandro, A.M.; Odorico, J.S.; Knechtle, S.J.; Pirsch, J.D.; Heisey, D.M.; Kirk, A.D.; Van der Werf, W.; Sollinger, H.W. (2000) Simultaneous pancreas-kidney transplantation and living related donor renal transplantation in patients with diabetes: is there a difference in survival? *Ann Surg*. Vol. 231, No. 3, (March 2000), pp. 417-23. ISSN 1528-1140.

Reddy, K.S.; Stablein, D.; Taranto, S.; Stratta, R.J.; Johnston, T.D.; Waid, T.H.; McKeown, J.W.; Lucas, B.A.; Ranjan, D. (2003) Long-term survival following simultaneous kidney-pancreas transplantation versus kidney transplantation alone in patients with type 1 diabetes mellitus and renal failure. *Am J Kidney Dis*. Vol. 41, No. 2, (February 2003), pp. 464-70, ISSN 0272-6386

Reddy, S., Ramsubeik, K., Vega, K., Frederico J., Palacio, C. (2010) Do HbA1c levels correlate with delayed gastric emptying in diabetic patients? *Journal of Neurogastroenterology and motility*. Vol. 16, No. 4, (October 2010), pp. 414-7, ISSN 1365-2982

Sato, H., Carvalho, G., Sato, T., Lattermann, R., Matsukawa, T., Schricker, T. (2010) The Association of preoperative glycaemic control, Intraoperative insulin sensitivity & outcomes after cardiac surgery. *Journal of Clinical Endocrinology & Metabolism*. Vol. 95, No. 9, (September 2010), pp. 4338-4344, ISSN 0021972X

Singh, R.P.; Stratta, R.J. (2008) Advances in immunosuppression for pancreas transplantation. *Curr Opin Organ Transplant*. Vol 13, No. 1, (February 2008), pp. 79-84, ISSN: 1531-7013.

Solez, K.; Colvin, RB.; Racusen, L.C. et al. (2007) Banff '05 Meeting Report: Differential diagnosis of chronic allograft injury and elimination of chronic allograft nephropathy ('CAN'). *Am J Transplant*. Vol. 7, No. 3, (March 2007), pp. 518–526. ISSN 1600-6143

Sollinger, H.W.; Belzer, F.O. Pancreas transplantation with urinary tract drainage. (1988) In: Groth, C.G., ed. Pancreatic Transplantation. 131-146, WB Saunders Company, ISBN 0. 7216 1614 3, Philadelphia, PA

Starzl, T.E.; Tzakis, A.G. (1988) Pancreatico-duodenal transplantation with enteric exocrine drainage. In: Groth CG, ed. Pancreatic Transplantation, (Ed.). pp. 119-129, WB Saunders Company, ISBN 0. 7216 1614 3 ,Philadelphia, PA

Stephanian, E.; Gruessner, R.W.; Brayman, K.L.; Gores, P.; Dunn, D.L.; Najarian, J.S.; Sutherland D.E. (1992) Conversion of exocrine secretions from bladder to enteric drainage in recipients of whole pancreaticoduodenal transplants. *Ann Surg*. Vol. 216, No. 6, (December 1992), 663-72, ISSN 1528-1140

Stockland, A.H.; Willingham, D.L.; Paz-Fumagalli, R.; Grewal, H.P.; McKinney, J.M.; Hughes, C.B.; Walser, E.M. (2009) Pancreas transplant venous thrombosis: role of endovascular interventions for graft salvage. *Cardiovasc Intervent Radiol*. Vol. 32, No. 2, (March 2009), pp. 279-83, ISSN: 1432-086

Stratta, R.J.; Taylor, R.J.; Lowell, J.A.; et al. (1993) Randomized trial of sandostatin prophylaxis for preservation

injury after pancreas transplantation. *Transplant Proc*, Vol. 25, No. 6, (December 1993), pp. 3190-2, ISSN: 0041-1345.

Stratta, R.J. (1999) Review of immunosuppressive usage in pancreas transplantation. *Clin Transplant*. Vol. 13, No. 1 (February 1999), p. 1-12, ISSN 1399-0012

Stratta, R.J.; Gaber, A.O.; Shokouh-Amiri, M.H. Reddy, K.S; Egidim, M.F.; Grewal, H.P.; Gaber, L.W. (2000) A prospective comparison of systemic-bladder versus portal-enteric drainage in vascularized pancreas transplantation. *Surgery*. Vol. 127, No. 2, pp. 217-26, (February 2000), ISSN 0002-9610

Stratta, R.J.; Alloway, R.R.; Lo, A.; Hodge, E.E. PIVOT Investigators. (2003) One year outcomes in simultaneous kidney-pancreas transplant recipients receiving an alternative regimen of daclizumab. Program and abstracts of American Transplant Congress 2003: The Fourth Joint American Transplant Meeting; May 30-June 4, 2003; Washington, DC. Abstract 662.

Sugitani A, Gritsch HA, Shapiro R, Bonham CA, Egidi MF, Corry RJ. (1998) Surgical complications in 123 consecutive pancreas transplant recipients: comparison of bladder and enteric drainage Transplant Proc. Vol. 30, No. 2, (March 1998), pp. 293-4, ISSN 0041-1345

Sutherland, D.E.R.; Goetz, F.C.; Najarian, J.S. (1988) Experience with single pancreatic transplantation compared with pancreas transplantation after kidney transplantation; and with transplantation with pancreas graft living related compared with cadaveric donors. In: Groth, C.G., ed. Pancreatic Transplantation. 175-189, WB Saunders Company, ISBN 0. 7216 1614 3 Philadelphia, Ph

Sureshkumar, K.K.; Patel, B.M.; Markatos, A.; Nghiem, D.D.; Marcus, R.J. (2006) Quality of life after organ transplantation in type 1 diabetics with end-stage renal disease. *Clin Transplant*. Vol. 20, No. 1, (January-February 2006), pp. 19-25, ISSN 0902-0063

The Diabetes Control and Complications Trial Research Group. (1993) The effect of intensive treatment of diabetes on the development andprogression of long-term complications in insulin-dependent diabetes mellitus. *N Engl J Med.* Vol. 30, No. 27, pp. 977–986, (September 1993), ISSN 1533-4406

Troppmann, C.; Gruessner, A.C.; Dunn, D.L.; Sutherland, D.E.; Gruessner, R.W. (1998) Surgical complications requiring early relaparotomy after pancreas transplantation: a multivariate risk factor and economic impact analysis of the cyclosporine era. *Ann Surg*. Vol. 227, No. 2, (February 1998), pp. 255-68, ISSN: 1528-1140

UK Transplant. September 2003. *National Protocol for assessment of kidney and pancreas transplant patients*. 28 February 2011, Available from: <http://www.uktransplant.org.uk/ukt/about_transplants/organ_allocation/pancreas/assessment_of_kidney_and_pancreas_tx_patients.doc>

United Network for Organ Sharing, 2010. Richmond, VA. Available from http://www.unos.org/Data/. Accessed 16 March 2010

Waki, K.; Terasaki, P.I.; Kadowaki, T. (2010) Long-Term Pancreas Allograft Survival in Simultaneous Pancreas-Kidney Transplantation by Era UNOS registry analysis. *Diabetes Care.* Vol. 33 , No. 8, (August 2010), pp. 1789-1791, ISSN 1935-5548

Ward, J.D. Diabetic Peripheral Neuropathy, In: Alberti, K.G.M.M.; Zimmet, P.; DeFronzo, R.A.; Keen, H. *International Textbook of Diabetes mellitus,* second edition, vol2, 1478-1496, John Wiley and Son, ISBN 0471939307, Canada

Watkins, P.J.; Edmonds, M.E.(1997) Autonomic Neuropathy, In: Alberti, K.G.M.M.; Zimmet, P.; DeFronzo, R.A.; Keen, H. *International Textbook of Diabetes mellitus,* second edition, vol. 2, pp. 1497-1506, John Wiley and Son, ISBN 0471939307, Canada

Watkins, P.J.; (2003) ABC of diabetes: Cardiovascular disease, hypertension, and lipids. *BMJ*. Vol. 326, No. 7405, (Jul 2003), pp. 874 , ISSN 0959-8138

Weimann, A.; Braga, M.; Harsanyi, L.; Laviano, A.; Ljungqvist, O.; Soeters, P.; DGEM (German Society for Nutritional Medicine); Jauch, K.W.; Kemen, M.; Hiesmayr, J.M.; Horbach, T.; Kuse, E.R.; Vestweber, K.H.; ESPEN (European Society for Parenteral and Enteral Nutrition). (2006) ESPEN Guidelines on Enteral Nutrition:

Surgery including organ transplantation. *Clin Nutr.* Vol. 25, No. 2, (April 2006), pp. 224-44. ISSN 1938-3207

Wiesbauer F, Heinze G, Regele H, Hörl WH, Schernthaner GH, Schwarz C, Kainz A, Kramar R, Oberbauer, R. (2010). Glucose control is associated with patient survival in diabetic patients after renal transplantation. *Transplantation,* Vol. 15, No. 5, (March 2010), pp. 612-619, ISSN 1534-0608

Wiseman, A.C. (2010) The role of kidney-pancreas transplantation in diabetic kidney disease. *Curr Diab Rep.* Vol. 10, No. 5, (October 2010), pp. 385-91, ISSN 1539-0829

Wong, T.Y.; Liew, G.; Tapp, R.J. *et al.* (2008). Relation between fasting glucose and retinopathy for diagnosis of diabetes: three population-based cross-sectional studies. *Lancet.* Vol. 371, No. 9614, (March 2008), pp. 736–43, ISSN 1474-547X.

Writing Team for the Diabetes Control and Complications Trial/ Epidemiology of Diabetes Interventions and Complications Research Group. (2003) Sustained effect of intensive treatment of type 1 diabetes mellitus on development and progression of diabetic nephropathy: the Epidemiology of Diabetes Interventions and Complications (EDIC) study. *JAMA* Vol. 22, No. 6, (October 2003), pp. 2159–2167, ISSN 00987484

Young, B.Y.; Gill, J.; Huang, E.; Takemoto, S.K.; Anastasi, B.; Shah, T.; Bunnapradist, S. (2009) Living donor kidney versus simultaneous pancreas-kidney transplant in type I diabetics: an analysis of the OPTN/UNOS database *Clin J Am Soc Nephrol.* Vol. 4, No. 4, (April 2009), pp. 845-52, ISSN 1555-905

6

Cardiovascular Diseases in Kidney Transplantation

Roberto Marcén and Sara Jiménez
Department of Nephrology. Ramón y Cajal Hospital,
University of Alcalá de Henares, Madrid
Spain

1. Introduction

Cardiovascular diseases that include atherosclerotic diseases; coronary artery disease, cerebrovascular disease and peripheral vascular disease, and cardiac functional diseases; congestive heart failure, left ventricular hypertrophy and arrhythmias, are very common in the general population and are the first cause of mortality (Wilson &Culleton, 1998, Culleton & Wilson, 1998). Moreover, patients with chronic renal failure have an increased risk of cardiovascular disease compared with the general population, and after stratification by age and gender, cardiovascular mortality is 10 to 20 times more frequent independently of treatment; predialysis, dialysis or after kidney transplantation (Foley et al, 1998). Kidney transplantation is the best therapy of end-stage renal disease by reducing cardiovascular mortality (McDonald &Russ, 2002, Ojo et al, 2000, Wolfe et al, 1999). But even after transplantation, a recipient of 25 to 35 years of age has a 10 times higher risk of cardiovascular mortality than an individual of similar sex and gender without renal failure (Foley et al, 1998). Among the cardiovascular diseases, atherosclerotic diseases are the most frequently studied and are associated with patient outcome. Ischaemic heart disease was the cause of 53% of total mortality in a study performed in Scandinavia 15 years ago (Lindholm et al, 1995) and these findings were still prevalent in a later report (Aakhus et al, 2004). However, several authors have recently emphasized the importance of functional cardiopathies such as congestive heart failure on patient outcome (Rigatto et al, 2002).
The high incidence of cardiovacular events and mortality in renal transplant recipients has been attributed to the increased presence of traditional (Ojo, 2006) and nontraditional risk factors (Ducloux et al, 2004, De Mattos et al, 2006). As traditional risk factors do not fully explain the high cardiovascular risk it has been postulated that some of these risk factors, age, diabetes and smoking, could have a higher deleterous impact in transplant recipients than in the general population (Kasiske et al, 2000a). Other authors consider that transplant related (De Mattos et al, 2006) and nontraditional or emergent factors, hyperhomcysteinemia and inflammation, could play a predominant role in the appearance of cardiovascular events (Ducloux et al, 2004). Progressive chronic graft dysfunction and death with functioning graft are the most important causes of graft loss (Matas et al, 2002, Collins et al, 2008) and cardiovascular diseases are the leading cause of mortality in renal transplant recipients dying with a functioning graft (Pilmore et al, 2010). Consequently decreasing

cardiovascular mortality could improve patient and graft outcomes (Howard et al, 2002, Marcén et al, 2001, Morales, 2008, Vanrenterghem et al, 2008).
The present chapter reviews the cardiovascular diseases which affect renal transplant recipients and their impact on patient mortality, the risk factors associated with these complications and the therapeutical strategies to improve patient and graft outcomes.

2. Cardiovascular diseases

Renal transplant recipients are not healthy individuals. They have a past history of chronic renal failure and dialysis therapy, both having negative impact on cardiovascular risk and they present variable chronic renal failure stages. All cardiovascular diseases; atheriosclerotic and functional cardiopathies can affect transplant recipients (Table 1).

Atheroesclerotic diseases	Functional cardiopathies
Coronary artery diseases	Congestive heart failure
Cerebrovascular diseases	Left ventricular hypertrophy
Peripheral vascular diseases	Arrhythmias

Table 1. Most common cardiovascular diseases affecting transplant recipients

As in the general population, cardiovascular diseases are important causes of morbidity and mortality in renal transplant recipients. Heart diseases and cerebrovascular diseases accounted for about 35% mortality in our Unit (Figure 1).

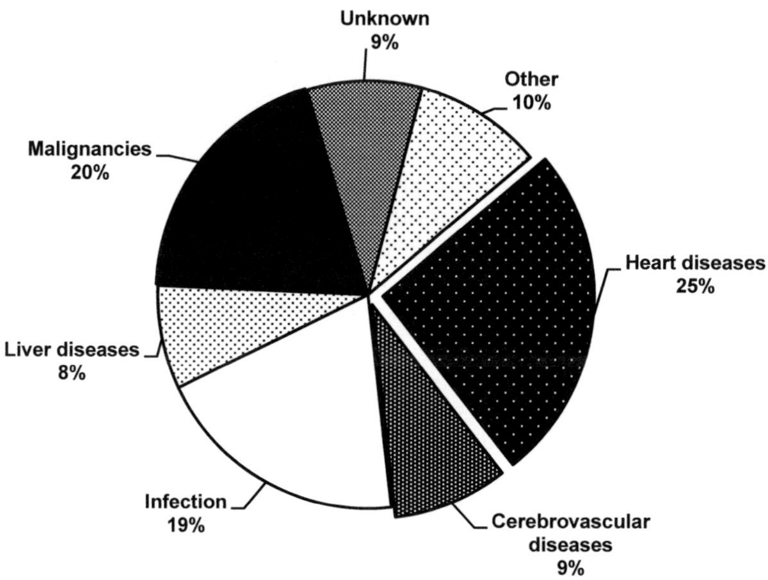

Fig. 1. Causes of mortality in 224 renal transplant recipients with functioning graft (Ramón y Cajal Hospital)

2.1 Atherosclerotic diseases

2.1.1 Coronary artery disease

Coronary artery disease is the most frequent atherosclerotic disease in the general population and a leading cause of cardiovascular mortality. It is generally admitted that coronary artery disease is between 2 and 6 times more frequent in renal transplant recipients than in the general population (Aarkhus et al, 1999, Kasiske, 1988, Lentine et al, 2005a, Marcén et al, 2006, Massy, 2001). A very high number of events occurring during the first weeks after transplantation have been attributed to surgical stress, immunosuppression and silent disease while the patient was on dialysis (Kasiske et al, 2000, 2005, Lentine et al, 2005, Marcén et al, 2006). In a retrospective study from the USA, the prevalence of coronary artery disease, defined as acute myocardial infarction, coronary revascularization procedures, or death due to coronary disease, was 23% at 15 years of follow-up and it was the cause of 18.7% of mortality (Kasiske et al, 1996). In a multicenter, retrospective study performed in Spain, the prevalence of coronary artery disease was 6.8% at 5 years (Marcén et al, 2006) and very similar findings have been reported from France (Doucloux et al, 2004), two low risk countries. Data from the United Network for Organ Sharing (UNOS) and United States Renal Data System (USRDS) registry showed that the prevalence of acute myocardial infarction was between 6% to 11 % at 3 years a 17% lower than that observed on waiting list patients (Kasiske et al, 2006, Lentine et al, 2005). Moreover, myocardial infarction has a poor prognosis and is the cause of high mortality (Herzog et al, 1998, 2000, Morales, 2008).
The diagnostic criteria and therapeutical measures must be those used in the general population and in patients with chronic renal failure (Murphy et al, 1998). As a high percentage of events occur in the first weeks or months after the procedure, efforts have to be made to prevent and treat coronary artery disease before transplantation. Several algorithms have been proposed in which patients are classified according to cardiovascular risk (Lentine et al, 2008b, Wang & Kasiske, 2010), but we have not yet the ideal diagnostic procedure for asymptomatic patients.

2.1.2 Cerebrovascular diseases

Cerebrovascular diseases include transient cerebral ischaemia, when focal neurologic symptoms resolve in 24 hours, and persistent neurological deficits documented by computed tomography or nuclear magnetic resonance. Patients with chronic renal disease have more severe atherosclerotic lesions in carotic arteries than the general population (Kennedy et al 2001). This could explain the 5 to 10 times higher risk of having ischaemic or haemorragic events when compared with the general population (Seliger et al, 2002, 2003a,b). In renal transplant recipients the annual incidence was from 0.5% to 2.3% (Abedini et al, 2009a, Aull-Watschinger et al, 2008, Cosio et al, 2005, Lentine et al, 2008a, Oliveras et al,2003), and ischaemic events predominated in a proportion of 2-3:1 compared with haemorragic events (Aull-Watschinger et al, 2008, Oliveras et al, 2003). In a long-term study, by actuarial analysis, 15% of patients who survived with a functioning graft for 15 years experienced a major crebrovascular event (Kasiske et al, 1996). The evolution of cerebrovascular diseases is poor and a mortality rate around of 50% three months after the event has been reported (Oliveras et al, 2003). In retrospective studies, cerebrovascular diseases were the cause of 5% to 8% of total mortality (Aull-Watschinger et al, 2008, Howard et al, 2002). Only the Assessment of Lescol in Renal Transplantation (ALERT) study has prospectively investigated these complications, the incidence was 8.8% during the 6.7 year follow-up period, and 21% of the cerebrovascular events, 48% of haemorragic and 8% of ischaemic, were fatal and accounted for 9.9% of total mortality (Abedini et al, 2009a).

2.1.3 Peripheral vascular disease

The incidence and clinical outcome of this complication have been seldom studied in renal transplant recipients. The diagnostic criteria include: intermitent claudication, ulceration with long-vessel disease on flow studies, amputations, by-pass or percutaneous angioplasty. The frequency reported was variable. In an old study, in which only amputation or revascularization procedures were included, the cumulative incidence was 15% at 15 years (Kasiske et al, 1996). In other studies, the incidence increased with the length of follow-up, from 2.1% at 1 year to 5.9% at 10 years (Sung et al, 2000). Data from the UNOS registry have shown a cumulative incidence of 20% in diabetic and 5% in nondiabetic patients at 3 years (Snyder et al, 2006). As the disease develops along years it is difficult to distinguish risk factors due to transplantation from those present before. The need of amputation is low about 2 to 3% (Sung et al, 2000). The disease by itself is not a cause of mortality but patients suffering from it have an increased risk of death with a functioning graft (Snyder et al, 2006, Sung et al, 2000).

3. Functional heart diseases

3.1 Congestive heart failure

Congestive heart disease is defined as dysnea plus at least two of the following characteristics; increased yugular venous pressure, basal lung rales, lung hypertension in radiography or pulmonary edema (Harnett et al, 1995). In dialysis patients, congestive heart failure is 36 times more frequent than in the general population and it is a mortality risk factor (Collins 2002, Stack &Bloemberg, 2001). Congestive heart disease has been studied less than coronary artery disease in the renal transplant population and it is associated with coronary artery disease in 30% of cases (Rigatto, 2003a,b). Its annual incidence was 3-5 times that of the general population, reached a cumulative incidence of 18.3% at 3years and was associated with poor graft function (Abbott et al, 2003b, Lentine et al, 2005, Rigatto, 2003a,b). It has a high impact on mortality, similar to that of coronary artery disease (Lentine et al, 2005).

3.2 Left ventricular hypertrophy

There are two types of left ventricular hypertrophy; concentric ventricular hypertrophy and dilatation with or without hypertrophy. The first one is associated with volume overload and the second with aortic insuficiency or severe anemia. Both types are more frequent in patients in renal failure than in the general population, reaching 20-50% in patients with chronic renal failure (Levin et al, 1996, Tucker et al, 1997) and up to 70% in those on dialysis (Foley et al, 1995, McGregor et al, 1998). Several prospective studies have shown that left ventricular hypertrophy improved during the first two years after transplantation but it was still present in about 40% of renal transplant recipients (Rigatto et al, 2000, Teruel et al, 1987). Factors related with no improvement were: age, left ventricular morphology, duration and severity of hypertension and time averaged pulse pressure (Rigatto et al, 2000). Moreover, renal transplant also improved ventricular function in most patients even in those with severe impairment (Parfrey et al 1995, Wali et al, 2005). However these findings have been recently questioned when cardiac structure was assessed by magnetic resonance

(Patel et al, 2008). Parameters of ventricular hypertrophy or impaired cardiac function were associated with increased risk of cardiovascular events and cardiovascular mortality in renal transplant recipients (Aull-Watschinger et al, 2008, McGregor et al, 2000). In a nonrandomized study, conversi6n from CNI to sirolimus regressed left ventricular mass thickness regardless of blood pressure changes, thus suggesting non-hemodynamic-effect mechanisms on the left ventricular mass (Paoletti et al, 2008).

3.3 Arrhythmias

Atrial fibrilation is the most common cardiac rythm disorder in the general population and in patients on dialysis (Harnett et al 1995, Zebe 2001). Data from renal transplant recipients, despite being a high risk population due to the pre-transplant history and the high prevalence of risk factors related to this complication such as hypertension and obesity, have only been recently reported. Registry studies from the USA have shown a cumulative prevalence around 7 % at 3 years (Abbott et al, 2003a, Lentine et al, 2006). Risk factors for postransplantation atrial fibrilation include older age, male gender, renal failure for hypertension, and coronary artery disease. As in the general population atrial fibrilation was associated with an increased cardiovascular mortality, up to 3 times higher than patients without the disease (Abbott et al, 2003, Lentine et al, 2006).

4. Cardiovascular risk factors

Three types of cardiovascular risk factors are generally identified in transplant recipients (Table 2). 1) Traditional risk factors are those which in the general population are associated with cardiovascular diseases, and their treatment decreases the incidence of these complications. They include; older age, hypertension, hypercholesterolemia, diabetes mellitus, tobacco smoking and obesity. Their incidence is mostly increased in advanced CKD stages (Ansell et al, 2007, Karthikeyan et al, 2004, Marcén et al, 2005). 2) Risk factors associated with the transplant; anaemia, graft dysfunction and related complications, proteinuria, and immunosuppression. Finally,3), non-traditional or emergent factors such as hyperhomocysteinemia and chronic inflammation.

Traditional risk factors	Transplant related factors	Nontraditional or emergent factors
Age Sex Hypertension Dislipidemia Diabetes Smoking Obesity	Anaemia Graft dysfunction Proteinuria Immunosuppression	Hyperhomocysteinemia Inflammation

Table 2. Cardiovascular risk factors

4.1 Traditional risk factors

4.1.1 Age and sex

Older age is a nonmodifiable cardiovascular risk factor in the general population. In renal transplant recipients it was associated with an increased risk for cardiovascular atherosclerotic diseases; ischemic heart disease, cerebrovascular disease, and peripheral vascular disease (Kasiske et al, 1996, Kasiske et al, 2006, Marcén et al, 2006, Oliveras et al, 2003, Rigatto et al, 2002, Snyder et al, 2006), and also for functional heart diseases; congestive heart failure, left ventricular hypertrophy and arrhythmias (Abbott et al, 2003, Lentine et al 2006, Rigatto et al, 2000, Rigatto et al, 2002). Male gender is a risk factor for ischemic heart disease and peripheral vascular disease (Kasiske, 1988, Rigatto et al, 2002, Kasiske et al, 2006, Marcén et al, 2006, Snyder et al, 2006) and female gender for cerebrovascular disease and congestive heart failure (Abbott et al, 2003, Lentine et al, 2008a).

4.1.2 Hypertension

It is a common complication in renal transplant recipients. Its prevalence varies between 70 and 90%. There are several causes and mechanisms of high blood pressure and many patients have several of them. A previous history of hypertension, artery graft stenosis, the own recipient kidneys, overweight, chronic graft dysfunction and immunosuppressive agents such as calcineurin inhibitors (CNIs), cyclosporine and tacrolimus, are the conditions generally associated with post-transplant hypertension (Koomans & Ligtenberg, 2001, Zhang et al, 2003). Among CNIs, cyclosporine seems to increase blood pressure more than tacrolimus (Ligtenberg et al, 2001). It has been associated with an increased risk of ischemic heart disease, congestive heart failure, left ventricular hypertrophy (Rigatto 2002) and with mortality (Kasiske et al 2004, Fernández-Fresnedo et al, 2005).

One characteristic of post-transplant hypertension is the lack of control despite treatment. In a study of 1295 patients, only 12.4% had a normal blood pressure one year after grafting and more than 95% of them were on antihypertensive therapy (Kasiske et al, 2004). Others found in their series a higher number of patients with normal blood pressure without therapy (26.0%) but they also reported that 32.0% of patients had uncontrolled blood pressure while they were on treatment (Tutone et al, 2005). Cross-sectional studies have shown that between 60 to 100% of patients according to the stage of graft failure had a blood pressure above 130/80 mm Hg and most of them were on antihypertensive therapy (Karthikeyan et al, 2004, Marcén et al, 2009a).

There are not specific blood pressure levels for renal transplant recipients and the reference values are those of the general population. As the renal transplant recipients are considered a high risk population for cardiovascular diseases, a blood pressure of 130/80 mm Hg has been recommended. Treatment includes changing life style, reducing the diet sodium intake, physical activity, low consumption of alcohol and antihypertensive agents (Choubanian et al, 2003). There are no specific antihypertensive agents to treat post-transplant hypertension and all agents can be used. The prescription has to be done taking into account the characteristic of each patient (KDIGO, 2009, Park & Luan, 2005). Most patients need to be treated with several antihypertensive agents. Studies in which angiotensin converting enzyme inhibitors or angiotensin receptor blockers have been compared with other antihypertensive agents have shown controversial results, and there are no studies in which the superiority of one agent over the others on patient survival has been definitively established (Opelz et al, 2006, Hiremath et al, 2007). There are not randomized, prospective studies that have demonstrated the beneficial effects of controlling blood pressure in renal transplant recipients, but it has been assumed that they would be similar to those obtained in the general population. However, retrospective registry studies have shown that decreasing blood pressure even several years after hypertension appearance was associated with a better patient outcome (Opelz et al, 2005).

4.1.3 Dyslipidemia

Lipid disorders are more common in renal transplant recipients than in the general population and include high levels of cholesterol and triglycerides. Also frequent are high levels of LDL-cholesterol, lipoprotein (a) and apolipoprotein B, while HDL-cholesterol can be high, normal or low. Hypercholesterolemia, total serum cholesterol above 200 mg/dl and LDL-cholesterol above 100 mg/dl, have been observed in up to 90 % of patients (Aakhus et al, 1996, Hricik et al, 1994). Several factors have been associated with hyperlipidemia; genetic predisposition, body weight gain, graft dysfunction, proteinuria, diabetes, immunosuppressive and antihypertensive agents (Massy & Kasiske, 1996).

Among immunosuppressive agents, corticosteroids, CNIs and mammalian target of rapamycin inhibitors (mTORs), sirolimus and everolimus, are those most frequently associated with hyperlipidemia. The mechanisms of corticosteroid-induced hyperlipidemia are through promoting insulin resistence and hyperinsulinism, reduction of lipoprotein lipase activity, overproduction of triglycerides and secretion of VDLD-cholesterol (Hricik et al, 1994). CNIs inhibit bile acid synthesis and binding of the drugs to the LDL-cholesterol receptor with reduction of its activity. Also a decrease in lipoprotein lipase activity and impairment of LDL-cholesterol catabolism may be involved (Moore et al, 2001). These effects seem to be more prominent with cyclosporine than with tacrolimus (Ligtenberg et al, 2001, Moore et al, 2001, Vincenti et al, 2002). mTORs are the agents with stronger hyperlipidemic effect (Kasiske et al, 2008), which is more accentuated in those patients also treated with cyclosporine than in those treated with tacrolimus (Ciancio et al, 2004). The pathogenesis of mTOR dyslipidemia is unclear. A reduced catabolism of apo B100 could be the cause of increased triglycerides and cholesterol and decreased lipoprotein lipase activity and increased free fatty acid levels may be contributing factors. Their effects are dose dependent and rapidly reversible (Kasiske et al, 2008, Webster et al, 2006).

As in the general population, hypercholesterolemia and low HDL-cholesterol levels are associated with ischemic heart disease (Kasiske, 1988 Kasiske et al, 1996, Kasiske et al, 2006, Marcén et al, 2006, Rigatto et al, 2002). The treatment of this complication may follow the recommendations given to the general population and confirmed by the transplant guidelines (KDIGO, 2009). It is important to begin with a rich diet of monosaturated fats, but diet therapy does not control hyperlipidemia and lipid-lowering agents have to be added. 3-Hydroxy-3methylglutaryl coenzyme A reductase inhibitors (statins) are the elective pharmacologic agents in hypercholesterolemic patients. Fluvastatin, pravastatin and atorvastatin seem to have a more favourable safety profile over simvastatin and lovastatin. In patients with hypertriglyceridemia, gemfibrocil is the pharmacological agent of choice. Some observational studies have shown an association between statin therapy and better patient outcome (Cosio et al, 2002a, Wiesbauer et al, 2008). However, the Assessment of Lescol in Renal Transplantation (ALERT) study did not show differences in the primary compound end point, despite a reduction of 32% in the LDL-cholesterol blood levels at 5 years follow-up, between recipients treated with fluvastatin compared with those on placebo (Holdaas et al, 2003). A later evaluation of the study showed the benefits of the treatment but only when statin therapy started in the first two years after transplantation and in low-risk recipients (Holdaas et al 2005, Jardine et al 2004). In case of statin intolerance or hyperlipidemia of difficult control, ezetimibe that blocks the cholesterol absorption in the brush border, alone or combined with statins, is an efficient and safe alternative (Buchanan et al 2006, Langone & Chuang, 2006).

4.1.4 Diabetes

In the renal transplant recipients, two types of diabetes mellitus can be distinguished, diabetes mellitus as the cause of end-stage renal disease and new onset diabetes mellitus (NODAT). The prevalence of diabetes mellitus as the cause of renal failure is variable among countries. In the USA, more than 20% of the patients on the waiting list or transplanted have diabetes mellitus as the cause of renal failure (Collins et al, 2008). The incidence of NODAT varies between 2% to 50% in the first posttransplantation year according to the criteria used in its definition (Montori et al, 2002). When the American Diabetes Association criteria were used, the incidence of NODAT at 12 months was 13% and of glucose intolerance of 33% in a study performed at the Mayo Clinic (Cosio et al, 2005). Similar findings have been observed in a prospective study from Spain (Marcén et al, 2006). As the term NODAT does not include states of impaired fasting glucose and impaired glucose tolerance which pose a cardiovascular threat similar to overt diabetes, the term transplant associated hyperglycemia (TAH) has been proposed (Crutchlow & Bloom, 2008). The most common risk factors associated with NODAT or TAH include: race, blacks or hispanics, older age, obesity, family history, hepatitis C virus infection and some immunosuppressive agents such as corticosteroids, CNIs (tacrolimus) and mTORs (Crutchlow & Bloom, 2007, Montori et al, 2002).
The effects of immunosuppresive agents on glucose metabolism have been widely reviewed (Heisel et al, 2004, Miller, 2002, Morales & Dominguez, 2006). Both CNIs, cyclosporine and tacrolimus, cause NODAT by inducing insulin resistance or by impaired insulin secretion (Hornum et al, 2010). Early trials designed to compare the efficacy and security of cyclosporine and tacrolimus, and registry data showed a higher incidence of NODAT in patients treated with tacrolimus (Kasiske et al, 2003, Mayer et al, 1997, Vincenti et al, 2002) and more recent studies have confirmed these findings (Vincenti et al 2007). Also mTORs are associated with an increased risk of NODAT (Johnston et al, 2008). These agents induce hyperglucemia by impairing insulin-mediated suppression of hepatic glucose production, by ectopic triglyceride deposition leading to insulin resistance, or by direct β cell toxicity (Crutchlow & Bloom, 2007).
Single centre and registry studies have shown the association of NODAT with acute myocardial infarction, cerebrovascular events and mortality (Cosio et al 2002b, 2005, 2008, Kasiske et al 2003, Lentine et al, 2005, 2008). The treatment has the objective of preventing the symtoms due to uncontrolled hyperglucemia and the microvascular complications as the transplant recipients develop identical complications as the nontransplanted diabetic patients (Burroughs et al, 2007). The guidelines of the American Diabetes Association and the Joint Nacional Committee on Prevention, Detection, Evaluation, and Treatment of High Blood Pressure for patients with type 2 diabetes have been recommended (Haffner SM 2003).

4.1.5 Tobacco

The effects of tobacco on the health in the general population are well known. It is a risk factor of cardiovacular diseases, malignancies and respiratory diseases (Bartecchi et al, 1994). About 25% of the renal transplant population are active smokers after transplantation (Cosio et al 1999, Kasiske & Klinger, 2000, Zitt et al, 2007). In transplant recipients, tobacco was associated with cardiovascular diseases and mortality (Kasiske & Klinger, 2000). It has been reported that the negative impact of tobacco on health disappeared after five years, and some authors emphasize that efforts have to be made to convince the patients about the benefits of avoiding smoking. There are few data about the influence of transplant on toxic habits, but some studies suggest that transplantation constituted a strong reason to give up smoking (Banas et al, 2008).

4.1.6 Obesity

Obesity is a growing health problem in the general population. Epidemiological studies have shown its association with a higher morbidity and mortality due to cardiovascular diseases (Allison et al, 1999). Transplant recipients have a tendency to gain body weight mostly in the first year after grafting. In a study performed in our Unit, the mean body weight gain in the first year was 5 kg or 8.7 % of the body weight at the time of transplantation and the percentage of obese patients increased nearly two fold, from 6.5% to 11.7% (Marcén et al, 2007). Inappropriate dietary habits, decreased physical activity, and increased appetite as a result of well-being and corticosteroid therapy are among the causes of owerweight and obesity after transplantation.

Both body weight gain and obesity (body mass index >30 kg/m2) are associated with an increased risk for NODAT, hypertension, hyperlipidemia and metabolic syndrome which are cardiovascular risk factors (Armstrong et al, 2005, El-Agroudy et al 2004). The effects of weight gain and obesity on graft and patient outcome are controversial. Some authors do not find that the complication has any impact on patient mortality (Chang et al 2007, Marcén at al, 2007, Massarweh et al, 2005). However, other studies and registry data have shown their negative impact on patient survival due to an increased cardiovascular and infectious mortality (Aalten et al, 2006, El-Agroudy et al 2004, Meier-Kriesche et al, 2002). In our opinion, controlling weight gain and weight reduction in patients with marked obesity seems to be a goal to improve well-being and outcomes in renal transplant recipients.

4.2 Risk factors associated with transplantation

4.2.1 Anaemia

Post-transplant anaemia is a common complication that has only been recently studied and considered. Its prevalence depends greatly on the definition criteria and the time post-transplant. Nowadays, there is a trend toward the use of the World Health Organization criteria which define anaemia as serum haemoglobin less than 12 g/dl in women and less than 13 g/dl in men. The prevalence of anaemia is about 90% during the first posttransplant weeks and decreases to 25% to 35% at 12 months and remains stable or slightly increases thereafter (Kamar et al, 2008, Vanrenterghem et al, 2003, Yorgin et al, 2002). In cross-sectional studies the prevalence of anaemia reached more than one third of patients and it was severe, serum haemoglobin below 11 g/dl, in about 10% (Karthikeyan et al, 2004, Marcen et al, 2009a, Molnar et al, 2007, Vanrenterghem et al, 2003). The origen of anaemia is multifactorial and graft function is the most important factor (Shah et al, 2006, Vanrenterghem et al, 2003, Yorgin et al, 2002). However, it does not completely explain post-transplant anaemia, as renal transplant recipients have more severe anaemia for each chronic renal disease stage when compared with nontransplantation subjects (Chadban et al, 2007). Several immunosuppressive agents such as azathioprine, mycophenolate mofetil (MMF), enteric coated mycophenolic acid (EC-MPA) and mTORs may cause anemia due to bone marrow toxicity or to disorders on iron homeostasis (Augustine et al, 2004, Fishbane et al, 2009, Vanrenterghem et al, 2003, Wang et al, 2004). The combination of MMF or EC-MPA with mTORs is specially toxic for the bone marrow (Hricik, 2003, Rigatto, 2006). Other

medications as angiotensin converting enzyme inhibitors and angiotensin receptor blockers are known to cause anaemia and should be cautiously used.
Recent studies have shown an association between anaemia and graft survival, cardiovascular diseases and mortality. Post-transplant anaemia seems to be a risk factor of congestive heart failure and of left ventricular hypertrophy but not of ischaemic heart disease (Borrow et al, 2008, Rigatto et al, 2002, 2003b). In addition, anaemia has been associated with increased mortality in some studies (Chhabra et al, 2008, Imoagene-Oyedeji et al, 2006, Kamar et al, 2008, Molnar et al, 2007) but not in others (Winkelmayer et al, 2006). The treatment of anaemia must follow the recommendations given for patients with chronic kidney disease in the Kidney Disease Outcomes Quality Initiative (KDOQI) guidelines (KDIGO, 2009). Iron supplementation and erythropoiesis stimulant agents should be administered to maintain serum haemoglobin between 11 and 12 g/dl.

4.2.2 Graft dysfunction

Renal function measured by the estimated glomerular filtration rate (eGFR) is a cardiovascular risk factor in the general population (Go et al, 2004). An important number of renal transplant recipients have different stages of renal failure (Figure 2), and at least two thirds have chronic renal failure defined by an eGFR below 60 ml/min/1.73m2 (Ansell et al, 2007, Karthikeyan et al, 2004, Marcén et al, 2005). As cardiovascular diseases are the leading cause of renal transplant recipient mortality, it seems logical to think in the existence of some links between premature cardiovascular death and poor graft function. Registry and prospective studies have demonstrated a correlation betwen serum creatinine and cardiovascular events or cardiovascular mortality (Fellstrom et al, 2005, Meier-Kriescheet al, 2003, Pilmore et al, 2010, Soveri et al, 2006). However, for other authors the increased cardiovascular risk of patients with poor graft function is mostly due to the effects of hypertension and anaemia than to graft failure itself (Rigatto et al, 2002). Moreover, uncontrolled hyperparathyroidism mostly in recipients with poor graft function may be a risk factor for progression of coronary artery calcification (Mazzaferro et al, 2009). The treatment of renal dysfunction includes the control of hypertension and dyslipidemias (Arias et al, 2005, Opelz et a, 2005, Wiesbauer et al, 2008) as well as the use of non-nephrotoxic immunosuppressive agents as MMF, EC-MPA and belatacept and dose reduction or withdrawal of CNIs.
The prevalence of proteinuria in the renal transplant recipients is between 7.5 and 45% (Knoll, 2009). It is a risk factor of progressive renal function loss and of cardiovascular disease in nontransplantation patients. Retrospective studies have reported that proteinuria is an important predictor of cardiovascular events and mortality in renal transplant recipients (Fernandez-Fresnedo et al, 2002, Roodnat 2001). It is important to note that proteinuria is frequently associated with graft dysfunction, hypertension and obesity and the effects of proteinuria on cardiovascular events could be mediated by these conditions or viceversa. Treatment of proteinuria includes control of hypertension, maintaning blood pressure levels below 120/80 mm Hg, of dyslipidemias and of overweigth, and avoiding immunosuppressive agents associated with proteinuria as mTORs (Amer & Cosio, 2009). Angiotensin converting enzime inhibitors and angiotensin receptor blockers are the elective agents of treatment of hypertension in patients with proteinuria because of their antiproteinuric effects. However, these agents can deteriorate graft function and increase the severity of anaemia, both cardiovascular risk factors as well. Moreover, there are no definitive studies which support the effectiveness of this treatment.

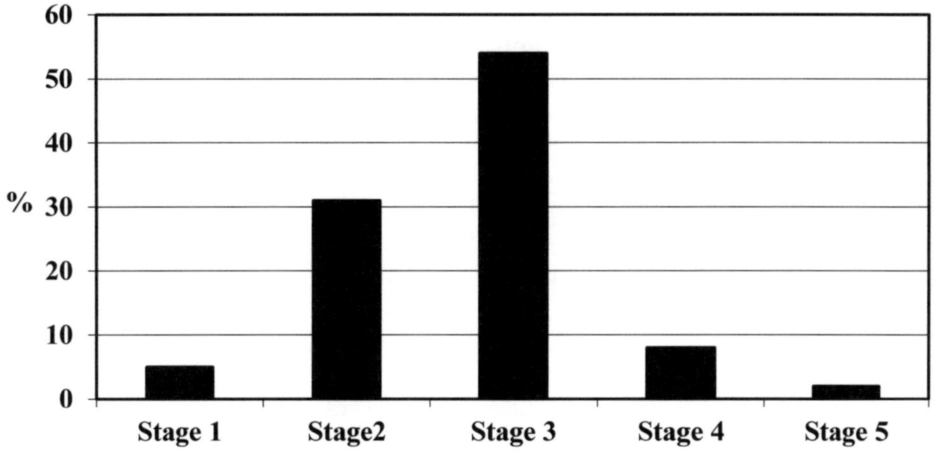

Fig. 2. Distribution of chronic kidney disease stages at 12 months in 447 renal transplant recipients (Ramón y Cajal Hospital)

4.2.3 Immunosuppression

The effects of immunosuppressive agents in cardiovascular risk factors have been previously reviewed (Miller, 2002, Marcén, 2009b, Morales & Dominguez-Gil, 2006). In addition, the impact of these agents on each cardiovascular risk factor has already been described. Corticosteroids and CNIs are the agents with worst cardiovascular risk profile, increasing the incidence and severity of traditional risk factors such as hypertension, hyperlipidemia, diabetes and obesity. CNIs also are nephrotoxic and cause graft function impairment. mTORs increase the risk of anaemia, hyperlipidemia, diabetes and proteinuria (Webster et al, 2006, Schena et al, 2009). MMF and EC-MPA may increase the risk of anaemia but have no impact in the other cardiovascular risk factors. Combinations of CNIs with MMF and EC-MPA or with mTOR allow corticosteroid withdrawal without harm. On the other hand, MMF and EC-MPA and mTORs alone or in combination can be used for CNI dose reduction or withdrawal. All these strategies have been shown to be effective in improving cardiovascular risk but there are no prospective studies in which this improvement is followed by a lower incidence of cardiovascular events or mortality (Schena et al, 2009). Among the new immunosuppressive agents, belatacept improved short-term cardiovascular risk profile and graft function when compared with cyclosporine (Vincenti et al, 2010, Durrbach et al 2010). However, phase II trials with tasocitinib have shown no improvement in hyperlipidemia and blood pressure when compared with patients who received tacrolimus (Busque et al, 2009).

4.3 Emergent risk factors

4.3.1 Hyperhomocysteinemia

Homocystein is a sulfur amino acid produced in all cells, and hyperhomocysteinemia has been considered a cardiovascular risk factor in the general population. Hyperhomocysteinemia is present in around 60% to 70% of renal transplant recipients. Homocystein levels are related with graft function, folic acid levels, serum albumin, age, and treatment with CNIs (Bostom et al, 1999, Ducloux et al, 2000, Friedman et al, 2002). The impact of homocystein levels on cardiovascular events is controversial. Some authors found an association between the homocystein levels and cardiovascular diseases (Ducloux et al, 2000, 2004) and a prospective study has shown that homocystein levels above 12 µmol/l were associated with 2.44 times increased mortality (Winkelmayer et al, 2005). Other authors have not found this association (Hagen et al, 2001). The treatment consists in the administration of folic acid supplements (5 mg/day) even with normal folic acid levels (Fernandez-Miranda et al, 2000). The efficacy of this therapy in the prevention of cardiovascular events has been examined in the Folic Acid for Vascular Outcome Reduction in Transplantation (FAVORIT). This trial should contribute to answer this question (Bostom et al, 2009).

4.3.2 Inflammation

C-reactive protein (CRP) is an acute phase marker of inflammation. It is produced by the liver under control of several citokines. In the general population, C-reactive protein is associated with obesity and poor renal function (Stuveling et al, 2003). It is also a negative predictor of acute myocardial infarction, cerebrovascular disease and cardiovascular mortality (Ridker et al, 1997). In renal transplant recipients, its levels are associated with graft function, waist circumference and smoking (Van Ree et al, 2005). The association between graft function and C-reactive protein levels could be explained by the situation of chronic low-grade inflammation, by being a marker of graft-mediated immune response or by a decreased renal excretion. As in the general population, it has been considered a risk factor of cardiovascular disease and mortality (Ducloux et al 2004, Winkelmayer et al 2004). Data from the ALERT study have confirmed the previous findings, baseline levels of CRP as well as of IL-6, another inflammation marker, were independently associated with major cardiovascular events and all-cause mortality (Abedini et al, 2009b). Results from a retrospective study have shown an association between MMF therapy and less inflammation than other immunosuppressive agents (Wong et al, 2007).

5. Therapeutical strategies

The management of each particular cardiovascular disease in renal transplant recipients should be similar to that used in the general population. In addition, clinical trials have demonstrated that cardiovascular events and cardiovascular mortality have been reduced by controlling blood glucose, lipid levels and blood pressure in the general population. As interventional studies are lacking in the transplant population, it seems reasonable to extrapolate these findings to transplant recipients. However, transplant recipients present differences from the general population, one of them is the high incidence of graft dysfunction. Preserving graft function has to be a goal in the management of transplant recipients and this could be partly accomplished by controlling the traditional cardiovascular risk factors and by a prudent use of immunosuppressive agents. CNIs minimization or withdrawal may be individually considered. Additional interventions such as treatment of anaemia with erytropoyesis stimulating agents could help in the prevention of cardiovascular diseases but the optimal haemoglobin threshold has to be determined. The benefits of lowering homocysteine levels have not been proved. In addition, long-term interventional studies should be performed in order to improve graft and patient outcomes (Table 3).

Control of cardiovascular risk factors	Preserving graft function	Treating emergent factors
Blood pressure Dislipidemias Diabetes Smoking Obesity Anaemia	Minimization/avoidance of CNIs Control of proteinuria	Folic acid supplements Aspirin

Table 3. Prevention and treatment of cardiovascular diseases after transplantation.

6. Summary

Cardiovascular diseases are common after transplantation. Coronary vascular disease, cerebrovascular disease and congestive heart failure are the diseases most commonly associated with mortality. The increased incidence of cardiovascular events could be partly explained by the high prevalence of traditional risk factors which are not adequately controlled and by the presence of renal dysfunction. Pretransplant evaluation of candidates, control of traditional risk factors and preservation of graft function should be the measures taken to improve patient outcome. The control of traditional risk factors has been effective in the reduction of cardiovascular events in the general population and there are no reasons to believe that it does not work in the transplant population. In addition, adequate control of traditional risk factors could preserve progression of graft failure. A prudent use of immunosuppressive agents could also help to improve the cardiovascular risk profile and graft function. The benefits of additional interventions need to be proved.

7. References

Aakhus, S., Dahl, K. & Widerøe, TE. (1863). Hyperlipidaemia in renal transplant patients. *J Intern Med*. Vol.239, No.5, (May 1996), pp.407-415. ISSN: 0954-6820.

Aakhus, S., Dahl, K. & Wideroe, TE. (1986). Cardiovascular morbidity and risk factors in renal transplant patients. *Nephrol Dial Transplant*. Vol. 14, No.3, (March 1999) pp.648-654. ISSN: 0931-0509.

Aakhus, S., Dahl, K. & Wideroe, TE. (1987). Cardiovascular disease in stable renal transplant patients in Norway: morbidity and mortality during a 5-yr follow-up. *Clin Transplant*. Vol. 18, No.5, (October 2004), pp.596-604. ISSN: 0902-0063.

Aalten, J., Christiaans, MA., de Fijter, H., Hené, R., van der Heijde, JH., Roodnat. J., Surachno, J. & Hoitsma, A. (1988). The influence of obesity on short- and long-term graft and patient survival after renal transplantation. *Transplant Int*. Vol.19, No.11 (November 2006), PP. 901-907. ISSN.0934-0874.

Abbott, KC., Reynols, JC., Taylor, AJ. & Agodoa, LY. (2001). Hospitalized atrial fibrillation after renal transplantation in the United States. *Am J Transplant* . Vol. 3, No.4, (June 2003a), pp.471-476. ISSN: 1600-6135.

Abbott, KC., Yuan, CM., Taylor, AJ., Cruess, DF. & Agodoa, LY. (1990). Early renal insufficiency and hospitalized heart disease after renal transplantation in the era of modern immunosuppression. *J Am Soc Nephrol* Vol.14, No.9, (November 2003b), pp.2358-2365, ISSN: 1046-6673.

Abedini, S., Holme, I., Fellstrom, B., Jardine, A., Cole, E., Maes, B. & Holdaas, H. on behalf of the ALERT study group. (1963). Cerebrovascular events in renal transplant recipients. *Transplantation*. Vol.87, No.1, (January 2009a), pp.112-7. ISSN: 0041-1337.

Abedini, S., Holme, I., März, W., Weihrauch, G., Fellstróm, B., Jardine, A., Cole, E., Maes, B., Neumayer, H-H., Gronhagen-Riska, C., Ambühl, P. & Holdaas, H on behalf of the ALERT study group. (2006). Inflammation in renal transplantation. *Clin J Am Soc Nephrol* Vol.4, No.7, (July 2009b), pp. 1246-1254. ISSN: 1555-9041.

Allison, DB., Fontaine, KR., Manson, JE., Stevens, J. & Vantallie, TB. (1883). Annual deaths attibutable to obesity in the United States. *JAMA* Vol.282, No.16, (October 1999), pp.1530-1538, ISSN. 0098-7484.

Amer, H. & Cosio, FG. (1990). Significance and management of proteinuria in kidney transplant recipients. *J Am Soc Nephrol.* Vol.20, No.12, (December 2009), pp. 2490-2492, ISSN: 1046-6673.

Ansell, D., Udayarej, UP., Steenkamp, R. & Dudley, CRK. (2001). Chronic renal failure in kidney transplant recipients. Do they receive optimum care?: data from the UK renal registry. *Am J Transplant* Vol.7, No.5, (May 2007), pp.1167-1176. ISSN:1600-6135.

Arias, M., Fernández-Fresnedo, G., Rodrigo, E., Ruiz, JC., González-Cotorruelo, J. & Gómez-Alamillo, C. (1972). Non-Immunologic intervention in chronic allograft nephropathy. *Kidney Int* Vol.99 (December 2005), pp.S118-S123, ISSN: 0085-2538.

Armstrong, KA., Campbell, SB., Hawley, CM., Nicol. DL., Johnson, DW. & Isbel, NM. (2001). Obesity is associated with worsening cardiovascular risk factor profiles and proteinuria progression in renal transplant recipients *Am J Transplant* . Vol.5, No.11, (November 2005), pp.2710-2718, ISSN.1600-6135.

Augustine, JJ., Knauss, TC., Schulak, JA., Bodziak, KA., Siegel, C. & Hricik, DE. (2001). Comparative effects of sirolimus and mycophenolate mofetil on erythropoiesis in kidney transplant patients. *Am J Transplant.* Vol.4, No.12, (December 2004), pp.2001-2006, ISSN.1600-6135.

Aull-Watschinger, S., Konstantin, H., Demetriou, D., Schillinger, M., Habicht, A., Hörl, WH. & Watschinger, B. (1986). Pre-transplant predictors of cerebrovascular events after kidney transplantation. *Nephrol Dial Transplant* Vol. 23, No. 4 (April 2008), pp. 1429-1435, ISSN: 0931-0509.

Banas, MC., Banas, B., Wolf, J., Hoffman, U., Krüger, B., Böger, CA., Orth, SR. & Krämer, BK. (1986). Smoking behaviour of patients before and after renal transplantation. *Nephrol Dial Transplant* Vol.23, No.4, (April 2008), pp.1442-1446, ISSN.0931-0509.

Bartecchi, CE., MacKenzie, TD. & Schrier, RW. (1812). The human cost of tobacco use (first of two parts). *New Engl J Med.* Vol.330, No.13 (March 1994), pp.907-912, ISSN. 0028-4793.

Borrows, R., Loucaidou, M., Chusney, G., Borrows, S., Tromp, JV., Cairns, T., Griffith, M., Hakim, N., McLean, A., Palmer, A., Papalois, V. & Taube, D. (1986). Anaemia and congestive heart failure early post-renal transplantation. *Nephrol Dial Transplant.* Vol.23, No.5, (May 2008), pp.3:1728-1734, ISSN.0931-0509.

Bostom, AG., Gohh, RY., Beaulieu, AJ., Han, H., Jacques, PF., Selhub, J., Dworkin, L. & Rosenberg, IH. (1963). Determinants of fasting plasma total homocysteine levels among chronic stable renal transplant recipients. *Transplantation.* Vol.68, No.2, (July 1999), pp.257-261, ISSN: 0041-1337.

Bostom, AG., Carpenter, MA., Hunsicker, L., Jacques, PF., Kusek, JW., Levey, AS., McKenney, JL., Mercier, RY., Pfeffer, MA. & Selhub, J. (1981). Baseline characteristics of participants in the folic acid for vascular outcome reduction in transplantation (FAVORIT) trial. *Am J Kidney Dis.* Vol.53, No.1, (January 2009), pp.121-128, ISSN: 0272-6386.

Buchanan, C., Smith, L, Corbett, J., Nelson, E. & Shihab F. (2001). A retrospective analysid of ezetimibe treatment in renal transplant recipients. *Am J Trasplant* Vol.6, No.4, (April 2006), pp.770-774, ISSN: 1600-6135.

Burroughs, TE., Swindle, J., Takemoto, S., Lentine, KL., Machnicki, G., Irish, WD., Brennan, DC. & Schnitzler, MA. (1963). Diabetic complications associated with new-onset diabetes mellitus in renal transplant recipients. *Transplantation* Vol.83, No.8 (April 2007), pp.1027-1034, ISSN. 0041-1337.

Busque, S., Leventhal, J., Brennan, DC., Steinberg, S., Klintmalm, G., Shah, T., Mulgaonkar, S., Bromberg, JS., Vincenti, F., Harharan, S., Slakey, D., Peddi, VR., Fisher, RA., Lawendy, N., Wang, C. & Chan, G. (2001). Calcineurin-inhibitor-free immunosuppression based on the JAK inhibitor CP-690,550: a pilot study in the novo kidney allograft recipients. *Am J Transplant.* Vol.9, No.8 (August 2009), pp.1936-1945, ISSN: 1600-6135.

Chadban, SJ., Baines, L., Polkingghome, K., Jefferys, A., Dogra, S., Kanganas, C., Irish, A., Eris, J. & Walker, R. (1981). Anemia after kidney transplantation is not completely explained by reduced kidney function. *Am J Kidney Dis.* Vol.49, No.2, (February 2007), pp.301-309, ISSN.0272-6386.

Chhabra, D., Grafals, M., Skaro, AI., Parker, M. & Gallon, L. (2006). Impact of anemia after renal transplantation on patient and graft survival and on rate of acute rejection. *Clin J Am Soc Nephrol.* Vol.3, No.4, (July 2008), pp.1168-1174, ISSN.1555- 9041.

Chang, SH., Coates, PT. & McDonald, SP. (1963). Effects of body mass index at transplant on outcomes of kidney transplantation. *Transplantation.* Vol.84, No.8, (October 2007), pp.981-987, ISSN. 0041-1337.

Chobanian, AV., Bakris, GL., Black, HR., Cushman, WC., Green, LA., Izzo, JL. Jones, DW., Materson, BJ., Oparil, S., Wright, JT. & Roccella, EJ. (1883). Seventh report of the joint national comittee on prevention, detection, evaluation, and treatment of high blood pressure. The JNC 7 report. *JAMA.* Vol. 289, No.19, (December 2003), pp.2560-2572, ISSN: 0098-7484.

Ciancio, G., Burke, GW., Gaynor, JJ., Mattiazzi, A., Roth, D., Kupin, W., Nicolas, M., Ruiz, P., Rosen, A. & Miller, J. (1963). A randomized long-term trial of tacrolimus/sirolimus versus tacrolimus/mycophenolate mofetil, versus cyclosporine (NEORAL)/ sirolimus in renal transplantation II. Survival, function, and protocol compliance at 1 year. *Transplantation* Vol.77, No.2, (January 2004), pp.252-258, ISSN: 0041-1337.

Collins AJ. (1972). Impact of congestive heart failure and other cardiac diseases on patients outcomes. *Kidney Int.* Suppl 81 (October 2002), pp.S3-7, ISSN: 0085-2538.

Collins, AJ., Foley, RN., Herzog, C., Chavers, BM., Gilbertson, D., Ishani, A., Kasiske, BL., Liu, J., Mau, LW., McBean, M., Murray, A., St Peter, W., Guo, H., Li, Q., Li, S., Li, S., Peng, Y., Qiu, Y., Roberts, T., Skeans, M., Snyder, J., Solid, C., Wang, C., Weinhandl, E., Zaun, D., Arko, C., Chen, SC., Dalleska, F., Daniels, F., Dunning, S., Ebben, J., Frazier, E., Hanzlik, C., Johnson, R., Sheets, D., Wang, X., Forrest, B., Constantini, E., Everson, S., Eggers, PW. & Agodoa L. (2008). (1981). Excerpts from the United States Renal Data System 2007 annual data report. *Am J Kidney Dis.* Vol. 51, 1 Suppl 1, (January 2008), pp.S1-320, ISSN: 0272-6386.

Cosio, FG., Falkenhaim, MF., Pesavento, TE., Yim, S., Alamir, A., Henry, ML. & Ferguson, RM. (1987). Patient survival after renal transplantation.II. The impact of smoking . *Clin Transplant* Vol.13, No.4, (August 1999), pp.336-341. ISSN. 0902-0063.

Cosio, FG., Pesavento, TE., Pelletier, RP., Henry, M., Ferguson, RM., Kim, S. & Lemeshow, S. (1981). Patient survival after renal transplantation III: the effects of statins, *Am J Kidney Dis* Vol.40, No.3, (September 2002a), pp.638-643. ISSN. 0272-6386.

Cosio, FG., Pesavento, TE., Kim, S., Osei, K., Henry, M. & Ferguson, RM. (1972). Patient survival after renal transplantation:IV. Impact of post-transplant diabetes. *Kidney Int*. Vol.62, No.4 (October 2002b), pp. 1440-1446. ISSN. 0085-2538.

Cosio, FG., Kudva, Y., van der Velde, M., Larson, TS., Textor, SC., Griffin, MD. & Stegall, MD. (1972) New onset hyperglycemia and diabetes are associated with increased cardiovascular risk after kidney transplantation. *Kidney Int* . Vol.67, No.6, (June 2005), pp. 2415-2421. ISSN: 0085-2538.

Cosio, FG., Hickson, LJ., Griffin, MD., Stegall, MD. & Kudva, Y. (2001). Patient survival and cardiovascular risk after kidney transplantation: the challenge of diabetes. *Am J Transplant* Vol.8, No.3, (March 2008), pp.593-599, ISSN. 1600-6135.

Crutchlow MF & Bloom RD. (2006). Transplant-associated hyperglycemia:a new look at an old problem. *Clin J Am Soc Nephrol* Vol.2, No.2, (March 2007), pp.343-355, ISSN: 1555-9041

Culleton, BF. & Wilson, PWF. (1990). Cardiovascular disease: risk factors, secular trends, and therapeutic guidelines. *J Am Soc Nephrol.* Vol.9, 12 suppl, (December 1998), pp:S5-S15, ISSN: 1046-6673.

De Mattos, AM., Prather, J., Olyaei, AJ., Shibagaki, Y., Keith, DS., Mori, M., Norman, DJ. et Becker, T. (1972). Cardiovascular events following renal transplantation: role of traditional and transplant-specific risk factors. *Kidney Int.* Vol. 70, No. 4, (August 2006), pp.757-764, ISSN: 0085-2538.

Ducloux, D., Motte, G., Challier, B., Gibey, R. & Chalopin, JM. (1990). Serum total homocysteine and cardiovascular ocurrence in chronic stable renal transplant recipients: a prospective study. *J Am Soc Nephrol.* Vol.11, No.1, (January 2000), pp.134- 137, ISSN: 1046-6673.

Ducloux, D., Kazory, A. & Chalopin, JM. (1972). Predicting coronary heart disease in renal transplant recipients: a prospective study. *Kidney Int* . Vol. 66, No.1, (July 2004), pp.441-447, ISSN: 0085-2538.

Durrbach, A., Pestana, JM., Pearson, T., Vincenti, F., García, CD., Campistol, J., Rial, MdeC., Florman, S., Block, A., Di Russo, G., Xing, J., Garg, P. & Grinyo, J. (2001). A phase III study of belatacept versus cyclosporine in kidney transplants from extended criteria donors (BENEFIT-EXT study). *Am J Transplant*. Vol.10, No.3, (March 2010), pp.547-557, ISSN: 1600- 6135.

El-Agroudy, AE., Wafa, EW., Greith, OE., El-Dein, ABS. & Ghoneim, MA. (1963). Weight gain after renal transplantation is a risk factor for patient and graft outcome. *Transplantation*. Vol15, No.77, (May 2004), pp.1381-1385. ISSN.0041-1337.

Fellström, B., Jardine, AG., Soveri, I., Cole, E., Neumayer, HH., Maes, B., Gimpelewicz, C. & Holdaas, H. (1963). Renal dysfunction as a risk factor for mortality and cardiovascular disease in renal transplantation: experience from the Assessment of Lescol in Renal Transplant trial. *Transplantation* Vol.79; No.7, (August 2005), pp. 1160-1163, ISSN: 0041-1337.

Fernández-Fresnedo, G., Escallada, R., Rodrigo, E., De Francisco, AL., Cotorruelo, JG., Sanz De Castro, S., Zubimendi, JA., Ruiz, JC. & Arias, M. (1963). The risk of cardiovascular disease associated with proteinuria in renal transplant patients. *Transplantation*. Vol.76, No.8, (April 2002), pp.1345-1348, ISSN: 0041-1337.

Fernández-Fresnedo, G., Escallada, R., Martin de Francisco, AL., Ruiz, JC., Rodrigo, E., Sanz de Castro, S., GonzalezCotorruelo, .J & Arias, M. (2001). Association between pulse pressure and cardiovascular disease in renal transplant patients. Am J Transplant Vol.5, No.2, (February, 2005), pp.394-398, ISSN: 1600-6135.

Fernandez-Miranda, C., Gómez, P., Díaz-Rubio, P., Estenoz, J., Carillo, JL., Andrés, A. & Morales, JM. (1987). Plasma homocysteine levels in renal transplanted patients on cyclosporine or tacrolimus therapy: effect of treatment with folic acid. *Clin Transplant*. Vol.14, No.2, (April 2000), pp.110-114, ISSN: 0902-0063.

Fishbane, S., Cohen, DJ., Coyne, DW., Djamali, A., Singh, AK. & Wish, JB. (1972). Posttransplant anemia: the role of sirolimus. *Kidney Int* . Vol.76, No.4, (August 2009), pp.376-382, ISSN.0085-2538.

Foley, RN., Parfrey, PS., Harnett, JD., Kent, GM., Murray, DC. & Barré, PE. (1990). The prognostic importance of left ventricular geometry in uremic cardiomyopathy. *J Am Soc Nephrol*. Vol.5, No.12, (June 1995), pp. 2024-2031, ISSN: 1046-6673.

Foley, RN. Parfrey, PS. & Sarnak, MJ (1981). Clinical epidemiology of cardiovascular disease in chronic renal disease. *Am J Kidney Dis*. Vol.32, No.5, suppl.3, (November 1998), pp.S112-S119, ISSN: 0272-6386.

Friedman, AN., Rosenberg, IH., Selhub, J., Levey, AS. & Bostom, AG. (2001). Hyperhomocysteinemia in renal transplant recipients. *Am J Trasnsplant* . Vol.2, No.4, (April 2002), pp.308-313, ISSN: 1600-6135.

Go, AS., Chertow, GM., Fan, D., McCulloch, CE. & Hsu, C. (1812). Chronic kidney disease and the risks of death, cardiovascular events, and hospitalization. *N Engl J Med* Vol.351; No.13, (September 2004), pp.1296-1305, ISSN: 0028-4793.

Haffner, SM. (1978). Management of dyslipidemia in adults with diabetes. *Diabetes Care* Vol26, Suppl 1, (January 2003), pp.S83- S86. ISSN. 0149-5992.

Hagen, W., Födinger, M., Heinz, G., Buchmayer, H., Hörl, WH. & Sunder-Plassman, G. (1972). Effect of MTHFR genotypes and hyperhomocysteinemia on patient and graft survival in kidney transplant recipients. *Kidney Int* . Vol.78, (February 2001), pp.S253-S257, ISSN: 0085-2538.

Harnett, JD., Foley, RN., Kent, GM., Barre, PE., Murray, D. & Parfrey, PS. (1972). Congestive heart failure in dialysis patients: prevalence, incidence, prognosis and risk factors. *Kidney Int* . Vol.47, No.3, (March 1995), pp.884-890, ISSN: 0085-2538.

Heisel O, Heisel R, Balshaw R & Keown P. (2001). New onset diabetes mellitus in patients receiving calcineurin inhibitors: a systematic review and meta-analysis. *Am J Transplant* Vol.4, No.4, (April 2004), pp.583-595, ISSN: 1600-6135.

Herzog, CA., Ma, JZ & Collins AJ (1812). Poor long-term survival after acute myocardial infarction among patients on long-term dialysis. *N Enl J Med*. Vol. 339, No.12, (September 1998), pp. 799-805, ISSN: 0028-4793.

Herzog, CA., Ma, JZ. & Collins, AJ. (1981). Long term survival of renal transplant recipients in the United States after acute myocardial infarction. *Am J Kidney Dis*. Vol. 36, No. 1, (July 2000), pp.145-153, ISSN: 0272-6386.

Hiremath, S., Ferguson, D., Doucette, S., Mulay, AV. & Knoll, GA. (2001). Renin angiotensin system blockade in kidney transplantation: a systematic review of the evidence. *Am J Transplant*. Vol.7, No.10, (October 2007), pp. 2350-2360, ISSN: 1600-6135.

Holdaas, H., Fellström, B., Jardina, AG., Holme, I., Nyberg, G., Fauchald, P., Frönhagen-Riska, C., Madsen, S., Neumayer, H-H., Cole, E., Maes, B., Ambühl, P., Olsson,

AG., Haertmann, A., Solbu, DO. & Pedersen, TR. on behalf of the Assessment of Lescol in renal transplantation (ALERT) Study Investigators. (1823). Effect of fluvastatin on cardiac outcomes in renal transplant recipients: a multicentre, randomised, placebo-controlled trial. *Lancet* Vol.361, No.9374, (June 2003), pp:2024-2031, ISSN: 0140-6736.

Holdaas, H., Fellström, B., Jardine, AG. Nyberg, G., Grönhagen-Riska, C., Madsen, S., Neumayer, HH., Cole, E., Maes, B., Ambühl, P., Logan, JO., Staffler, B. & Gimpelewicz, C.(1986). Beneficial effect of early initiation of lipid-lowering therapy following renal transplantation. *Nephrol Dial Transplant* Vol.20, No.5, (May 2005), pp.974-980, ISSN: 0931-0509.

Hornum M, Jorgensen KA, Hansen JM, Nielsen FT, Christensen KB, Mathiesen ER &Feldt-Rasmussen B. (1990). New-onset diabetes mellitus after kidney transplantation in Denmark. *Clin J Am Soc Nephrol* Vol.5, No.4, (April, 2010), pp.709-716, ISSN. 1555-9041.

Howard, RJ., Patton, PR., Reed, AI., Hemming, AW., Van der Werf, WJ., Pfaff, WW., Srinivas, TR. & Scornik JC. (1963). The changing causes of graft loss and death after kidney transplantation. *Transplantation*. Vol. 73, No. 12, (April 2002), pp.1923-1928, ISSN: 0041-1337.

Hricik, DE. (1981). Posttransplant hyperlipidemia: the treatment dilemma. *Am J Kidney Dis*. Vol.23, No.5, (May 1994), pp.766-771, ISSN: 0272-6386.

Hricik, DE. (2001). Anemia after kidney transplantation-is the incidence increasing?. *Am J Transplant*. Vol.3, No.7, (July 2003), pp.771-772, ISSN.1600-6135.

Imoagene-Oyedeji, AE., Rosas, SE., Doyle, AM., Goral, S. & Bloom, RD. (1990). Posttransplantation anemia at 12 months in kidney recipients treated with mycophenolate mofetil: risk factors and implications for mortality. *J Am Soc Nephrol*. Vol.17, No.11, (November 2006), pp.3240-7, ISSN.1046-6673.

Jardine, AG., Holdaas, H., Fellström, B., Cole, E., Nyberg, G., Grönhagen-Riska, C., Madsen, S., Neumayer, HH., Maes, B., Ambühl, P., Olsson, AG., Holme, I., Fauchald, P., Gimpelwicz, C. & Pedersen, TR. (2001). Fluvastatin prevents cardiac death and myocardial infarction in renal transplant recipients: Pos-hoc subgroup analyses of the ALERT study. *Am J Transplant* Vol4, No.6 (June 2004), pp.988-995, ISSN: 1600-6135.

Johnston, O., Rose, CL., Webster, AC. & Gill, JS. (1990). Sirolimus is associated with new-onset diabetes in kidney transplant recipients. *J Am Soc Nephrol* Vol.19, No.7, (July 2008), pp.1411-1418, ISSN.1046-6673.

Kamar, N. & Rostaing, L. (1963). Negative impact of one-year anemia on long-term patient and graft survival in kidney transplant patients receiving calcineurin inhibitors and mycophenolate mofetil. *Transplantation*. Vol.85, No.8, (April 2008), pp.1120-1124, ISSN.0041-1337.

Karthikeyan, V., Karpinski, J., Nair, RC. & Knol,l G. (2001). The burden of chronic kidney disease in renal transplant recipients. *Am J Transplant*. Vol.4, No.2, (February 2004), pp.262-269. ISSN.1600-6135.

Kasiske, BL. (1946). Risk factors fos accelerated atheroesclerosis in renal transplant recipients. *Am J Med*. Vol. 84, No. 6, (January 1988), pp. 985-992, ISSN: 0002-9343.

Kasiske, BL., Guijarro, C., Massy, ZA., Wiederkehr, MR. & Ma, JZ. (1990). Cardiovascular disease after renal transplantation. *J Am Soc Nephrol*. Vol.7, No. 1, (January 1996), pp.158-165, ISSN: 1046-6673.

Kasiske, BL., Chakkera, HA & Roel J. (1990). Explained and unexplained ischemic heart disease risk after renal transplantation. *J Am Soc Nephrol*. Vol. 11 No. 11, (September 2000a) pp. 1735-1743. ISSN. 1046-6673.

Kasiske, BL. & Klinger, D. (1990). Cigarrette smoking in renal transplant recipients. *J Am Soc Nephrol* Vol.11, No.4, (April 2000b), pp. 753-759. ISSN. 1046-6673.

Kasiske, BL., Synder, JJ., Gilberston, D. & Matas, AJ. (2001). Diabetes mellitus after kidney transplantation in the United States. *Am J Transplant* Vol.3, No.2, (February 2003), pp.178-185, ISSN.1600-6135.

Kasiske, BL., Anjum, S., Shah, R., Skogen, J., Kandaswamy, C., Danielson, B., O'Shaughnessy, EA., Dahl, DC., Silkensen, JR., Sahadevan, M. & Snyder, JJ. (1981). Hypertension after kidney transplantation. *Am J Kidney Dis* Vol.43, No.6, (April 2004), pp. 1071-1081, ISSN: 0272-6386.

Kasiske, BL., Malik, MA. & Herzog, CA. (1963). Risk-stratified screening for ischemic heart disease in kidney transplant candidates. *Transplantation*. Vol. 80, No. 6, (September 2005), pp. 815-20. ISSN: 0041-1337.

Kasiske, BL., Maclean, JR. & Snyder JJ. (1990). Acute myocardial infarction and kidney transplantation. *J Am Soc Nephrol*. Vol. 17, No.3, (March 2006), pp. 900-907, ISSN: 1046-6673.

Kasiske, BL., de Mattos, A., Flechneer, SM., Gallon, L., Meier-Kriesche, H-U., Weir, MR. & Wilkinson, A. (2001). Mammalian target of rapamycin inhibitor dyslipidemia in kidney transplant recipients. *Am J Transplant* Vol.8, No7, (July 2008), pp. 1384-1392, ISSN: 1600-6135.

KDIGO clinical practice guideline for the care of kidney transplant recipients. (2001). *Am J Transplant*. Vol.9, Suppl 3 (November 2009), pp.S1-155. ISSN.1600-6135.

Kennedy, R., Case, C., Fathi, R., Johnson, D., Isbel, N. & Marwick, TH. (1946). Does renal failure cause an atherosclerotic milieu in patients with end-stage renal disease? *Am J Med*. Vol.110, No.3, (February 2001), pp.:198-204, ISSN: 0002-9343.

Knoll, GA. (1981). Proteinuria in kidney transplant recipients: prevalence, prognosis and evidence-based management. *Am J Kidney Dis*. Vol.54, No.6 (December 2009), pp.1131-1144, ISSN: 0272-6386.

Koomans, HE. & Ligtenberg, G. (1963). Mechanism and consequences of arterial hypertension after renal transplantation. *Transplantation* Vol.72, 6 Suppl, (September 2001), pp.S9-S12, ISSN: 0041-1337.

Langone, AJ. & Chuang, P. (1963). Ezetimibe in renal transplant patients with hyperlipidemia resistant to HMG-CoA reductase inhibitors. *Transplantation* Vol.81, No.5, (March 2006), pp.804-807, ISSN: 0041-1337.

Lentine, KL., Brennan, DC. & Schnitzler, MA. (1990). Incidence and predictors of myocardial infarction after kidney transplantation. *J Am Soc Nephrol*. Vol. 16, No. 2, (February 2005), pp.496-506. ISSN. 1046-6673.

Lentine, KL., Schnitzler, MA., Abbott, KC., Li. L., Burroughs, TE., Irish, W. & Brennan, DC. (1981). De novo congestive heart failure after kidney transplantation: a common condition with poor prognostic implications. *Am J Kidney Dis* Vol.46, No.4, (October 2005), pp.720-733, ISSN. 0272-6386.

Lentine, KL., Schnitzler, MA., Abbott, KC. Li, L., Xiao, H., Burroughs, TE., Takemoto, SK., Willoughby, LM., Gavard, JA. & Brennan, DC. (2006). Incidence, predictors, and associated outcomes of atrial fibrillation after kidney transplantation. *Clin J Am Soc Nephrol* Vol.1, No.2, (March 2006), pp.288-296, ISSN: 1555-9041.

Lentine, KL., Rocca Rey, LA., Kolli, S., Bacchi. G., Schnitzler, MA., Abbott, KC., Xiao, H. & Brennan, DC. (2006). Variations in the risk for cerebrovascular events after kidney transplant compared with experience on the waiting list and after graft failure. *Clin J Am Soc Nephrol* Vol. 3, No.4, (July 2008a), pp. 1090-1101. ISSN. 1555-9041.

Lentine, KL., Schnitzler, MA., Brennan, DC., Snyder, JJ., Hauptman, PJ., Abbott, KC., Axelrod, D., Salvalaggio, PR. & Kasiske, B. (2006). Cardiac evaluation before kidney transplantation: a practice patterns analysis in Medicare-insured dialysis patients. *Clin J Am Soc Nephrol.* Vol.3, No.4, (April 2008b), pp. 1115-24. ISSN. 1555-9041.

Levin, A., Singer, J., Thompson, CR., Ross, H. & Lewis, M. (1981). Prevalent left ventricular hypertrophy in the predialysis population : identifying opportunities for intervention. *Am J Kidney Dis* . Vol.27, No.3, (March 1996), pp. 347-354, ISSN: 0272-6386.

Ligtenberg, G., Hene, RJ., Blankestijn, PJ. & Koemans, HA (1990). Cardiovascular risk factors in renal transplant recipients: cyclosporin A versus tacrolimus. *J Am Soc Nephrol* Vol.12, No.2, (February 2001), pp.368-373, ISSN: 1046-6673..

Lindholm, A., Albrechtsen, D., Frodin, L., Tufveson, G., Persson, NH. & Lundgran, G. (1963). Ischemic heart disease-major cause of death and graft loss alter transplantation in Scandinavia. *Transplantation.* Vol. 60, No. 5, (September 1995), pp.451-457, ISSN: 0041-1337.

Marcén, R., Pascual, J., Teruel, JL. Villafruela. JJ., Rivera, ME., Mampaso, F., Burgos, FJ. & Ortuño, J. (1963). Outcome of cadaveric renal transplant patients treated for 10 years with cyclosporine. Is chronic allograft nephropathy the major cause of graft loss?. *Transplantation.* Vol.72, No.1, (July 2001), pp.57-62, ISSN: 0041-1337.

Marcén, R., Pascual, J., Tenorio, M., Ocaña, J., Teruel, JL., Villafruela, JJ., Fernández, M., Burgos & FJ., Ortuño, J. (1969). Chronic kidney disease in renal transplant recipients. *Transplant Proc.* Vol.37, No.9, (November 2005), pp.3718-3720, ISSN:0041- 1345.

Marcén, R., Morales, JM., del Castillo, D., Campistol, JM., Serón, D., Valdés, F., Anaya, F., Andrés, A., Arias, M., Bustamante, J., Capdevila, L., Escuin, F., Gil-Vernet, S., González-Molina, M., Lampreave, I., Oppenheimer, F., & Pallardó, L., for the Spanish Renal Forum. (1969). Posttransplant diabetes mellitus in renal allograft recipients: a prospective multicenter study at 2 years. *Transplant Proc* Vol.38, No.10, (December 2006), pp:3530-3532. ISSN: 0041-1345.

Marcén, R., Morales, JM., Arias, M., Fernández-Juarez, G., Fernández-Fresnedo, G., Ahdrés, A., Rodrigo, E., Pascual, J., Dominguez, B. & Ortuño, J. (1990). Ischemic heart disease after renal transplantation in patients on cyclosporine in Spain. *J Am Soc Nephrol.* Vol.17, 12 Suppl 3, (December 2006), pp.S286-S290, ISSN: 1046-6673.

Marcén, R., Fernández, A., Pascual, J., Teruel, JL., Villafruela, JJ., Rodríguez, N., Martins, J., Burgos, FJ. & Ortuño, J. (1969). High body mass index and posttransplant weigth gain are not risk factors for kidney graft and patient outcomes. *Transplant Proc* . Vol.39, No.7, (September 2007), pp.:2205-2207, ISSN. 0041-1345.

Marcén, R., del Castillo, D., Capdevila, L., Fernandez-Fresnedo, G., Rodrigo, E., Cantarell, C., Fernandez-Rodriguez, A., Lópes- Silva, MO., Camps, J., Aljama, P., Ortuño, J. & Arias, M. (1963). Achieving chronic kidney disease treatment targets in renal transplant recipients: results from a cross-sectional study in Spain. *Transplantation* Vol. 87, No.9, (May 2009a), pp. 1340-1346. ISSN.0041-1337.

Marcén, R. (1971). Immunosuppressive drugs in kidney transplantation. Impact on patient survival, and incidence of cardiovascular disease, malignancy and infection. *Drugs*. Vol.69, No.16, (November 2009b), pp. 2227-2243. ISSN.0012- 6667.

Massarweh, NN., Clayton, JL., Mangum, CA., Florman, SS. & Slakey, DP. (1963). High body mass index and short-and long- term renal allograft survival in adults. *Transplantation*. Vol.80, No.10, (November 2005), pp.1430-1434, ISSN. 0041-1337.

Massy, ZA. (1963). Hyperlipidemia and cardiovascular disease after organ transplantation. *Transplantation*. Vol.72, suppl.6, (September 2001), pp.S13-S15, ISSN: 0041-1337.

Massy, ZA. & Kasiske, BL. (1990). Post-transplant hyperlipidemia: mechanism and management. *J Am Soc Nephrol*. Vol.7, No.7, (July 1996), pp.971-977, ISSN: 1046-6673.

Matas, AJ., Humar, A., Gillingham, KJ., Payne, WD., Gruessner, RWG., Kandaswamy, R., Dunn, DL., Najasrian, JS. & Sutherland, DER. (1972). Five preventable causes of kidney graft loss in the 1990s: A single-center analysis. *Kidney Int* Vol. 62, No. 2, (August 2002), pp.704-714, ISSN: 0085-2538.

Mayer, AD., Dmitrewski, J., Squifflet, JP., Besse, T., Grabensee, B., Klein, B., Eigler, FW., Heemann, U., Pichlmayr, R., Behrend, M., Vanrenterghem, Y., Donck, J., van Hooff, J., Christiaans, M., Morales, JM., Andres, A., Johnson, RW., Short, C., Buchholz, B., Rehmert, N., Land, W., Schleibner, S., Forsythe, JL., Talbot, D., & Pohanka, E., (1963). Multicenter randomized trial comparing tacrolimus (FK506) and cyclosporine in the prevention of renal allograft rejection. A report of the European tacrolimus multicenter renal study group. *Transplantation* Vol.64, No.3 (August 1997), pp.436-443, ISSN. 0041-1337.

Mazzaferro, S., Pascquali, M., Taggi, F., Baldinelli, M., Conte, C., Muci, ML., Pirozzi, N., Carbone, I., Francone, M. & Pugliese, F. (2006). Progression of coronary artery calcification in renal transplantation and the role of secondary hyperparathyroidism and inflammation. *Clin J Am Soc Nephrol* Vol.4, No.3 (March 2009), pp.685-690, ISSN: 1555-9041.

McDonald, SP. & Russ, GR. (1986). Survival of recipients of cadaveric kidney transplants compared with those receiving dialysis treatment in Australia an New Zealand 1991-2001. *Nephrol Dial Transplant*. Vol.17, No.12, (December 2002) pp.2212-2219, ISSN: 0931-0509.

McGregor, E., Jardine, AG., Murray, LS., Dargie, HJ., Rodger, RS., Junor, BJ., McMillan, MA. & Briggs JD. (1986). Pre-operative echocardiographic abnormalities and adverse outcome following renal transplantation. *Nephrol Dial Transplant*. Vol.13, No.6, (June 1998), pp.1499-505, ISSN: 0931-0509

McGregor, E., Steward, G., Rodger, SC. & Jardine AG. (1986). Early echocardiographic changes and survival following transplantation. *Nephrol Dial Transplant*. Vol.15, No.1, (January 2000), pp.93-93, ISSN: 0931-0509.

Meier-Kriesche, HU., Vaghela, M., Thambuganipalle, R., Friedman, G., Jacobs, M. & Kaplan, B. (163). The effect of body mass index on long-term renal allograft. *Transplantation*. Vol.68, No.9, (November 1999), pp.1294-1297, ISSN: 0041-1337.

Meier-Kriesche, HU., Arndorfer, JA. & Kaplan, B. (1963). The impact of body mass index on renal transplant outcomes: a significant independent risk factor for graft failure and patient death. *Transplantation*. Vol.73, No.1, (January 2002), pp.70-74, ISSN.0041-1337.

Meier-Kriesche, HU., Baliga, R. & Kaplan, B. (1963). Decreased renal function is a strong risk factor for cardiovascular death after renal transplantation. *Transplantation* Vol.75, No.8 (April 2003), pp.1291-1205, ISSN: 0041-1337.

Miller LW. (2001). Cardiovascular toxicities of immunosuppressive agents. *Am J Transplant.* Vol.2, No.9, (October 2002), pp.807- 818, ISSN: 1600-6135.

Molnar, MZ., Czira, M., Ambrus, C., Kovacs, AC., Pap, J., Remport, A., Szeifer, L. & Mucsi, I. (2001). Anemia is associated with mortality in kidney-transplanted patients- a prospective cohort study. *Am J Transplant.* Vol.7, No.4, (April 2007), pp. 818-824, ISSN.1600-6135.

Montori, VM., Basu, A., Erwin, PJ., Velosa, JA., Gabriel, SE.& Kudva, YC.(1978). Posttransplantation diabetes. A systematic review of the literature. *Diabetes Care* Vol. 25, No.3, (March, 2002), pp.538-592, ISSN: 0149-5992.

Moore, R., Hernandez, D. & Valantine, H. (1990). Calcineurin inhibitors and post-transplant hyperlipidaemias. *Drugs Saf* Vol.24, No.10, (2001), pp.755-766.

Morales, JM. & Dominguez-Gil, B. (1990). Impact of tacrolimus and mycophenolate mofetil combination on cardiovascular risk profile after transplantation. *J Am Soc Nephrol* Vol.17, 12 Suppl 3, (December 2006), pp.S296-S303, ISSN: 1046-6673.

Morales, JM., Marcén, R., Andrés, A., González- Molina, M., del Castillo, D., Cabello, M., Capdevila, L., Campistol, JM., Oppenheimer, F., Serón, D., Gil-Vernet, S., Lampreave, I., Valdés, F., Anaya, F., Escuin, F., Arias, M., Pallardó, L. & Bustamente J. (1972). Renal transplantation in the moderm immunosuppresive era in Spain: four-year results from a multicenter database focus on post-transplant cardiovascular disease. *Kidney Int Suppl.* Vol.111, (December 2008), pp. S94-S99, ISSN: 0085-2538.

Murphy, SW., Foley, RN. & Parfrey, PS. (1981). Screening and treatment for cardiovascular disease in patients with chronic renal disease. *Am J Kidney Dis.* Vol.32, 5 Suppl 3, (November 1998), pp.S184-S199, ISSN: 0272-6386..

Ojo, AO., Hanson, JA., Wolfe, RA., Leichtman, AB., Agodoa, LY. & Port FK. (1972). Long-term survival in renal transplant recipients with graft function. *Kidney Int* . Vol. 57, No.1, (January 2000), pp. 307-313, ISSN: 0085-2538.

Ojo, AO. (1963). Cardiovascular complications after renal transplantation and their prevention. *Transplantation.* Vol.82, No.5, (September 2006), pp.603-611, ISSN: 0041-1337.

Oliveras, A., Roquer, J., Puig, JM., Rodriguez, A., Mir, M., Orfila, A., Masramon, J. & Loveras, J. (1987). Stroke in renal transplant recipients: epidemiology, predictive risk factors and outcome. *Clin Transplant* Vol. 17, No.1, (February 2003), pp.1-8, ISSN:0902-0063.

Opelz, G., Döhler, B. for the Collaborative Transplant Study. (2001). Improved long-term outcomes after renal transplantation associated with blood pressue control. *Am J Transplant.* . Vol.5, No.11, (November 2005), pp.2725-2731, ISSN: 1600.6135.

Opelz, G., Zeier, M., Laux, G., Morath, C. & Döhler, B. (1990). No improvement of patients or graft survival in transplant recipients treated with angiotensin-converting enzyme inhibitors or angiotensin II type 1 receptor blockers: a collaborative transplant study report. *J Am Soc Nephrol* . Vol.17, No.11, (November 2006), pp.3257-3262, ISSN: 1046-6673.

Paoletti, E., Amidore, M., Cassottana, P., Gherzi, M., Marsano, L. & Cannella, G. (1981). Effects of sirolimus on left ventricular hypertrophy in kidney transplant recipients:

a 1-year nonrandomized controlled trial. *Am J Kidney Dis* . Vol.52, No.2, (August 2008), pp.324-330, ISSN: 0272-6386.

Parfrey, PS., Harnett, JD., Foley, RN., Kent, GM., Murray, DC., Barre, PE. & Guttmann. RD. (1963). Impact of renal transplantation on uremic cardiomyopathy. *Transplantation* . Vol. 60. No. 9, (November 1995), pp. 908-914, ISSN: 0041- 1337.

Park, JM. & Luan, FL. (1990). Management of hypertension in solid-organ transplantation. *Prog Transplant*. Vol.15, No.1, (March 2005), pp. 17-22, ISSN: 1526-9248.

Patel, RK., Mark, PB., Jonhston, N., McGregor, E., Dargie, H. &, Jardine AG. (2006). Renal transplantation is not associated with regression of left ventricular hypertrophy: a magnetic resonance study. *Clin J Am Soc Nephrol* . Vol.3, No.6, (November 2008), pp.1807-1811, ISSN: 1555-9041.

Pilmore, H., Dent, H., Chang, S., McDonald, SP. & Chadban SJ. (1963). Reduction in cardiovascular death after kidney transplantation. *Transplantation*. Vol. 89, No. 7, (April 2010), pp.851-857. ISSN: 0041-1337.

Ridker, PM., Cushman, M., Stampfer, MJ., Tracy, RP. & Hennekens, CH. (1812). Inflammation , aspirin, and the risk of cardiovascular disease in apparently healthy men. *N Engl J Med* . Vol.336, No.14, (April 1997), pp.973-979, ISSN: 0028-4793.

Rigatto, C., Foley, RN., Kent, GM., Guttman, R. & Parfrey, PS. (1963). Long-term changes in left ventricular hypertrophy after renal transplantation. *Transplantation* . Vol.70, No.4, (August 2000), pp. 570-575, ISSN: 0041-1337.

Rigatto, C., Parfrey, P., Foley, R., Negrijn, C., Tribula, C. & Jeffey J. (1990). Congestive heart failure in renal transplant recipients: risk factors, outcomes, and relationship with ischemic heart disease. *J Am Soc Nephrol* . Vol.13, No.4, (April 2002), pp. 1084-1090. ISSN.1046-6673.

Rigatto, C. (1990). Clinical epidemiology of cardiac disease in renal transplant recipients. *Semi in Dial* Vol.16, No.2, (March-April 2003a), pp. 106-110, ISSN: 1525-139X.

Rigatto, C., Foley, R., Jeffery, J., Negrijn, C., Tribula, C. & Parfrey P. (1990). Electrocardiographic left ventricular hypertrophy in renal transplant recipients: prognostic value and impact of blood pressure and anemia. *J Am Soc Nephrol* Vol. 14. No. 2, (February 2003b), pp.462-468. ISSN.1046-6673.

Rigatto, C. (2001). Anemia, renal transplantation and the anemia paradox. *Semin Nephrol.* Vol.26, No.4, (July 2006), pp.307- *312.*ISSN 0270-9295.

Roodnat, JI., Muldr, PGH., Rischen-Vos, J., van Riemsdijk, IC., van Gelder, T., Zietse R., Izermans, JN. & Weimar, W. (1963). Proteinuria after renal transplantation affects not only graft survival but also patient survival. *Transplantation*. Vol.72, No.3, (August 2001), pp.438-444, ISSN: 0041-1337.

Schena, FP., Pascoe, MD., Aberu, J., del Carmen, Rial, M., Oberbauer, R., Brennan, DC., Campistol, JM., Racusen, L., Polinsky, MS., Goldberg-Alberts, R., Li, H., Scarola, J. & Neylan, JF. for the sirolimus CONVERT trial study group. (1963). Conversion from calcineurin inhibitors to sirolimus maintenance therapy in renal allograft recipients: 24-months efficacy and safety results from the CONVERT trial. *Transplantation*. Vol.87, No.2 (January 2009), pp.233-242, ISSN: 0041-1337.

Seliger, SL., Weiss, NS., Gillen, DL., Kestenbaum, B., Ball, A., Sherrard, DJ. & Stehman-Breen, CO. (1972). HMG-CoA reductase inhibitors are associated with reduced mortality in ESRD patients. *Kidney Int.* Vol.61, No.1, (January 2002), pp.297-304, ISSN:0085-2538.

Seliger, SL., Gillen, DL., Longstreth, WT., Kestenbaum, B. & Stehman-Breen CO. (1972). Elevated risk of stroke among patients with end-stage renal disease. *Kidney Int.* Vol. 64, No.2, (August 2003), pp.603-609, ISSN:0085-2538.

Seliger, SL., Gillen, DL., Tirschwell, D., Wasse, H., Kestenbaum, BR. & Stehman-Breen CO. (1990). Risk factors for incident stroke among patients with end-stage renal disease. *J Am Soc Nephrol* Vol. 14, No.10 (October 2003), pp.2623-2631, ISSN: 1046-6673.

Shah, N., Al-Khoury, S., Afzali, B., Covic, A., Roche, A., Msarsh, J., Macdougall, IC. & Goldsmirhm DJA. (1963). Posttransplantation anemia in adult renal allograft recipients: prevalence and predictors. *Transplantation* Vol.81, No.8 (April 2006), pp.1112-1118, ISSN.0041-1337.

Snyder, JJ., Kasiske, BL. & Mac Lean, R. (1990). Peripheral arterial disease and renal transplantation. *J Am Soc Nephrol* Vol.17, No.7, (July 2006), pp.2056-2068, ISSN: 1046-6673.

Soveri, I., Holdaas, H., Jardine, A., Gimpelewicz, C., Staffler, B. & Fellström, B. (1986). Renal transplant dysfunction-importance quantified in comparison with traditional risk factors for cardiovascular disease and mortality. *Nephrol Dial Transplant* Vol.21, No.8, (August 2006), pp.2282-2289. ISSN:0931-0509.

Stack, AG. & Bloembergen, WE. (1981). A cross-sectional study of the prevalence and clinical correlates of congestive heart failure among incident U.S. dialysis patients. *Am J Kidney Dis* Vol. 38, No. 5, (November 2001), pp. 992-1000, ISSN: 0272- 6386.

Stuveling, EM., Hillege, HL., Bakker, SJ., Gans, RO., De Jong, PE. & de Zeeuw, D. (1972). C-reactive protein is associated with renal function abnormalities in a non-diabetic population. *Kidney Int* . Vol.63, No.2, (February 2003), pp.654-661, ISSN: 0085-2538.

Sung, RS., Althoen, M., Howell, TA. & Merion, RM. (1963). Peripheral vascular occlusive disease in renal transplant recipients: risk factors and impact on kidney allograft survival. *Transplantation.* Vol.70, No.7, (October 2000), pp. 1049-1054, ISSN: 0041-1337.

Teruel, JL., Rodriguez Padial, L., Quereda, C., Yuste, P., Marcen, R. & Ortuño, J. (1963). Regression of left ventricular hypertrophy after renal transplantation. A prospective study. *Transplantation.* Vol.43, No.2, (February 1987), pp.307-309, ISSN: 0041-1337

Tucker, B., Fabbian, F., Giles, M., Thuraisingham, RC., Raine, AE. & Baker LR. (1997). Left ventricular hypertrophy and ambulatory blood pressure monitoring in chronic renal failure. *Nephrol Dial Transplant* Vol.12, No.4, (April 1997), pp. 724-728, ISSN: 0272-6376.

Tutone, VK., Mark, PB., Steward, GA., Tan, CC., Geddes, CC. & Jardine AG. (1987). Hypertension, antihypertensive agents and outcomes following renal transplantation. *Clin Transplant* Vol.19, No. 2, (April 2005), pp.181-192, ISSN: 0902-0063.

Van Ree, RM., de Vries, APJ., Oterdoom ,LH., The, TH., Gansevoort, RT., van der Heide, JJH., van Son, WJ., Ploeg, RJ., de Jong, PE., Gans, ROB. & Bakker, SJL. (1986).Abdominal obesity and smoking are important determinants of C-reactive protein in renal transplant recipients. *Nephrol Dial Transplant* . Vol.20, No.11 (November 2005), pp.2524-2531, ISSN: 0931-0509.

Vanrenterghem, Y., Ponticelli, C., Morales, JM., Abramowicz, D., Baboolal, K., Eklund, B., Kliem, V., Legendre, C., Morais Sarmento, AL. & Vincenti, F. (2001). Prevalence and management of anemia in renal transplant recipients: a European survey. *Am J Transplant*. Vol.3, No.7, (July 2003), pp.835-845, ISSN.1600-6135.

Vanrenterghem, YFC., Claes, K., Montagnino, G., Fieuws, S., Maes, B., Villa, M. & Ponticelli, C. (1963). Risk factors for cardiovascular events after successful renal transplantation. *Transplantation*. Vol. 85, No.2, (January 2008), pp. 209-216, ISSN: 0041-1337.

Vincenti, F., Jensik, SC., Filo, RS., Millar, J. & Pirsch, J. (1963). A long-term comparison of tacrolimus (FK506) and cyclosporine in kidney transplantation: evidence for improved allograft survival at five years. *Transplantation* Vol.73, No.5 (March 2005), pp. 775-782. ISSN. 0041-1337.

Vincenti, F., Friman, S., Scheuermann, E., Rostaing, L., Jenssen, T., Campistol, JM., Uchida, K.., Pescovitz, MD., Marchetti, P., Tuncer, M., Citterio, F., Wiecek, A., Chadban, S., El-Shahawy, M., Budde, K. & Goto, N. on behalf of the DIRECT investigators. (2001). Results of an international, randomised trial comparing glucose metabolism disorders and outcome with cyclosporine versus tacrolimus. *Am J Transpl* Vol.7, No.6, (June 2007), pp. 1506-1514, ISSN.1600-6135.

Vincenti, F., Charpentier, B., Vanrenterghen, Y., Rostaing, L., Bresnahan, B., Darji, P., Massari, P., Mondragon-Ramirez, GA., Agarwal, M., Di Russo, G., Lin, CS., Garg, P. & Larsen, CP. (2001). A phase III study of belatacept-based immunosuppression regimens versus cyclosporine in renal transplant recipients (BENEFIT study). *Am J Transplant*. Vol.10, No.3, (March 2010), pp.535-546, ISSN: 1600-6135.

Wali, RK., Wang, GS., Gottlieb, SS., Bellumkonda, L., Hansalia, R., Ramos, E., Drachenberg, C., Papadimitriou, J., Brisco, MA., Blahut, S., Fink, JC., Fisher, ML., Bartlett, ST. & Weir MR. (1983). Effect of kidney transplantation on left ventricular systolic dysfunction and congestive heart failure in patients with end-stage renal disease. *J Am Coll Cardiol*, Vol. 45, No.7 (April 2005), pp.1051-1060, ISSN: 0735-1097.

Wang, K., Zhang, H., Li, Y., Wei, Q., Li, H., Yang, Y. & Lu, Y. (1969). Safety of mycophenolate mofetil versus azathioprine in renal transplantation: a systematic review. *Transplant Proc.* Vol.36, No7, (September 2004), pp.2068-2070, ISSN.0041-1345.

Wang, JH. & Kasiske, BL. (1992). Screening and management of pretransplant cardiovascular disease. *Curr Opin Nephrol Hypertens.* Vol.19, No.6, (November 2010), pp.586-591, ISSN: 1473-6543.

Webster, AC., Lee, VWS., Chapman, JR. & Craig, JC. (1963). Target of rapamycin inhibitors (sirolimus and everolimus) for primary immunosuppression of kidney transplant recipients; a systemsatic review meta-analysis of randomized trials. *Transplantation* Vol.81, No.9, (May 2006), pp. 1234-1248, ISSN: 0041-1337.

Wiesbauer, F., Heinze, G., Mitterbauer, C., Harnoncourt, F., Hörl, WH. & Oberbauer, R. (1990). Statin use is associated with prolonged survival of renal transplant recipients. *J Am Soc Nephrol* Vol.19, No.11, (November 2008), pp. 2211-2218, ISSN: 1046-6673.

Wilson, PWF. & Culleton, BF. (19981). Epidemiology of cardiovascular disease in the United States. *A J Kidney Dis.* Vol 32, No5, suppl 3. (November 1998), pp.S56-S65, ISSN: 0272-6386.

Winkelmayer, WC., Lorenz, M., Kramar, R., Fodinger, M., Hörl, WH. & Sunder-Plassmann, G. (2001). C-reactive protein and body mass index independently predict mortality in kidney transplant recipients. *Am J Transplant.* Vol.4, No.7, (July 2004), pp.1148-1154, ISSN: 1600-6135.

Winkelmayer, WC., Kramar, R., Curhan, GC., Chandraker, A., Endler, G., Födinger, M., Hörl, WH. & Sunder Plassmann, G. (1990). Fasting plasma total homocysteine levels and mortality and allograaft loss in kidney transplant recipients: a prospective study. *J Am Soc Nephrol* . Vol.16, No.1, (January 2005), pp.255-260, ISSN: 1046-6673.

Winkelmayer, WC., Chandraker, A., Brookhart, MA., Kramar, R. & Sunder-Plassmann, G. (1986). A prospective stydy of anaemia and long-term outcomes in kidney transplant recipients. *Nephrol Dial Transplant*. Vol.21, No.12, (December 2006), pp.3559-3566, ISSN.0931-0509.

Wolfe, RA., Ashby, VB., Milford, EL., Ojo, AO., Ettenger, RE., Agodoa, LY., Held, PJ. & Port, FK. (1812). Comparison of mortality in all patients on dialysis, patients on dialysis awaiting transplantation, and recipients of a first cadaveric transplant. *N Engl J Med*. Vol. 341, No.23 (December 1999), pp.1725-1730, ISSN: 0028-4793.

Wong, BM., Huang, M., Zaltzman, JS. & Prasad, GV. (1963). Mycophenolate mofetil and C-reactive protein in renal transplant recipients. *Transplantation*. Vol.83, No.1, (January 2007), pp.48-53, ISSN: 0041-1337.

Yorgin, PD., Scandling, JD., Belson, A., Sanchez, J., Alexander, SR. & Andreoni, KA. (2001). Late post-transplant anemia in adult renal transplant recipients. An under-recognized problem? *Am J Transplant*. Vol.2, No.5, (May 2002), pp.429-435, ISSN.1600-6135.

Zhang, R., Leslie, B., Boudreaux, JP., Frey, D. & Reisin E. (1827). Hypertension after kidney transplantation: impact, pathogenesis and therapy. Am J Med Sci Vol: 325, No.4, (April 2003), pp.202-208, ISSN: 1538-2990.

Zebe H. (1986). Atrial fibrillation in dialysis patients. *Nephrol Dial Transplant*. Vol. 16, No.5, (June 2001), pp. 765-8, ISSN: 0931- 0509.

Zitt, N., Kollerits, B., Neyer, U., Mark, W., Heininger, D., Mayer, G., Kronenberg, F., & Lhotta, K. (1986). Cigarette smoking and chronic allograft nephropathy. *Nephrol Dial Transplant*. Vol.22, No.10, (October 2007), pp.3034-3034, ISSN. 0931-0509

7

Obesity and Kidney Transplantation

Alex Chang[1], Susan Hou[1] and Holly Kramer[1,2]
[1]*Loyola University Medical Center, Department of Medicine, Division of Nephrology and Hypertension*
[2]*Department of Preventive Medicine and Epidemiology, USA*

1. Introduction

Worldwide, countries continue to face an epidemic of obesity, the number one risk factor for diabetes and hypertension. Obesity likely mediates, at least in part, the majority of kidney disease among industrialized societies. Due to the rising prevalence of obesity, the incidence of chronic kidney disease (CKD) and end-stage kidney disease (ESKD) will likely not decrease over the next several decades, but may in fact increase. The impact of obesity is especially important for kidney transplantation because many obese individuals are precluded from kidney transplantation due to concerns over the potential medical and surgical complications associated with their body habitus. Because higher BMI appears to be associated with decreased mortality among patients receiving dialysis, clinicians may be reluctant to counsel obese patients to lose weight. To understand the impact of obesity on transplantation, the discussion needs to begin with a review of how obesity impacts mortality in populations with CKD. This chapter will then discuss trends in obesity among adults receiving dialysis, controversies surrounding the preclusion of morbidly obese individuals from transplantation, and behavior modifications and surgical interventions and their respective risks and benefits for obesity management.

2. BMI and mortality in the general population

Body mass index (BMI) (the weight in kilograms divided by the square of the height in meters) has been widely used to estimate overweight and obesity. Weight indexed for height was first used by life insurance companies to estimate life expectancy in the early part of the twentieth century (1, 2). In 1997, the World Health Organization (WHO) created categories for underweight (BMI<18.5 kg/m^2), overweight (BMI 25.0-29.9 kg/m^2), and obesity stages I (BMI 30.0-34.9 kg/m^2) , II (BMI 35.0-39.9 kg/m^2), and III (≥40 kg/m^2) (Table 1) (3). Controversy exists as to whether these BMI categories are applicable for assessing mortality risk in all age and racial/ethnic groups. However, in the general U.S. population, studies have consistently shown that a BMI ≥ 35 kg/m^2 heightens mortality risk in young and middle-aged individuals (4-6) but this risk declines with advancing age (7). A meta-analysis of studies limited to adults 65 years or older concluded that federal guidelines for ideal weight (BMI 18.7-25 kg/m^2) may be too restrictive for populations over the age of 70 years due to lack of evidence that overweight in the elderly confers excess mortality risk (8).

BMI	(kg/m²)
Underweight	<18.5
Normal	18.5-24.9
Overweight	25.0-29.9
Class I Obesity	30.0-34.9
Class II Obesity	35.0-39.9
Class III Obesity	≥40
Waist circumference	**(cm)**
Increased risk	Men ≤ 102 Women ≤ 88
Decreased risk	Men >102 Women >88

*Adapted from World Health Organization 1998 guidelines for obesity classification (3)

Table 1. Classification of Underweight, Overweight, and Obesity by BMI and Waist Circumference*

3. Abdominal obesity in the general population

The indexing of weight for height (BMI) includes fat mass and fat-free mass and provides no information about body composition or regional adiposity. Abdominal fat remains a strong predictor of mortality even after adjustment for sensitive measures of total body fat. In fact, the increased cardiovascular risk associated with obesity is mainly mediated by abdominal fat (9). Visceral adipose tissue produces cytokines including tumor necrosis factor alpha, which can cause insulin resistance by the suppression of adiponectin. Abdominal obesity can amplify this problem by the high influx of portal fatty acids, cytokines, and hormones into the liver from omental adipocytes, resulting in increased hepatic synthesis of apolipoprotein B and very low density lipids (10). Although abdominal fat can be measured directly by using dual-energy X-ray absorptiometry, computed tomography, or magnetic resonance imaging, waist circumference correlates highly with abdominal fat and can be measured easily and fairly reliably (11-13). The definition of abdominal adiposity (waist circumference ≥102 cm in men and ≥88 cm in women) is based on a Scottish study which found that this threshold for waist circumference effectively identified obese (BMI ≥30kg/m²) individuals in addition to adults with BMI < 30 kg/m² in the setting of a high waist/hip ratio (Table 1) (14). While waist circumference thresholds for abdominal adiposity may differ by racial/ethnic groups (i.e. > 87cm and > 83cm in Japanese men and women, respectively) (15), individuals with abdominal adiposity are more likely to have hypertension, diabetes, dyslipidemia, and the metabolic syndrome than individuals without abdominal adiposity, even after adjusting for BMI class (16, 17). Furthermore, abdominal adiposity is associated with increased mortality risk regardless of BMI or racial/ethnic group (16-18).

4. Obesity trends in CKD stages 1-5

Rates of obesity worldwide have increased dramatically over the past 20 years. In the U.S., prevalence of obesity has doubled from 15 to 30% while morbid obesity prevalence increased by four-fold (19). Overall, obesity trends in adults with ESKD mirror those in the general population. Not surprisingly, during years 1995-2002, the mean BMI among patients initiating dialysis increased from 25.7 to 27.5 kg/m^2 (20). The percentage of incident ESKD patients who had stage II obesity (BMI>35 kg/m^2) during this timeframe increased from 9.4% to 15.4%. Likewise, the percentage of patients listed for kidney transplantation who were obese (BMI≥30kg/m^2) increased from 11.6% to 25.1% between the years 1987 and 2001 (21).

5. Adiposity measures and mortality in adults with CKD

Using BMI measures as a proxy of adiposity in CKD patients may not account for differences in body composition or muscle wasting. Indeed, studies using BMI to study adverse outcomes in the CKD population have shown conflicting results from the general population (22-24). Similarly, in studies of adults with CKD who are not receiving dialysis, BMI has not been found to be an independent predictor of cardiovascular disease or all-cause mortality (25,26). To examine associations between abdominal adiposity as measured by the waist-hip ratio (WHR) and BMI with cardiovascular events, Elsayed et al pooled data from the Atherosclerosis Risk in Communities Study and the Cardiovascular Health (ARIC) Study (27). A total of 1,669 adults with CKD were followed for a mean of 9.3 years. Mean age was 70.3 years and mean estimated glomerular filtration rate (eGFR) was 51.1 ml/min/m^2. The highest WHR group had a 36% increased hazard of cardiovascular events compared to the lowest WHR group. Obesity (BMI>30 kg/m^2) was not associated with cardiovascular events when compared to those with an ideal BMI (18.5-24.9 kg/m^2).

Among adults receiving dialysis, numerous studies have reported a survival benefit with higher BMI compared to BMI in the ideal (18.5-24.9 kg/m^2) and low (< 18.5 kg/m^2) range (28-31). It has been posited that fat may play a protective role in these patients who often suffer from protein-energy malnutrition and inflammation (28). However, BMI represents both muscle mass and abdominal and peripheral fat. Higher muscle mass reflects better physical functioning, which is extremely important for predicting mortality in patients with co-morbid conditions such as ESKD. An Italian study of 537 dialysis patients examined associations of waist circumference, waist-to-hip ratio (WHR), and BMI with cardiovascular and total mortality (32). The inverse relationship between BMI and mortality was reaffirmed whereas waist circumference and WHR were directly associated with increased cardiovascular and total mortality. After adjustment for cardiovascular risk factors, every 10-cm higher waist circumference conferred an excess 26% risk for death and an excess 38% risk for cardiovascular death (32). The association between BMI and mortality in patients receiving dialysis has also been shown to be modified by muscle mass as reflected by 24-hour creatinine excretion (33).

Few studies have examined the link between adiposity measures and mortality in adult kidney transplant recipients. Kovedsky examined BMI and waist circumference in 993 kidney transplant recipients in Hungary (34). Mean age was 50.9 years, 21% were diabetic, and mean eGFR rate was 50.9 ml/min/1.73 m^2. Individuals with higher BMI or waist circumference were more likely to be diabetic, less likely to smoke, and more likely to have had delayed graft function. While risk of mortality declined with higher BMI, a 15 cm higher waist circumference was associated with greater than 2-fold increase in all-cause mortality after adjustment for BMI (34).

In summary, BMI may be inadequate by itself to assess mortality risk associated with adiposity. Waist circumference reflects visceral adiposity burden and is directly associated with mortality among individuals with co-morbid conditions such as ESKD while BMI appears to be inversely related to mortality (30-32, 34). Many centers currently exclude patients with BMI >35 kg/m^2 from kidney transplantation until they are able to lose weight (35, 36). Use of waist circumference in the evaluation of kidney transplant candidates may provide more accurate information regarding the pre- and post-transplantation risks associated with obesity.

6. Access to kidney transplantation and barriers due to obesity

Obesity is currently an important barrier keeping many individuals from being listed for kidney transplantation (37). A study of the UNOS database from 1995-2006 evaluated the association between BMI and time to transplantation (38). Individuals with severe obesity (BMI 35-40 kg/m^2) and morbid obesity (BMI 40-60 kg/m^2) at time of initial listing were 28% and 44% less likely, respectively, to receive a deceased-donor kidney transplant compared to individuals with an ideal BMI (18.5-24.9 kg/m^2) (38). This study could not account for the number of obese individuals who were never listed at all due to their weight, and likely underestimates the impact obesity may have on access to transplantation. Indeed, 15% of transplant centers did not list a single severely obese (BMI 35-40 kg/m^2) patient during the 11-year period of the study (38). While this study cannot prove causality, it seems likely that body habitus is a major deciding factor when determining whether a person may be listed for transplantation. Certainly, economic pressures favor kidney transplantation for "low-risk" non-obese patients in which complication rates and hospital stay may be lower. Moreover, obesity is considered a reversible risk factor, and losing weight prior to transplant is thought to be beneficial, especially considering how common weight gain is after kidney transplantation (37). Obese kidney transplant recipients are at increased risk for short-term complications including delayed wound healing, longer surgical times, and delayed graft function (39, 40). Data on whether obese transplant recipients are at higher risk for long-term adverse outcomes remains controversial, but the majority of larger studies suggest poorer long-term outcomes among obese individuals compared to non-obese individuals (40-42).

The decision by some transplant centers to use BMI thresholds for the exclusion of patients from kidney transplantation should consider both societal and individual level concerns. From an individual-level perspective, kidney transplantation offers a clear survival benefit over dialysis regardless of obesity status (43,44). Among obese adults receiving dialysis for ESKD during years 1995-1999, both living and deceased donor kidney transplant recipients had decreased mortality risk of 61% and 77%, respectively, compared to those remaining on the kidney transplant waiting list. Due to the excess surgical risks and graft failure among obese individuals, one option would be to limit opportunities for cadaveric kidneys. However, evidence for this is contentious. Excluding obese individuals due to increased risk ignores the fact that co-morbid conditions such as diabetes pose similar risk as obesity yet these conditions do not preclude transplantation (40). Transplantation centers should also consider the extra time an obese patient spends on dialysis while trying to lose weight in order to be listed for transplantation. Unfortunately, weight loss is usually unsuccessful for individuals with severe obesity (45).

7. Obese kidney transplant patients

7.1 Post-operative complications

For all surgical procedures, obesity can complicate the post-operative period with delayed wound healing, increased rates of ventral hernias, and longer operating times and hospitalizations. In transplant recipients, obesity is also associated with heightened risk of infections, and post-transplant diabetes (49-53). One single-center study which included 2013 adult kidney transplants performed between 1984 and 1998, superficial or deep wound infections occurred in 4.8%, whereas 3.6% developed either a fascial dehiscence or hernia of the wound (54). Those with BMI ≥ 30 kg/m² had a 340% increased risk for a wound infection and 182% increased risk for a fascial dehiscence or incisional hernia compared to those with BMI < 30 kg/m².

Delayed graft function (DGF), defined as the need for dialysis therapy in the first week after kidney transplantation, places a recipient at increased risk for chronic rejection and decreased graft survival. Only a minority of single-center studies have shown that obesity increases risk for decreased graft survival after kidney transplantation (46-53) but this may be due to small sample sizes in these single-center studies. In a large study which included 51,927 kidney transplant recipients, severe obesity (BMI > 35 kg/m²) was associated with a 51% increased risk of DGF compared to the transplant recipients with a BMI between 22-24 kg/m² (41). These findings were supported by a study which included data from 27,377 kidney transplant recipients (40).

Overall mortality, regardless of obesity status, is substantially reduced with kidney transplantation (43,44). However, compared to non-obese kidney transplant recipients, obese transplant recipients appear to have an increased risk of graft loss although not all studies agree (39-56). Overall, BMI > 35 kg/m² appears to increase graft failure risk by approximately 20-30% compared to recipients who are not obese while no excess risk is seen among transplant recipients with a BMI between 30-35 kg/m² (40,41). The magnitude of the association between morbid obesity and graft failure is similar to the increased risk of graft failure associated with diabetes (40). Overall mortality after kidney transplantation does not appear to be associated with obesity itself. However, obese patients may have co-morbid conditions which influence survival (40).

7.2 Weight loss interventions for obese adults with CKD

7.2.1 Who should lose weight

The management of obesity requires identification of individuals who will benefit from weight loss. All obese patients (BMI ≥ 30 kg/m²) should be counseled to modify their lifestyles (diet and physical activity) to induce weight loss but goals must be individualized (57). In adults with CKD, abdominal obesity, measured by waist circumference should be considered an indication for weight loss considering the increased risk of cardiovascular and total mortality associated with increased waist circumference (27, 32, 34). Weight loss in patients with diabetic and non-diabetic kidney diseases has been shown to reduce proteinuria (58, 59). However, there is a paucity of data regarding the long-term outcomes of intentional weight loss in adults with CKD. Perhaps the strongest evidence supporting weight loss in this population comes from surgical intervention studies in the morbidly obese. Successful weight loss dramatically improves blood pressure, proteinuria, and in some cases, stabilizes GFR (60-63). However, surgical interventions for obesity carry significant risks as discussed later.

Regardless of the small survival benefits associated with obesity observed among patients receiving dialysis, kidney transplantation greatly improves longevity and survival is substantially higher among obese kidney transplant recipients compared to individuals remaining on the waiting list (38). In fact, obesity should be considered the most important modifiable mortality risk factor if a patient receiving dialysis is not listed for kidney transplantation solely due to obesity (45). Weight loss goals for obese patients receiving dialysis who are seeking kidney transplantation must be assessed individually and goals should account for the obesity-related co-morbid conditions and nutritional status of that individual. Moreover, interventions should also account for the patient's body composition because increasing muscle mass may improve overall fitness and survival (31, 45).

7.2.2 Weight gain after kidney transplantation

Weight gain after kidney transplantation is very common, with studies showing increased weight between 8-14 kg one year post-transplant (37, 39, 64). Johnson et al showed that a 10% weight gain correlated with increased serum cholesterol and triglyceride levels which may heighten cardiovascular risk (49, 65). In a study of 3,899 white Australian and New Zealand adults, weight gain of 10% to 19.9% during the first year after transplantation and stable weight (0% to 4.9% gain) during the second year after transplantation were associated with the best outcomes while weight loss over the first two years after transplantation was associated with the worst outcomes (66). A 20% weight gain above the pre-transplant weight during the first year with continued weight gain during the second year after transplantation was associated with increased graft loss and mortality compared to transplant recipients who maintained their weight after the second year.

Certain individuals may be at higher risk for excessive weight gain after kidney transplantation than others. Certainly the improved appetite and sense of well-being may lead to augmented caloric intake. A study of renal transplant recipients from a racially diverse center between 1983 and 1998 reported that African Americans were at higher risk for weight gain (67), and these results have been supported by several other studies (47, 49, 50, 64). Part of this race disparity may be due to socioeconomic status because accounting for income level attenuates the association between race and weight gain after kidney transplantation (64). Weight gain patterns after transplantation seem to mirror the general population as the majority of studies have shown that younger age, female sex and low income-status increase the probability of weight gain (47, 49, 50, 64). Patients who are obese at the time of kidney transplantation appear to have similar (67) or greater weight gain (47, 64) compared to non-obese kidney transplant recipients.

Immunosuppressant medications have varying adverse cardiovascular risk profiles. Corticosteroids can cause excessive weight gain and redistribution of fat to undesired areas (face and back) as well as worsen blood pressure, glucose and lipid metabolism (68). Overall, steroid doses used for kidney transplantation are much lower than in the past with some transplant protocols minimizing or avoiding steroid use. However, minimization or avoidance of steroid use in kidney transplantation must be counterbalanced with adequate immunosuppression, which often requires lymphocyte depleting agents or anti-IL2 strategies coupled with the use of other immunosuppressive medications (69). One study examined 95 kidney transplant recipients enrolled in National Institutes of Health clinical transplant trials (70). Regardless of therapy received, weight increased by 5 kg (not BMI) on average among all patients at one year post-transplant. Another small retrospective study compared patterns of weight gain among 301 kidney transplant recipients receiving chronic corticosteroid therapy to patients who had early corticosteroid withdrawal (within 7 days post-transplant) (71). A 33% lower rate of weight gain among the early corticosteroid withdrawal group was observed. In contrast, a Dutch study which included 123 patients found no difference in one year post-transplant weight gain between patients who were and were not maintained on low dose steroids (72). In a study of 334 transplant patients at a single institution, average weight gain in patients treated with a steroid taper to 10 mg/day over the course of a year was 28.5% lower compared to the group in whom the steroid dose was tapered to 5mg/day at 6 months (73). The benefits of corticosteroid-sparing regimens on weight gain as well as long-term outcomes are yet uncertain and deserve further study.

7.3 Weight management before and after kidney transplantation

7.3.1 Lifestyle modifications

A multidisciplinary approach to weight management is necessary to maximize weight loss. This approach should utilize all members of the kidney transplant or CKD team including dieticians, nurses, psychologists, social workers and physicians. These members should work together to identify specific needs, motivations, and barriers for each individual patient who requires weight loss. For most patients, a combined approach including diet, exercise and behavior modifications, similar to methods used in the general population, should be applied. Preclusion of kidney transplantation due to obesity generally focuses on BMI thresholds > 35 kg/m^2. Patients with this level of obesity will frequently fail traditional methods for weight loss and surgical interventions should be considered after a trial of lifestyle changes. In the following paragraphs, we describe traditional dietary changes for weight loss and the benefits of exercise in patients with CKD. This is then followed by a discussion of the risks and benefits of weight loss drugs and bariatric surgery.

7.3.2 Dietary interventions for patients not receiving dialysis

Dietary modification remains the most important component of any weight loss intervention and dietary interventions have been shown to be effective in ameliorating weight gain after kidney transplantation (74-76). As weight gain is quite common after kidney transplantation, dietary counseling prior to kidney transplantation with frequent follow-up after transplantation should be done. To aid in developing a plan, a diet history should be obtained and patients can take part in this plan by keeping a food diary for several days. Review of medications that may contribute to weight gain should be completed. While numerous diets exist, none can be universally recommended for patients with CKD including the kidney transplant recipient (77). A conservative approach is to restrict caloric intake by approximately 500 kcal/day, which in the absence of physical activity changes, will lead to a weight loss of 1 pound per week (74). More restrictive diets (<1,200 kcal/day) require more intensive monitoring of the nutritional status and well-being of the patient.

With the exception of protein intake, there are no exact recommendations for specific nutrient and dietary composition for patients with CKD. The American Heart Association guidelines for a healthy lifestyle provide no specific recommendations for diet and state that the exact percentage of carbohydrates, proteins, and fat within a given meal will not in itself influence weight management (78). Addressing portion size and reducing energy intake to less than energy expenditure is the only reliable way to facilitate weight loss (78). High protein diets for weight loss are quite popular and can be successful for some individuals, but data on long-term safety is lacking (79). High protein diets should be avoided in adults with CKD due to concerns that higher protein intake can accelerate loss of GFR (80). Accordingly, the National Kidney Foundation-Kidney Disease Outcomes Quality Initiative (NKF-KDOQI) guidelines recommend that protein intake not exceed 0.8g/kg/day with 50 to 75% of the protein derived from lean poultry, fish, and vegetables (81). This level of protein intake is substantially lower than the average protein intake in many individuals in the U.S. and other countries where protein intake may exceed 1.2 gm/kg/day. Diets such as the Dietary Approaches to Stop Hypertension (DASH) diet emphasize the consumption of fresh fruits and vegetables, whole grains, and low dairy while minimizing red meat intake, sodium intake and processed foods. The DASH diet may provide additional benefits beyond those associated with weight loss (82). However, the DASH diet contains higher levels of protein (1.4 g/kg/d), potassium (4500mg/d), and phosphorus (1.7g/d) than recommended by the NKF-KDOQI guidelines for the CKD patient (74). Specific nutritional recommendations for CKD and kidney transplant recipients remain poorly defined, and more research needs to be done to better define an optimal diet before making specific recommendations. Thus, diet interventions for the CKD patient must be individualized and focus should be on portion size reduction. Identification of excess snacking times (e.g. night time) and intake of nutrient poor yet high calorie foods will help the individual patient reduce their caloric intake. In general, the weight loss goals should not exceed 1 pound per week.

7.3.3 Dietary interventions for patients receiving dialysis

Studies to support dietary recommendations for patients receiving dialysis to promote weight loss are substantially limited. Current guidelines for patients receiving dialysis recommend protein intake of 1.2g/kg/day and 30 to 35 kcal/kg/day for stable patients (81). However, in order to lose weight, obese patients must reduce caloric consumption to less than caloric expenditure. Nutritional plans should be individualized to ensure that the unique nutritional requirements of patients receiving dialysis are met. Food diaries and dietary histories can be used to help identify sources of empty calories. There is no strong evidence to suggest any particular dietary intervention to promote weight loss in patients receiving dialysis. One conservative approach is to start with 25 kcal/kg/d based on the adjusted body weight (ideal body weight - [dry total body weight - ideal body weight]/4) and then adjustments can be made based on the patient's weight loss (45). However, this method is not as reliable as using direct measures of resting energy expenditure to determine caloric needs. Additional research is needed to determine safe and effective interventions for weight loss in this patient population.

7.3.4 Dietary interventions for kidney transplant recipients

Several studies have examined dietary interventions to ameliorate weight gain after kidney transplantation. One single-center study gave 11 consecutive kidney transplant recipients individualized, intensive dietary advice for the first 4 months after transplantation (76). These individuals were then compared to 22 patients who received kidney transplants 4 years prior to the study and had not received dietary advice post-transplantation. Baseline characteristics of the two groups were similar with mean BMI of about 24 kg/m^2 in both groups. The group who received dietary advice showed no statistically significant change in weigh four months after transplantation compared to their pre-transplant weight. In contrast, the group with no dietary intervention had a significant weight gain of 7kg four months after transplantation and

11.8 kg at one year after transplantation (76). Another study enrolled 34 overweight and obese (mean BMI 33 kg/m^2) kidney transplant recipients who were highly motivated to lose weight in a weight loss program (83). During the initial visit, the negative impact of obesity after kidney transplantation was discussed and participants wrote down and reviewed a detailed 3-day history of their own dietary habits but no dietary advice was given. After six months of follow-up, only 27% of those in the weight loss program had weight gain compared to 80% of controls (83). While these two studies were not randomized controlled clinical trials, the study results support a beneficial role for dietary counseling after kidney transplantation. Transplant centers should utilize an approach whereby all potential kidney transplant recipients receive some individualized counseling on lifestyle (diet and physical activity) both before and after kidney transplantation. The use of dietary histories and food diaries are encouraged because it will enable the patient to participate in the development of plans to facilitate changing their own dietary habits.

8. Exercise

Increasing physical activity may promote modest weight loss and improve physical functioning. Patients with CKD are overall a sedentary population with markedly reduced peak maximal oxygen and reduced physical functioning compared to individuals with normal kidney function (84, 85). A study of ambulatory patients new to dialysis found that physical activity scores for these patients were below the 5th percentile of healthy individuals and estimated that 95% of patients initiating dialysis have very low fitness levels (84). Decreased physical activity is associated with excess mortality in adults with CKD (85, 86). Exercise in patients with CKD improves functional aerobic capacity, muscular strength, and blood pressure (87, 88). However, currently there is insufficient evidence to make specific exercise recommendations for patients with CKD. In addition, the co-existence of multiple co-morbid conditions in this patient population limits the capacity to exercise. In any case, considering the poor physical functioning demonstrated in the majority of patients receiving dialysis, exercise should be encouraged if possible (84). Low-to-moderate-intensity aerobic exercise three times per week should be recommended to all patients able to do so, just as it is recommended for the general population (89). The risk of cardiac events during exercise has not been quantified in patients with CKD, but the risks are likely no greater than those occurring during diagnostic tests for cardiovascular disease (3.6 myocardial infarctions per 10,000 tests) (90, 91).

9. Pharmacologic agents for weight loss

Dietary change remains difficult for the majority of individuals and some patients may request weight loss medications to augment weight loss. It should be noted that weight loss medications will only modestly improve weight loss and these drugs are frequently accompanied by substantial side effects. These possible risks and benefits must be discussed with the patient when considering the use of weight loss medications. Moreover, the safety of any weight loss drug should be strongly scrutinized given that two weight loss medications, sibutramine and rimonabant, were removed from the U.S. and European markets due to concerns about heightened risk of cardiovascular disease and suicide, respectively (92, 93). This illustrates the need for extreme caution with any weight loss medication.

In the U.S., the only medication currently approved by the FDA for long-term use is orlistat, which can promote modest weight loss but is accompanied by frequent gastrointestinal side effects. Short-term agents that are FDA-approved such as phentermine or diethylpropion should be avoided in kidney transplant recipients or individuals with CKD due to associated conditions such as hypertension, and cardiovascular disease risk. Thus, the only weight loss medication that potentially could be safe in populations with CKD is orlistat. Orlistat reversibly inhibits gastric and pancreatic lipases and blocks approximately 30% of gastrointestinal absorption of triglycerides. Only a small amount of orlistat is systemically absorbed with 800 mg of orlistat daily yielding minimal plasma concentrations of the drug (94). A small non-randomized trial of orlistat was conducted among patients with stages 3-5 CKD (95). These participants followed a low-fat renal-specific diet, and exercise was encouraged (95). Orlistat was given at the standard dose of 120 mg three times daily and patients were followed for two years. An average of 8.3 kg weight loss was noted and this loss occurred mostly during the initial six month period of the study. However, the weight loss was maintained after two years of follow-up. Gastrointestinal adverse events were common including flatulence, diarrhea, and fatty stools, with 43% reporting at least one side effect in the initial month of therapy. After six months of orlistat use, only 10% reported side effects (95). Thus, orlistat augments weight loss, but only modestly.

Among kidney transplant recipients, orlistat use may complicate the immunosuppressant regimen. Orlistat interferes with cyclosporine absorption because cyclosporine is highly lipid-soluble. To prevent this issue, orlistat should not be taken within a two-hour window of taking cyclosporine and cyclosporine levels should be closely monitored (96, 97). Another concern is the increased risk of oxalate nephropathy with this drug. Although rare, acute kidney injury due to renal oxalosis has been reported in an adult with CKD taking orlistat for weight loss (98). Patients should also be advised that fat intake must be limited to less than 30% of total calories otherwise the patient may experience fecal incontinence. Fat-soluble vitamin deficiencies can also occur with use of orlistat and it is recommended that patients be supplemented with fat-soluble vitamins when taking orlistat (99).

Other pharmacologic agents such as serotonin reuptake inhibitors and buproprion are not approved for long-term use of weight maintenance in the general population, and have not been well-studied in adults with CKD. Over-the-counter dietary supplements should also be discouraged due to a dearth of evidence regarding efficacy, safety, and possible interactions with immunosuppressive medications.

10. Surgical options

Surgical options for weight management should only be considered after lifestyle interventions fail to yield adequate weight loss. These surgical options include procedures that divert food from the stomach into lower parts of the gastrointestinal tract to limit food absorption and reduce the size of the stomach leading to early satiety (Roux-en-Y diversion) and gastric banding (100). An adjustable gastric band placed around the upper part of the stomach may be inflated or deflated by injecting or removing saline through a port underneath the skin (100). Given the procedure is performed by an experienced surgeon, mortality risk is < 2% with gastric banding and approximately 3% with gastric diversion procedures. However, mortality risk may be higher in patients with a BMI≥ 50 kg/m^2 (101, 102). Regardless of the type of procedure, the majority of weight loss occurs during the first year after surgery with greater weight loss consistently occurring with gastric diversion procedures (70.1%) vs. gastric banding (47.5%) (101, 102). Advantages of gastric banding include less hospitalization time and fewer short-term complications (see Table 2) (103). However, long-term complications of gastric banding are higher than gastric diversion procedures albeit less severe. For instance, intragastric band erosion is caused by chronic ischemia of the gastric wall due to the constrictive effects of the band. The gastric band can also migrate and lead to severe abdominal pain and vomiting. A recent report of long-term followup at a center in Belgium reported that approximately 1 out of every 3 patients who underwent gastric banding experienced gastric band erosion with almost half required band removal (104).

	Roux-en-Y Gastric Bypass	Laparoscopic Adjustable Gastric Banding
Mortality	<1%	<1%
Resolution of type 2 diabetes	++	+
Maintenance of weight loss after 2 years	+++	+
Length of hospitalization	2-8 days	1-3 days
Short-term complications	More common	Less common
Long-term complications	Less common, but more serious (i.e. bowel obstruction, marginal ulcer, incisional hernia, nutrient deficiency)	More common, but less serious (i.e. band slippage with pouch dilation, band erosion, port problems)
Reoperation rates§	10-20%	20-60%
Vitamin deficiencies (B vitamins, fat soluble vitamins)	++ (may require substantial supplementation)	+ (often corrected with multivitamin supplement)

*Adapted from Tice et al. (102)
§Reoperation rates from studies with long-term follow-up >24 months (102, 121-123)
Table 2. Comparison of Roux-en-Y Gastric Bypass and Laparoscopic Adjustable Gastric Banding*

Patients receiving dialysis may obtain substantial weight loss allowing for kidney transplantation (105-107), but information on risk and long-term benefits remains limited. Using Medicare claims data during years 1991-2004 linked with the United States Renal Data System, investigators evaluated post-bariatric surgery mortality risk and outcomes (108). On average, patients lost 30-60% of their total pre-surgery body weight. Overall 30-day mortality risk was similar for patients listed for a kidney transplant and for kidney transplant recipients (3.5%). Allograft failure was reported in a patient 30 days after the kidney transplant (108). The largest single-center series of kidney transplant patients reported outcomes for 10 kidney transplant recipients who underwent gastric bypass surgery for excessive weight gain leading to morbid obesity after transplantation (109).

Mean age was 44 years and the gastric bypass surgeries occurred on average 5.3 years after transplantation. In this group, there were no fatalities within the first 30 days after bariatric surgery and patients on average lost 70.5% of their excess weight above ideal weight (109).

Clearly, the substantial weight loss after bariatric surgery can lead to resolution of diabetes and less need for blood pressure lowering medications in adults without CKD. In fact, 98% and 48% of adults with obesity and diabetes no longer have type 2 diabetes two years after undergoing gastric diversion and gastric banding, respectively, for obesity management (102). Other obesity related co-morbid conditions may resolve as well such as fatty liver, hypercholesterolemia and sleep apnea (101). These long-term benefits likely apply to patients with CKD, but the surgical risks may be heightened in this population. Gastric band erosion has been reported in a kidney transplant recipient treated with gastric banding for weight management (110). While these surgical complications are not unique to the transplant population, the presence of immunosuppressant agents could worsen the side effects of bariatric surgery.

Nutritional deficiencies are common after bariatric surgery for weight loss and this may be complicated by poor nutritional choices of the individual patient. Patients may become deficient in iron, calcium, B vitamins and fat soluble vitamins (101). An important complication of gastric bypass surgery includes increased oxalate absorption due to decreased intestinal absorption of fatty acids, and this could lead to kidney stones, renal oxalosis, acute kidney injury, allograft loss and even oxalate-induced anemia (111-115). The Roux-en-Y surgery results in a smaller gastric pouch which may not produce as much acid, and as a result, the higher stomach pH and the smaller surface area of both stomach and small intestine may impact the absorption of some drugs (116, 117). It should be noted that increased cyclosporine dosing may be required after gastric diversion procedures (117). The pharmacokinetics of tacrolimus, mycophenolate, and sirolimus may also change after gastric diversion, and higher doses of several immunosuppressants may be needed after gastric bypass (116). Obese patients often require lower doses of cyclosporine per body weight compared to lean recipients (118, 119) and dosing for cyclosporine based on ideal body weight is recommended (118-120). Given the excessive weight loss which occurs rapidly after bariatric surgery, levels of immunosuppressant drugs including mycophenolate mofetil, should be followed closely after gastric bypass surgery, especially during the first 18 months after bariatric surgery.

Due to the lack of information on long-term consequences of bariatric surgery, no specific recommendations can be made for patients with CKD or kidney transplant recipients. Thus, the decision to utilize bariatric surgery for weight management needs to be individualized. Most importantly, clinicians must ensure that these patients are informed of the associated risks before they proceed with surgical interventions for obesity management.

Regardless of obesity status, kidney transplantation is associated with improved survival and decreased morbidity compared to dialysis. Thus, obesity may be viewed as the most important modifiable mortality risk factor for patients precluded from kidney transplantation due to obesity status. Weight management should include a multi-disciplinary approach with dietary advice on caloric restriction and encouragement to increase physical activity. Patients should actively take part in the development of the obesity management plan (e.g. keep food diary). If lifestyle interventions fail to yield adequate weight loss, then surgical options should be considered. Clinicians should discuss frankly the potential risk of bariatric surgery for weight management. Transplant centers should also incorporate dietary counseling both before and after kidney transplantation to ameliorate weight gain after transplantation which may heighten cardiovascular risk. Future research should address the use of both BMI and waist circumference to improve risk stratification and obesity interventions for patients before and after kidney transplantation.

11. References

[1] Metropolitan Life Insurance Company. New weight standards for men and women. Stat Bull Metropol Life Insur Co 1959;40:1–4.

[2] Kuczmarski RJ, Flegal KM. Criteria for definition of overweight in transition: background and recommendations for the united states. Am J Clin Nutr. 2000 Nov;72(5):1074-81.

[3] WHO: Obesity: Preventing and managing the global epidemic: Report of a WHO Consultation on Obesity, Geneva, June 3-5, 1997. Geneva, Switzerland, World Health Organization, 1998.

[4] Adams KF, Schatzkin A, Harris TB, Kipnis V, Mouw T, Ballard-Barbash R, et al. Overweight, obesity, and mortality in a large prospective cohort of persons 50 to 71 years old. N Engl J Med. 2006 Aug 24;355(8):763-78.

[5] Fontaine KR, Redden DT, Wang C, Westfall AO, Allison DB. Years of life lost due to obesity. JAMA. 2003 Jan 8;289(2):187-93.

[6] Peeters A, Barendregt JJ, Willekens F, Mackenbach JP, Al Mamun A, Bonneux L, et al. Obesity in adulthood and its consequences for life expectancy: A life-table analysis. Ann Intern Med. 2003 Jan 7;138(1):24-32.

[7] Stevens J, Cai J, Pamuk ER, Williamson DF, Thun MJ, Wood JL. The effect of age on the association between body-mass index and mortality. N Engl J Med. 1998 Jan 1;338(1):1-7.

[8] Heiat A, Vaccarino V, Krumholz HM. An evidence-based assessment of federal guidelines for overweight and obesity as they apply to elderly persons. Arch Intern Med. 2001 May 14;161(9):1194-203.

[9] Bigaard J, Frederiksen K, Tjonneland A, Thomsen BL, Overvad K, Heitmann BL, et al. Waist circumference and body composition in relation to all-cause mortality in middle-aged men and women. Int J Obes (Lond). 2005 Jul;29(7):778-84.

[10] Haslam DW, James WP. Obesity. Lancet. 2005 Oct 1;366(9492):1197-209.

[11] Rankinen T, Kim SY, Perusse L, Despres JP, Bouchard C. The prediction of abdominal visceral fat level from body composition and anthropometry: ROC analysis. Int J Obes Relat Metab Disord. 1999 Aug;23(8):801-9.

[12] Reeder BA, Senthilselvan A, Despres JP, Angel A, Liu L, Wang H, et al. The association of cardiovascular disease risk factors with abdominal obesity in canada. canadian heart health surveys research group. CMAJ. 1997 Jul 1;157 Suppl 1:S39-45.

[13] Pouliot MC, Despres JP, Lemieux S, Moorjani S, Bouchard C, Tremblay A, et al. Waist circumference and abdominal sagittal diameter: Best simple anthropometric indexes of abdominal visceral adipose tissue accumulation and related cardiovascular risk in men and women. Am J Cardiol. 1994 Mar 1;73(7):460-8.

[14] Lean ME, Han TS, Morrison CE. Waist circumference as a measure for indicating need for weight management. BMJ. 1995 Jul 15;311(6998):158-61.

[15] Narisawa S, Nakamura K, Kato K, Yamada K, Sasaki J, Yamamoto M. Appropriate waist circumference cutoff values for persons with multiple cardiovascular risk factors in japan: A large cross-sectional study. J Epidemiol. 2008;18(1):37-42.

[16] Janssen I, Katzmarzyk PT, Ross R. Body mass index, waist circumference, and health risk: Evidence in support of current national institutes of health guidelines. Arch Intern Med. 2002 Oct 14;162(18):2074-9.
[17] Balkau B, Deanfield JE, Despres JP, Bassand JP, Fox KA, Smith SC,Jr, et al. International day for the evaluation of abdominal obesity (IDEA): A study of waist circumference, cardiovascular disease, and diabetes mellitus in 168,000 primary care patients in 63 countries. Circulation. 2007 Oct 23;116(17):1942-51.
[18] Koster A, Leitzmann MF, Schatzkin A, Mouw T, Adams KF, van Eijk JT, et al. Waist circumference and mortality. Am J Epidemiol. 2008 Jun 15;167(12):1465-75.
[19] Mokdad AH, Ford ES, Bowman BA, Dietz WH, Vinicor F, Bales VS, et al. Prevalence of obesity, diabetes, and obesity-related health risk factors, 2001. JAMA. 2003 Jan 1;289(1):76-9.
[20] Kramer HJ, Saranathan A, Luke A, Durazo-Arvizu RA, Guichan C, Hou S, et al. Increasing body mass index and obesity in the incident ESRD population. J Am Soc Nephrol. 2006 May;17(5):1453-9.
[21] Friedman AN, Miskulin DC, Rosenberg IH, Levey AS. Demographics and trends in overweight and obesity in patients at time of kidney transplantation. Am J Kidney Dis. 2003 Feb;41(2):480-7.
[22] Kalantar-Zadeh K, Kopple JD. Obesity paradox in patients on maintenance dialysis. Contrib Nephrol. 2006;151:57-69.
[23] Kalantar-Zadeh K, Kopple JD, Kilpatrick RD, McAllister CJ, Shinaberger CS, Gjertson DW, et al. Association of morbid obesity and weight change over time with cardiovascular survival in hemodialysis population. Am J Kidney Dis. 2005 Sep;46(3):489-500.
[24] Kovesdy CP, Czira ME, Rudas A, Ujszaszi A, Rosivall L, Novak M, et al. Body mass index, waist circumference and mortality in kidney transplant recipients. Am J Transplant. 2010 Dec;10(12):2644-51.
[25] Madero M, Sarnak MJ, Wang X, Sceppa CC, Greene T, Beck GJ, et al. Body mass index and mortality in CKD. Am J Kidney Dis. 2007 Sep;50(3):404-11.
[26] Kwan BC, Murtaugh MA, Beddhu S. Associations of body size with metabolic syndrome and mortality in moderate chronic kidney disease. Clin J Am Soc Nephrol. 2007 Sep;2(5):992-8.
[27] Elsayed EF, Tighiouart H, Weiner DE, Griffith J, Salem D, Levey AS, et al. Waist-to-hip ratio and body mass index as risk factors for cardiovascular events in CKD. Am J Kidney Dis. 2008 Jul;52(1):49-57.
[28] Kalantar-Zadeh K, Kopple JD. Obesity paradox in patients on maintenance dialysis. Contrib Nephrol. 2006;151:57-69.
[29] Kalantar-Zadeh K, Kopple JD, Kilpatrick RD, McAllister CJ, Shinaberger CS, Gjertson DW, et al. Association of morbid obesity and weight change over time with cardiovascular survival in hemodialysis population. Am J Kidney Dis. 2005 Sep;46(3):489-500.
[30] Kalantar-Zadeh K, Kuwae N, Wu DY, Shantouf RS, Fouque D, Anker SD, et al. Associations of body fat and its changes over time with quality of life and prospective mortality in hemodialysis patients. Am J Clin Nutr. 2006 Feb;83(2):202-10.

[31] Johansen KL, Young B, Kaysen GA, Chertow GM. Association of body size with outcomes among patients beginning dialysis. Am J Clin Nutr. 2004 Aug;80(2):324-32.
[32] Postorino M, Marino C, Tripepi G, Zoccali C, CREDIT (Calabria Registry of Dialysis and Transplantation) Working Group. Abdominal obesity and all-cause and cardiovascular mortality in end-stage renal disease. J Am Coll Cardiol. 2009 Apr 14;53(15):1265-72.
[33] Beddhu S, Pappas LM, Ramkumar N, Samore M. Effects of body size and body composition on survival in hemodialysis patients. J Am Soc Nephrol. 2003 Sep;14(9):2366-72.
[34] Kovesdy CP, Czira ME, Rudas A, Ujszaszi A, Rosivall L, Novak M, et al. Body mass index, waist circumference and mortality in kidney transplant recipients. Am J Transplant. 2010 Dec;10(12):2644-51.
[35] Holley JL, Monaghan J, Byer B, Bronsther O. An examination of the renal transplant evaluation process focusing on cost and the reasons for patient exclusion. Am J Kidney Dis. 1998 Oct;32(4):567-74.
[36] Scandling JD. Kidney transplant candidate evaluation. Semin Dial. 2005 Nov-Dec;18(6):487-94.
[37] Potluri K, Hou S. Obesity in kidney transplant recipients and candidates. Am J Kidney Dis. 2010 Jul;56(1):143-56.
[38] Segev DL, Simpkins CE, Thompson RE, Locke JE, Warren DS, Montgomery RA. Obesity impacts access to kidney transplantation. J Am Soc Nephrol. 2008 Feb;19(2):349-55.
[39] Johnson DW, Isbel NM, Brown AM, Kay TD, Franzen K, Hawley CM, et al. The effect of obesity on renal transplant outcomes. Transplantation. 2002 Sep 15;74(5):675-81.
[40] Gore JL, Pham PT, Danovitch GM, Wilkinson AH, Rosenthal JT, Lipshutz GS, et al. Obesity and outcome following renal transplantation. Am J Transplant. 2006 Feb;6(2):357-63.
[41] Meier-Kriesche HU, Arndorfer JA, Kaplan B. The impact of body mass index on renal transplant outcomes: A significant independent risk factor for graft failure and patient death. Transplantation. 2002 Jan 15;73(1):70-4.
[42] Chang SH, Coates PT, McDonald SP. Effects of body mass index at transplant on outcomes of kidney transplantation. Transplantation. 2007 Oct 27;84(8):981-7.
[43] Pelletier SJ, Maraschio MA, Schaubel DE, Dykstra DM, Punch JD, Wolfe RA, et al. Survival benefit of kidney and liver transplantation for obese patients on the waiting list. Clin Transpl. 2003:77-88.
[44] Glanton CW, Kao TC, Cruess D, Agodoa LY, Abbott KC. Impact of renal transplantation on survival in end-stage renal disease patients with elevated body mass index. Kidney Int. 2003 Feb;63(2):647-53.
[45] Kramer H, Tuttle KR, Leehey D, Luke A, Durazo-Arvizu R, Shoham D, et al. Obesity management in adults with CKD. Am J Kidney Dis. 2009 Jan;53(1):151-65.
[46] Bennett WM, McEvoy KM, Henell KR, Valente JF, Douzdjian V. Morbid obesity does not preclude successful renal transplantation. Clin Transplant. 2004 Feb;18(1):89-93.
[47] Drafts HH, Anjum MR, Wynn JJ, Mulloy LL, Bowley JN, Humphries AL. The impact of pre-transplant obesity on renal transplant outcomes. Clin Transplant. 1997 Oct;11(5 Pt 2):493-6.

[48] Howard RJ, Thai VB, Patton PR, Hemming AW, Reed AI, Van der Werf WJ, et al. Obesity does not portend a bad outcome for kidney transplant recipients. Transplantation. 2002 Jan 15;73(1):53-5.
[49] Johnson CP, Gallagher-Lepak S, Zhu YR, Porth C, Kelber S, Roza AM, et al. Factors influencing weight gain after renal transplantation. Transplantation. 1993 Oct;56(4):822-7.
[50] Merion RM, Twork AM, Rosenberg L, Ham JM, Burtch GD, Turcotte JG, et al. Obesity and renal transplantation. Surg Gynecol Obstet. 1991 May;172(5):367-76.
[51] Modlin CS, Flechner SM, Goormastic M, Goldfarb DA, Papajcik D, Mastroianni B, et al. Should obese patients lose weight before receiving a kidney transplant? Transplantation. 1997 Aug 27;64(4):599-604.
[52] Marks WH, Florence LS, Chapman PH, Precht AF, Perkinson DT. Morbid obesity is not a contraindication to kidney transplantation. Am J Surg. 2004 May;187(5):635-8.
[53] Yamamoto S, Hanley E, Hahn AB, Isenberg A, Singh TP, Cohen D, et al. The impact of obesity in renal transplantation: An analysis of paired cadaver kidneys. Clin Transplant. 2002 Aug;16(4):252-6.
[54] Halme L, Eklund B, Salmela K. Obesity and renal transplantation. Transplant Proc. 1995 Dec;27(6):3444-5.
[55] Holley JL, Shapiro R, Lopatin WB, Tzakis AG, Hakala TR, Starzl TE. Obesity as a risk factor following cadaveric renal transplantation. Transplantation. 1990 Feb; 49(2): 387-9.
[56] Meier-Kriesche HU, Vaghela M, Thambuganipalle R, Friedman G, Jacobs M, Kaplan B. The effect of body mass index on long-term renal allograft survival. Transplantation. 1999 Nov 15;68(9):1294-7.
[57] Snow V, Barry P, Fitterman N, Qaseem A, Weiss K, Clinical Efficacy Assessment Subcommittee of t5he American College of Physicians. Pharmacologic and surgical management of obesity in primary care: A clinical practice guideline from the american college of physicians. Ann Intern Med. 2005 Apr 5;142(7):525-31.
[58] Morales E, Valero MA, Leon M, Hernandez E, Praga M. Beneficial effects of weight loss in overweight patients with chronic proteinuric nephropathies. Am J Kidney Dis. 2003 Feb;41(2):319-27.
[59] Praga M, Hernandez E, Andres A, Leon M, Ruilope LM, Rodicio JL. Effects of body-weight loss and captopril treatment on proteinuria associated with obesity. Nephron. 1995;70(1):35-41.
[60] Palomar R, Fernandez-Fresnedo G, Dominguez-Diez A, Lopez-Deogracias M, Olmedo F, Martin de Francisco AL, et al. Effects of weight loss after biliopancreatic diversion on metabolism and cardiovascular profile. Obes Surg. 2005 Jun-Jul;15(6):794-8.
[61] Navarro-Diaz M, Serra A, Romero R, Bonet J, Bayes B, Homs M, et al. Effect of drastic weight loss after bariatric surgery on renal parameters in extremely obese patients: Long-term follow-up. J Am Soc Nephrol. 2006 Dec;17(12 Suppl 3):S213-7.
[62] Serra A, Granada ML, Romero R, Bayes B, Canton A, Bonet J, et al. The effect of bariatric surgery on adipocytokines, renal parameters and other cardiovascular risk factors in severe and very severe obesity: 1-year follow-up. Clin Nutr. 2006 Jun;25(3):400-8.

[63] Chagnac A, Weinstein T, Herman M, Hirsh J, Gafter U, Ori Y. The effects of weight loss on renal function in patients with severe obesity. J Am Soc Nephrol. 2003 Jun;14(6):1480-6.
[64] Clunk JM, Lin CY, Curtis JJ. Variables affecting weight gain in renal transplant recipients. Am J Kidney Dis. 2001 Aug;38(2):349-53.
[65] Kasiske BL. Cardiovascular disease after renal transplantation. Semin Nephrol. 2000 Mar;20(2):176-87.
[66] Chang SH, McDonald SP. Post-kidney transplant weight change as marker of poor survival outcomes. Transplantation. 2008 May 27;85(10):1443-8.
[67] Baum CL, Thielke K, Westin E, Kogan E, Cicalese L, Benedetti E. Predictors of weight gain and cardiovascular risk in a cohort of racially diverse kidney transplant recipients. Nutrition. 2002 Feb;18(2):139-46.
[68] Marcen R. Immunosuppressive drugs in kidney transplantation: Impact on patient survival, and incidence of cardiovascular disease, malignancy and infection. Drugs. 2009 Nov 12;69(16):2227-43.
[69] Augustine JJ, Hricik DE. Steroid sparing in kidney transplantation: Changing paradigms, improving outcomes, and remaining questions. Clin J Am Soc Nephrol. 2006 Sep;1(5):1080-9.
[70] Elster EA, Leeser DB, Morrissette C, Pepek JM, Quiko A, Hale DA, et al. Obesity following kidney transplantation and steroid avoidance immunosuppression. Clin Transplant. 2008 May-Jun;22(3):354-9.
[71] Rogers CC, Alloway RR, Buell JF, Boardman R, Alexander JW, Cardi M, et al. Body weight alterations under early corticosteroid withdrawal and chronic corticosteroid therapy with modern immunosuppression. Transplantation. 2005 Jul 15;80(1):26-33.
[72] van den Ham EC, Kooman JP, Christiaans MH, Nieman FH, van Hooff JP. Weight changes after renal transplantation: A comparison between patients on 5-mg maintenance steroid therapy and those on steroid-free immunosuppressive therapy. Transpl Int. 2003 May;16(5):300-6.
[73] Marcic S, kramer H, luke A, holt DR, hou SH. risk factors for weight gain following renal transplantation. abstract presented at 37th annual meeting of the american society of nephrology; october 29-november 1, 2004; st. louis, MO. .
[74] Eckel RH. Clinical practice. nonsurgical management of obesity in adults. N Engl J Med. 2008 May 1;358(18):1941-50.
[75] Guida B, Trio R, Laccetti R, Nastasi A, Salvi E, Perrino NR, et al. Role of dietary intervention on metabolic abnormalities and nutritional status after renal transplantation. Nephrol Dial Transplant. 2007 Nov;22(11):3304-10.
[76] Patel MG. The effect of dietary intervention on weight gains after renal transplantation. J Ren Nutr. 1998 Jul;8(3):137-41.
[77] Packard DP, Milton JE, Shuler LA, Short RA, Tuttle KR. Implications of chronic kidney disease for dietary treatment in cardiovascular disease. J Ren Nutr. 2006 Jul;16(3):259-68.
[78] Lichtenstein AH, appel LJ, brands M, et al, for the American Heart Association Nutrition Committee: Diet and lifestyle recommendations revision 2006: A scientific statement from the American Heart Association Nutrition Committee [erratum in Circulation 114:E629, 2006]. Circulation 114:82-96, 2006.

[79] Kennedy ET, Bowman SA, Spence JT, Freedman M, King J. Popular diets: Correlation to health, nutrition, and obesity. J Am Diet Assoc. 2001 Apr;101(4):411-20.
[80] Levey AS, Adler S, Caggiula AW, England BK, Greene T, Hunsicker LG, et al. Effects of dietary protein restriction on the progression of advanced renal disease in the modification of diet in renal disease study. Am J Kidney Dis. 1996 May;27(5):652-63.
[81] National kidney foundation: K/DOQI clinical practice guidelines for nutrition in chronic renal failure.am JKidney dis 35:S1-S140, 2000 (suppl 2).
[82] Appel LJ, Moore TJ, Obarzanek E, Vollmer WM, Svetkey LP, Sacks FM, et al. A clinical trial of the effects of dietary patterns on blood pressure. DASH collaborative research group. N Engl J Med. 1997 Apr 17;336(16):1117-24.
[83] Jezior D, Krajewska M, Madziarska K, Regulska-Ilow B, Ilow R, Janczak D, et al. Weight reduction in renal transplant recipients program: The first successes. Transplant Proc. 2007 Nov;39(9):2769-71.
[84] Johansen KL, Kutner NG, Young B, Chertow GM. Association of body size with health status in patients beginning dialysis. Am J Clin Nutr. 2006 Mar;83(3):543-9.
[85] Johansen KL. Exercise and chronic kidney disease: Current recommendations. Sports Med. 2005;35(6):485-99.
[86] Beddhu S, Baird BC, Zitterkoph J, Neilson J, Greene T. Physical activity and mortality in chronic kidney disease (NHANES III). Clin J Am Soc Nephrol. 2009 Dec;4(12):1901-6.
[87] Moinuddin I, Leehey DJ. A comparison of aerobic exercise and resistance training in patients with and without chronic kidney disease. Adv Chronic Kidney Dis. 2008 Jan;15(1):83-96.
[88] Boyce ML, Robergs RA, Avasthi PS, Roldan C, Foster A, Montner P, et al. Exercise training by individuals with predialysis renal failure: Cardiorespiratory endurance, hypertension, and renal function. Am J Kidney Dis. 1997 Aug;30(2):180-92.
[89] Office of the US surgeon general. physical activity and health a report of the surgeon general. washington, DC: US department of health and human services, national center for chronic disease prevention and health promotion, 1996. .
[90] Copley JB, Lindberg JS. The risks of exercise. Adv Ren Replace Ther. 1999 Apr;6(2):165-71.
[91] Haskell WL. Cardiovascular complications during exercise training of cardiac patients. Circulation. 1978 May;57(5):920-4.
[92] FDA. FDA drug safety communication: FDA recommends against the continued use of Meridia (sibutramine). http://www.fda.gov/Drugs/DrugSafety/PostmarketDrugSafetyInformationforPatientsandProviders/ucm191652.htm (accessed March 26, 2011).
[93] European Medicines Agency. Public statement on Zimulti: Withdrawal of the marketing authorisation in the European Union. http://www.ema.europa.eu/ema/index.jsp?curl=pages/news_and_events/news/2009/11/news_detail_000125.jsp&jsenabled=true (accessed March 26, 2011).
[94] Henness S, Perry CM. Orlistat: A review of its use in the management of obesity. Drugs. 2006;66(12):1625-56.
[95] MacLaughlin HL, Cook SA, Kariyawasam D, Roseke M, van Niekerk M, Macdougall IC. Nonrandomized trial of weight loss with orlistat, nutrition education, diet, and

exercise in obese patients with CKD: 2-year follow-up. Am J Kidney Dis. 2010 Jan;55(1):69-76.
[96] Zhi J, Moore R, Kanitra L, Mulligan TE. Pharmacokinetic evaluation of the possible interaction between selected concomitant medications and orlistat at steady state in healthy subjects. J Clin Pharmacol. 2002 Sep;42(9):1011-9.
[97] Nagele H, Petersen B, Bonacker U, Rodiger W. Effect of orlistat on blood cyclosporin concentration in an obese heart transplant patient. Eur J Clin Pharmacol. 1999 Nov;55(9):667-9.
[98] Singh A, Sarkar SR, Gaber LW, Perazella MA. Acute oxalate nephropathy associated with orlistat, a gastrointestinal lipase inhibitor. Am J Kidney Dis. 2007 Jan;49(1):153-7.
Finer N, James WP, Kopelman PG, Lean ME, Williams G. One-year treatment of obesity: A randomized, double-blind, placebo-controlled, multicentre study of orlistat, a gastrointestinal lipase inhibitor. Int J Obes Relat Metab Disord. 2000 Mar;24(3):306-13.
[99] Phurrough S, salive M, brechner R, tillman K, harrison S, O'Connor D: Decision memo for bariatric surgery for the treatment of morbid obesity 2006. available at http://www.cms.hhs.gov/mcd/viewdecisionmemo.asp ?id_160. accessed march 22, 2011.
[100] Bouldin MJ, Ross LA, Sumrall CD, Loustalot FV, Low AK, Land KK. The effect of obesity surgery on obesity comorbidity. Am J Med Sci. 2006 Apr;331(4):183-93.
[101] Buchwald H, Avidor Y, Braunwald E, Jensen MD, Pories W, Fahrbach K, et al. Bariatric surgery: A systematic review and meta-analysis. JAMA. 2004 Oct 13;292(14):1724-37.
[102] Tice JA, Karliner L, Walsh J, Petersen AJ, Feldman MD. Gastric banding or bypass? A systematic review comparing the two most popular bariatric procedures. Am J Med. 2008 Oct;121(10):885-93.
[103] Himpens J, Cadiere GB, Bazi M, Vouche M, Cadiere B, Dapri G. Long-term outcomes of laparoscopic adjustable gastric banding. Arch Surg. 2011 Mar 21.
[104] Koshy AN, Coombes JS, Wilkinson S, Fassett RG. Laparoscopic gastric banding surgery performed in obese dialysis patients prior to kidney transplantation. Am J Kidney Dis. 2008 Oct;52(4):e15-7.
[105] Newcombe V, Blanch A, Slater GH, Szold A, Fielding GA. Laparoscopic adjustable gastric banding prior to renal transplantation. Obes Surg. 2005 Apr;15(4):567-70.
[106] Takata MC, Campos GM, Ciovica R, Rabl C, Rogers SJ, Cello JP, et al. Laparoscopic bariatric surgery improves candidacy in morbidly obese patients awaiting transplantation. Surg Obes Relat Dis. 2008 Mar-Apr;4(2):159,64; discussion 164-5.
[107] Modanlou KA, Muthyala U, Xiao H, Schnitzler MA, Salvalaggio PR, Brennan DC, et al. Bariatric surgery among kidney transplant candidates and recipients: Analysis of the united states renal data system and literature review. Transplantation. 2009 Apr 27;87(8):1167-73.
[108] Alexander JW, Goodman H. Gastric bypass in chronic renal failure and renal transplant. Nutr Clin Pract. 2007 Feb;22(1):16-21.
[109] Buch KE, El-Sabrout R, Butt KM. Complications of laparoscopic gastric banding in renal transplant recipients: A case study. Transplant Proc. 2006 Nov;38(9):3109-11.

[110] Asplin JR, Coe FL. Hyperoxaluria in kidney stone formers treated with modern bariatric surgery. J Urol. 2007 Feb;177(2):565-9.
[111] Nelson WK, Houghton SG, Milliner DS, Lieske JC, Sarr MG. Enteric hyperoxaluria, nephrolithiasis, and oxalate nephropathy: Potentially serious and unappreciated complications of roux-en-Y gastric bypass. Surg Obes Relat Dis. 2005 Sep-Oct;1(5):481-5.
[112] Nasr SH, D'Agati VD, Said SM, Stokes MB, Largoza MV, Radhakrishnan J, et al. Oxalate nephropathy complicating roux-en-Y gastric bypass: An underrecognized cause of irreversible renal failure. Clin J Am Soc Nephrol. 2008 Nov;3(6):1676-83.
[113] Sinha MK, Collazo-Clavell ML, Rule A, Milliner DS, Nelson W, Sarr MG, et al. Hyperoxaluric nephrolithiasis is a complication of roux-en-Y gastric bypass surgery. Kidney Int. 2007 Jul;72(1):100-7.
[114] Bernhardt WM, Schefold JC, Weichert W, Rudolph B, Frei U, Groneberg DA, et al. Amelioration of anemia after kidney transplantation in severe secondary oxalosis. Clin Nephrol. 2006 Mar;65(3):216-21.
[115] Rogers CC, Alloway RR, Alexander JW, Cardi M, Trofe J, Vinks AA. Pharmacokinetics of mycophenolic acid, tacrolimus and sirolimus after gastric bypass surgery in end-stage renal disease and transplant patients: A pilot study. Clin Transplant. 2008 May-Jun;22(3):281-91.
[116] Alexander JW, Goodman HR, Gersin K, Cardi M, Austin J, Goel S, et al. Gastric bypass in morbidly obese patients with chronic renal failure and kidney transplant. Transplantation. 2004 Aug 15;78(3):469-74.
[117] Orofino L, Pascual J, Quereda C, Burgos J, Marcen R, Ortuno J. Influence of overweight on survival of kidney transplant. Nephrol Dial Transplant. 1997 Apr;12(4):855.
[118] Kasap B, Soylu A, Turkmen M, Kavukcu S, Bora S, Gulay H. Effect of obesity and overweight on cyclosporine blood levels and renal functions in renal adolescent recipients. Transplant Proc. 2006 Mar;38(2):463-5.
[119] Flechner SM, Kolbeinsson ME, Tam J, Lum B. The impact of body weight on cyclosporine pharmacokinetics in renal transplant recipients. Transplantation. 1989 May;47(5):806-10.
[120] Rodrigo E, de Cos MA, Sanchez B, Ruiz JC, Pinera C, Fernandez-Fresnedo G, et al. High initial blood levels of tacrolimus in overweight renal transplant recipients. Transplant Proc. 2005 Apr;37(3):1453-4.
[121] Sjöström L, Narbro K, Sjöström CD, Karason K, et al. Swedish Obese Subjects Study. Effects of bariatric surgery on mortality in Swedish obese subjects. N Engl J Med. 2007 Aug 23;357(8):741-52.
[122] Suter M, Calmes JM, Paroz A, Giusti V. A 10-year experience with laparoscopic gastric banding for morbid obesity: high long-term complication and failure rates. Obes Surg. 2006 Jul;16(7):829-35.
[123] Mittermair RP, Obermüller S, Perathoner A, Sieb M, Aigner F, Margreiter R. Results and complications after Swedish adjustable gastric banding-10 years experience. Obes Surg. 2009 Dec;19(12):1636-41.

8

The Impact of Donor Type and Quality on Renal Transplant Outcomes

Hung Do Nguyen[1], Kenneth Yong[1,2], Rebecca Croke[1] and Wai H Lim[1,2]
[1]*Sir Charles Gairdner Hospital, Department of Renal Medicine, Western Australia*
[2]*University of Western Australia, Western Australia*
Australia

1. Introduction

Renal transplantation improves survival of patients with end-stage kidney disease (ESKD) (Wolfe, McCullough et al. 2009). In most countries, including the United States and Australia, there continues to be a growing disparity between the limited availability of deceased-donor kidneys compared to potential transplant candidates. In contrast, live-donor kidney transplantation has been steadily increasing over time. It has been well established that the type (live or deceased donor kidneys) and quality (donor age and presence of donor comorbidities) of donor kidneys have a significant impact on renal allograft outcomes. In this chapter, we will focus on both live-donor and deceased donor kidney transplantation and the impact of donor factors and types on graft and patient outcomes. With the continuing shortage of deceased donor kidneys coupled with a growing number of older transplant candidates, there has been a greater acceptance of using older donor kidneys, including increased utility of expanded criteria donor (ECD) and donation after cardiac death (DCD) kidneys. We will look at the impact of using ECD and DCD kidneys on graft and patient survival, and to identify modifiable factors that may improve transplant outcomes in recipients receiving ECD and DCD kidneys. Finally, we will discuss whether the implementation of utility-based allocation strategies for deceased donor kidneys is an appropriate way forward to provide a balance between utility and equity in the distribution of deceased donor kidneys.

2. Live-donor kidney transplantation

Since its introduction over 50 years ago, live-donor kidney transplantation is associated with better graft and patient outcomes compared with deceased donor kidney transplantation. The majority of live-related kidney transplantation is from siblings and parents, although spousal donation is becoming increasingly more common. There have been many live donor factors that have been identified which could affect transplant outcomes and this will be discussed in greater details in this chapter.

2.1 Trends In live donor transplantation

Live-donor renal transplantation has increased considerably over time, with some countries like the United States and Australia reporting an increase of at least 50% over the past decade(Horvat, Shariff et al. 2009). Even in countries without a deceased donor renal transplant program such as the Middle East and Asia, live-donor renal transplantation continues to grow substantially(Ghods and Savaj 2006; Horvat, Shariff et al. 2009). It is currently estimated that live-donor renal transplantation accounts for over 40% of total renal transplant numbers worldwide. According to the Australia and New Zealand Dialysis and Transplant (ANZDATA) Registry report, the proportion of live-donor renal transplantation has increased from 31% in 1998 to 44% in 2008 (Figure 1)(Campbell, McDonald et al. 2009). Similar increases have been reported in other countries including Europe and the United States (De Meester 1998; Oosterlee and Rahmel 2008; Horvat, Shariff et al. 2009; US Organ Procurement and Transplantation Network and Scientific Registry of Transplant Recipients 2009; ERA-EDTA Registry 2010).

Within the United States, Europe and Australia, the increased rates of live-donor renal transplantation are directly attributable to growth of live-unrelated donor (LURD) kidney transplants (Oosterlee and Rahmel 2008; Campbell, McDonald et al. 2009; US Organ Procurement and Transplantation Network and Scientific Registry of Transplant Recipients 2009; ERA-EDTA Registry 2010). In Australia, the proportion of LURD has increased substantially from 31% of overall live-donor transplants in 2000 to 50% in 2008. The majority of live-related donor (LRD) kidney transplants are from parental or sibling donors, whereas spousal donation accounts for the majority of LURD transplants. Furthermore, the adoption of laparoscopic donor nephrectomy techniques coupled with low rates of short- and long-term complications of kidney donation has also contributed significantly to the expansion of live-donor transplantation (Bia, Ramos et al. 1995; Schweitzer, Wilson et al. 2000).

Finally, there is greater acceptance of older live-donors over the past decade despite donor age having been shown to affect renal transplant outcomes. In the United States, the proportion of older donors >50 years age has increased by almost 7% between 1999 and 2008, with similar proportional increase in other countries (US Organ Procurement and Transplantation Network and Scientific Registry of Transplant Recipients 2009).

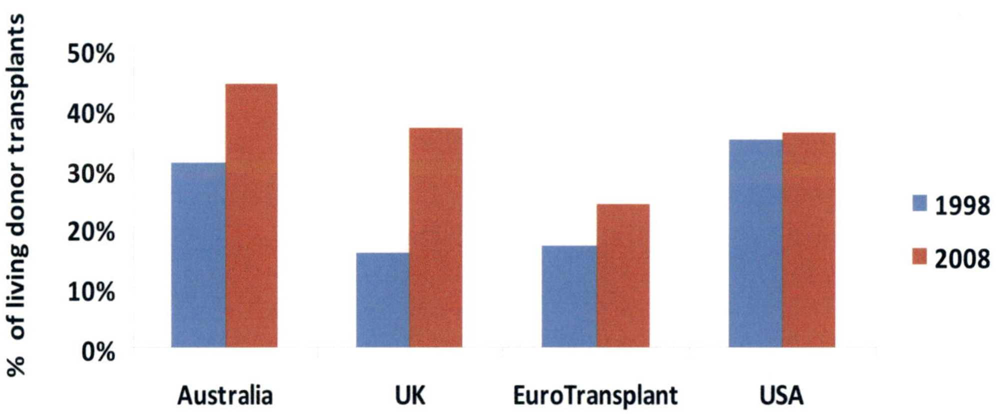

Fig. 1. Living donor transplants as proportion of total transplants.

2.2 Outcome of live compared to deceased-donor kidney transplantation

Live-donor transplantation is associated with superior graft and patient outcomes compared with deceased-donor transplantation (Table 1) (Terasaki, Cecka et al. 1995; Gjertson and Cecka 2000; Campbell, McDonald et al. 2009; US Organ Procurement and Transplantation Network and Scientific Registry of Transplant Recipients 2009). In addition, the introduction of pre-emptive live-donor renal transplantation provides ESKD patients the option of avoiding dialysis (Mange, Joffe et al. 2001; Meier-Kriesche and Kaplan 2002; Liem and Weimar 2009). Finally, it has been established by several large single centre and registry studies that the superior outcomes of live-donor transplantation occur independently of human leukocyte antigen (HLA)-matching and donor or recipient characteristics (Terasaki, Cecka et al. 1995; Gjertson and Cecka 2000; Fuggle, Allen et al. 2010).

Large registry analyses from the United States, Europe and Australia have demonstrated a significant graft and/or patient survival advantage and possibly reduction in rejection risk in pre-emptive live-donor transplants compared to non-pre-emptive live-donor transplants, possibly related to avoidance of dialysis exposure (Donelly, Oman et al. 1995; Mange, Joffe et al. 2001; Milton, Russ et al. 2008). However, one study suggested that short duration of dialysis of <90 days prior to transplant had comparable graft survival to pre-emptive transplant recipients (Milton, Russ et al. 2008). Interestingly, unlike pre-emptive live-donor transplantation, pre-emptive deceased donor transplantation does not appear to be associated with improved graft or patient survival compared to non-pre-emptive deceased donor transplantation (Kessler, Ladriere et al. 2011).

		1 year graft / patient survival	5 year graft / patient survival	10 year graft / patient survival
Australia	Live	96.8% / 98.7%	87.5% / 94.1%	68.8% / 86.7%
	Deceased	91.6% / 96.4%	80.8% / 89.0%	58.6% / 72.6%
United States	Live	95.7% / 98.3%	80.4% / 90.2%	57.0% / 76.5%
	Deceased	90.5% / 95.2%	67.3% / 80.7%	41.0% / 60.6%

Table 1. Unadjusted 1, 5 and 10-year graft and patient survival rates following primary living and deceased donor transplantation in Australia & United States in 2008 (Campbell, McDonald et al. 2009; US Organ Procurement and Transplantation Network and Scientific Registry of Transplant Recipients 2009).

2.3 Effect of donor characteristics on live-donor kidney transplant outcomes

2.3.1 Donor gender

A disproportionately greater number of female donors have been observed in live-donor programs in most countries, including the United States and Australia(Kayler, Meier-Kriesche et al. 2002; Campbell, McDonald et al. 2009). In Australia, female donors accounted for 53% and 62% of overall LRD and LURD donors respectively, the latter likely to reflect the growth in spousal donation (Campbell, McDonald et al. 2009). The reason for the greater proportion of female donors remains unclear although differences in medical (higher rates of cardiovascular disease in men) and psychosocial (financial issues and differing perception towards donation between genders) factors may be contributing (Bloembergen, Port et al. 1996; Schaubel, Stewart et al. 2000; Zimmerman, Donnelly et al. 2000).

In deceased donor kidney transplants, female donors have been shown to be associated with higher rates of rejection, poorer post-transplant graft function and possibly reduced graft and patient survival (Vereerstraeten, Wissing et al. 1999; Zeier, Dohler et al. 2002). In live-donor kidney transplantation, large single centre studies have suggested that female donors are associated with a greater risk of rejection and poorer post-transplant graft function (Oien, Reisaeter et al. 2005; Oien, Reisaeter et al. 2007), but this association has not been observed in large registry analyses (Kayler, Rasmussen et al. 2003; Lim, Chang et al. 2007). The failure to account for differences in donor-recipient body mass in these studies may in part explain the conflicting results between studies. It is plausible that the inverse association between female donors and post-transplant graft function may be attributed to 'inadequate' nephron mass from smaller female donors into larger male recipients with subsequent hyperfiltration injury and decline in renal function (Brenner, Cohen et al. 1992; Brenner, Lawler et al. 1996). Supporting this explanation, *Poggio et al* demonstrated that donors with larger kidney volume (typically donors with larger body sizes and male donors), as determined by 3D helical computed tomography scanning, were associated with lower rejection risk and improved post-transplant radionuclide glomerular filtration rate (GFR) (Poggio, Hila et al. 2006). However, selective transplantation of donor and recipient pairs based on size-matching remains debatable.

2.3.2 Donor-recipient relationship

A number of large single centre studies and registry analyses including United Network of Organ Sharing (UNOS) and ANZDATA have demonstrated similar graft and patient outcomes between LRD and LURD transplants, even though LURD were more likely to be older donors and often have poorer HLA-matching (Figure 8)(Terasaki, Cecka et al. 1995; Gjertson and Cecka 2000; Humar, Durand et al. 2000; Lim, Chang et al. 2007). Early studies have indicated that husband-to-wife (Terasaki, Cecka et al. 1997; Rosenberg, Jones et al. 2004) and child-to-mother live-donor transplants were associated with an increased risk of rejection and graft failure (Cecka 1995; Mahanty, Cherikh et al. 2001), possibly related to prior exposure to donor HLA antigens during pregnancy (Miles, Schaubel et al. 2008; Fuggle, Allen et al. 2010). In a recent ANZDATA analysis of 1989 primary live-donor renal transplants between 1995 and 2004, *Lim et al* reported that the risk of graft and patient survival was similar between LRD and LURD transplants. In this study, parental donors were associated with an increased risk of acute rejection at 6 months (odds ratio [OR] 1.69, 95% confidence interval [CI] 1.13-2.53) and lower GFR at 1 and 3 years post-transplant, but this did not translate to inferior graft or patient survival (Lim, Chang et al. 2007). In contrast, husband-to-wife and child-to-mother transplants were not associated with poorer graft outcomes in this study. Analysis of the UNOS database suggested that in recipients with genetic-predisposed ESKD such as focal segmental glomerulosclerosis (FSGS), type I diabetes and polycystic kidney disease (PKD), LRD kidney transplants may be associated with poorer graft outcomes compared with LURD transplants but this association remains debatable (Futagawa, Waki et al. 2005).

2.3.3 Expanded-criteria live donors

As with deceased donors, certain live donor characteristics have been identified that may have a significant impact on renal allograft outcomes. The identification of these donor characteristics in the assessment of potential live donor-recipient pairing may help in the selection of the most appropriate live donor to achieve the best graft outcomes. A large retrospective chart review of 264 live donor-recipient pairs transplanted between 1997 and 2003 at Cleveland clinic demonstrated that older donor age ≥45 years (compared with <45 years), donor radionuclide GFR ≤110mL/min (compared with >110mL/min), donor systolic blood pressure ≥120mmHg (compared with <120mmHg) and donor cholesterol ≥200mg/dL (compared with <200mg/dL) were associated with a greater risk of acute rejection, delayed graft function (DGF), poorer post-transplant graft function and/or graft loss at 2 and 3 years post-transplantation in the adjusted model. What was interesting about this study were the additive negative effects of increasing number of donor factors on graft function. In this study, there was no association between donor uric acid, fasting glucose, gender or race and graft outcomes (Issa, Stephany et al. 2007). Other studies have demonstrated a similar strong independent relationship between live donor GFR and post-transplant graft function (Poggio, Hila et al. 2006).

The recent meta-analyses by *Iordanous Y et al* of living expanded criteria kidney donors demonstrated that older live donors were associated with poorer composite outcomes of graft and patient survival compared to younger donors (meta-analysis of 12 studies, 72% vs. 80%, unadjusted relative risk [RR] of survival 0.89, 95% CI 0.83-0.95). However, the association between donor age and survival appeared to diminished over time (1980 - RR 0.79, 95% CI 0.65-0.96 compared to 1990 - RR 0.91, 95% CI 0.85-0.99), possibly related to the use of more potent immunosuppression (Iordanous, Seymour et al. 2009). The relationship between donor hypertension or lipid level and graft outcomes in this study remains unclear. Studies examining the association between donor obesity and donor urinary abnormalities (i.e. presence of proteinuria and/or haematuria pre-donation) are lacking. When examining live donor-recipient age difference, *Ferrari P et al* demonstrated that live donor-recipient pairs with ≥30 years age difference had similar graft and patient outcomes as those with lesser donor-recipient age difference suggesting large discrepancy in donor-recipient age difference should not discourage the decision for transplantation (Ferrari, Lim et al. 2011).

It is important to acknowledge that these are retrospective studies and therefore do not clearly establish causality between live donor factors and renal graft outcomes. Nevertheless, identifying unfavorable live donor characteristics could complement the assessments of recipients in stratifying their post-transplant risk of graft dysfunction or failure.

3. ABO-incompatible and desensitization programs

The complexity of live- and deceased donor transplantation has evolved over the years such that many transplanting centres are performing ABO-incompatible transplants and desensitizing highly allo-sensitized transplant candidates to improve their transplant potential. Other innovative programs that have been established to enhance live-donor transplantation include the paired kidney exchange program (as a strategy to overcome incompatible transplants) and tumour-resected kidney transplant program whereby patients with small renal tumours are considered for kidney donation following radical nephrectomy and resection of renal tumour.

3.1 ABO-incompatible live-donor transplants

Alexandre et al first described transplantation across the blood group barrier in 1987, but there has since been a broad expansion of this program worldwide (Alexandre G 1987). With the greater availability of more potent immunosuppression coupled with the capability to measure isohemagglutinin antibodies, the outcomes of ABO-incompatible live-donor kidney transplantation are comparable to compatible live-donor kidney transplantation (Crew and Ratner 2010). However, there continues to be an early significant risk of antibody-mediated rejection (AMR). The concept of blood group incompatible transplantation involves the removal of isohemagglutinin antibodies (i.e. antibodies formed against blood group antigen A and/or B) to low levels using immunoabsorption technique (ABO antibody-specific) or plasmapheresis (not ABO antibody-specific) thereby avoiding hyperacute rejection following transplantation. Although splenectomy was once considered standard practice pre-blood group incompatible transplantation to prevent early AMR, the introduction of anti-CD20 antibody rituximab has largely eliminated the need for splenectomy achieving equivalent outcomes. However, the need for pre-transplant rituximab remains debatable (Tanabe, Ischida et al. 2009).

Tanabe et al recently reported on the outcome of 800 ABO-incompatible kidney transplants in Japan performed since 1989. The reported 5-year graft and patient survival in this cohort was 79% and 90% respectively (Tanabe K 2007). Acute AMR occurred in up to 30% of transplant recipients resulting in early graft loss in 10% of recipients with refractory AMR (Crew R 2010). Although acute AMR may be treated successfully with further immunoabsorption or plasmapheresis, recipients who develop AMR have poorer graft survival (AMR and no AMR - graft survival of 84% and 100% at 3 years and 49% and 95% at 8 years) and a greater risk of developing transplant glomerulopathy, especially in recipients with concurrent pre-transplant donor specific antibodies (DSA) (Einecke, Sis et al. 2009; Toki, Ishida et al. 2009). Acute AMR is less common after 3 months post-transplant, presumably related to the development of accommodation, a phenomenon of persistent anti-donor antibody in the absence of allograft injury (Dehoux and Gianello 2009).

3.2 ABO-incompatible deceased donor transplants

In 1991, an Organ Procurement Transplant Network (OPTN)/UNOS variance has approved a voluntary national allocation of blood group A2 and A2B deceased donor kidneys into blood group B and O transplant candidates to improve their transplant potential, although this allocation practice had already been adopted into clinical practice by the Midwest Transplant Network since 1986 (Nelson, Shield et al. 2002). As a result of this practice, 31% more blood group B transplant candidates with low anti-A IgG titres received a transplant achieving comparable graft survival as those who had received blood group B kidneys using conventional immunosuppression (10 year graft survival was 72% and 69% respectively) (Bryan, Nelson et al. 2004; Bryan, Winklhofer et al. 2005). Recent analysis of the United States Renal Data System (USRDS) database between 1995 and 2006 demonstrated that blood group O and B recipients (n=238) who had received blood group A2 kidneys had significantly shorter waiting-time compared to blood group compatible transplants (n=149,880). Graft loss and patient survival were similar in blood group A2 to B or O recipients and blood group compatible recipients (Hurst, Sajjad et al. 2010). These favourable reports suggest that this strategy should be considered in allocation programs to enhance the transplant potential of appropriate blood group B and O transplant candidates with low anti-A titres.

3.3 Desensitization of highly-sensitized patients for live-donor transplantation

There is an increasing number of transplant candidates who are allo-sensitized to HLA as a result of previous exposure to HLA antigens, typically following blood transfusions, prior transplantation and pregnancy. The presence of high levels of class I and/or II DSA (i.e. anti-HLA antibodies with reactivity against the potential donor leading to positive complement-dependent cytotoxicity [CDC] cross-match) is associated with poorer graft outcomes, including the development of acute and chronic AMR, transplant glomerulopathy and late graft loss (Eng, Bennett et al. 2008; Gloor, Winters et al. 2010; Eng, Bennett et al. 2011; Mujtaba, Goggins et al. 2011). A study by *LeFaucheur et al* demonstrated that the presence of DSA significantly reduces graft survival rates compared to recipients without DSA (1 year graft survival - 81% and 94% respectively and 8 years graft survival 47% and 78% respectively) (Lefaucheur, Suberbielle-Boissel et al. 2008) (Table 2). In addition, recent study by *Mujtaba M et al* demonstrated that the 3-year graft survival in highly-sensitized patients with lower total DSA (i.e. total mean fluorescent intensity [MFI] of <9500) was 100% compared to 76% in those with higher total DSA (i.e. total MFI >9500; p = 0.022) (Mujtaba, Goggins et al. 2011).

Studies reporting the utilization of desensitization technique to allow transplantation in highly-sensitized transplant candidates have focused predominantly on live-donor transplantation, which allows early planning and implementation of treatment at a suitable time. With the greater understanding of HLA antigens and anti-HLA antibodies, innovative techniques have been established to allow live-door transplantation across a 'positive CDC cross-match' barrier. Combinations of rituximab, plasmapheresis and/or intravenous immunoglobulin (IVIg) have been used successfully to desensitize highly allo-sensitized transplant candidates, therefore allowing live-donor transplantation to occur safely (Jordan, Vo et al. 2003; Gloor and Stegall 2010). The typical desensitization regimens involve either a single high dose of IVIg or combination plasmapheresis with low dose IVIg, although the latter may be more effective in achieving a negative CDC cross-match (Gloor, DeGoey et al. 2003; Stegall, Gloor et al. 2006). The addition of rituximab remains debatable and unsubstantiated and splenectomy has largely been eliminated from most desensitization protocols (Locke, Zachary et al. 2007). Current literature indicates that transplantation could safely proceed if DSA intensity is lowered sufficiently to render a negative CDC cross-match and/or an IgG titre of ≤16 by isohemagglutination. Following successful transplantation, ongoing monitoring of DSA and early recognition of AMR is crucial to avoid early graft loss. On re-exposure to donor antigens against which the recipient is sensitized, memory B lymphocytes in their spleen, bone marrow and lymph nodes undergo an amnestic reaction leading to the development of antibody-producing cells, which can produce high levels of DSA within days or weeks suggesting positive cross-match kidney transplantation requires both pre- and post-transplantation interventions to continually suppress DSA levels. Despite advances in desensitization techniques, AMR and transplant glomerulopathy occur in over 30% and 45% respectively in live donor positive cross-match kidney transplantations (Gloor J 2010).

3.4 Desensitization of highly-sensitized patients on deceased donor wait-list

Desensitization of deceased donor transplant wait-list candidates with multiple anti-HLA antibodies to enhance their transplant potential remains debatable due to the uncertain availability of deceased donor kidneys and these patients may remain on the deceased donor transplant wait-list indefinitely (Table 2). *Vo et al* reported the successful transplantation of 6 highly sensitized patients who received deceased donor kidneys following desensitization with IVIg (2g/kg on days 0 and 30) and rituximab (1g on days 7 and 22) over a 4-week period. These patients were on the deceased donor wait-list for 144±89 months (range 60-324 months), but had waited only an additional 5±6 months for a transplant. These patients achieved excellent graft and patient outcomes despite having a greater risk of acute rejection (Vo, Lukovsky et al. 2008). The same group reported an additional 45 successful deceased donor transplants in highly sensitized patients using a similar but modified desensitization approach using one instead of two doses of rituximab. In this cohort, desensitized patients waited for an additional 4.2±4.5 months before receiving a deceased donor graft. Overall graft failure and death at 2 years were 80% and 91% respectively, but almost 30% of graft loss was directly attributed to AMR (Vo, Peng et al. 2010).

	Number of patients	AMR incidence (%)	1-year DCGS (%)	2-year DCGS (%)
Lefaucheur et al (2008)	43	35	89	89
Thielke et al (2009)	51	32	93	81
Magee et al (2008)	28	39	92	89
Gloor et al (2010)	119	41	89	89
Haririan et al (2009)	41	12	90	85
Vo et al (2008)	16	30	94	Not reported
Vo et al (2010)#	76	29	87	84

Table 2. Incidence of antibody mediated rejection (AMR) and death-censored graft survival (DCGS) following positive-crossmatch kidney transplantation. #Stratified by donor type – DCGS at 1 and 2 years for live donor (LD) 90% and 90%; for deceased donor (DD) 82% and 80%.

4. Innovative live-donor programs

4.1 Paired kidney exchange

Blood group or cross-match incompatibility between a potential donor-recipient pair is often a major barrier for kidney transplantation. Paired kidney exchange (PKE), which was first described in 1986 (Rapaport F 1986), circumvents the incompatibility by allowing a live-donor to direct the donated kidney to a different but compatible recipient, with the intent that another donor will donate to the first donor's designated recipient (Delmonico 2004). Most PKE programs involves the use of computer-generated algorithms to create potential donor-recipient pairings using virtual databases containing patient characteristics along with blood group types and degree of sensitization (de Klerk, Keizer et al. 2005). There are several alternatives to the conventional 2-way or 3-way kidney paired donation types, such that an altruistic donor could create a domino paired donation (i.e. kidneys from altruistic donor set off a chain of simultaneous transplants terminating in a donation to a candidate on the deceased donor wait-list) (Gentry, Montgomery et al. 2011). Although overcoming incompatibility remains the primary focus of PKE, donor and recipients pairs may participate in the exchange in the hope of finding a better HLA-matched kidney or younger kidney amongst other reasons. Match rates for incompatible pairs can be as high as 50% (de Klerk M 2006) and as a result can increase transplant activity even in small populations by almost 10% (Ferrari P 2009). Successful PKE programs have been established in the Netherlands, South Korea, United Kingdom, United States and more recently Australia.

4.2 Tumour-resected kidney transplant program

Transplantation of donor kidneys following *ex-vivo* resection of small kidney tumours is a novel source of donor kidneys that was first described in 1995 (Penn I 1995). Although these kidneys are clearly outside the standard criteria for donor kidneys coupled with the small but potential transmission of donor-derived malignancy into recipients, the success of such program in many countries is encouraging.

The largest reported case series of utilizing donor kidneys with small renal cancers comes from Australia. In this single-centre program, 43 patients were transplanted with kidneys removed from patients with <3cm incidentally detected renal cell cancer, majority of which were patients undergoing radical nephrectomy for presumed renal cell cancer. In this program, a vigorous informed consent was undertaken and only older transplant candidates >60 years of age or those with significant comorbidities were eligible to receive these kidneys (Nicol D 2008). In this program, patient survival at 1 and 5 years of recipients of tumour-resected kidney transplants was 92% and 88% respectively, compared to 98% and 74% patient survival for patients on the deceased donor wait-list (n=153) and 99% and 97% patient survival for recipients of LURD renal transplants (n=120; log rank score 10.4, P = 0.005) (Brook, Gibbons et al. 2010). There was one tumour recurrence occurring at 9 years post-transplantation, but it was unclear whether this was donor-derived. An additional 22 similar successful cases from United States and Japan were reported with no documented tumour recurrence (Buell J 2005; Mannami, Mannami et al. 2008).

5. Deceased donor kidney transplantation

There continues to be an enormous disparity between the availability of deceased-donor kidneys and potential recipients. This problem is further exacerbated by a greater acceptance of older ESKD patients for renal replacement therapy. In Australia, acceptance of ESKD patients aged 70-74 years for renal replacement therapy has increased from 390 per million population (pmp) in 2004, to 469 pmp in 2008 (McDonald, Excell et al. 2009). Furthermore, the proportion of potential transplant candidates aged >65 years on the deceased donor wait-list has increased by 21% between 2005 and 2008 (Chadban, McDonald et al. 2006; Campbell, McDonald et al. 2009). The Scientific Registry of Transplant Patients (SRTR) has recorded a similar increase of prevalent potential recipients aged ≥70 years on the deceased donor wait-list, rising from 114 in 1990 to 2544 in 2004 (Rao, Merion et al. 2007). There has been little increase in deceased donor rates worldwide. In Australia, deceased donor rates have remained low at 11 donors pmp in 2009 (10 pmp in 2005), compared to 34 pmp in Spain, 24 pmp in United States and 17 pmp in the United Kingdom (Excell, Hee et al. 2010; Fabre, Murphy et al. 2010). However, there has been an increase in acceptance of older donor kidneys in Australia, with the number of deceased donors aged ≥55 years increasing 1.8-fold between 2001-03 to 2007-09 (Excell, Hee et al. 2010). Kidneys from older donors are associated with poorer graft outcomes including late graft loss, chronic allograft nephropathy and higher risk of cardiovascular mortality (Meier-Kriesche, Cibrik et al. 2002; Oppenheimer, Aljama et al. 2004); this is partially offset by the reduction in mortality associated with reduced wait-list time. In addition, female-to-male donation, major donor kidney weight/recipient weight inadequacy, cerebrovascular accidents (CVA) as the cause of donor death and the presence of donor comorbidities such as diabetes have an adverse impact on graft and/or patient survival (Feldman, Fazio et al. 1996; Giral, Nguyen et al. 2005; Ahmad, Cole et al. 2009; Shaheen, Shaheen et al. 2010). However, utilization of kidneys from deceased donors who had developed acute renal failure prior to organ procurement does not appear to have an unfavorable effect on graft outcome (Deroure, Kamar et al. 2010). A continuous kidney donor risk index has been developed using registry data to quantify expected graft survival for any given set of donor characteristics relative to a healthy 40-year old donor and may be useful as a decision-making tool at the time of the deceased donor kidney offer (Rao, Schaubel et al. 2009). However, the significance of such index in the different transplant eras or population groups remains unclear. In the remaining chapter, we will focus primarily on the use and outcomes of ECD and DCD donor kidneys, which have become important source of deceased donor kidneys over the last decade.

5.1 Expanded-criteria donor (ECD) kidneys (Table 3)

With the ongoing shortage of deceased donor kidneys coupled with the continued growth of potential transplant candidates, there has been an increase utilization of ECD kidneys. Compared with non-ECD kidneys, ECD kidneys are associated with poorer graft outcomes. Between 2005 and 2009 in Australia, there has been a 1.3-fold increase in the number of ECD kidneys (Excell, Hee et al. 2006; Excell, Hee et al. 2010)

In 2002, OPTN/UNOS Board of Directors established a definition of ECD kidneys, which was based on a retrospective review of 29,068 recipients from SRTR database (Port FK 2002). The term ECD kidneys was assigned based on a ≥70% greater risk of developing graft failure when compared to younger donor kidneys (aged between 10 and 39 years) and defined as any donor aged ≥60 years, or any donor aged 50-59 years, with two of the following three donor criteria: CVA death, terminal creatinine >133μmol/L, or hypertension (Metzger, Delmonico et al. 2003). Although the concept of ECD focuses primarily on advanced donor age, other risk factors such as CVA, hypertension, diabetes and high serum creatinine were also taken into account (Cosio, Qiu et al. 1996; Ojo, Leichtman et al. 2000). Multiple studies have demonstrated that recipients of ECD kidneys have better survival compared to potential recipients on the waiting-list but long-term outcomes associated with ECD grafts remains unclear (Wolfe, Ashby et al. 1999; Ojo, Hanson et al. 2001).

Further modification of the definition of ECD kidneys has been proposed in an attempt to further improve the stratification and identification of donor kidneys with increased risk of early graft dysfunction or graft loss. In 2001, *Nyberg et al* devised the Deceased Donor Score (DDS), which incorporated several donor-derived factors that have been shown to independently affect graft outcomes (Nyberg SL 2001; Nyberg SL 2003). However, this score has not been adopted widely for clinical application.

In a retrospective study of 2845 French transplant recipients aged ≥60 years, ECD kidneys were associated with poorer graft survival compared to non-ECD kidneys (Savoye, Tamarelle et al. 2007). The difference in graft survival was 6.2% at 12 months and 14.2% at 5 years (adjusted relative risk [RR] of graft failure associated with ECD kidneys compared to non-ECD kidneys was 1.98, $p<0.01$). Nonetheless, survival of ECD recipients was superior to potential recipients remaining on the waiting list (adjusted RR of potential recipients on waiting-list compared to recipients of ECD and non-ECD kidneys were 2.32 and 3.78 respectively, $p<0.0001$). Similarly, analysis of the SRTR between 1990 and 2005 demonstrated that recipients aged ≥70 years receiving ECD or non-ECD deceased donor kidneys had a 56% lower mortality risk compared to wait-listed dialysis patients aged ≥70 years (RR 0.59; 95%CI 0.53, 0.65; $p<0.0001$), and this benefit persisted in elderly patients with diabetes and hypertension (Rao, Merion et al. 2007). As the unadjusted 1-year graft and death-censored graft survival (DCGS) of elderly transplant recipients were 81% and 90% respectively; and were 67% and 85% respectively at 3years, this suggested that a considerable proportion of these recipients die with functioning grafts.

A retrospective analysis of ANZDATA of 4466 deceased donor transplants between 1991 and 2005 reported poorer outcomes in recipients of ECD kidneys, compared to non-ECD kidneys (Collins, Chang et al. 2009). Compared to non-ECD kidneys, ECD kidneys were associated with poorer graft function and a greater risk of DGF, acute rejection and death-censored graft failure (DCGF).

The observed reduction in graft survival in recipients of ECD kidneys is likely related to an increase in glomerulosclerosis with the associated reduction in functional nephron mass, which has been shown to correlate with an increased risk of DGF, graft loss and poorer graft function (Gaber, Moore et al. 1995). On average, the adjusted graft survival of ECD kidneys is 8% lower at 1 year and up to 20% lower at 3-5 years compared to non-ECD kidneys (Ojo AO 2001).

Although ECD kidneys are associated with poorer outcomes compared to non-ECD kidneys, the contribution of donor age, especially the upper acceptable age limit on graft outcomes amongst ECD grafts remains unclear. In a retrospective analysis of the UNOS/OPTN database, the impact of donor age on 9580 ECD kidneys were examined (Chavalitdhamrong, Gill et al. 2008). There was no association between donor age and acute rejection, although ECD kidneys from donors aged ≥70 years had poorer function at 12 months compared to grafts from younger ECD donors. In an adjusted model, ECD kidneys from donors aged ≥70 years were associated with an increased risk of graft failure and patient death compared to ECD kidneys from donors aged 50-69 years (hazard ratio [HR] 1.37 and 1.37 respectively, $p<0.01$). When stratified by recipient age, ECD kidneys from donors aged ≥70 years (compared to ECD 50-69 years) were associated with an increased risk of DCGF for recipients aged 41-60 years (HR 1.48, 95%CI 1.06, 2.06; $p=0.02$) but not for older recipients aged >60 years (HR 1.12, 95%CI 0.86, 1.46; $p=0.40$), suggesting that older ECD kidneys may have a smaller unfavourable impact in older recipients. In contrast, an Italian study demonstrated that 3-year graft and patient survival was similar in recipients receiving ECD kidneys from donors >75 years and <75 years (Collini, Kalmar et al. 2009). This inconsistent finding may be explained by the greater use of double kidneys (from donors >75 years) in the Italian study.

As ECD kidneys are more susceptible to peri-transplant insults, strategies to reduce cold ischemic time, improve donor kidney preservation (Burdick JF) and preventing or reducing reperfusion injury using agents such as superoxide dismutase (Land W) or platelet-

activating factor receptor antagonists (Grino JM) may be beneficial. However, these strategies have not translated to improvement in renal graft outcomes. Initial avoidance of calcineurin-inhibitors (CNI) in early post-transplant period has been suggested to reduce the risk of DGF in recipients of ECD kidneys but this approach has not been adopted widely.
Although there is a lack of consensus amongst transplant physicians and surgeons regarding the allocation of ECD kidneys, most would advocate selective utilization of these kidneys for older recipients (particularly avoiding recipients <40 years) (Merion, Ashby et al. 2005; Schold and Meier-Kriesche 2006), for recipients with extended wait-time (Carter, Chan et al. 2005; Cecka, Cohen et al. 2006) or to consider dual graft transplantation into a single recipient to avoid unnecessary discard of older donor kidneys (Waiser, Schreiber et al. 2000; Tan, Alfrey et al. 2004).

	Donor/recipient groups	**Graft outcome**	**Patient outcome**
Collins M et al 2009 *ANZDATA (n=4466)*	 Non-ECD <50y Non-ECD 50-59y ECD 50-59y ECD ≥60y	*1/5y DCGS** 94% / 88% 91% / 84% 87% / 81% 87% / 71%	*1/5y patient survival** 97% / 92% 97% / 90% 97% / 89% 96% / 87%
Collini A et al 2009 *Single centre (n=192)*	 ECD >75y ECD <75y	*1/3y graft survival* 73% / 64% 82% / 71%	*10y patient survival* 81% / 81% 92% / 90%
Savoye E et al 2009 *Single centre (n=2845)*	 Expanded criteria 0^ Expanded criteria 1^ Expanded criteria 2^ Expanded criteria 3^	*1/5y graft survival#* 93% / 83% 87% / 74% 87% / 65% 83% / 55%	*1/5y patient survival* ECD – 97% / 67% Non-ECD – 98% / 91%
Chavalitdhamrong D et al 2008; OPTN/UNOS database (n=9580)	 ECD 50-69y ECD ≥70y	*3/5y graft survival** 69% / 55% 62% / 44%	*3/5y patient survival** 82% / 71% 75% / 58%

Table 3. Effect of expanded criteria donor on renal transplant outcomes. *$p<0.05$; #analysis in patients aged ≥60 years, ^expanded criteria risk factors including donor aged >60 years, donor hypertension, donor diabetes, donor death from cerebrovascular accident. Abbreviation: ANZDATA – Australia and New Zealand Dialysis and Transplant Registry, ECD – expanded criteria donor, OPTN – Organ Procurement Transplant Network, UNOS – United Network of Organ Sharing, y – year(s). Adapted from Lim et al (Nephrol Dial Transplant 2010).

5.2 Donation after cardiac death donor kidneys

Over the last decade, the number of brain-death donors has steadily declined, in part attributed to changes in neurosurgical practice (Jüttler, Schwab et al. 2007). However, the use of DCD donor kidneys has increased substantially. In Australia, the number of DCD donors has increased from 1 to 42 between 2000 and 2009 (Excell, Hee et al. 2010), whereas in the United Kingdom, the proportion of DCD of all deceased donors has increased by 29% between 2000 and 2009 (Transplant 2010). The prolonged warm ischaemic period that invariably accompanies DCD kidney transplants is likely to explain the greater incidence of

DGF (Locke, Segev et al. 2007). As a result, DCD kidneys are more likely to be allocated locally to minimize cold ischaemic time. Recent analysis of the UK transplant registry demonstrated that compared with brain-death donor kidney transplants, recipients of controlled DCD donor kidneys of Maastricht category 3 (defined as donors awaiting cardiac arrest following withdrawal of life-sustaining treatment in intensive care unit (Kootstra, Daemen et al. 1995)) was associated with a significantly greater risk of DGF but lower risk of acute rejection up to 3 months post-transplant (Figure 2). For primary but not repeat renal allograft recipients of DCD kidneys, overall 5-year graft survival was comparable to primary and repeat renal allograft recipients of brain-death donor kidneys in unadjusted and adjusted models. Repeat renal allograft recipients of DCD kidneys have a greater risk of primary non-function compared to primary renal allograft recipients of DCD kidneys. Increasing donor and recipient age, as well as prolonged cold ischaemic time but not the presence of DGF or HLA-matching were associated with poorer graft outcomes in primary renal allograft recipients of DCD kidneys (Summers, Johnson et al. 2010). With comparable transplant outcomes between brain-death and controlled DCD donor kidneys, DCD kidneys are considered an acceptable source of donor kidneys although particular attention in reducing cold ischaemic time and avoidance of large donor-recipient age differences and avoidance of allocating DCD kidneys to repeat renal allograft recipients may be appropriate.

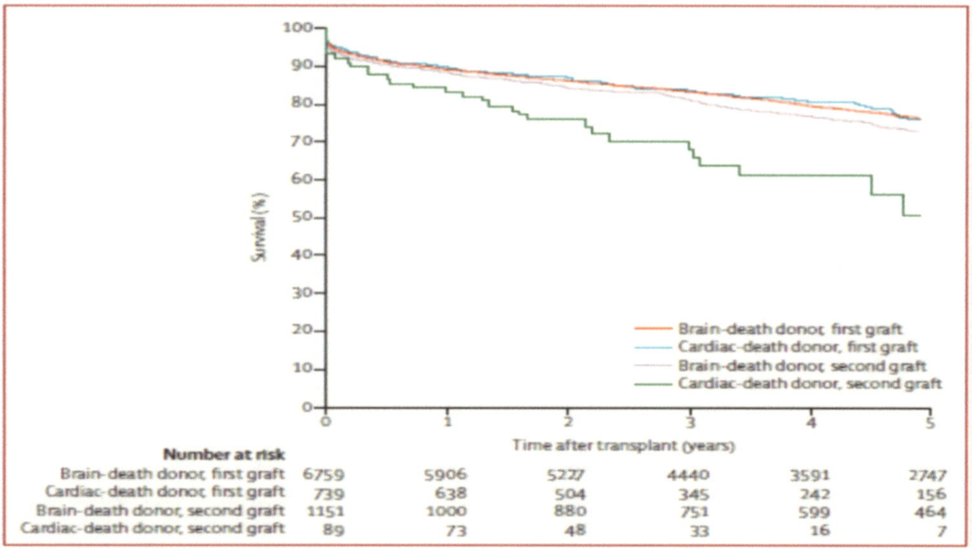

Fig. 2. Kaplan-Meier survival estimates comparing brain-death and cardiac-death donor grafts, stratified by primary and repeat grafts (adapted from Summers et al 2010).

5.3 Utility-based allocation strategies to maximise overall functioning graft years

Allocating younger donor kidneys to older potential recipients has raised concerns amongst many transplant physicians and surgeons, as many older recipients will die with functioning grafts. If these younger kidneys were re-allocated from older to younger recipients, a proportion may have continued to function for a substantial period in younger recipients. As older recipients have reduced life expectancies, adopting an allocation strategy that better matches the life expectancy of the donor kidney with that of the recipient may be more appropriate (Meier-Kriesche, Schold et al. 2005). Allocation strategies that have been examined included the concept of donor-recipient age-matching and the creation of a kidney allocation score (KAS) to improve the utility of deceased donor kidneys. These strategies will be discussed in this chapter.

5.3.1 Age-matching

Allocation of deceased donor kidneys according to donor-recipient age-matching avoids the allocation of younger donor kidneys to older recipients and older donor kidneys to younger recipients according to a single donor and recipient age cut-off value. The Eurotransplant Seniors Program (ESP) is an example of an age-matching allocation model that has been successfully implemented in the allocation of deceased donor kidneys.

5.3.1.1 Eurotransplant seniors program

The foundation of ESP, which was established in 1999, was to preferentially allocate older donor kidneys ≥65 years to ABO-compatible, unsensitized older recipients ≥65 years receiving a primary graft (Cecka, Cohen et al. 2006). The ESP was designed to match the functional potential of donor kidneys ≥65 years to the functional requirements of older recipients aged ≥65 years. Although a degree of age-matching already occurred prior to the development of ESP such that the very young donor kidneys were seldom allocated to older recipients, this may be explained by younger healthier potential recipients near the top of the list declining a suboptimal donor graft, and therefore retain their place on the waiting list until a younger donor kidney becomes available. Similar practice also occurs in countries such as the United States and Australia where age-matching is not part of the standard allocation process (Segev 2009; Lim, Chang et al. 2010).

In ESP, donor kidneys were distributed locally to reduce cold ischaemic time, in an attempt to reduce the risk of DGF. Consequently, this program has not only resulted in an improvement in transplant access in older recipients by reducing wait-list times, younger recipients had also benefited from this program with improved access to younger donor kidneys (Smits, Persijn et al. 2002). Compared to 'old-to-any' (i.e. recipients of any age receiving a donor kidney ≥65 years) and 'any-to-old' (i.e. recipients aged between 60-64 years receiving donor kidneys of any age) transplants (allocated via Eurotransplant Kidney Allocation System [ETKAS]), recipients of ESP had significantly lower risk of DGF; presumably related to the reduction in cold ischaemic time. However, ESP recipients had a greater risk of acute rejection, presumably related to a greater degree of HLA-mismatch(es), which was ignored in the allocation of ESP kidneys. One and 5-year DCGS in ESP recipients were similar to 'old-to-any' recipients (1 year - 83% and 81% respectively; 5 years - 67% for both groups) but were inferior compared to 'any-to-old' recipients (1 year 90% and 5 years 81%) (Table 4). When stratified by donor age, the 1 and 5-year graft survival in the ESP group was 75% and 47% compared to 74% and 53% for 'any-to-old' recipients with older donors aged ≥60 years ($p=0.38$) and 85% and 67% for 'any-to-old' recipients with younger donors aged <60 years ($p<0.001$) suggesting older recipients receiving older donor kidneys allocated through the ETKAS system had similar outcome as ESP recipients. Although the risk of DGF was reduced in ESP recipients, this remained an important predictor of graft outcomes indicating that DGF may have a greater adverse impact on graft outcome in older recipients receiving older donor kidneys. It is conceivable that strategies to reduce the risk of DGF in ESP recipients (e.g. attempts to further reduce cold ischaemia) may lead to an improvement in graft and patient outcomes. An important and often overlooked finding in this study is that younger recipients of older donor kidneys have poorer survival, similar to that of the 'any-to-old' recipients allocated through the ETKAS system (Table 4).

Eurotransplant Senior DR-compatible Program is a new future initiative of the ESP to preferentially allocate kidneys to recipients with 0 HLA-DR mismatches and therefore potentially reducing the risk of rejection (de Fijter 2009). The outcome of this approach will be prospectively evaluated in the coming years.

5.3.1.2 Simulated age-matching allocation of deceased donor kidneys

In Australia, utilization of older donors has steadily increased, with donors aged ≥55 years increasing from 134 to 241 between 2001-03 and 2007-09 (i.e. an increase of 16% of overall donors) (Excell, Hee et al. 2010). A recent ANZDATA registry study of 4616 renal transplant recipients has demonstrated that the adoption an age-matching allocation model would lead to substantial improvement in the number of functioning graft years and associated cost savings (Lim, Chang et al. 2010). In this study, recipients ≥55 years had more than a 2.5-fold increased risk of death with functioning graft compared to recipients <55 years (HR 2.84, 95%CI 1.97, 4.10 for 0-1 year; HR 2.78, 95%CI 2.19, 3.53 for 1-8 years and HR 4.44, 95%CI 3.10, 6.35 for >8 years; all p-values <0.01). However, the risk of early (<1 year) and late (>8 years) DCGF was similar in younger and older recipients. Compared with younger donor grafts, older donor grafts ≥60 years were associated with a significant increased risk of DCGF, death with functioning graft and poorer post-transplant graft function. The application of an age-matching allocation model to this cohort would result in an additional 262 mean functioning graft years, which equates to $11.8-21.7 million dialysis cost savings (cost per patient per year on dialysis $45,000-$83,000) (Cass, Chadban et al. 2006). Similarly, analysis of the SRTR database of 74,998 deceased donor transplants performed between 1990 and 2002 demonstrated that if older recipients aged 60-64 years received younger donor grafts aged 15-50 years, the application of age-matching allocation would have increased graft life by 27,500 years, with estimated cost savings in excess of 1 billion dollars (Meier-Kriesche, Schold et al. 2005). However, at an individual level, the absolute impact of age-matching appears less impressive. In the ANZDATA study by *Lim et al*, Younger recipients of younger donor kidneys would on average have an additional 3 functioning graft years compared to older recipients receiving younger donor kidneys (11.6 vs 8.7 mean graft years respectively) and the negative impact of older donor kidneys on functioning graft years appears to be greater for younger compared to older recipients (9.3 vs 7.1 mean graft years respectively) (Table 4).

Retrospective analysis of the OPTN database demonstrated that for every 1 year increase in donor age, the risk of graft failure (HR 1.01, p<0.001) and death with functioning graft (HR 1.004, p<0.001) was increased substantially (Moers, Kornmann et al. 2009). The negative impact of donor age on graft survival appears maximal between donors aged between 36 to 40 years (Keith, Demattos et al. 2004). In a simulated age-matching allocation system, the reallocation of older donor grafts ≥65 years from younger recipients <65 years (old-to-young) to older recipients ≥65 years (old-to-old) would result in an absolute reduction in 10-year graft survival by 8% (from 21% to 13%, p<0.001), whereas reallocation of donor kidneys <65 years from recipients ≥65 years (young-to-old) to younger recipients <65 years (young-to-young) would result in an improvement in 10-year graft survival by 7% (19% to 26%, p=0.40). Unlike the ANZDATA study, there was no net benefit of implementing an old-for-old allocation system with regards to overall functional graft years (Table 4).

5.3.2 Kidney allocation score

In 2004, a subcommittee of the UNOS/OPTN recommended that the establishment of a Kidney Allocation Score (KAS) based on Life Years From Transplant (LYFT - measures transplant utility), combined with panel reactive antibody (PRA), Donor Profile Index (DPI - measures donor quality) and dialysis time (measures transplant equity) could potentially lead to an increase in the total number of life years gained from a restricted number of available deceased donor kidneys (Wolfe, McCullough et al. 2009; OPTN 2010). LYFT is defined as the additional years of life that a potential transplant recipient could expect to gain as a consequence of the transplant as compared to not receiving a transplant. LYFT is calculated from an equation generated by statistical modeling of historical data combining

	Donor/ recipient groups	Graft outcome	Patient outcome
Frei U et al 2008 ESP/ETKAS^ (n=3539)	D/R ≥55 (ESP) D ≥65 / R - any age D - any age / R 60-64	*5y patient DCGS** 67% 67% 81%	*5y patient survival** 60% 71% 74%
Lim W et al 2010 ANZDATA (n=4616)	D <60 / R <55 D <60 / R ≥55 D ≥60/ R <55 D ≥60 / R ≥55	*Mean graft years* 11.6 9.3 8.7 7.1	NR
Keith D et al 2004 OPTN Registry (n=50,322)	D 30-41/ R 0-40 D 30-41 / R ≥55 D ≥55 / R 0-40 D ≥55 / R ≥55	NR	*10y patient survival* 82% 45% 76% 35%
Moers C et al 2009 OPTN Registry (n=99,860)	D <65 / R <65 D <65 / R ≥65 D ≥65/ R <65 D ≥65 / R ≥65	*10y graft survival* NR 19% 21% NR	*DFG* NR 56% 40% NR
Waiser et al 2000 Single centre (n=1269)	D ≤55 / R ≤55 D ≤55 / R >55 D >55/ R ≤55 D >55/ R >55	*8y graft survival** 50% 53% 21% 57%	*DFG* 11% 27% 2% 26%

Table 4. Effect of age-matching allocation on graft and patient outcomes. *p<0.05; ^Prospective data. Abbreviation: ESP - Eurotransplant Senior Program, ETKAS - Eurotransplant Kidney Allocation System, ANZDATA - Australia and New Zealand Dialysis and Transplant Registry, OPTN - Organ Procurement Transplant Network, D - donor, R - recipient, DCGS - death-censored graft survival, DFG - death with functioning graft, y - year(s), NR - not reported. Adapted from Lim et al (Nephrol Dial Transplant 2010).

the observed biological effects of patient and donor characteristics on survival. The equation created had a C-value of 0.75, that is the equation predicted the potential transplant recipients with the longer lifetime 75% of the time, although the equation may be inaccurate for the prediction of lifetimes for potential transplant candidates with characteristics that differ from the historical group. A C-value of 0.75 is comparable to the model for end-stage liver disease (MELD) with a C-value of 0.64, commonly used by many transplanting centres to prioritize patients for liver transplantation based on expected survival (Sharma, Schaubel et al. 2008). In addition, based on DPI, the kidneys with the longest survival potential will be allocated according to the combined score of LYFT (80% of total score) and dialysis time/PRA (20% of total score), whereas kidneys with lesser potential for long-term survival will be allocated according to dialysis time and PRA, such that better donor kidneys are allocated to younger potential recipients, who will have the longest expected LYFT. Older potential recipients, who will have a lower expected LYFT and potential recipients with the longest dialysis time will be less likely to receive better donor kidneys but may have an advantage in being allocated shorter-lived kidneys more rapidly (i.e. shorter waiting-time). If deceased donor kidney allocation was based on the KAS, there would a total expected increase in LYFT of 2642 years during a single year of allocation as compared with the current allocation system in the United States.

A perception that organ allocation is occurring in an inequitable manner could potentially reduce organ donor rates. Nevertheless, the utilization of KAS may improve allocation based solely on age-matching, with other patient factors such as diabetes, which are known to adversely affect graft and patient survival, are taken into account in the calculation of LYFT (Machnicki, Pinsky et al. 2009).

5.3.3 Positives and negatives of implementing utility-based allocation models

It remains unclear whether the implementation of utility-based allocation models will achieve a better balance between utility and equity. While kidney transplantation is more cost effective than dialysis, it will take considerable time for the expected lower long-term cost to offset the high initial cost associated with transplantation. In older recipients who are more likely to die with a functioning graft, the expense of transplantation may not be acceptable, on an economic basis, especially with a high-quality donor kidney.

Although adoption of an allocation model based on LYFT is likely to increase functioning graft years, this model is difficult to implement and may even be perceived as being discriminatory to potential 'high-risk' potential recipients (e.g. indigenous and highly sensitised potential recipients) who will have a higher predicted graft loss, resulting in a lower LYFT (Young and Gaston 2000; Young and Gaston 2005). The applicability of LYFT based on historical data to more recent eras and patient cohorts, where there may be differing clinical practices and use of novel immunosuppressive agents remains uncertain. In addition, the optimal weighting of DPI, dialysis time or other factors in the calculation of KAS remains undecided. Although not directly considered in the KAS and age-matching allocation models, KAS may indirectly take into consideration social equity and possibly quality of life, assuming that younger recipients receiving younger donor kidneys will have a longer lifespan and therefore greater contribution to society compared to older recipients (Laupacis, Keown et al. 1996). In contrast, age-matching allocation is simpler but chronological age is often a poor estimate of physiological age and therefore, allocation policy based solely on age-matching could potentially disadvantage a number of healthy older potential recipients.

6. Conclusion

With the continuing shortage of deceased donor organs coupled with the increased utilization of marginal live and deceased donors including ECD and DCD donor kidneys, there have been considerable interest in examining the outcomes of these grafts. Over the last decade, there has been an expansion of innovative transplant programs, including paired exchange and tumour-resected kidney transplant programs, which has helped to overcome incompatible transplants and increase donor kidney pool respectively. In this chapter, understanding the association between live and deceased donor characteristics and transplant outcomes will assist clinicians and potential recipients in the informed process of donor selection as well as the prediction of graft outcomes following transplantation.

7. References

Ahmad, M., E. Cole, et al. (2009). "Impact of deceased donor diabetes mellitus on kidney transplant outcomes: a propensity score-matched study." Transplantation 88(2): 251-60.

Alexandre G, S. J., De Bruyère M, Latinne D, Reding R, Gianello P, Carlier M, Pirson Y (1987). "Present experiences in a series of 26 ABO-incompatible living donor renal allografts." Transplant Proceedings 19(6): 4538-4542.

Bia, M. J., E. L. Ramos, et al. (1995). "Evaluation of living renal donors. The current practice of US transplant centers." Transplantation 60(4): 322-7.

Bloembergen, W. E., F. K. Port, et al. (1996). "Gender discrepancies in living related renal transplant donors and recipients." J Am Soc Nephrol 7(8): 1139-44.

Brenner, B. M., R. A. Cohen, et al. (1992). "In renal transplantation, one size may not fit all." J Am Soc Nephrol 3(2): 162-9.

Brenner, B. M., E. V. Lawler, et al. (1996). "The hyperfiltration theory: a paradigm shift in nephrology." Kidney Int 49(6): 1774-7.

Brook, N., N. Gibbons, et al. (2010). "Outcomes of transplants from patients with small renal tumours, live unrelated donors and dialysis wait-listed patients." Transpl Int 23(5): 476-83.

Bryan, C., P. Nelson, et al. (2004). "Transplantation of A2 and A2B kidneys from deceased donors into B waiting list candidates increases their transplantation rate." Clin Transpl: 127-33.

Bryan, C., F. Winklhofer, et al. (2005). "Improving access to kidney transplantation without decreasing graft survival: long-term outcomes of blood group A2/A2B deceased donor kidneys in B recipients." Transplantation 80(1): 75-80.

Buell J, H. M., Thomas M, Munda R, Alloway R, First M, Woodle E (2005). "Donor kidneys with small renal cell cancers: can they be transplanted?" Transplant Proceedings 37(2): 581-582.

Burdick JF, R. J., McBride MA, Kauffman HM, Bennett LE (1997). "National impact of pulsatile perfusion on cadaveric kidney transplantation." Transplantation 64(12): 4.

Campbell, S., S. McDonald, et al. (2009). Transplant Waiting List. The Thirty Second Report Australia and New Zealand Dialysis and Transplant Registry. S. McDonald, L. Excell and B. Livingston. Adelaide.

Campbell, S., S. McDonald, et al. (2009). Chapter 8 : Transplantation. ANZDATA Registry 32nd Annual Report. Adelaide, South Australia, Australia and New Zealand Dialysis and Transplant Registry (ANZDATA).

Carter, J., S. Chan, et al. (2005). "Expanded criteria donor kidney allocation: marked decrease in cold ischemia and delayed graft function at a single center." Am J Transplant 5(11): 2745-53.

Cass, A., S. Chadban, et al. (2006). Economic impact of end-stage kidney disease in Australia. K. H. Australia.

Cecka, J., B. Cohen, et al. (2006). "Could more effective use of kidneys recovered from older deceased donors result in more kidney transplants for older patients?" Transplantation 81(7): 966-70.

Cecka, J. M. (1995). "Living donor transplants." Clin Transpl: 363-77.

Chadban, S., S. McDonald, et al. (2006). Transplant Waiting List. The Twenty Ninth Report: Australia and New Zealand Dialysis and Transplant Registry. S. McDonald, S. Chang and L. Excell. Adelaide.

Chavalitdhamrong, D., J. Gill, et al. (2008). "Patient and graft outcomes from deceased kidney donors age 70 years and older: an analysis of the Organ Procurement Transplant Network/United Network of Organ Sharing database." Transplantation 85(11): 1573-9.

Collini, A., P. Kalmar, et al. (2009). "Renal transplant from very old donors: how far can we go?" Transplantation 87(12): 1830-6.

Collins, M., S. Chang, et al. (2009). "Outcomes of transplantation using kidneys from donors meeting expanded criteria in Australia and New Zealand, 1991 to 2005." Transplantation 87(8): 1201-9.

Cosio, F., W. Qiu, et al. (1996). "Factors related to the donor organ are major determinants of renal allograft function and survival." Transplantation 62(11): 1571-6.

Crew, R. and L. Ratner (2010). "ABO-incompatible kidney transplantation: current practice and the decade ahead." Curr Opin Organ Transplant 15: 526-30.

Crew R, R. L. (2010). "ABO-incompatible kidney transplantation: current practice and the decade ahead." Current Opinion in Organ Transplantation 15: 526-530.

de Fijter, J. (2009). "An old virtue to improve senior programs." Transpl Int 22(3): 259-68.

de Klerk, M., K. Keizer, et al. (2005). "The Dutch national living donor kidney exchange program." Am J Transplant 5(9): 2302-5.

de Klerk M, W. M., Haase-Kromwijk B, Claas F, Weimar W (2006). "A highly efficient living donor kidney exchange program for both blood type and crossmatch incompatible donor-recipient combinations." Transplantation 82(12): 1616-1620.

De Meester, J. (1998). Kidney: Donation, Waiting Lists and Transplants. Eurotransplant International Foundation Annual Report 1998 [internet]. B. Cohen, G. Persijn and J. De Meester. Leiden (Netherlands), Eurotransplant.

Dehoux, J. and P. Gianello (2009). "Accomodation and antibodies." Transpl Immunol 21: 106-10.

Delmonico, F. (2004). "Exchanging kidneys - advances in living-donor transplantation." N Engl J Med 350(18): 1812-14.

Deroure, B., N. Kamar, et al. (2010). "Expanding the criteria of renal kidneys for transplantation: use of donors with acute renal failure." Nephrol Dial Transplant 25(6): 1980-6.

Donelly, P., P. Oman, et al. (1995). "Predialysis living donor renal transplantation: Is it still the 'gold standard' for cost, convenience and graft survival." Transplant Proc 27: 1444-6.

Einecke, G., B. Sis, et al. (2009). "Antibody-mediated microcirculation injury is the major cause of late kidney transplant failure." Am J Transplant 9(11): 2520-31.

Eng, H., G. Bennett, et al. (2011). "Donor HLA Specific Antibodies Predict Development and Define Prognosis in Transplant Glomerulopathy." Hum Immunol.

Eng, H., G. Bennett, et al. (2008). "Anti-HLA donor-specific antibodies detected in positive B-cell crossmatches by Luminex predict late graft loss." Am J Transplant 8(11): 2335-42.

ERA-EDTA Registry (2010). ERA-EDTA Annual Report 2008 [internet]. Amsterdam (Netherlands).

Excell, L., K. Hee, et al. (2006). ANZOD Registry Report 2006. Australia and New Zealand Organ Donation Registry. L. Excell, K. Hee and G. Russ. Adelaide.

Excell, L., K. Hee, et al. (2010). ANZOD Registry Report 2010. Australia and New Zealand Organ Donation Registry. L. Excell, K. Hee and G. Russ. Adelaide.

Excell, L., K. Hee, et al. (2010). ANZOD Registry Report 2010. ANZOD Registry Report. L. Excell, K. Hee and G. Russ. Adelaide, Australia and New Zealand Organ Donation Registry.

Fabre, J., P. Murphy, et al. (2010). "Presumed consent: a distraction in the quest for increasing rates of organ donation." BMJ 341: c4873.

Feldman, H., I. Fazio, et al. (1996). "Recipient body size and cadaveric renal allograft survival." J Am Soc Nephrol 7(1): 151-7.

Ferrari, P., W. Lim, et al. (2011). "Effect of donor-recipient age difference on graft function and survival in live-donor kidney transplantation." Nephrol Dial Transplant 26(2): 702-8.

Ferrari P, W. C., Christiansen F (2009). "Paired kidney donations to expand the living donor pool: the Western Australian experience." The Medical Journal of Australia 190(12): 700-703.

Frei, U., J. Noeldeke, et al. (2008). "Prospective age-matching in elderly kidney transplant recipients--a 5-year analysis of the Eurotransplant Senior Program." Am J Transplant 8(1): 50-7.

Fuggle, S. V., J. E. Allen, et al. (2010). "Factors affecting graft and patient survival after live donor kidney transplantation in the UK." Transplantation 89(6): 694-701.

Futagawa, Y., K. Waki, et al. (2005). "Living-unrelated donors yield higher graft survival rates than parental donors." Transplantation 79(9): 1169-74.

Gaber, L., L. Moore, et al. (1995). "Glomerulosclerosis as a determinant of posttransplant function of older donor renal allografts." Transplantation 60(4): 334-9.

Gentry, S., R. Montgomery, et al. (2011). "Kidney paired donation: fundamentals, limitations, and expansions." Am J Kidney Dis 57(1): 144-51.

Ghods, A. J. and S. Savaj (2006). "Iranian Model of Paid and Regulated Living-Unrelated Kidney Donation." Clinical Journal of the American Society of Nephrology 1(6): 1136-1145.

Giral, M., J. Nguyen, et al. (2005). "Impact of graft mass on the clinical outcome of kidney transplants." J Am Soc Nephrol 16(1): 261-8.

Gjertson, D. W. and J. M. Cecka (2000). "Living unrelated donor kidney transplantation." Kidney Int 58(2): 491-9.

Gloor, J., S. DeGoey, et al. (2003). "Overcoming a positive crossmatch in living-donor kidney transplantation." Am J Transplant 3(8): 1017-23.

Gloor, J. and M. Stegall (2010). "Sensitized renal transplant recipients: current protocols and future directions." Nat Rev Nephrol 6(5): 297-306.

Gloor, J., J. Winters, et al. (2010). "Baseline donor-specific antibody levels and outcomes in positive crossmatch kidney transplantation." Am J Transplant 10(3): 582-9.

Gloor J, W. L., Cornell L, Fix L, DrGoey S, Knauer R, Cosio F, Gandhi M, Kremers W, Stegall M (2010). "Baseline donor-specific antibody levels and outcomes in positive crossmatch kidney transplantation." American Journal of Transplantation 10: 582-589.

Grino JM (1994). "BN 52021: a platelet activating factor antagonist for preventing post-transplant renal failure. A double-blind, randomized study. The BN 52021 Study Group in Renal Transplantation." Annals of Internal Medicine 121(5): 12.

Horvat, L. D., S. Z. Shariff, et al. (2009). "Global trends in the rates of living kidney donation." Kidney Int 75(10): 1088-98.

Humar, A., B. Durand, et al. (2000). "Living unrelated donors in kidney transplants: better long-term results than with non-HLA-identical living related donors?" Transplantation 69(9): 1942-5.

Hurst, F., S. Sajjad, et al. (2010). "Transplantation of A2 Kidneys into B and O Recipients Leads to Reduction in Waiting Time: USRDS Experience." Transplantation 89: 1396-1402.

Iordanous, Y., N. Seymour, et al. (2009). "Recipient outcomes for expanded criteria living kidney donors: the disconnect between current evidence and practice." Am J Transplant 9(7): 1558-73.

Issa, N., B. Stephany, et al. (2007). "Donor factors influencing graft outcomes in live donor kidney transplantation." Transplantation 83(5): 593-9.

Jordan, S., A. Vo, et al. (2003). "Intravenous immune globulin treatment inhibits crossmatch positivity and allows for successful transplantation of incompatible organs in living-donor and cadaver recipients." Transplantation 76(4): 631-6.

Jüttler, E., S. Schwab, et al. (2007). "Decompressive Surgery for the Treatment of Malignant Infarction of the Middle Cerebral Artery (DESTINY): a randomized, controlled trial." Stroke 38(9): 2518-25.

Kayler, L. K., H. U. Meier-Kriesche, et al. (2002). "Gender imbalance in living donor renal transplantation." Transplantation 73(2): 248-52.

Kayler, L. K., C. S. Rasmussen, et al. (2003). "Gender imbalance and outcomes in living donor renal transplantation in the United States." Am J Transplant 3(4): 452-8.

Keith, D., A. Demattos, et al. (2004). "Effect of donor recipient age match on survival after first deceased donor renal transplantation." J Am Soc Nephrol 15(4): 1086-91.

Kessler, M., M. Ladriere, et al. (2011). "Does pre-emptive kidney transplantation with a deceased donor improve outcomes? Results from a French transplant network." Transpl Int 24(3): 266-75.

Kootstra, G., J. Daemen, et al. (1995). "Categories of non-heart-beating donors." Transplant Proc 27: 2893-94.

Land W, S. H., Schleibner S, Illner WD, Abendroth D, Rutili G, Arfors KE, Messmer K (1994). "The beneficial effect of human recombinant superoxide dismutase on acute and chronic rejection events in recipients of cadaveric renal transplants." Transplantation 57(2): 7.

Laupacis, A., P. Keown, et al. (1996). "A study of the quality of life and cost-utility of renal transplantation." Kidney Int 50(1): 235-42.

Lefaucheur, C., C. Suberbielle-Boissel, et al. (2008). "Clinical relevance of preformed HLA donor-specific antibodies in kidney transplantation." Am J Transplant 8(2): 324-31.

Liem, Y. S. and W. Weimar (2009). "Early living-donor kidney transplantation: a review of the associated survival benefit." Transplantation 87(3): 317-8.

Lim, W., S. Chang, et al. (2010). "Donor-recipient age matching improves years of graft function in deceased-donor kidney transplantation." Nephrol Dial Transplant 25(9): 3082-9.

Lim, W. H., S. H. Chang, et al. (2007). "Parental donors in live-donor kidney transplantation associated with increased rejection rates and reduced glomerular filtration rates." Transplantation 84(8): 972-80.

Locke, J., D. Segev, et al. (2007). "Outcomes of kidneys from donors after cardiac death: implications for allocation and preservation." Am J Transplant 7: 1797-807.

Locke, J., A. Zachary, et al. (2007). "The utility of splenectomy as rescue treatment for severe acute antibody mediated rejection." Am J Transplant 7(4): 842-6.

Machnicki, G., B. Pinsky, et al. (2009). "Predictive ability of pretransplant comorbidities to predict long-term graft loss and death." Am J Transplant 9(3): 494-505.

Mahanty, H. D., W. S. Cherikh, et al. (2001). "Influence of pretransplant pregnancy on survival of renal allografts from living donors." Transplantation 72(2): 228-32.

Mange, K. C., M. M. Joffe, et al. (2001). "Effect of the use or nonuse of long-term dialysis on the subsequent survival of renal transplants from living donors." N Engl J Med 344(10): 726-31.

Mannami, M., R. Mannami, et al. (2008). "Last resort for renal transplant recipients, 'restored kidneys' from living donors/patients." Am J Transplant 8(4): 811-8.

McDonald, S., L. Excell, et al. (2009). New patient commencing treatment in 2008. Australia and New Zealand Dialysis and Transplant Registry. S. McDonald, L. Excell and B. Livingston. Adelaide: 1-12.

Meier-Kriesche, H., D. Cibrik, et al. (2002). "Interaction between donor and recipient age in determining the risk of chronic renal allograft failure." J Am Geriatr Soc 50(1): 14-7.

Meier-Kriesche, H., J. Schold, et al. (2005). "Kidneys from deceased donors: maximizing the value of a scarce resource." Am J Transplant 5: 1725-30.

Meier-Kriesche, H. U. and B. Kaplan (2002). "Waiting time on dialysis as the strongest modifiable risk factor for renal transplant outcomes: a paired donor kidney analysis." Transplantation 74(10): 1377-81.

Merion, R., V. Ashby, et al. (2005). "Deceased-donor characteristics and the survival benefit of kidney transplantation." JAMA 294(21): 2726-33.

Metzger, R., F. Delmonico, et al. (2003). "Expanded criteria donors for kidney transplantation." Am J Transplant 3(Suppl 4): 114-25.

Miles, C. D., D. E. Schaubel, et al. (2008). "The role of donor-recipient relationship in long-term outcomes of living donor renal transplantation." Transplantation 85(10): 1483-8.

Milton, C., G. Russ, et al. (2008). "Pre-emptive renal transplantation from living donors in Australia: Effect on allograft and patient survival." Nephrology 13: 535-40.

Moers, C., N. Kornmann, et al. (2009). "The influence of deceased donor age and old-for-old allocation on kidney transplant outcome." Transplantation 88(4): 542-52.

Mujtaba, M., W. Goggins, et al. (2011). "The strength of donor-specific antibody is a more reliable predictor of antibody-mediated rejection than flow cytometry crossmatch analysis in desensitized kidney recipients." Clin Transplant 25(1): E96-102.

Nelson, P., C. r. Shield, et al. (2002). "Increased access to transplantation for blood group B cadaveric waiting list candidates by using A2 kidneys: time for a new national system?" Am J Transplant 2(1): 94-9.

Nicol D, P. J., Wall D, Griffin A, Campbell S, Isbel N, Hawley C, Johnson D (2008). "Kidneys from patients with small renal tumours: a novel source of kidneys for transplantation." British Journal of Urology International 102(2): 188-192.

Nyberg SL, M. A., Kremers WK, Thostenson JD, Larson TS, Prieto M, Ishitani MB, Sterioff S, Stegall MD (2003). "Improved scoring system to assess adult donors for cadaver renal transplantation." Am J Transplant 2(6): 6.

Nyberg SL, M. A., Rogers M, Harmsen WS, Velosa JA, Larson TS, Prieto M, Ishitani MB, Sterioff S, Stegall MD (2001). "Donor scoring system for cadaveric renal transplantation." Am J Transplant 1(2): 8.

Nyengaard JR, B. T. (1992). "Glomerular number and size in relation to age, kidney weight, and body surface in normal man (abstract)." The Anatomical Record 232(2): 7.

Oien, C. M., A. V. Reisaeter, et al. (2007). "Living donor kidney transplantation: the effects of donor age and gender on short- and long-term outcomes." Transplantation 83(5): 600-6.

Oien, C. M., A. V. Reisaeter, et al. (2005). "Gender imbalance among donors in living kidney transplantation: the Norwegian experience." Nephrol Dial Transplant 20(4): 783-9.

Ojo, A., J. Hanson, et al. (2001). "Survival in recipients of marginal cadaveric donor kidneys compared with other recipients and wait-listed transplant candidates." J Am Soc Nephrol 12(3): 589-97.

Ojo, A., A. Leichtman, et al. (2000). "Impact of pre-existing donor hypertension and diabetes mellitus on cadaveric renal transplant outcomes." Am J Kidney Dis 36(1): 153-9.

Ojo AO, H. (2001). "Survival in recipients of marginal cadaveric donor kidneys compared with other recipients and wait-listed transplant candidates." Journal of the American Society of Nephrology 12(3): 9.

Oosterlee, A. and A. Rahmel, Eds. (2008). Eurotransplant International Foundation Annual Report 2008 [internet]. Leiden (Netherlands), Eurotransplant.

Oppenheimer, F., P. Aljama, et al. (2004). "The impact of donor age on the results of renal transplantation." Nephrol Dial Transplant 19(Suppl 3): iii11-iii15.

OPTN. (2010). "Kidney allocation policy development." http://optn.transplant.hrsa.gov/kars.asp.

Penn I (1995). "Primary kidney tumors before and after renal transplantation." Transplantation 59(4): 480-485.

Poggio, E., S. Hila, et al. (2006). "Donor kidney volume and outcomes following live donor kidney transplantation." Am J Transplant 6(3): 616-24.

Port FK, B.-G. J., Metzger RA, Dykstra DM, Gillespie BW, Young EW, Delmonico FL, Wynn JJ, Merion RM, Wolfe RA, Held PJ (2002). "Donor characteristics associated with reduced graft survival: An approach to expanding the pool of kidney donors." Transplantation 74(9): 5.

Rao, P., R. Merion, et al. (2007). "Renal transplantation in elderly patients older than 70 years of age: results from the Scientific Registry of Transplant Recipients." Transplantation 83(8): 1069-74.

Rao, P., D. Schaubel, et al. (2009). "A comprehensive risk quantification score for deceased donor kidneys: the kidney donor risk index." Transplantation 88(2): 231-6.

Rapaport F (1986). "The case for a living emotionally related international kidney donor exchange registry." Transplant Proceedings 18(3 (Suppl. 2)): 5-9.

Rosenberg, J. C., B. Jones, et al. (2004). "Accelerated rejection following offspring-to-mother and husband-to-wife transplants." Clin Transplant 18(6): 729-33.

Savoye, E., D. Tamarelle, et al. (2007). "Survival benefits of kidney transplantation with expanded criteria deceased donors in patients aged 60 years and over." Transplantation 84(12): 1618-24.

Schaubel, D. E., D. E. Stewart, et al. (2000). "Sex inequality in kidney transplantation rates." Arch Intern Med 160(15): 2349-54.

Schold, J. and H. Meier-Kriesche (2006). "Which renal transplant candidates should accept marginal kidneys in exchange for a shorter waiting time on dialysis?" Clin J Am Soc Nephrol 1(3): 532-8.

Schweitzer, E. J., J. Wilson, et al. (2000). "Increased rates of donation with laparoscopic donor nephrectomy." Ann Surg 232(3): 392-400.

Segev, D. (2009). "Evaluating options for utility-based kidney allocation." Am J Transplant 9: 1513-8.

Shaheen, M., F. Shaheen, et al. (2010). "Impact of recipient and donor nonimmunologic factors on the outcome of deceased donor kidney transplantation." Transplant Proc 42(1): 273-6.

Sharma, P., D. Schaubel, et al. (2008). "Re-weighting the model for end-stage liver disease score components." Gastroenterology 135(5): 1575-81.

Smits, J., G. Persijn, et al. (2002). "Evaluation of the Eurotransplant Senior Program. The results of the first year." Am J Transplant 2: 664-70.

Stegall, M., J. Gloor, et al. (2006). "A comparison of plasmapheresis versus high-dose IVIG desensitization in renal allograft recipients with high levels of donor specific alloantibody." Am J Transplant 6: 346-51.

Summers, D., R. Johnson, et al. (2010). "Analysis of factors that aff ect outcome after transplantation of kidneys donated after cardiac death in the UK: a cohort study." Lancet 376: 1303-11.

Tan, J., E. Alfrey, et al. (2004). "Dual-kidney transplantation with organs from expanded criteria donors: a long-term follow-up." Transplantation 78(5): 692-6.

Tanabe K (2007). "Japanese experience of ABO-incompatible living kidney transplantation." Transplantation 84(12 Suppl): S4-7.

Tanabe, K., H. Ischida, et al. (2009). "Evaluation of two different preconditioning regimens for ABO-incompatible living kidney donor transplantation. A comparison of splenectomy vs. rituximab-treated non-splenectomy preconditioning regimens." Contrib Nephrol 162: 61-74.

Terasaki, P. I., J. M. Cecka, et al. (1997). "Spousal and other living renal donor transplants." Clin Transpl: 269-84.

Terasaki, P. I., J. M. Cecka, et al. (1995). "High survival rates of kidney transplants from spousal and living unrelated donors." N Engl J Med 333(6): 333-6.

Toki, D., H. Ishida, et al. (2009). "Acute antibody-mediated rejection in living ABO-incompatible kidney transplantation: long-term impact and risk factors." Am J Transplant 9(3): 567-77.

Transplant, N. H. S. B. a. (2010). "Transplant activityin the UK, 2008-2009." from http://www.organdonation.nhs.uk/ukt/statistics/transplant_activity_report/current_activity_reports/ukt/2008_09/transplant_activity_uk_2008-09.pdf.

US Organ Procurement and Transplantion Network and Scientific Registry of Transplant Recipients (2009). US Organ Procurement and Transplantion Network and the Scientific Registry of Transplant Recipients Annual Report 2009: Transplant Data 1999-2008, US Department of Health and Human Services.

Vereerstraeten, P., M. Wissing, et al. (1999). "Male recipients of kidneys from female donors are at increased risk of graft loss from both rejection and technical failure." Clin Transplant 13(2): 181-6.

Vo, A., M. Lukovsky, et al. (2008). "Rituximab and intravenous immune globulin for desensitization during renal transplantation." N Engl J Med 359: 242-51.

Vo, A., A. Peng, et al. (2010). "Use of intravenous immune globulin and rituximab for desensitization of highly HLA-sensitized patients awaiting kidney transplantation." Transplantation 89: 1095-102.

Waiser, J., M. Schreiber, et al. (2000). "Age-matching in renal transplantation." Nephrol Dial Transplant 2000(15).

Wolfe, R., V. Ashby, et al. (1999). "Comparison of mortality in all patients on dialysis, patients on dialysis awaiting transplantation, and recipients of a first cadaveric transplant." N Engl J Med 341(23): 1725-30.

Wolfe, R., K. McCullough, et al. (2009). "Predictability of survival models for waiting list and transplant patients: calculating LYFT." Am J Transplant 9(7): 1523-7.

Young, C. and R. Gaston (2000). "Renal transplantation in black Americans." N Engl J Med 343(21): 1545-52.

Young, C. and R. Gaston (2005). "Understanding the influence of ethnicity on renal allograft survival." Am J Transplant 5: 2603-4.

Zeier, M., B. Dohler, et al. (2002). "The effect of donor gender on graft survival." J Am Soc Nephrol 13(10): 2570-6.

Zimmerman, D., S. Donnelly, et al. (2000). "Gender disparity in living renal transplant donation." Am J Kidney Dis 36(3): 534-40.

9

Donor Quality Scoring Systems and Early Renal Function Measurements in Kidney Transplantation

Quirino Lai et al.*
Department of General surgery and Organ transplantation,
Sapienza University of Rome, Rome
Italy

1. Introduction

Over the last years, an extensive improvement in the use of non-standard kidney allografts from deceased donors has been observed due to a chronic scarcity in the number of available donors. However, use of these donors seems to give worse results, higher delayed graft function (DGF) and rejection rates and briefer graft survivals.
Nevertheless, a standardized definition of non-standard donor is still under debate.
On these grounds, several studies have focalized on the importance of events immediately before or early post-transplant in determining allograft outcome: introduction of scores based on peri-operative features capable to predict graft function may yield huge implications for organ allocation policies, as well as for immediate and late clinical and immunological management of recipients. In fact, if pre-KT information could accurately predict suboptimal early graft function, the success of various mechanical, immunosuppressive and organ allocation strategies may be improved.
The aim of this review is to analyze the different pre- and post-transplant score systems, detecting their role in the clinical practice and comparing them in terms of prognostic ability.

2. Donor quality scoring systems

In the last decades, several different scoring systems based on donor, recipient and transplant parameters have been proposed with the intent to predict early and late post-KT graft function.
Despite several of these scores have been validated on large cohorts or have been adopted by national allocation systems, no one of them has been already internationally recognized as the best model for graft function prediction.
We analyzed these scores, stratifying them in three groups according to the different parameters by which they are composed: demographic and serological variables, histological graft variables, donor and histological graft variables.

---

* Francesco Nudo, Vincenzo Morabito, Giovanni Battista Levi Sandri, Fabio Melandro, Lucia Parlati, Nicola Guglielmo, Marco Di Laudo, Manuela Garofalo, Luca Poli, Renzo Pretagostini and Pasquale B Berloco

2.1 Demographic and serological variables

Several scores exclusively based on donor features or composed by a combination of parameters obtained by donor, transplant and donor-recipient match have been created. Some of these scores are commonly adopted in the care practice: we reported the most commonly used.

2.1.1 ECD

In March 2001, a consensus meeting who took place in Crystal City introduced a new definition of expanded criteria donor (ECD) (Rosengard et al, 2002). Under the work group's proposed plan, the Organ Procurement and Transplantation Network (OPTN), through its contract with the United Network for Organ Sharing (UNOS) developed a standard policy for national kidney allocation in the United States. In November 2001, the OPTN/UNOS Board of Directors adopted the new ECD definition and the new allocation system became operative in October 2002. The new definition of ECD derived from four different donor risk factors for graft failure: age, history of hypertension, cerebrovascular accident as a cause of death and final pre-procurement creatinine > 1.5 mg/dL.

Different combinations of these four parameters characterized each donor kidney and a relative risk of graft loss was determined for each donor profile (**Figure 1**).

	RR			
	Normal creatinine		High creatinine	
Age (years)	No HTN	HTN	No HTN	HTN
Cause of death was not cerebrovascular accident				
0–9	1.40**	1.59**	1.52**	–
10–39	1.00	1.14**	1.09*	1.24**
40–49	1.17**	1.33**	1.28**	1.45**
50–59	1.41**	1.60**	1.53**	**1.74****
60+	**1.90****	**2.16****	**2.07****	**2.36****
Cause of death was cerebrovascular accident				
0–9	1.60**	**1.82****	**1.74****	**1.98****
10–39	1.14**	1.30**	1.24**	1.41**
40–49	1.34**	1.52**	1.46**	1.66**
50–59	1.61**	**1.83****	**1.75****	**1.99****
60+	**2.17****	**2.47****	**2.37****	**2.69****

Source: SRTR data analyses as of August 1, 2002.
HTN = donor hypertension. Numbers in boldface indicate RR > 1.7.
*$p < 0.05$, **$p < 0.0005$.

Fig. 1. Relative risks (RR) of graft loss by four donor characteristics. Taken from Metzger et al., 2003.

The ECD kidney was then arbitrarily defined as any kidney whose relative risk of graft failure exceeded 1.7 when compared to a reference group of ideal donor kidneys (age 10–39 years, no hypertension, no cerebrovascular accident as cause of death and terminal predonation creatinine level < 1.5 mg/dL).

The definition of ECD status is the following (**Table 1**):

a. Donor age older than 59 years;
b. Donor age between 50 and 59 years with, additionally two of the following: death caused by cerebrovascular accident (CVA); terminal creatinine more than 1.5 mg/dL; history of hypertension.

	Donor age categories (years)				
Donor condition	**< 10**	**10-39**	**40-49**	**50-59**	**≥ 60**
CVA + HTN + Creat > 1.5				X	X
CVA + HTN				X	X
CVA + Creat > 1.5				X	X
HTN + Creat > 1.5				X	X
CVA					X
HTN					X
Creat > 1.5					X
None of the above					X

Source: OPTN.
CVA = cerebrovascular accident was cause of death.
HTN = history of hypertension.
Creat > 1.5 = Creatinine > 1,5 mg/dL.

Table 1. ECD for kidney donors. Taken from Rosengard et al., 2002 (with modifications).

A multicentre study (Metzger et al., 2003) based on OPTN/SRTR data showed a progressive increase in ECD utilization across the years, confirming the worse results obtained from these donors in terms of both patient and graft survivals.
Nevertheless, a more rational definition of ECD has given major opportunities to patients who had presented limited access to KT to be transplanted.
A monocentre analysis (Stratta et al., 2004) reported an effective increased volume of KTs within 1 year after the adoption of ECD policy; moreover, the authors observed similar results in terms of graft function and morbidity among recipients who received organs from standard or ECD. A systematic approach to ECD kidneys based on nephron mass matching and nephron sparing measures showed to provide optimal short-term outcomes and renal function comparable to standard kidneys.

2.1.2 DDS

Using ECD, a better allocation policy was obtained. On the other hand, the binary nature of the ECD definition may have underappreciated the variability of the quality of the organ.
On these grounds, (Nyberg et al., 2001) a more granulated scoring system (deceased donor score, DDS) was developed. DDS was based on seven different donor variables easily available at the moment of procurement. The end measure for the development of the score was the 6-month creatinine clearance value.
The variables analyzed were:
Cause of death (0-6 points), history of hypertension (0-6), renal creatinine clearance before procurement (0-6), age (0-6), history of diabetes mellitus (0-3), cold ischemia time (0-3) and severity of renal artery plaque (0-3).

The population enrolled for the study (241 cadaveric KT recipients) was stratified in four groups: grade A (0-5 points), grade B (6-10), grade C (11-15) and grade D (16-32).
Adoption of this score permitted an effective stratification of the population, showing that information available at the time of organ harvesting may estimate early graft function after cadaveric renal transplantation.
The same Authors (Nyberg et al., 2003) improved on their original scoring system studying the data 34.324 KT patients reported in the OPTN/SRTR registry. The five donor variables adopted were:
Age (0-25 points), history of hypertension (0-4), creatinine clearance before procurement (0-4), cause of death (0-3), HLA mismatch (0-3).
The entire population was stratified in four different grades according to the cumulative donor score: grade A (0-9 points), grade B (10-19), grade C (20-29) and grade D (30-39).
The influence of donor score on both graft function and survival was most severe above 20 points (**Figure 2**).

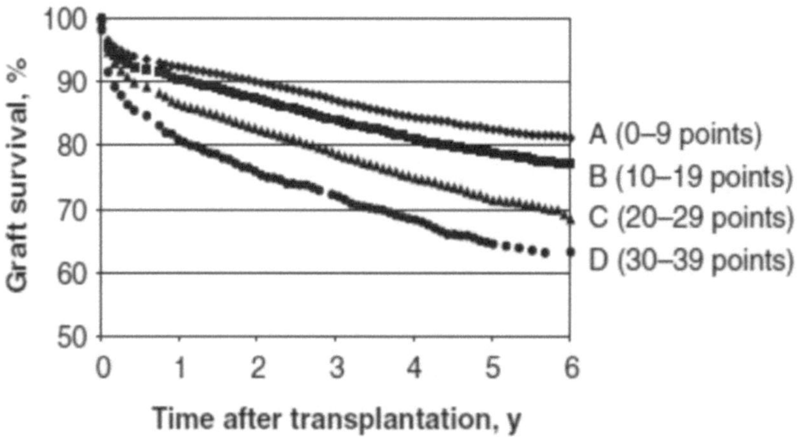

Fig. 2. Nyberg score grading significantly influences graft survival after transplantation. The greatest 6-year graft survival difference was observed between grades B and C, suggesting a cutoff for 'marginal' kidneys of approximately 20 points. Taken from Nyberg et al., 2003.

Afterwards, according to Nyberg score, this threshold value designates "marginal" kidneys.

2.1.3 DGF nomogram

According to the most commonly adopted definition, DGF is the need for dialysis in the first week after transplantation.
A multicentre study (Irish et al., 2003) analyzed data obtained from 13.846 patients reported in the United States Renal Data System (USRDS) registry from 1995 to 1998. Using a multivariable logistic regression analysis, factors contributing to DGF were analyzed.
The pre-KT donor and recipient factors analyzed were:
Donor: age, history of hypertension, terminal creatinine, donation after cardiac death, death caused by anoxia or CVA; cold ischemia time; HLA mismatch; combined organ transplantation.
Recipient: gender, race, diabetes, history of previous transplantation, history of transfusion, history of dialysis before transplantation, peak panel reactive anti-HLA antibodies.

A nomogram quantifying the relative contribution of each risk factor was created, providing a useful tool for developing a pretransplantation index of the likelihood of DGF occurrence (**Figure 3**).
Seven years later, a new analysis (Irish et al., 2010) was performed on 24.337 patients transplanted during the period 2003-2006. The authors developed a novel nomogram and a web-based calculator (http://www.transplantcalculator.com/DGF) as an easily accessible tool for predicting DGF.
Comparing risk factors in the modern (2003-2006) and in the earlier era (1995-1998), weight of immunological factors attenuated, while impact of donor renal function increased by 2-fold. The most significant factors associated with DGF were cold ischemia time, donor creatinine, body mass index, donation after cardiac death and donor age.

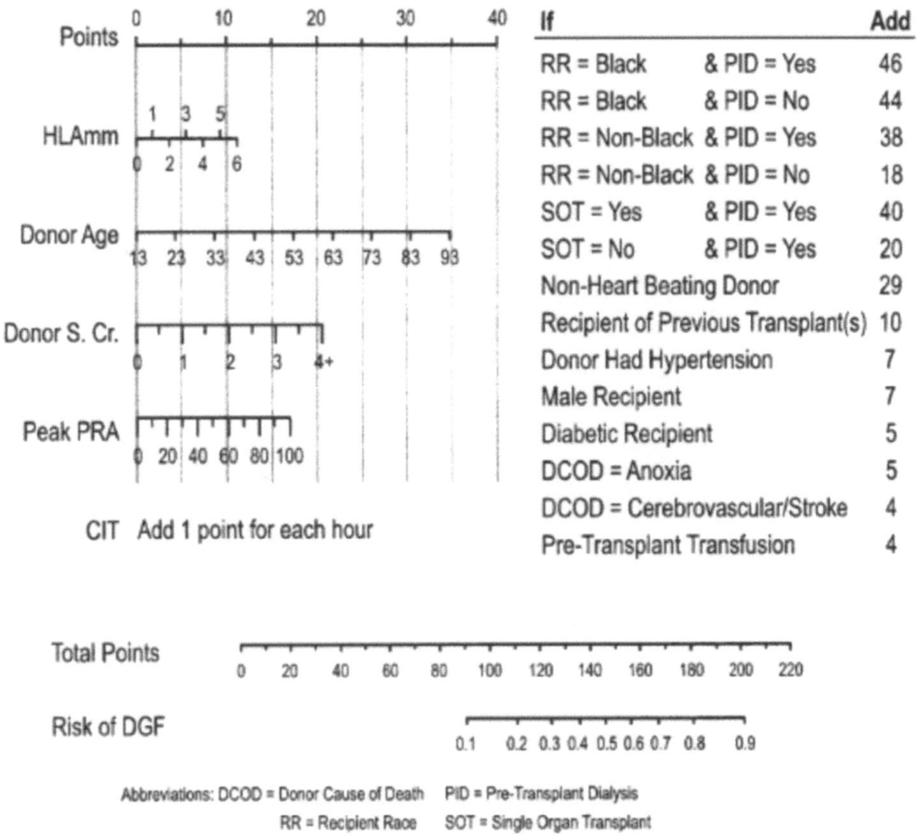

Fig. 3. Nomogram for estimating the risk of delayed graft function (DGF) in adult renal transplant recipients. HLAmm, HLA mismatch; S.Cr., serum creatinine; PRA, panel-reactive antibody; CIT, cold ischemia time; RR, recipient race; PID, pre-transplantation dialysis; DCOD, donor cause of death; SOT, single-organ transplant. Taken from Irish et al., 2003.

2.1.4 Pessione score

A retrospective analysis of a cohort of 7.209 deceased KT recipients transplanted in France from 1996 to 2000 was performed and a new scoring system (Pessione et al.. 2003) was ideated.

After multivariate analysis, only three parameters resulted as significant independent risk factors for graft failure:

Cerebrovascular cause of death, history of hypertension and elevated serum creatinine (> 150 micromol/L).

Donor age > 60 years was a statistically significant, but dependent, risk factor. The increased risk of graft loss in patients who presented the cumulative effect of donor risk factors was greater in recipients aged more than 60 years (one risk factor: RR = 1.8; two risk factors: RR = 2.7) (**Figure 4**).

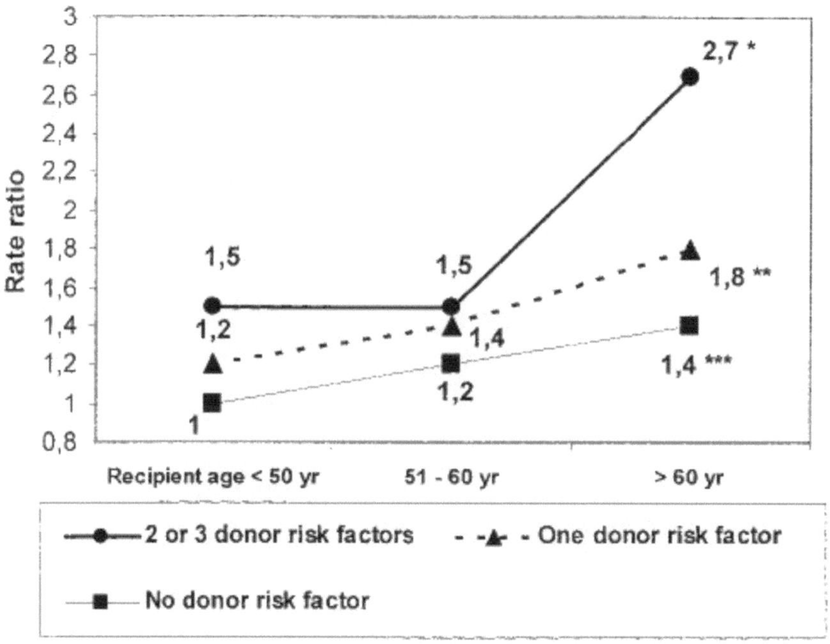

Fig. 4. Rate ratios of graft failure according to the absence or the presence of one or >2 significant donor risk factors in the different recipient age groups. *p-value = 0.008 (vs. patients <60 yr), ** p-value = 0.04 (vs. patients <60 yr), *** p-value = NS (vs. patients <60 yr). Taken from Pessione et al., 2003.

2.1.5 DRS

Donor risk score (DRS) (Schold et al., 2005) represents a model in which not only significant donor features, but also donor-recipient matches and cold ischemia time are adopted.

The variables used for the creation of the score were:

Donor race; donor history of hypertension; donor history of diabetes; donor death due to CVA; cold ischemia time; HLA mismatch; donor/ recipient cytomegalovirus (CMV) match.

The following grades based on accumulated "points" have been proposed: grade I (0-0.234), grade II (0.234-0.524), grade III (0.524-0.853), grade IV (0.853-1.17), and grade V (>1.17).

Adopting this model, the projected half-lives by donor grade, calculated utilizing data beyond 2-year posttransplant, were: grade I = 10.7 years; II = 10.0 years; III = 7.9 years; IV = 5.7 years; V = 4.5 years.
Comparing DRS with ECD and Nyberg score, the first one was the best model in graft loss stratification (**Figure 5**).

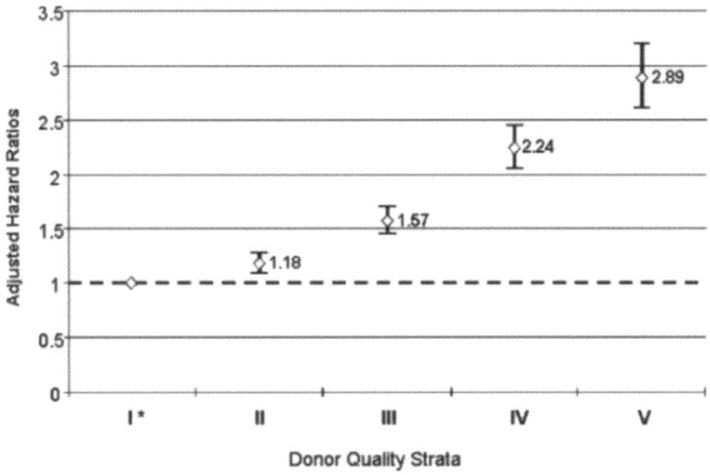

Fig. 5. Multivariate estimates for graft loss by donor grade. *Grade I donor serves as the reference group in the model. Taken from Schold et al., 2005.

2.1.6 KDRI

Kidney donor risk index (KDRI) (Rao et al., 2009) was proposed as a continuous combining donor and transplant variables to quantify graft failure risk. The authors analyzed 69.440 patients using national data from 1995 to 2005.
The fourteen proposed KDRI donor and transplant factors, each found to be independently associated with graft failure or death, were:
Donor: age, race, history of hypertension, history of diabetes, serum creatinine, cerebrovascular cause of death, height, weight, donation after cardiac death, hepatitis C virus status;
Transplant: human leukocyte antigen-B and DR mismatch, cold ischemia time, double or en bloc transplant.
The KDRI reflected the rate of graft failure relative to that of a healthy 40-year-old donor. Transplants of kidneys in the highest KDRI quintile (>1.45) had an adjusted 5-year graft survival of 63%, compared with 82% and 79% in the two lowest KDRI quintiles (<0.79 and 0.79-<0.96, respectively) (**Figure 6**).

2.1.7 DGF score

An analysis on a monocentre cohort of Italian KTs (Pretagostini et al., 2009) was performed with the intent to define the risk factors for the development of DGF.
The authors found five different donor and transplant parameters most commonly observed in non standard donors:
Donor age ≥ 60 years (P = 0.005), Creatinine Clearance < 40 mL/min (P = 0.025), history of diabetes mellitus (P = 0.026), history of hypertension (P = 0.017), and cold ischemia time > 15 hours (P < 0.0001).

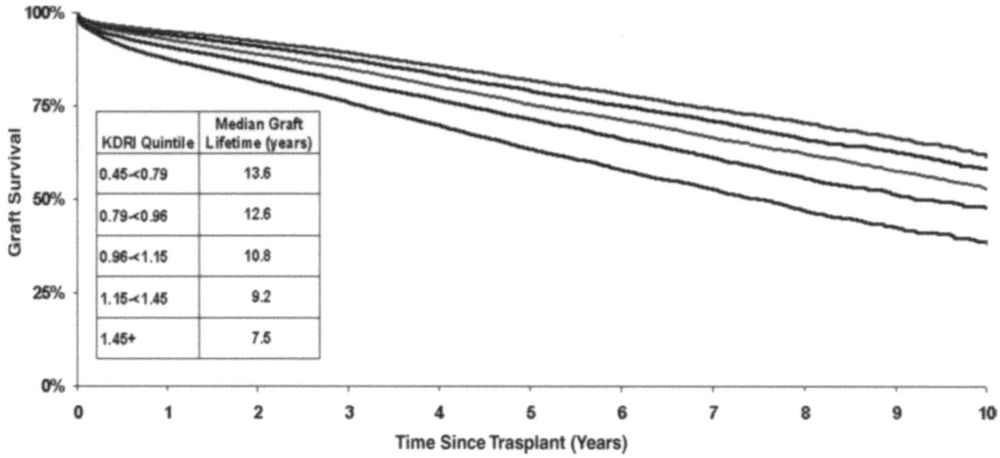

Fig. 6. Adjusted graft survival by KDRI quintile. Each survival pertains to a recipient who is aged 50 years, non-diabetic, and at the reference level of all other recipient factors. Extrapolation was used for the first and second quintile. Taken from Rao et al., 2009.

2.2 Histological graft variable

Above clinical features, another adopted approach fo4r the identification of high-risk kidneys is to use a pre-KT biopsy in order to characterize potential kidney grafts, help predict the graft outcome and provide a reference point for analysis of subsequent biopsies. Several different histological parameters have been correlated with poor outcomes (i.e. percentage of sclerotic glomerules, degree of tubulointerstitial and chronic vascular lesions). Starting from these considerations, all these histological changes were integrated into histological scoring systems with the intent to consent a better allocation of kidneys from elder donors. All the histological scores reported in literature in the last decades were based on the previously proposed semiquantitative analysis of renal histology (Pirani & Salinas-Madrigal, 1975).

2.2.1 Remuzzi score

The results of a consensus created by an international panel of pathologists (Remuzzi et al., 1999) consented the creation of a new score, This method was presented for the evaluation of kidneys procured from donors older than 60 years of age. This new method quantified the number of nephrons for each kidney with the intent to estimate if the grafts should be available for KT and whether single or dual transplantation should be used. This panel suggested a biopsy-based score ranging from a minimum of 0 (indicating the absence of renal lesions) to a maximum of 12 (indicating the presence of marked changes in the renal parenchyma) (**Table 2**).

The four different parameters considered in the scoring system were:

Glomerular global sclerosis (0-3), tubular atrophy (0-3), interstitial fibrosis (0-3) and arterial and arteriolar narrowing (0-3).

Kidneys with a score of 3 or lower were predicted to contain enough viable nephrons to be used as single transplants. Those with a score of 4, 5, or 6 could be used as dual transplants, on the assumption that the sum of the viable nephrons in the two kidneys approached the number in one ideal kidney. Kidneys with a score of 7 or greater were discarded, since it

was assumed that they would deliver an insufficient dose of nephrons, even in a dual transplantation.
The validity of the score was tested (Remuzzi et al., 2006) analyzing a prospective cohort study of 62 patients who received one or two histologically evaluated kidneys from donors older than 60 years of age.
The outcomes of these grafts were compared with the outcomes among 248 matched recipients of single kidney grafts that had not been histologically evaluated and were either from 124 donors with age ≤ 60 years or from 124 donors older than 60 years.

Pretransplant biopsy protocol: semiquantitative method of evaluation of slides #
Glomerular global sclerosis Based on three sections (the first, middle, and last sections, if available); the number of globally sclerosed glomerules expressed as a percentage. 0 none globally sclerosed 1+ < 20% global glomerulosclerosis 2+ 20 to 50% global glomerulosclerosis 3+ > 50% global glomerulosclerosis
Tubular atrophy 0 absent 1+ < 20% of tubuli affected 2+ 20 to 50% of tubuli affected 3+ > 50% of tubuli affected
Interstitial fibrosis 0 absent 1+ < 20% of renal tissue replaced by fibrous connective tissue 2+ 20 to 50% of renal tissue replaced by fibrous connective tissue 3+ > 50% of renal tissue replaced by fibrous connective tissue
Arterial and arteriolar narrowing For the vascular lesions, if the changes are focal, the most severe lesion present gives the final grade. 0 absent 1+ increased wall thickness but to a degree that is less than the diameter of the lumen 2+ wall thickness that is equal or slightly greater to the diameter of the lumen 3+ wall thickness that far exceeds the diameter of the lumen with extreme luminal narrowing or occlusion
Final grade (range from 0 to a total of 12) 0 to 3 mild OK for single transplant 4 to 6 moderate OK for double transplant 7 to 12 severe should not be transplanted
Only biopsies with ≥ 25 glomerules considered for slide evaluation. Kidneys with evidence of acute tubular necrosis are not considered for the double transplant. Biopsies are graded as mild if they have 0 to 3 points in total provided they are less than 3 in any one category. Biopsies are graded as moderate if they have 4 to 6 points in total provided they do not have 3 points in more than one category.

Table 2. Histological score proposed by Remuzzi et al., 1999 (with modifications).

Analyzing long-term graft survival, excellent results were observed using the grafts previously selected by biopsy.
Graft survival in recipients of histologically evaluated kidneys did not differ significantly from that of grafts from younger donors previously evaluated with biopsy. On the other side, survivals were strongly superior to that of elder grafts not pre-operatively evaluated with biopsy.
Adopting this score, long-term survival of single or dual kidney grafts from donors older than 60 years of age were similarly excellent, showing that systematic hystological approach may help to expand the donor-organ pool for kidney transplantation without a contemporaneous lack of results .

2.2.2 Karpinski score

A New study based on histological aspects (Karpinski et al., 1999) was performed on 57 allografts procured by 34 elderly donors (age ≥ 60 years) with hypertension and/or vascular disease.
Graft survival of these patients was compared with the results of 57 control recipients selected to have similar baseline demographics but receiving transplants from younger donors.
Donor renal pathology was scored 0-3 (none to severe disease) in four areas (**Table 3**):
Glomerulosclerosis, tubular atrophy, interstitial fibrosis and vascular disease.
Vascular disease was composed by two different parameters (e.g. arteriolar narrowing and arterial sclerosis).
The number of sclerotic glomerules was expressed as a percent of the total number of glomerules available for evaluation.
For the vascular lesions, both arteries were evaluated separately. However, for the final vascular score, the most severe lesion of either arterioles or arteries determined the final grade. Each of the 4 compartments was given a score from 0 to 3; the total score was expressed out of 12.
A donor vessel score of 3/3 was associated with a 100% incidence of delayed graft function and poor 1-year graft function.

2.3 Donor and histological graft variables

A new model (Anglicheau et al., 2008) in which both histological and clinical variables were combined was developed in France. Before this study, in fact, a definitive role of pre-implantation biopsies versus clinical scores had not been extensively studied in marginal donors.
Pre-KT biopsies of 313 grafts from donors aged more than 50 years were analyzed.
Authors evaluated the ability in predicting 1-year poor graft function (estimated glomerular filtration rate [eGFR] < 25 mL/min/1.73 m2) of several donor clinical and histological features.
In multivariate analysis, the clinical and histological features that resulted statistically significant were:
Clinical parameters = donor hypertension and a serum Creatinine level ≥150 lmol/L before organ recovery.
Histological parameters: glomerulosclerosis, arteriolar hyalinosis, Pirani and CADI score.
However, the model who presented the highest performance in predicting low eGFR was achieved using a composite score that included donor serum creatinine (≥150 lmol/L or <150 lmol/L), donor hypertension and glomerulosclerosis (≥10% or <10%) (**Figure 7**).

Pretransplant biopsy protocol: semiquantitative method of evaluation of slides #
Glomerular wcore 0 none globally sclerosed 1+ < 20% global glomerulosclerosis 2+ 20 to 50% global glomerulosclerosis 3+ > 50% global glomerulosclerosis
Tubular score 0 absent 1+ < 20% of tubuli affected 2+ 20 to 50% of tubuli affected 3+ > 50% of tubuli affected
Interstitial score 0 absent 1+ < 20% of cortical parenchyma replaced by fibrous connective tissue 2+ 20 to 50% of cortical parenchyma replaced by fibrous connective tissue 3+ > 50% of cortical parenchyma replaced by fibrous connective tissue
Vascular score Arteriolar narrowing (or hyaline arteriolosclerosis)## 0 absent 1+ increased wall thickness but to a degree that is less than the diameter of the lumen 2+ wall thickness that is equal or slightly greater to the diameter of the lumen 3+ wall thickness that far exceeds the diameter of the lumen with extreme luminal narrowing or occlusion Arterial sclerosis (or intimal fibrous thickening-fibroplasia)## 0 absent 1+ increased wall thickness but to a degree that is less than the diameter of the lumen 2+ wall thickness that is equal or slightly greater to the diameter of the lumen 3+ wall thickness that far exceeds the diameter of the lumen with extreme luminal narrowing or occlusion
Only biopsies with at least 20 glomerules are considered for slide evaluation. ## For the vascular lesions, both arteries are evaluated separately. However, for the final vascular score, the most severe lesion of either arterioles or arterie determines the final grade.

Table 3. Scoring system proposed by Karpinski et al., 1999 (with modifications).

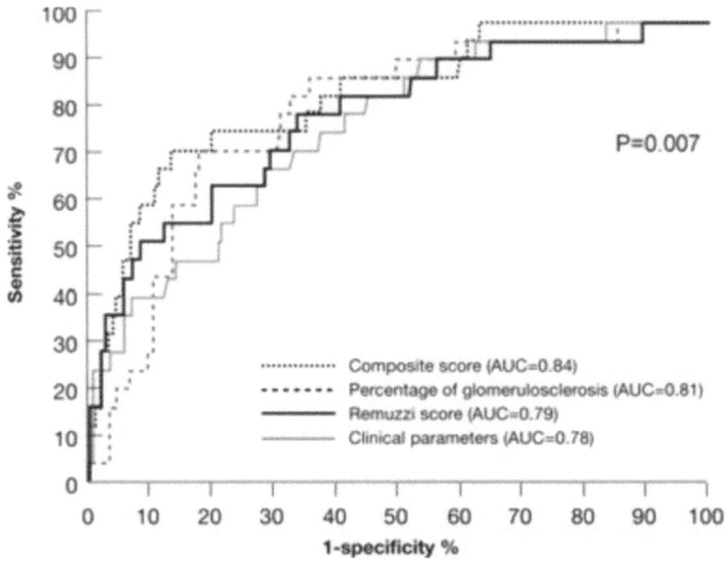

Fig. 7. Receiver operating characteristics (ROC) curves for clinical, histopathological and composite scoring systems as predictors of low eGFR at 1-year posttransplant. Global test: p-value = 0.007; composite score vs glomerulosclerosis: p-value = NS; composite score vs Pirani score: p-value = 0.001; composite score vs clinical parameters: p-value = 0.009). Taken from Anglicheau et al., 2008.

3. Measures of early graft function

Many measures of early graft function have been reported in Literature. Many of them were proposed with the intent to give a better definition of DGF. In fact, DGF is both an outcome and a predictor of the subsequent course of a renal transplant. Commonly adopted definition of DGF is the requirement for dialysis within the first week after KT (Daly et al., 2005). However, postoperative requirement of dialysis represents a very subjective and not standardized clinical decision. Recently, efforts have been made to quantify DGF more scientifically, adopting different scores based on urine output, serum creatinine levels, fluid overload and uremic status of the patient.
A comprehensive review of the literature (Yarlagadda et al., 2008) reported 18 different definitions for DGF (**Table 4**).

Definitions	No. of studies	No. of patients
Dialysis-based definitions		
Need for dialysis in the first week after transplant	41	259.251
Need for dialysis in the first week after transplant once hyperacute rejection, vascular and urinary tract complications were ruled out	2	760
Need for dialysis after transplant	2	737
Need for dialysis in the first 10 days after transplant	1	41
Absence of life-sustaining renal function that requires dialysis on two or more occasions within the first week after transplant	1	547

Definitions	No. of studies	No. of patients
Need for dialysis in the first 7 days after transplant with specific exclusion of single early post-operative dialysis performed for hyperkalemia	1	319
Return to maintenance hemodialysis within the first 4 days after transplantation	1	263
Creatinine-based definitions		
Serum creatinine increased or remained unchanged or decreased <10%/day during 3 consecutive days after the transplant	5	1471
Creatinine reduction ratio <30% and /or urine creatinine on Day 2 <1000 mg	2	401
Serum creatinine >2.5 mg/dL on Day 7 or the need for post-transplant hemodialysis	1	99
Time required for the kidney to reach Crcl>10 mL/min greater than 1 week.	1	843
Failure of creatinine to decline in the first 48 h in the absence of rejection	1	291
Combination		
Failure of serum creatinine to fall below pre-transplant levels, within 1 week regardless of the urine output	1	158
Patients with rise in serum Cr at 6–8 h post-operatively or <300 cc of urine despite adequate volume and diuretics	1	143
Dialysis requirement after transplant or a serum creatinine 150 μmol/L at Day 8	1	112
Urine output <1 L in 24 h and <25% fall in serum creatinine from baseline in first 24 h post-transplant	1	244
Urine output <75 mL/h in first 48 h or failure of serum Cr to decrease by 10% in the first 48 h	1	66
Need for dialysis in the first week after transplant or failure of serum creatinine to decrease within 24 h after transplant	1	104

Table 4. Different DGF definitions. Taken from Yarlagadda et al., 2008 (with modifications).

In the same study, 10 proposal of diagnostic technique to identify DGF were also proposed (**Figure 8**). Starting from these grounds, we have stratified the early measures of graft function in three different categories: creatinine-based definition, urine-based definition and combined definition.

3.1 Creatinine-based definition

a. Serum creatinine level of > 3 mg/dL on the fifth day after surgery (Humar et al., 2000).

b. CCR2 and 24-h UC2

This score was created (Govani et al., 2002) combining the creatinine reduction ratio between days 1 and 2 (CRR2) and the 24-h urinary creatinine levels at post-KT day 2 (UC2)

Equation: CRR2(%) = ([Cr1–Cr2]×100)/Cr1). (Cr1 = serum creatinine level at post-KT day 1; Cr2 = serum creatinine level at post-KT day 2).

The cut-off value for poor function corresponded to a CCR2 ≤ 30%.

c. CCR2

CCR2 was also adopted (Rodrigo et al., 2004; Salahudeen et al., 2004) as unique criterion for the definition of early graft function. The reported Authors used the same threshold value of 30%.

d. CCR7

Creatinine reduction ratio at day 7 (CCR7) (Johnston et al., 2007) was proposed as score of initial graft function.

Equation: $CRR7(\%) = ([Cr0 - Cr7] \times 100)/Cr0)$. *(Cr0 = serum creatinine levels immediately before KT and no later than 6 hours after last dialysis; Cr7 = serum creatinine levels at post-KT day 7).*

The cut-off value for poor function corresponded to a CCR7 ≤ 70% (**Figure 9**).

e. Number of days to achieve a creatinine clearance of > 10 mL/min, calculated by the Gault-Cockroft formula (Giral-Classe et al., 1998).
f. Serum creatinine level increased, remained unchanged or decreased by less than 10% per day immediately after surgery during three consecutive days for > 1 week (Boom et al., 2000).

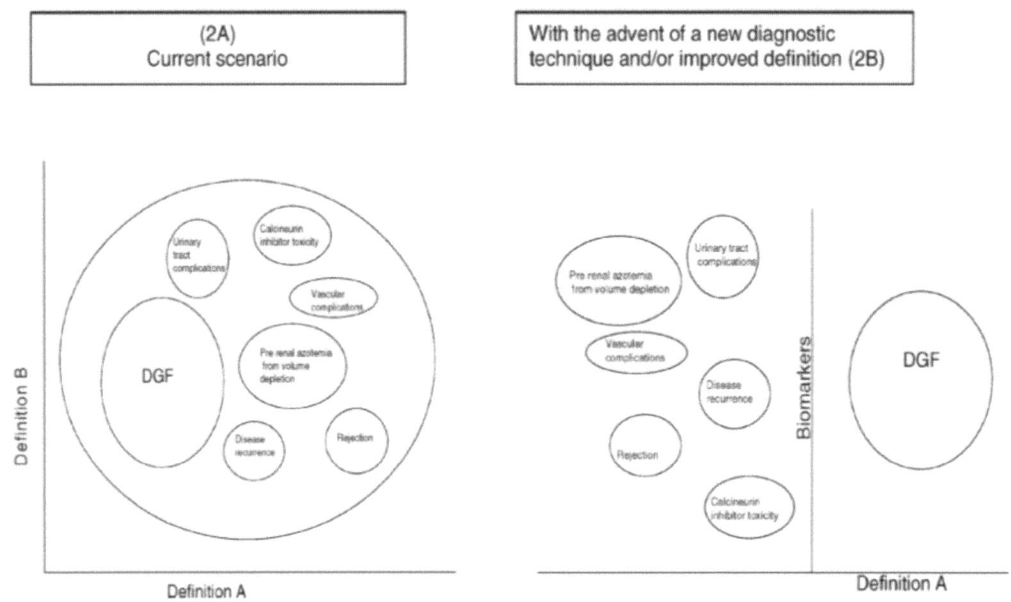

Fig. 8. Different clinical conditions that present as early graft dysfunction. (**A**) Current definitions do not allow us to distinguish DGF from other causes of graft dysfunction. (**B**) With an improved definition and/or diagnostic technique patients with DGF can be correctly classified. Taken from Yarlagadda et al., 2008.

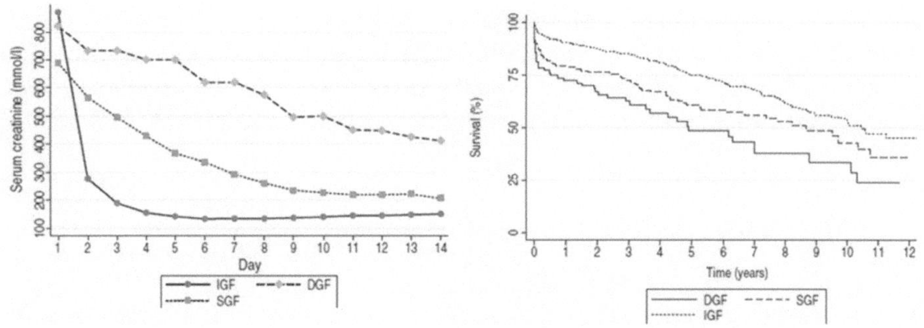

Fig. 9. *Left:* Decline in creatinine within 2 weeks post-KT. *Right:* graft survival curves. IGF: initial good function (CCR7 > 70%), DGF: delayed graft function (need for dialysis), SGF: scarce graft function (CCR7 ≤ 70% no dialysis). Taken from Johnston et al., 2007.

3.2 Urine-based definition

UO7

Urine output at post-KT day 7 (UO7) was recently proposed (Lai et al., 2010).
Equation: UO7 = total urine output on day 7 post-transplantation (mL)/weight (kg)/24 hours.
UO7 presented an elevated power for the prediction of 1-year graft function: at ROC analysis, UO7 presented an elevated area under the curve (0.811) (**Figure 10**). A cut-off value of 500 mL/24 h showed high sensitivity (98.5%).

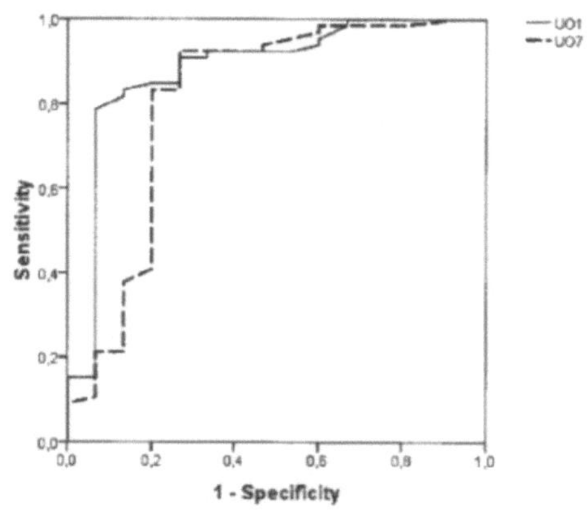

Fig. 10. ROC curves for post-KT day 1 urine output (UO1) and day 7 urine output (UO7) according to 1-year graft function (eGFR ≥ 30 mL/min/1.73 m2). Taken from Lai Q et al, 2009.

3.3 Combined definition

a. Cr7 and UO1

A score based on the combination of serum creatinine at post-KT day 7 (Cr7) and urine output at post-KT day 1(UO1) was proposed (Schnuelle et al., 2007).

Equation: UO1 = total 1st postoperative day urine output (mL)/weight (kg)/24 hours.

Kaplan-Maier survival estimates indicated a threshold effect of UO1 and Cr7, which could dissect the risk of graft failure. The thresholds referring to the 2nd quintile corresponded to a UO1 > 630 ml and a Cr7 <2.5 mg/dl. Combination of both of the parameters predicted a 5-year graft survival probability >90%, according to a hazard ratio of 0.21 (95% CI 0.09–0.46) (**Figure 11**).

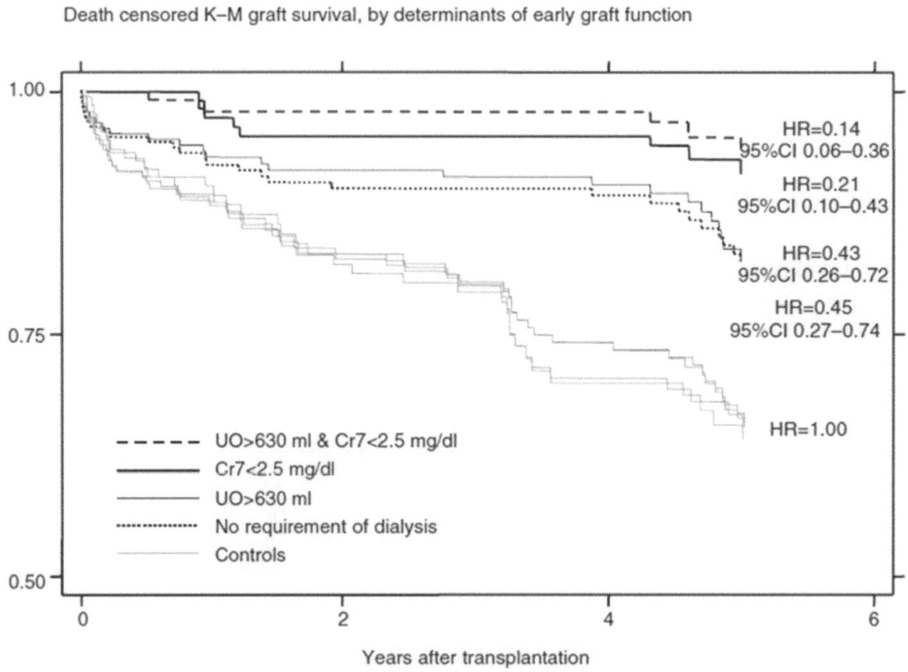

Fig. 11. Summary plot of 5-year graft survival estimates, by surrogates of early graft function as categorized by freedom from dialysis post-transplant, urine output exceeding 630 ml post-transplant, decline of serum creatinine below 2.5 mg/dl during the 1st week, and the combination of the latter criteria. Survival curves of the respective controls not meeting these requirements are displayed in light-colored lines. Taken from Schnuelle et al., 2007.

b. A definition of DGF obtainable within 6 hours after KT was proposed (Gonwa et al., 2002). It was based on a rising serum creatinine level above that before surgery or a urine output of < 300 mL within 6 h of transplantation, despite diuretics and adequate volume. Adoption of a very early definition of no-graft function was adopted with the intent to choose the correct immunosuppressive therapeutic approach to the patients.
c. A new model for the definition of DGF was created (Halloran & Hunsicker, 2001) by the combination of urine output of < 1 L in the first 24 h or a decrease in serum creatinine of < 20-30%.
d. DGF was recently defined (Lai et al., 2009) as the presence of one of the following conditions: at least 1-day persistent oligoanuria (≤ 500 mL/24 h) during the first week or an increased, unchanged, or decreased by ≤ 30% 7-day serum creatinine as compared with the pre-KT value.

4. Comparison among the scoring systems

Many researches have been performed on the identification of pre- or early post-operative clinical predictors of graft function; however, the great majority of them were based on isolated studies, usually in the populations from which they were initially derived. Moreover, only a small number of papers have focalized on their attention on the comparison among the different scoring systems.

For example, a previously reported study (Schold et al., 2005) compared preoperative scores (ECD, DDS and DRS), showing DRS was the best model for the prediction of graft survival at multivariable analysis. In the same period, another study (Nyberg et al., 2005) showed the superiority of DDS respect to ECD.

The first comparative analysis of preoperative and early post-operative scores (Moore et al., 2007) tested the ability of these clinical variables to predict suboptimal early function variably assessed by: DGF (dialysis requirement during the first week), DGF duration, slow graft function (creatinine > 3 mg/dl on day 5) and creatinine reduction ratio on day 2.

Multiple regression analysis was performed on 217 consecutive renal transplant recipients: DGF nomogram, DDS and ECD were compared. All scoring systems showed associations with early graft function, although only DGF nomogram remained statistically significant in the multiple regression model. However, the overall utility of the DGF nomogram in DGF prediction was moderate.

Two years later, a new comparative study (Moore et al., 2009) focalized on its attention on the role of pre- and post-KT models for the prediction of graft dysfunction: primary outcome measures were creatinine at 12 months and the development of chronic kidney disease stage 4T. The preoperative donor quality scores tested were: ECD, DDS, DRS and DGF nomogram: the postoperative early function measures were: dialysis requirement and duration; extended DGF according to Boom definition (Boom et al., 2000); Cr5, Cr7, CRR2, CRR7 and UO1.

Among the donor scoring systems, DRS was best associated with subsequent 6-month and 1-year allograft function. The study suggested a sort of "hierarchy": DRS > ECD > DDS > DGF nonogram.

These results could be explained by the different ways the scores were initially developed. For example, DGF nomogram was developed with regard to dialysis requiring DGF specifically, DDS was focalized on 6-month creatinine clearance, while DRS and ECD had graft failure as the end measure. The "granulated" complexity of DRS and DDS scores may explain their superiority above ECD.

Among the early function measures, extended definition of DGF, Cr5 and dialysis duration showed greatest predictive power in the patient population overall and in the subgroups of patients who not required or required dialysis, respectively. DGF resulted superior to the standard DGF definition: however, its importance lied in the simultaneous comparison of donor scores and early postoperative renal function to assess the best "baseline" indicator for later allograft dysfunction (**Figure 12**).

In another recent paper (Moore et al., 2010) dDGF (dialysis-based definition) and extDGF (extended; Boom et al., 2000) were compared (**Figure 13**). In the multivariable model, extDGF but not dDGF was significantly associated with graft failure (HR 1.47; p-value = 0.02). Similar results were observed for overall graft failure. The utility of extDGF as an early marker of late poor allograft outcomes suggested superiority over the traditional and often subjective dialysis-based definition.

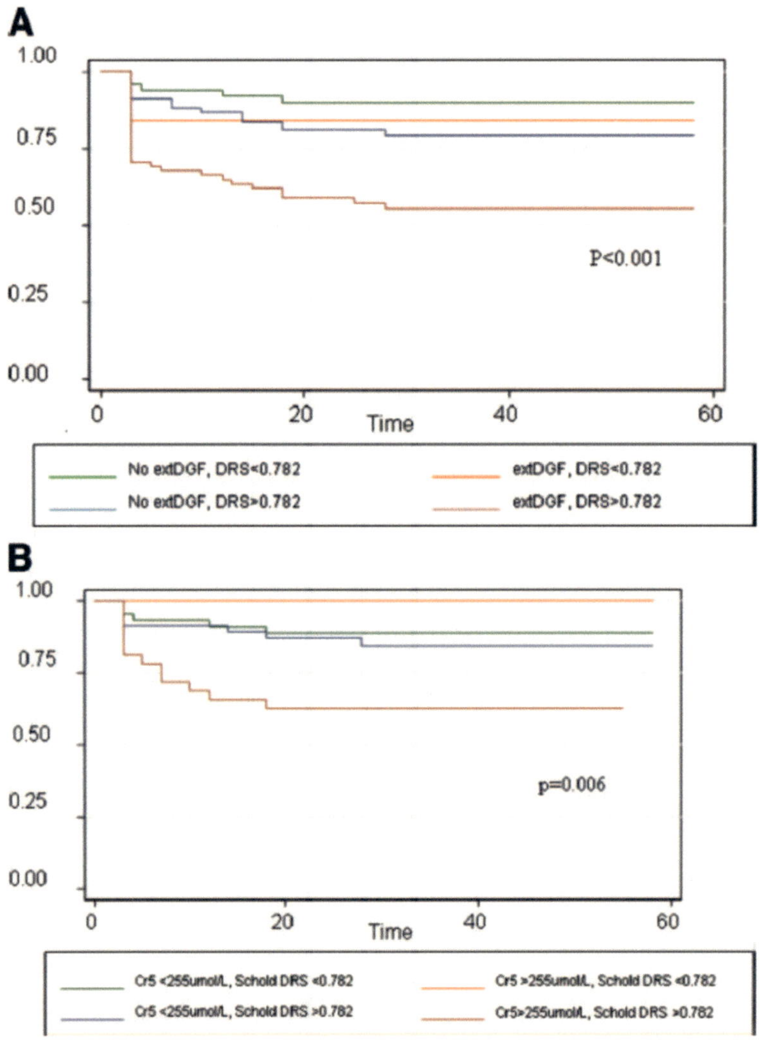

Fig. 12. (**A**) Kaplan-Meier survival curves for a combined variable of Donor Risk Score (DRS) and the extended definition of delayed graft function (extDGF) for time to stage 4T chronic kidney disease in all patients. (**B**) Kaplan-Meier survival curves for a combined variable of Donor Risk Score (DRS) and serum creatinine at day 5 (Cr5) for time to stage 4T chronic kidney disease in patients not requiring dialysis immediately postoperatively. Taken from Moore et al., 2009.

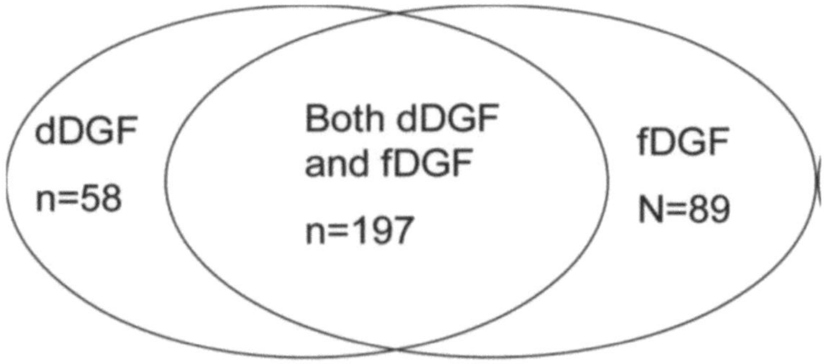

Fig. 13. Diagram shows distribution of early graft function. dDGF, dialysis-based definition of delayed graft function; fDGF (or extDGF), functional definition of delayed graft function. Taken from Moore et al., 2010.

Among creatinine-based models, Cr5 represented the "best" marker of early graft function in patients who didn't undergo a post-KT dialysis (Moore et al., 2009).
Indeed, the influence of pre- or post-KT dialysis on creatinine measurements independent of allograft excretory function was too great a confounder to allow meaningful interpretation of these parameters also in dialyzed patients.
Exclusive (Lai et al., 2010) or combined (Schnuelle et al., 2007) use of UO could be of some benefit in a better evaluation of these patients: however, more consistent large studies on this field are still required.
No comparative studies among clinical and histological scores have been reported. Studies are needed for a better understanding of the effective role of histological features and its comparison with pre- and immediately post-KT variables.

5. Conclusion

Donor scores, histological scores and early postoperative measures of renal allograft function may be of clinical utility in assessing the risk for subsequent renal dysfunction. This has relevance to organ allocation policy and also to the clinical management of individuals in the early postoperative period.
However, no one of the proposed criteria has still been internationally adopted.
Probably, a combined score based on pre- and post-operative clinical features and histological aspects may offer improved prognostication for graft outcome.
However, the first objective of a score must be its feasibility: its excessive "granulation" could transform it in a hardly adopted instrument in the care practice.
New studies focalized on the validation of previously proposed scores or for the development of new prognostication models are still required.

6. Acknowledgment

We thank the "Inter-University Consortium for Organ Transplantation".
We thank the "Kidney Transplant Group" of Sapienza University of Rome.

7. References

Anglicheau, D.; Loupy, A.; Lefaucheur, C.; Pessione, F.; Létourneau, I. & al. (2008). A simple clinico-histopathological composite scoring system is highly predictive of graft outcomes in marginal donors. *American Journal of Transplantation*, Vol.8, No.11, (November 2008), pp. 2325-2334.

Boom, H.; Mallat, MJ.; de Fijter, JW.; Zwinderman, AH. & Paul, LC. (2000). Delayed graft function influences renal function, but not survival. *Kidney International*, Vol.58, No.2, (August 2000), pp. 859-866.

Daly, PJ.; Power, RE.; Healy, DA.; Hickey, DP.; Fitzpatrick JM. & al. (2005). Delayed graft function: a dilemma in renal transplantation. *British Journal of Urology International*, Vol.96, No.4, (September 2005), pp. 498-501.

Giral-Classe, M.; Hourmant, M.; Cantarovich, D.; Dantal, J.; Blancho, G. & al. (1998). Delayed graft function of more than six days strongly decreases long-term survival of transplanted kidneys. *Kidney International*, Vol.54, No.3, (September 1998), pp. 972-978.

Gonwa, TA.; Mai, ML.; Smith, LB.; Levy, MF.; Goldstein, RM. & al. (2002). Immunosuppression for delayed or slow graft function in primary cadaveric renal transplantation. Use of low dose tacrolimus therapy with post-operative administration of anti-CD25 monoclonal antibody. *Clinical Transplantation*, Vol.16, No.2, (April 2002), pp. 144-149.

Govani, MV.; Kwon, O.; Batiuk, TD.; Milgrom, ML. & Filo RS. (2002). Creatinine reduction ratio and 24-hour creatinine excretion on posttransplant day two. Simple and objective tools to define graft function. *Journal of the American Society of Nephrology*, Vol.13, No.2, (June 2002), pp. 1645-1649.

Halloran, PF. & Hunsicker, LG. (2001) Delayed graft function. State of the art. Summit meeting, Scottsdale, Arizona, USA, November 10-11, 2000. *American Journal of Transplantation*, Vol.1, No.2, (July 2001), pp. 115-120.

Humar, A.; Payne, WD.; Sutherland, DE. & Matas, AJ. (2000). Clinical determinants of multiple acute rejection episodes in kidney transplant recipients. *Transplantation*, Vol.69, No.11, (June 2000), pp. 2357-2360.

Irish, WD.; McCollum, DA.; Tesi, RJ.; Owen, AB.; Brennan, DC. & al. (2003). Nomogram for predicting the likelihood of delayed graft function in adult cadaveric renal transplant recipients. *Journal of the American Society of Nephrology*, Vol.14, No.11, (November 2003), pp. 2967-2974.

Irish, WD.; Ilsley, JN.; Schnitzler, MA.; Feng, S. & Brennan, DC. (2010). A risk prediction model for delayed graft function in the current era of deceased donor renal transplantation. *American Journal of Transplantation*, Vol.10, No.10, (October 2010), pp. 2279-2286.

Johnston, O.; O'Kelly, P.; Spencer, S.; Donohoe, J.; Walshe, JJ. & al. (2006). Reduced graft function (with or without dialysis) vs immediate graft function – A comparison of longterm renal allograft survival. *Nephrology Dialysis Transplantation*, Vol.21, No.8, (August 2006), pp. 2270-2274.

Karpinski, J.; Lajoie, G.; Cattran, D.; Fenton, S.; Zaltzman, J. et al. (1999). Outcome of kidney transplantation from high-risk donors is determined by both structure and function. *Transplantation*, Vol.67, No.8, (April 1999), pp. 1162-1167.

Lai, Q.; Pretagostini, R.; Poli, L.; Melandro, F.; Ferretti, S. et al. (2009). Delayed graft function decreases early and intermediate graft outcomes after expanded criteria donor kidney transplants. *Transplantation Proceedings*, Vol.41, No.4, (May 2009), pp. 1145-1148.

Lai, Q.; Pretagostini, R.; Poli, L.; Levi Sandri, GB.; Melandro, F. et al. (2010). Early urine output predicts graft survival after kidney transplantation. *Transplantation Proceedings*, Vol.42, No.4, (May 2010), pp. 1090-1092.

Metzger, RA.; Delmonico, FL.; Feng, S.; Port, FK.; Wynn, JJ. & al. (2003). Expanded criteria donors for kidney transplantation. *American Journal of Transplantation*, Vol.3, Suppl.4, (2003), pp. 114-125.

Moore, J.; Tan, K.; Cockwell, P.; Krishnan, H.; McPake, D. & al. (2007). Predicting early renal allograft function using clinical variables. *Nephrology Dialysis Transplantation*, Vol.22, No.9, (September 2007), pp. 669-677.

Moore, J.; Ramakrishna, S.; Tan, K.; Cockwell, P.; Eardley, K. & al. (2009). Identification of the optimal donor quality scoring system and measure of early renal function in kidney transplantation. *Transplantation*, Vol.87, No.4, (February 2009), pp. 578-586.

Moore, J.; Shabir, S.; Chand, S.; Bentall, A.; McClean, A. & al. (2010). Assessing and comparing rival definitions of Delayed Renal Allograft Function for predicting subsequent graft failure. *Transplantation*, Vol.90, No.10, (September 2010), pp. 1113-1116.

Nyberg, SL.; Matas, AJ.; Rogers, M.; Harmsen, WS.; Velosa, JA. & al. (2001). Donor scoring system for cadaveric renal transplantation. *American Journal of Transplantation*, Vol.1, No.2, (July 2001), pp. 162-170.

Nyberg, SL.; Matas, AJ.; Kremers, WK.; Thostenson, JD.; Larson, TS. & al. (2003). Improved scoring system to assess adult donors for cadaver renal transplantation. *American Journal of Transplantation*, Vol.3, No.6, (June 2003), pp. 715-721.

Nyberg, SL.; Baskin-Bey, ES.; Kremers, W.; Prieto, M.; Henry, ML. & al. (2005). Improving the prediction of donor kidney quality: deceased donor score and resistive indices. *Transplantation*, Vol.80, No.7, (October 2005), pp. 925-929.

Pessione, F.; Cohen, S.; Durand, D.; Hourmant, M.; Kessler, M. & al. (2003). Multivariate analysis of donor risk factors for graft survival in kidney transplantation. *Transplantation*, Vol.75, No.3, (February 2003), pp. 361-367.

Pirani, CL. & Salinas-Madrigal L. (1975). Evaluation of percutaneous renal biopsy.; In: *Kidney pathology decentenial.; 1966-1975;* SC. Sommers; Norwalk CT (Ed.) ; Appleton-Century-Crofts: 1975.

Pretagostini, R.; Lai, Q.; Poli, L.; Levi Sandri, GB.; Travaglia, D. & al. (2009). Predictive characteristics of delayed graft function after expanded and standard criteria donor kidney transplantations. *Transplantation Proceedings*, Vol.41, No.4, (May 2009), pp. 1149-1151.

Rao, PS.; Schaubel, DE.; Guidinger, MK.; Andreoni, KA.; Wolfe, RA. & al. (2009). A comprehensive risk quantification score for deceased donor kidneys: the kidney donor risk index. *Transplantation*, Vol.88, No.2, (July 2009), pp. 231-236.

Remuzzi, G.; Grinyò, J.; Ruggenenti, P.; Beatini, M.; Cole, EH. & al. (1999). Early experience with dual kidney transplantation in adults using expanded donor criteria. Double Kidney Transplant Group (DKG). Journal of the *American Society of Nephrology*, Vol.10, No.12, (December 1999), pp. 2591-2598.

Remuzzi, G.; Cravedi, P.; Perna, A.; Dimitrov, BD.; Turturro, M. & al. (2006). Long-term outcome of renal transplantation from older donors. *New England Journal of Medicine*, Vol.354, No.4, (January 2006), pp. 343-352.

Rodrigo, E.; Ruiz, JC.; Piñera, C.; Fernández-Fresnedo, G.; Escallada, R. & al. (2004). Creatinine reduction ratio on post-transplant day two as criterion in defining delayed graft function. *American Journal of Transplantation*, Vol.4, No.7, (July 2004), pp. 1163-1169.

Rosengard, BR.; Feng, S.; Alfrey, EJ.; Zaroff, JG.; Emond, JC. & al. (2002). Report of the Crystal City meeting to maximize the use of organs recovered from the cadaver donor. *American Journal of Transplantation*, Vol.2, No.8, (September 2002), pp. 701-711.

Salahudeen, AK.; Haider, N. & May, W. (2004). Cold ischemia and the reduced long-term survival of cadaveric renal allografts. *Kidney International*, Vol.65, No.2, (February 2004), pp. 713-718.

Schnuelle, P.; Gottmann, U.; Köppel, H.; Brinkkoetter, PT.; Krzossok, S. & al. (2007). Comparison of early renal function parameters for the prediction of 5-year graft survival after kidney transplantation. *Nephrology Dialysis Transplantation*, Vol.22, No.1, (January 2007), pp. 235-245.

Schold, JD.; Kaplan, B.; Baliga, RS. & Meier-Kriesche, HU. (2005). The broad spectrum of quality in deceased donor kidneys. *American Journal of Transplantation*, Vol.5, No.4 Part.1, (April 2005), pp. 757-765.

Stratta, RJ.; Rohr, MS.; Sundberg, AK.; Armstrong, G.; Hairston, G. & al. (2005). Increased kidney transplantation utilizing expanded criteria deceased organ donors with results comparable to standard criteria donor transplant. *Annals of Surgery*, Vol.239, No.5, (May 2004), pp. 688-695.

Yarlagadda, SG.; Coca, SG.; Garg, AX.; Doshi, M.; Poggio, E. & al. (2008). Marked variation in the definition and diagnosis of delayed graft function: a systematic review. *Nephrology Dialysis Transplantation*, Vol.23, No.9, (September 2008), pp. 2995-3003.

10

Donor Characteristics in 1,000 Consecutive Simultaneous Pancreas-Kidney Transplants

Hans W. Sollinger, Jon S. Odorico,
Glen E. Leverson, Barbara J. Voss,
and Anthony M. D'Alessandro
Department of Surgery,
Division of Transplantation,
University of Wisconsin,
U.S.A.

1. Introduction

In 2003, Krieger et al. from our group published a manuscript which investigated the use of pancreas grafts for transplantation in different UNOS regions in the United States (1). It was reported that the utilization of pancreata showed a wide variation depending on the region. To approach some degree of standardization, we calculated the ratio of pancreata used for transplantation with the number of livers procured and transplanted. Using the data from our own institution, we had experienced that at least 70% of liver donors should provide acceptable pancreas grafts. The results of the study, however, demonstrated that in some regions, less than 20% of liver donors yielded pancreas grafts. Ensuing discussion revealed that the lack of established criteria to predict the outcome of pancreas transplantation based on available donor criteria was one of the reasons many centers, in particular less experienced programs, were hesitant to accept donors other than those expected to provide excellent pancreas grafts, and therefore, outcomes. Since then, few publications have addressed the correlation between available donor criteria and short- or long-term outcomes. One single center report analyzing outcomes in 61 simultaneous pancreas-kidney transplants (SPK) was published in 1995 by Douzdjian et al. (2), and a multi-center European report by Vinkers et al. (3) attempted to establish a donor quality score. During the preparation of this manuscript, the online version of a large-scale analysis using data from the Scientific Registry of Transplant Recipients (SRTR) in 9,401 transplants from 2000 to 2006 became available for review (4).

The purpose of this manuscript is to report the donor characteristics in 1,000 consecutively performed SPK transplants at a single center. Pancreas-kidney retrieval and donor management, as well as donor evaluation, were performed by the same organ procurement organization (UW OPO). Retrieval was performed by surgeons trained at our institution. Using only donor data easily available to OPO personnel and surgeons, we attempt here to provide straightforward guidelines regarding the acceptability of pancreas grafts. A unique feature of this study is the fact that long-term follow up is available up to 22 years.

2. Materials and methods

Between December 18, 1985 and December 3, 2007, 1,000 consecutive donor pancreatectomies were performed by the members of the University of Wisconsin transplant team and the University of Wisconsin OPO. In general, the retrieval team consisted of a transplant surgeon or a Board-certified/eligible surgeon, a transplant fellow and a procurement specialist. Over the 20-year interval, only a small number of surgeons and transplant specialists—all trained at our institution—were involved, keeping the surgical approach standardized. The principles of the donor operation have been previously described in detail (5). Our routine consisted of *in situ* flushing with UW solution (ViaSpan®, Bristol-Myers Squibb, Garden City, NY), after dissection of the pancreas and liver. A point was made not to exceed 2 liters of flush solution. The mesenteric vessels were always ligated. Donor demographics are shown in Table 1. Donor management was conducted by the intensive care staff of the referring hospital in consultation with OPO personnel. No OPO personnel was on site until the retrieval procedure. During organ retrieval, generous use of colloids was used to reduce pancreatic edema. All organs were stored in UW solution. Surgical implant technique, recipient management and immunosuppressive therapy have been previously described (6). It is of note that we never used any systemic anticoagulation in the recipients post-transplant.

Data for analysis was obtained from the UW OPO records and transferred into the UW Transplant database.

Histocompatibility testing was performed prior to all transplants, but no attempt was made to match donor and recipient as closely as possible. The only absolute requirement was a negative T-cell crossmatch using the NIH technique.

Statistical Analysis

For statistical analysis, continuous variables were summarized by reporting mean and standard deviation, and categorical variables were summarized by reporting percentages. Event rates were estimated using methods of Kaplan and Meier and compared between groups using a log rank test. $P<0.05$ was considered significant. All analyses were performed using SAS statistical software (SAS Institute, Inc., Cary, NC).

3. Results

For reporting purposes, the highest value among donor laboratory values was chosen for our calculations. BMI was determined by weight at the time of admission. Vasopressor use was defined as the use of any vasopressor at any time from the patient's admission to the time of the retrieval procedure. As expected, long-term outcomes for pancreas graft survival correlated with donor age (Figure 1). Donor age as previously reported by others appears to be a major risk factor. As previously reported by Fernandez, et al., young donors do extremely well despite higher technical difficulties (7). The youngest SPK donor in our experience was three years of age. These grafts should be placed into smaller recipients. BMI also had a significant correlation with inferior long-term outcomes (Figure 2). Obese donors, even in the younger age groups, have pancreata which are infiltrated by fatty tissue and respond poorly to preservation. In addition, fat necrosis after transplantation may lead to intra-abdominal fluid collections and subsequent abscess formation. Nevertheless, on occasion a donor with a high BMI may have a normal-appearing pancreas which can be safely used for transplantation.

Laboratory determinations such as amylase and lipase ($p>0.08$) have not shown any correlation with outcomes, as previously reported by Odorico et al. in a smaller cohort (8). In addition, maximum glucose levels have no predictive value. Glucose values often reflect the resuscitation effort and may be skewed by the co-administration of other drugs such as corticosteroids. In an unpublished study by our group, determination of HbA_1C in 100 consecutive donors did not elicit a single abnormal value which would allow the conclusion that medical history is sufficient to rule out diabetes or pre-diabetes. At the start of our program, we were hesitant to retrieve pancreata from donors with abdominal trauma and prior surgery, which frequently included splenectomy. With growing experience, we have learned to use these donors after careful inspection of the pancreas and duodenum. There is no difference in long-term outcomes ($p=0.6585$). Pancreatic grafts from young trauma victims are frequently very edematous, but return to normal texture after preservation in UW solution. Furthermore, the use of vasopressors is not associated with inferior long-term survival ($p=0.9196$).

4. Discussion

Data published by UNOS/SRTR reveal that the number of SPKs performed has not increased despite an increase in the number of potential pancreas donors by an average of 482 per year since 2003 (4). Most of these consented organs have not been recovered. The non-recovery rate among pancreata is at an all-time high of about 72% (4). Among the possible reasons are a) an older donor population; b) allocation criteria which lists kidney recipients and SPK recipients on the same list; and c) surgeons' fears of achieving inferior results, which in turn might result in termination of insurance coverage for the program. These fears are heightened by the fact that few objective criteria for donor selection exist. In 1998, Odorico et al. from our group analyzed donor factors affecting outcome after pancreas transplantation in 240 recipients (8). The relevant conclusions were that pancreata from donors >45 years of age are associated with a higher failure rate. This finding was consistent with the observations of Gruessner et al. reported in 1994 (9). Odorico et al. also conclude that serum amylase and glucose did not correlate with graft failure (8). Furthermore, in a small series of donation after cardiac death (DCD) donors, no difference in short-term outcomes was noted. Douzdjian et al. analyzed their single-center experience in 61 SPKs and found that duration of brain death before procurement, length of donor admission and donor age were the major factors associated with inferior outcomes (2). In accordance with our observations, serum glucose and serum amylase did not correlate with outcomes.

Recently, the online version of a manuscript by Axelrod et al. was available for review (10). SRTR data from over 9,401 pancreas donors were used to develop a Pancreas Donor Risk Index (PDRI). As pointed out by Krieger (1), the authors emphasize that pancreas utilization shows great regional variation in the United States and that donor selection is widely used as a key factor to successful pancreatic transplantation. The study is based on retrospective data from multiple centers using a variety of procurement techniques.

The uniqueness of this manuscript is that universal procurement and retrieval techniques were used and that the implant team primarily consisted only of a small group of uniformly trained surgeons. Our message is that the donor surgeon should not be discouraged from

exploring a donor with high amylase, lipase and glucose levels. Also, the use of vasopressors should not be a reason to decline. Data by Bellingham et al. demonstrate that the same criteria apply in DCD pancreas donors (11).
Using these simplified criteria (age and BMI) for evaluating prospective pancreas donors, together with visual inspection of the graft, suitable pancreas grafts can be chosen to achieve excellent long-term functional outcomes (12). Adequately trained OPO personnel and procurement surgeons will be able to use these simple guidelines in order to maximize potential utilization of pancreas donors.

	Mean (range)
Age (years)	29 (3-60)
Weight (kg)	72 (15-156)
Amylase (U/L)	99 (2-2,002)
Glucose (mg/dL)	189 (6 – 824)
Pancreas cold storage time (hours)	15 (0-43)
	N (%)
Gender: Male Female	 604 (62.5%) 363 (37.5%)
Race: Caucasian African-American Asian Native American	 944 (97.5%) 16 (1.7%) 6 (6.2%) 1 (0.1%)

Table 1. Donor demographics

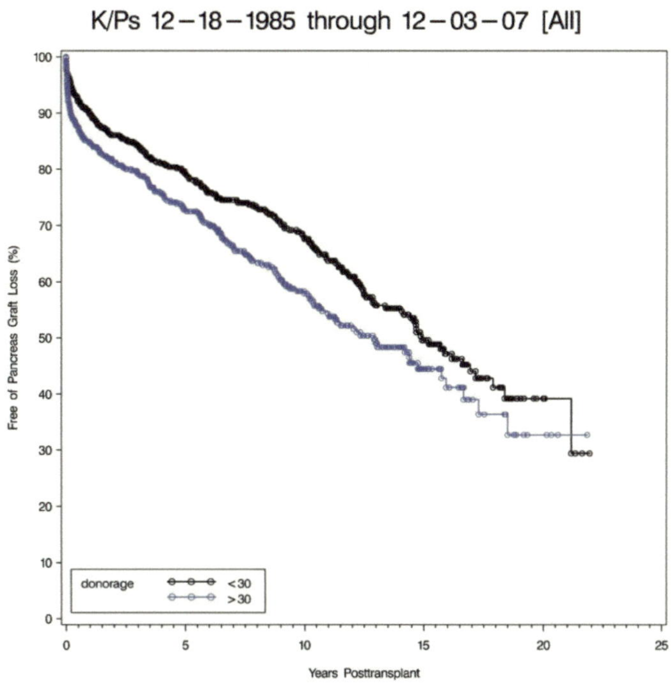

Fig. 1. Age and pancreas transplant outcome

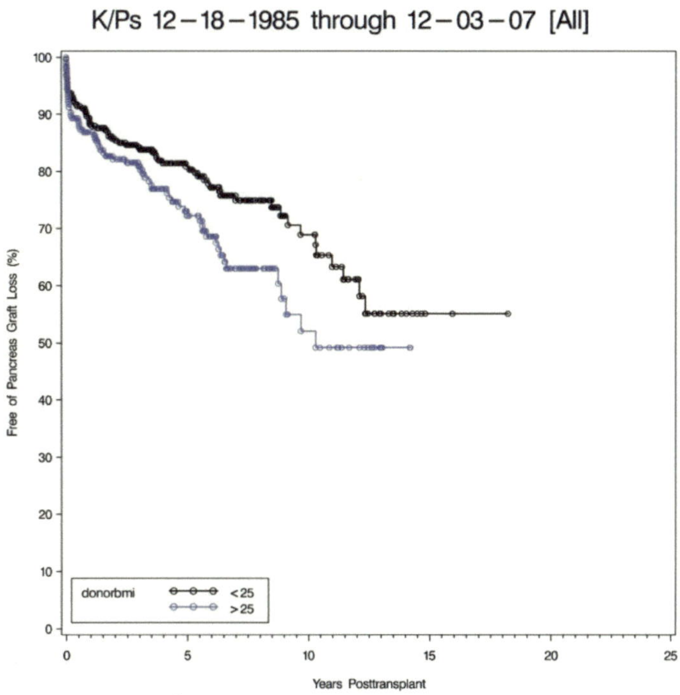

Fig. 2. BMI and pancreas transplant outcome

5. References

[1] Krieger NR, Odorico JS, Heisey DM, et al. Underutilization of pancreas donors. Transplantation 2003;75:1271-6.

[2] Douzdjian V, Gugliuzza KG, Fish JC. Multivariate analysis of donor and recipient risk factors for renal and pancreas allograft failure after pancreas-kidney transplantation. Transplant Proc 1995;27:3128-9.

[3] Vinkers MT, Rahmel AO, Slot MC, Smits JM, Schareck WD. How to recognize a suitable pancreas donor: a Eurotransplant study of preprocurement factors. Transplant Proc 2008;40:1275-8.

[4] Scientific Registry of Transplant Recipients [Internet]. www.ustransplant.org

[5] Sollinger HW, Odorico JS, Knechtle SJ, D'Alessandro AM, Kalayoglu M, Pirsch JD. Experience with 500 simultaneous pancreas-kidney transplants. Ann Surg 1998;228:284-96

[6] Sollinger HW, Odorico JS, Becker YT, D'Alessandro AM, Pirsch JD. One thousand consecutive simultaneous pancreas-kidney transplants at a single center with 22-year follow-up. Ann Surg 2009;250:618-30.

[7] Fernandez LA, Turgeon NA, Odorico JS, et al. Superior long-term results of simultaneous pancreas-kidney transplantation from pediatric donors. Am J Transplant 2004;4:2093-101.

[8] Odorico JS, Heisey DM, Voss BJ, et al. Donor factors affecting outcome after pancreas transplantation. Transplant Proc 1998;30:276-7.

[9] Gruessner RW, Troppmann C, Barrou B, et al. Assessment of donor and recipient risk factors on pancreas transplant outcome. Transplant Proc 1994;26:437.

[10] Axelrod DA, Sung RS, Meyer KH, Wolfe RA, Kaufman DB. Systematic Evaluation of Pancreas Allograft Quality, Outcomes and Geographic Variation in Utilization. Am J Transplant (in press).

[11] Bellingham J, Goodman J, Leverson G, et al. Ten-year outcomes of simultaneous pancreas-kidney transplantation from donation after cardiac death. Am J Transplant 2008;8(suppl. 2):201 (published abstract).

[12] Sollinger HW, Odorico JS, Becker YT, D'Alessandro AM, Pirsch JD. One thousand consecutive simultaneous pancreas-kidney transplants at a single center with 22-year follow-up. Ann Surg 2009;250:618-30.

11

Perioperative and Long-Term Safety of Living Kidney Donors

Masahiko Okamoto
Department of Organ Interaction Research Medicine
Kyoto Prefectural University of Medicine
Japan

1. Introduction

Because securing the safety of living kidney donor is essential to the continued success of this procedure, in this chapter we will review articles which focused not only on recipient outcome but also on living kidney donor to clarify what is known and what should be known in this field.

2. Indication for living kidney donor

For the perioperative and long-term safety, medical indication for living kidney donor is substantial issue. However, criteria for living kidney donor has been often derived empirically on a temporary basis and might vary by country, region and institute. Here, we summarize newly-developed guideline for the indication of living kidney donation which is internationally accepted such as the consensus of Amsterdam forum guideline (Delmonico F. 2005) and OPTN/UNOS guideline (Table 1). Then they were compared with the results of survey of US transplant center concerning evaluating living kidney donors (Mandelbrot DA, et al. 2007).

2.1 Age

There is no description of age limitation of living kidney donor in Amsterdam forum guideline. However age younger than 18 years old is attributed to contraindication in OPTN/UNOS guideline. Half of the institute did not set the upper limit of age, although widely accepted upper limit is 65 years old and some other institute set the cutoffs of 55, 60,70 and 75 years old (Mandelbrot DA, et al. 2007).

2.2 Obesity

Obesity was defined by a body mass index (BMI) of >30 kg/m^2. All potential donors should have BMI determined at initial evaluation because of data suggesting an association between obesity and kidney disease. In most guideline, BMI above 35 kg/m^2 is thought to be contraindication especially when other comorbid conditions are present. And obese patients should be encouraged to lose weight before kidney donation and should not to donate if they have other associated comorbid conditions. According to the survey of US transplant centers, about one-half of programs use a BMI cutoff of 35 kg/m^2, while 10%

exclude donors with BMI over 30 kg/m^2 and 20% exclude donors with BMI over 40 kg/m^2 (Mandelbrot DA, et al. 2007).

	Amsterudam Forum (2005)	OPTN/UNOS (2007)
Age	no description	<18 years old
Obesity	BMI>35kg/m^2	BMI>35kg/m^2
Renal function	GFR<80ml/min or 2SD below normal	CCr<80ml/min
Urinalysis abnormality	u-pro>300mg/day	u-pro>300mg/day
	persistant microhematuria	
Hypertension	BP>140/90 by ABPM	BP>130/90(50yo), anti-HT medication≥3
Diabetes	FBS≥126 or 2hr BS≥200	2hr BS≥140
Dyslipidemia	no excluison	no description
History of malignancy	depend on kind of malignancy	recent malignancy

BMI: Body mass index, GFR: Glomerular filtration rate, SD: Standard deviation, CCr: Creatinine clearance, BP: Blood pressure, ABPM: Ambulatory blood pressure monitoring, FBS: Fasting blood sugar, BS: Blood sugar

Table 1. Contraindication for living kidney donor

2.3 Renal function

The first substantial issue is which measurement should be adapted to estimate renal function of potential living donors. Creatinine clearance calculated by 24-hour urine collections has been used most frequently, however, may under- or overestimate glomerular filtration rate (GFR) in patients with normal or near normal renal function. Estimated GFR values are easy way but not standardized in this population. These methods may be replaced or supplemented by inulin clearance in cases of borderline GFR determination although it is a complicated method. In most program, a GFR<80 ml/minute or 2 standard deviations below normal (based on age, gender, and BSA corrected to 1.73/m^2) generally preclude donation (Delmonico F. 2005). According to the survey of US transplant center, few programs now have no specific cutoff, and no programs use 40 or 60 mL/min/1.73 m^2 as cutoffs (Mandelbrot DA, et al. 2007).

2.4 Proteinuria

Proteinuria should be assessed as a standard part of the donor work up. Dipstick measurements of proteinuria are not enough in the assessment of a prospective living donor. According to the survey of US transplant center, most programs use a 24-hour urine collection for protein. Some programs rely on a spot urine protein to creatinine ratio, and almost one-half of programs now use urinary albumin as a screen. As for cutoff level of proteinuria, more than 300 mg/24-hour of urineprotein is widely accepted as a contraindication to donation. Microalbuminuria determination is also reccomended, although its value as an international standard of evaluation for kidney donors has not been determined (Delmonico F. 2005).

2.5 Hematuria

Isolated microscopic hematuria may not be a contraindication to donation. Red blood cells (RBCs) with glomerular origin have a dysmorphic appearance observed by phase-contrast microscopy and automated RBC analysis. Patients with persistent microscopic hematuria should not be considered for kidney donation unless urine cytology and a complete urologic work up are performed. If urological malignancy and stone disease are excluded, a kidney biopsy may be indicated to rule out glomerular pathology such as IgA nephropathy.

2.6 Hypertension

Hypertension has been considered to be a contraindication in potential renal transplant donors. Some patients with easily controlled hypertension who meet other defined criteria may represent a low-risk group for development of kidney disease and may be acceptable as kidney donors. Hypertension exclusion criteria have become more flexible compared with previous survey (Bia MJ, et al. 1995). In recent survey, while 47% of programs exclude donors on any antihypertensive medication, 41% exclude donors if they are taking more than one medication, and 8% exclude donors taking more than two medications (Mandelbrot DA, et al. 2007). Blood pressure criteria tend to be looser if the donor is older, or if end organ damage is ruled out.

2.7 Diabetes

Diabetes is associated with an increased risk of postsurgical complications and future development of renal failure compared to the general population. Therefore, individuals with a history of diabetes or fasting blood glucose ≥126 mg/dl on at least two occasions or 2-hour glucose with OGTT ≥200 mg/dl are thought to be contraindication for living kidney donation in Amsterdam forum guideline. OPTN/UNOS guideline adapts more strict cutoff level where 2hr BS≥140 are considered to be contraindication for living kidney donation.
According to the survey of US transplant center, almost one-half of programs exclude donors based on elevated fasting blood glucose (FBG), but various cutoffs are used to define 'elevated' (from >100 mg/dl to >120mg/dl). Most programs exclude based on abnormal oral glucose tolerance test or Type II diabetes.

2.8 Dyslipidemia

Dyslipidemia should be included along with other risk factors in donor risk assessment, but dyslipidemia alone does not generally exclude kidney donation.

2.9 History of malignancy

Living kidney donors should be screened by standard medical guidelines to exclude malignancy. A prior history of malignancy may only be acceptable for donation if prior treatment of the malignancy does not decrease renal reserve or place the donor at increased risk for end stage renal disease (ESRD) and if prior treatment of malignancy does not increase the operative risk of nephrectomy. The history of melanoma, renal or urological malignancy, choriocarcinoma, hematologic malignancy, lung cancer, breast cancer and monoclonal gammopathy generally precludes living donation (Pham, PC, et al 2007).

3. Being donor with medical abnormality

Due to the extreme shortage of organ donors worldwide, the indications for live kidney donation have been expanding in terms of medical status, and now include patients with mild hypertension, older age, and mild decline of renal function. Individuals with isolated medical abnormalities (IMAs) are undergoing living donor nephrectomy more frequently. Knowledge of health risks for these living donors is important for donor selection, informed consent and follow-up. One systematical review with living kidney donors with preexisting IMA showed perioperative outcomes for donors with and without IMAs were similar (Young A, et al 2008). However, few studies reported longer term rates of hypertension, proteinuria or renal function. Studies were frequently retrospective and without a comparison group. Centers may accept some IMA donors considering the small risk of ESRD developing as result of the IMA (Bia MJ, et al. 1995). Some long-term follow-up study of IMA donors will be described below.

3.1 Being donor having hypertension

When seeing the relatively short-term outcomes of hypertensive donors, white subjects with moderate, essential hypertension and normal kidney function have no adverse effects regarding blood pressure, GFR, or urinary protein excretion during the first year after living kidney donation. Although further studies are essential to confirm long-term safety, these data suggest that selected hypertensive patients may be accepted for living kidney donation (Textor SC, et al. 2004).

One more study confirmed the long-term safety of hypertensive donors. When 674 live kidney donors were divided into two groups, survival rates in hypertension (HT)-group (N=54) by 20 years were equivalent as compared with non- HT group (N=620). Prevalence of renal dysfunction and ESRD were not increased in HT-group, while prevalence of HT and HT with medication was increased (Okamoto M. unpublished data). Those results demonstrated that those who have HT were able to donate their kidney safely with little major long-term morbidity by strict evaluation and careful postoperative follow-up.

3.2 Being donor having proteinuria

There were one long-term follow-up study of 70 renal outcome 25 years after donor nephrectomy in US single center (at the Cleveland Clinic). By this analysis patients with mild or borderline proteinuria before donation (0.160 g /24 hour) may represent a subgroup at particular risk for the development of significant proteinuria (>0.8 g /24 hour) 20 years or greater after donation (Goldfarb DA, et al. 2001).

3.3 Being donor having glucose intolerance

There were one report concerning long-term coutome of living kidney donors who donated kidneys having glucose intolerance (GI). In this study, 444 donor nephrectomies were divided into GI group and non-GI group according to the results of 75g-oral glucose tolerance test (75g-OGTT). Survival rates in the GI group up to 20 years were equivalent to those in the non-GI group. None of the patients with diabetes mellitus (75g-OGTT: DM pattern, n=27) had developed severe diabetic complications or ESRD at a mean follow-up point of 88±71 (range, 14-225) months. These results suggested that individuals who have GI without diabetic complication may be able to donate their kidney safely with little major morbidity if strict evaluation is performed before transplant (Okamoto M, et al. 2010).

3.4 Transplant outcomes from isolated medical abnormality (IMA) donors

According to the meta-analysis of 12 studies, recipients of kidneys from older donors had poorer 5-year patient and graft survival than recipients of kidneys from younger donors. However, few transplant outcomes were described for other IMA, namely, obesity, hypertension, reduced GFR, proteinuria and hematuria. This disconnect between donor selection and a lack of knowledge of recipient outcomes should give transplant decision-makers pause and sets an agenda for future research (Iordanous Y, et al. 2009).

4. Perioperative issue in living kidney donation

The first major concern regarding living kidney donation is the incidence of perioperative deaths and serious surgical complications. Although it is considered to be a relatively safe procedure, risk of death for the donor is generally estimated as being around 0.02-0.03%. Perioperative mortality and complications of donor nephrectomy including pulmonary embolism, pneumothorax, and less seriously, wound infection, unexplained fever and urinary tract infection will be described below.

4.1 Perioperative mortality

Donor safety is of paramount importance in living donor transplantation. Yet, living donor deaths actually occur (Ratner LE, et al. 2010). According to the survey of 171 United States kidney transplant centers, two donors (0.02%) out of 10,828 living donors died from surgical complications between 1999 and 2001 (Matas AJ, et al. 2003). However, in separate report from the various transplant center, there are little report of a donor death (Siebels M,et al. 2003, Jones KW, et al. 1997, Johnson EM, et al. 1997, Blohme I, et al. 1992).

4.2 Possible surgical complication

There are some surgical complication specific to living donor nephrectomy. Special care must be taken to prevent them.

4.2.1 Deep vein thrombosis/pulmonary embolism

Deep vein thrombosis/pulmonary embolism are most serious complication following living donor nephrectomy. Actually one specified death was caused by pulmonary embolism (Matas AJ, et al. 2003). We reported one case of pulmonary embolism which was diagnosed in relatively early period and successfully recovered with anti-coagulant therapy and transient mechanical ventilation (Ushigome H, et al. 2003). It is very important for surgeons to realize that this can develop in any case of living donor nephrectomy. Every effort should be made to prevent it by enough hydration, intermittent pneumatic compression (IPC) and, if necessary, prophylactic anti-coagulant therapy.

4.2.2 Pneumothorax

Pneumothorax also occurs because of anatomical reason, which sometime needs pleural drainage. The report from US single center (University of Minnesota) described 13 (1.5%) pneumothoraces (6 required intervention, 7 resolved spontaneously) among 871 living donor nephrectomies (Johnson EM, et al. 1997).

4.2.3 Bleeding

Bleeding is the most common cause of reoperation especially laparoscopic nephrectomy. According to the survey of United States kidney transplant centers, 26 donors (0.24%) out of 10,828 living donors needed reoperation because of bleeding (Matas AJ, et al. 2003). By a report of Swedish single center through a retroperitoneal approach, there were 5 cases (1.02%) of postoperative haemorrhage requiring reoperation out of 490 living donor nephrectomies (Blohme I, et al. 1992).

4.2.4 Incisional hernia

Incisional hernia can occur as in other laparotomic surgery and needs reoperation. According to the survey of United States kidney transplant centers, 22 donors (0.20%) out of 10,828 living donors needed reoperation because of hernia (Matas AJ, et al. 2003).

4.2.5 Femoral nerve compression

Femoral nerve compression may occur because it exists on the psoas muscle and it can be compressed by would retractor.

4.2.6 Wound infections, hematomas or seromas

Wound infections, hematomas or seromas happen most frequently after living donor nephrectomy as a minor complication. They usually resolve without major operation.

4.2.7 Pneumonias, atelectasis and urinary tract infections

Pneumonias and atelectasis also happens as a complication of general anesthesia. They tend to occur at an opposite site of nephrectomy because of lateral recumbent position. Urinary tract infections also happen as in other surgical procedure due to insertion of urethral catheter.

4.3 Risk factors for perioperative complications

Transplant professionals should avoid possible risk for living kidney donors. A couple of report analyzed the risk factor for them. According to analysis of live donors drawn from a mandated national registry of 80 347 live kidney donors in the United States between 1994 and 2009, surgical mortality was higher in men than in women (RR=3.0), in black vs. white and Hispanic individuals (RR=3.1), and in donors with hypertension vs. without hypertension (RR=27.4) (Segev DL, et al. 2010). The report from US single center (University of Minnesota) described that the analysis, by logistic regression, among 871 living donor nephrectomies identified significant risk factors for perioperative complications were male gender (vs. female), pleural entry (vs. no pleural entry), and weight > or = 100 kg (vs. < 100 kg) (Johnson EM, et al. 1997).

5. Long-term follow-up of living kidney donor -Survival, renal function, complication

The long-term consequences after kidney donation are not fully understood. However, most long-term follow-up studies of living kidney donors find no decrease in long-term survival. And most of the data suggested that the donors had normal renal function, with an incidence of hypertension comparable to that expected in the age-matched general population, while other demonstrated that donor nephrectomy is associated with mild proteinuria and hypertension. The Long-term follow-up study of living kidney donor concerning survival rate, renal function and various complications will be described including our Japanese experiences (Table 2).

Author	year	Subject	Tx done	No.	retrieval rate	HT	ESRD	die	Survival rate
Najarian JS	1992	single center	1963-1970	135	NA	32%	not stated	15	NA
Fehrman-Ekholm I	1997	single center	1964-1994	459	93%	35%	not stated	41	29% better
Fehrman-Ekholm I	2001	single center	1964-1995	451	77%	38%	1	49	NA
Goldfarb DA	2001	single center	1963-1975	180	38%	48%	2	24	NA
Ramcharan T	2002	single center	1963-1979	773	60%	similar	5	84	NA
Ellison MD	2002	UNOS registry		NA	NA	NA	56	NA	NA
Thiel GT	2005	naitonal registry	1993-2005	737	85%	35%	0	9	NA
Gossmann J	2005	single center	1973-2001	152	93%	30%	0	7	NA
Ibrahim HN	2009	single center	1963-2007	3698	NA	32%	11	268	Similar to NP
Okamoto M	2009	single center	1972-2006	601	80%	30.1%	4	55	better than NP

No.: total number of donor, HT: hypertension, ESRD: end-stage renal disease, UNOS: United Network for Organ Sharing, NA: not accessed, NP: Normal population

Table 2. Report of long-term outcome after living kidney donation

5.1 Long-term survival following living kidney donation

Most long-term follow up studies of living kidney donors find no decrease in long-term survival. By analysis of 430 previous living kidney donors in Swedish single center, the survival rate of 20 years was 29% better than the expected survival rate calculated by using national registers. They concluded that the better survival among donors is probably due to the fact that only healthy persons are accepted for living kidney donation (Fehrman-Ekholm I, et al. 1997). Moreover, the analysis of 481 previous Japanese living kidney donors also showed that the survival rate of kidney donors was better than the age- and gender-matched cohort from the general population, and the patterns and causes of death were similar with the general population (Okamoto M, et al. 2009). The study of larger numbers of donors as many as 3698 who donated kidneys during the period from 1963 through 2007 for a longer follow-up period in US single institute (University of Minnesota) also ascertained that the survival of kidney donors was similar to that of controls who were matched for age, sex, and race or ethnic group (Ibrahim, HN, et al. 2009). The overall evidence suggests that living kidney donors have survival similar to that of non-donors.

5.2 Hypertension following living kidney donation

Hypertension is thought to be one of major concerns following living kidney donation. However, a couple of study demonstrated no increase of hypertension after living donor nephrectomy. By a 15-year experience on 162 living donors in Italy, Long-term incidence of hypertension in living donors was similar to the general population (Sansalone CV, et al. 2006). Furthermore, the analysis of 402 donor nephrectomy in Sweden showed that, although hypertension was present in 38% of the donors, the age-adjusted prevalence of hypertension among donors was not higher than in the general population (Fehrman-Ekholm I, et al. 2001).

On the other hands, some study demonstrated increase of hypertension after living donor nephrectomy. Another analysis of 75 donors, in US single center (University of Missouri), showed that the prevalence of hypertension was significantly increased compared with age/sex matched data from epidemiological studies of the general population, especially in those over the age of 55 years (Saran R, et al. 1997). Also, in a live kidney donor cohort with a 93% retrieval rate of the 152 donors, mean blood pressure had increased from 125 ± 15/79 ± 11 to 134 ± 19/81 ± 9 mmHg ($p < 0.01$) which remained significantly below normal. (Gossmann J, et al. 2005). One Meta-analysis showed kidney donors may have a 5 mmHg increase in blood pressure within 5 to 10 years after donation over that anticipated with normal aging (Boudville N, et al. 2006). Future controlled, prospective studies with long periods of follow-up will better delineate the risk of hypertension following living kidney donation.

5.3 Proteinuria following living kidney donation

Most reported data suggested that proteinuria increased in living kidney donor population, although follow-up period and measurement of proteinuria and/or microalbuminuria differed by report.

German experience at a single center of 102 living kidney donors for 35 years showed microalbuminuria was found in 22.6% of the donors (Schostak M, et al. 2004). Another study showed, in a live kidney donor cohort with a 93% retrieval rate of the 152 donors, fifty six percent of donors developed proteinuria (>150 mg/day), but only 10% had albuminuria (Gossmann J, et al. 2005). By analysis of 402 outcome after donor nephrectomy in Sweden, significant proteinuria (> or =1.0 g/L) was found in 3% and slight proteinuria (<1.0 g/L) in 9% of the donors and proteinuria was associated with hypertension and a lower GFR (Fehrman-Ekholm I, et al. 2001).

One Meta-analysis, which analyzed a total of 5048 donors from forty-eight studies with an average follow-up of 7 years after donation (range 1-25 years), demonstrated that the average 24-h urine protein was 154 mg/day and concluded that kidney donation results in small increases in urinary protein. (Garg AX, et al. 2006).

5.4 Renal function following living kidney donation

Renal function is the greatest concerns at a long time after living kidney donation. In a report from Saudi Arabia of 25 living kidney donors, total kidney function measured as creatinine clearance showed significant drop by 36% of the pre donated value. However, remaining kidney clearance increased by an average of 34% of the pre donated level as measured by Tc 99m DTPA renography. Compensatory hypertrophy of the remaining kidney measured by ultrasound attributed to an increase in the renal volume of 15% (Shehab AB, et al. 1994). Other investigator shows 25% decrease of GFR with mean time after uninephrectomy of 11 years. (Gossmann J, et al. 2005), and 27% decrease of with mean patient follow-up of 25 years (Goldfarb DA, et al. 2001).

In a Swedish study, the average estimated GFR (12 years after donation) was 72±18% of the age-predicted value. The ratio of the estimated to the predicted GFR showed no correlation to the time since donation, indicating that there is no accelerated loss of renal function after donation (Fehrman-Ekholm I, et al. 2001). These results demonstrated that although living kidney donor lose GFR by 15-25%, they usually do not show the accelerated loss of renal function if they do not have risk factor for chronic renal disease (CKD). One unique study examined renal function >20 years after donation by comparing that with siblings. They showed no significant difference in serum creatinine (1.1±0.01 vs 1.1±0.03 mg/dl), blood urea nitrogen (17±0.5 vs 17±1.2 mg/dl) and creatinine clearance (82±2 vs 89±3.3 ml/min) between 57 donors (mean age 61±1) and 65 siblings (mean age 58±1.3) (Najarian JS, et al. 1992).

5.5 ESRD in previous donor

Although the Swiss Organ Living Donor Health Registry showed no ESRD in 737 living kidney donors between 1993 and January 2005 (Thiel GT, et al. 2005), there were considerable reports of ESRD of previous kidney donor as below.

In a survey which used the Organ Procurement and Transplantation Network (OPTN) database, a total of 56 previous living donors were identified as having been subsequently listed for cadaveric kidney transplantation. They concluded that living renal donation has long-term risks that may not be apparent in the short term and that the numbers reported underestimate the actual number of living donors with renal failure, because they include only patients listed for a kidney transplant. (Ellison MD, et al. 2002). In analysis of 402 donor nephrectomy in Sweden, no donor died in uremia or had dialysis treatment before death. However, three donors developed renal disease, and one was in dialysis treatment. In two of these cases, hereditary factors were possibly involved (Fehrman-Ekholm I, et al. 2001). In Mexican experience, they present four kidney donors who developed ESRD thereafter, three becoming kidney recipients (Gracida C, et al. 2001). Other two case reports described kidney donors who developed ESRD (Ladefoged J, et al. 1992, al Shohaib S, et al. 1995). By analysis of 464 outcomes after donor nephrectomy at University of Minnesota, 84 had died and 380 were alive. Of the 84 donors who had died, three were known to have had kidney failure. Of the 380 still alive, three had abnormal kidney function and two had undergone transplantation (Ramcharan T, et al. 2002).

One study carefully investigated the association between postoperative clinical courses and changes in renal function in eight donors who developed chronic kidney disease (CKD) stage 5 or ESRD. According to their findings, except for one donor who developed ESRD caused by a traffic accident, none of the donors developed progressive renal dysfunction immediately after donation. Their renal functions remained stable for a long period, but started to decline after developing new comorbidities, especially risk factors known as progression factors (proteinuria or hypertension) or accelerating factors (cardiovascular event or infection) of CKD (Kido R, et al. 2009). However, the overall evidence suggests that their risk of ESRD is not increased.

6. Ethical issue and quality of life (Q.O.L.) in living kidney donation

Most published reports have indicated healthy psychological status and improved quality of life (Q.O.L.) in living kidney donors. However, there have been some reports of depression and disrupted family relationships after kidney donation. The reasons of negative results were mainly related to poor outcome of the kidney recipient, or long-lasting major pain or disappointment about medical handling before and after organ donation. Ethical issue and Q.O.L. in living kidney donation will be described.

6.1 Ethical issue in living kidney donation

Not only medical aspect but also ethical aspect is very important part to continue living kidney transplantation. The general public's concerns of living kidney donation is the length of a hospital stay, out-of-pocket expenses, size and appearance of a scar, and the donor risk of developing kidney failure (Boulware LE, et al. 2002). In this respect, it is quite important process to inform prospective donor of these issues. Especially, a long-term medical risk with potential living donors is a vital aspect of informed consent. According to a survey of 203 practitioners in 35 countries, risks of hypertension, proteinuria or kidney failure requiring dialysis were frequently discussed (usually over 80% of practitioners discussed each medical condition). However, many practitioners do not believe these risks are increased after donation, with surgeons being less convinced of long-term sequelae compared with nephrologists. Thus, transplant professionals vary in the long-term risks they communicate to potential donors. (Housawi AA, et al. 2007).

Moreover, the expansion of living donor kidney transplantation to include significant numbers of donors with little to no preexisting relationship to the candidate has caused concern in the medical community regarding as donor psychological status, motivation, knowledge about donation and the potential for undue pressure to donate under some circumstances. (Dew MA, et al. 2007). Another rare but delicate issue in living-related kidney donation is discovering misattributed paternity. In a survey, the prevalence of misattributed paternity ranges between approximately 0.25% and 0.5% of all living kidney donations. Opinions about revealing this information were quite variable by practitioners (Young A, et al. 2009).

6.2 Quality of life (Q.O.L.) in living kidney donation

Same as medical risk, Q.O.L. in living kidney donors is substantial issue to continue this procedure. According to the experience in German single institute of 102 living kidney donors, everyday life was managed as well as before surgery after 2-4 wk by the highest percentage (42%) of patients, but working capacity was only regained after 1-3 months by a comparable percentage (44%). Forty-six percent had a very good and 33% a good feeling after the kidney donation. The relationship to the recipient had intensified in most cases. Ninety-one percent would again decide in favor of a donation (Schostak M, et al. 2004). By another survey, majority of living kidney donors had an excellent Q.O.L. As a group, they scored higher than the national norm on the SF-36, a standardized Q.O.L health questionnaire. However, 4% were dissatisfied and regretted the decision to donate. Further, 4% found the experience extremely stressful and 8% very stressful. Multivariate analysis found that relatives other than first degree and donors whose recipient died within 1 year of transplant were more likely to say they would not donate again if it were possible. Further, donors who had perioperative complications and female donors were more likely to find the overall experience more stressful (Johnson EM, et al. 1999).

Women considering kidney donation frequently ask whether a nephrectomy will impact their ability to have children (Nevis IF, et al. 2009). There is a single-center survey which described 490 pregnancies in 239 donors after donation. Compared to pregnancies before donation, pregnancies after donation had increased rates of gestational diabetes (0.7% vs. 2.7%), gestational hypertension (0.6% vs. 5.7%), preeclampsia (0.8% vs. 5.5%), prematurity (4.0% vs. 7.1%) and fetal loss (11.3% vs.19.2%). The authors reported that these incidences of adverse events observed in donors were similar or better than expected levels for the general population (Ibrahim H et al. 2009). Therefore, pregnancy after kidney donation is not necessarily contraindication although it is better to avoid.

7. Financial Issue in living kidney donation

Many nations have programs that help living donors with their financial costs while donors in other regions of the world are without support. Moreover some living kidney donors encounter difficulties obtaining life insurance, despite the surveys of insurance companies reporting otherwise.

7.1 Reimbursement for living kidney donation

The financial risk of living donation is theoretically well covered by different insurances. However, some of the donors had to cover some expenses by themselves (Wolters HH, et al. 2003). It is proposed to reimburse donor risk by a package of specific benefits (life insurance, health insurance and a small amount of cash) to minimize hazard and ensure donor interests. It will fund medical follow-up and enable data collection so that long-term risk can be accurately assessed (Gaston RS, et al. 2006).

One international research network examined legislation and programs that facilitate reimbursement, focusing on policy mechanisms, eligibility criteria, program duration and types of expenses reimbursed. According to their results, among 40 countries, reimbursement is expressly legal in 16, unclear in 18, unspecified in 6 and expressly prohibited in 1. Donor reimbursement programs exist in 21 countries; 6 have been enacted in the last 5 years. Lost income is reimbursed in 17 countries, while travel, accommodation, meal and childcare costs are reimbursed in 12 to 19 countries. Ten countries have comprehensive programs, where all major cost categories are reimbursed to some extent. These programs differ in operation and scope. Donors in other regions of the world are without support (Sickand M, et al. 2009). Effort should be taken to establish reimbursement system to facilitate living kidney donation where this procedure is performed.

7.2 Life insurance after living kidney donation

Being an organ donor may affect one's ability to obtain life, disability and health insurance. According to a systematic review, almost all companies would provide life and health insurance to living organ donors, usually with no higher premiums. However, concern about insurability was still expressed by 2%-14% of living organ donors in follow-up studies, and 3%–11% of donors actually encountered difficulties with their insurance (Yang RC, et al. 2007).

In another study, researchers contacted offices of life insurance companies in five major cities in Canada to obtain life insurance for fictitious living kidney donors and paired controls. As a result, all donor and control profiles received a quote, with no significant difference in the premium quoted. More time was spent on the phone for donor compared to control profiles, although difference was small. Age, gender, family history of kidney disease and new-onset hypertension had no further effect on donor insurability in regression analysis. They found no evidence that kidney donors were disadvantaged in the first step of applying for life insurance (Yang RC, et al. 2009).

8. Conclusion

Because securing the safety of donor is essential to the continued success of living kidney transplantation, we have reviewed important issues, namely, indication, donation with medical abnormality, perioperative problem, long-term follow-up, ethical issue, Q.O.L. and financial issue in living kidney donation. The background quite differ by region, therefore, it seems to be difficult to build a international standard. Regular follow-up of kidney donors is recommended in order to manage their complications effectively and to detect health problem early in those who may develop it. National registry is necessary to enable data collection so that long-term risk can be accurately assessed.

9. Reference

al Shohaib, S. (1992). Chronic renal failure following living-related kidney donation. *Nephron.* Vol. 71, No. 4, pp. 468, ISSN 0028-2766

Bia, MJ., Ramos, EL., Danovitch, GM., Gaston, RS., Harmon, WE., Leichtman, AB., Lundin, PA., Neylan, J. & Kasiske, BL. (1995). Evaluation of living renal donors. The current practice of US transplant centers. *Transplantation.* Vol. 60, No. 4, pp. 322-327, ISSN 0041-1337

Blohme, I., Fehrman, I. & Norden, G. (1992). Living donor nephrectomy. Complication rates in 490 consecutive cases. *Scand J Urol Nephrol.* Vol. 26, No. 2, pp. 149-53, ISSN 0036-5599

Boudville, N., Prasad, GV., Knoll, G., Muirhead, N., Thiessen-Philbrook, H., Yang, RC., Rosas-Arellano, MP., Housawi, A., Garg, AX. & Donor Nephrectomy Outcomes Research (DONOR) Network. (2006). Meta-analysis: risk for hypertension in living kidney donors. *Ann Intern Med.* Vol. 145, No. 3, pp. 185-196, ISSN 0003-4819

Boulware, LE., Ratner, LE., Sosa, JA., Tu, AH., Nagula, S., Simpkins, CE., Durant, RW. & Powe, NR. (2002). The general public's concerns about clinical risk in live kidney donation. *Am J Transplant.* Vol. 2, No. 2, pp. 186-193, ISSN 1600-6135

Delmonico, F. & Council of the Transplantation Society. (2005). A Report of the Amsterdam Forum On the Care of the Live Kidney Donor: Data and Medical Guidelines. *Transplantation.* Vol. 79, (6 Suppl), S53-66, ISSN 0041-1337

Dew, MA., Jacobs, CL., jowsey, SG., Hanto, R., Miller, C. & Delmonico, FL. (2007). Guidelines for the Psychosocial Evaluation of Living Unrelated Kidney Donors in the United States *Am J Transplant.* Vol. 7, No. 5, pp. 1047-1054, ISSN 1600-6135

Ellison, MD., McBride, MA., Taranto, SE., Delmonico, FL. & Kauffman, HM. (2002). Living kidney donors in need of kidney transplants: a report from the organ procurement and transplantation network. *Transplantation.* Vol. 74, No. 9, pp. 1349-1351, ISSN 0041-1337

Fehrman-Ekholm, I, Elinder, CG, Stenbeck, M, Tyden, G. & Groth, CG. (1997). Kidney donors live longer. *Transplantation.* Vol. 64, No. 7, pp. 976-978, ISSN 0041-1337

Fehrman-Ekholm, I., Duner, F., Brink, B., Tyden, G. & Elinder, CG. (2001). No evidence of accelerated loss of kidney function in living kidney donors: results from a cross-sectional follow-up. *Transplantation.* Vol. 72, No. 3, pp. 444-449, ISSN 0041-1337

Garg, AX., Muirhead, N., Knol,l G., Yang, RC., Prasad, GV., Thiessen-Philbrook., H, Rosas-Arellano, MP., Housawi ,A., Boudville, N. & Donor Nephrectomy Outcomes Research (DONOR) Network. (2006). Proteinuria and reduced kidney function in living kidney donors: A systematic review, meta-analysis, and meta-regression. *Kidney Int.* Vol. 70, No. 10, pp. 1801-1810, ISSN 0085-2538

Gaston, RS., Danovitch, GM., Epstein, RA., Kahn, JP., Matas, AJ. & Schnitzler, MA. (2006). Limiting financial disincentives in live organ donation: a rational solution to the kidney shortage. *Am J Transplant.* Vol. 6, No. 11, pp. 2548-2555, ISSN 1600-6135

Goldfarb, DA., Matin, SF., Braun, WE., Schreiber, MJ., Mastroianni, B., Papajcik, D., Rolin, HA., Flechner, S., Goormastic, M. & Novick, AC. (2001). Renal outcome 25 years after donor nephrectomy. *J Urol.* Vol. 166, No. 6 pp. 2043-2047, ISSN 0022-5347

Gossmann, J., Wilhelm, A., Kachel, HG., Jordan, J., Sann, U., Geiger, H., Kramer, W. & Scheuermann, EH. (2005). Long-term consequences of live kidney donation follow-up in 93% of living kidney donors in a single transplant center. *Am J Transplant.* Vol. 5, No. 10, pp. 2417-2424, ISSN 1600-6135

Gracida, C., Espinoza, R. & Cancino, J. (2004). Can a living kidney donor become a kidney recipient? *Transplant Proc.* Vol. 36, No. 6, pp. 1630-1631, ISSN 0041-1345

Housawi, AA., Young, A., Boudville, N., Thiessen-Philbrook., H, Muirhead, N., Rehman, F., Parikh, CR., Al-Obaidli, A., El-Triki, A. & Garg, AX. Donor Nephrectomy Outcomes Research (DONOR) Network. (2007). Transplant professionals vary in the long-term medical risks they communicate to potential living kidney donors: an international survey. *Nephrol Dial Transplant.* Vol. 22, No. 10, pp. 3040-3045, ISSN 0931-0509

Ibrahim, H., Akkina, S., Leister, E., Gillingham, K., Cordner, G., Guo, H., Bailey, R., Rogers, T. & Matas, AJ. (2009). Pregnancy outcomes after kidney donation. *Am J Transplant.* Vol. 9, No. 4, pp. 825–834, ISSN 1600-6135

Ibrahim, HN., Foley, R., Tan, L., Rogers, T., Bailey, RF., Guo, H., Gross, CR & Matas, AJ.(2009). Long-term consequences of kidney donation. *N Engl J Med.* Vol. 360, No. 5, pp. 459-469, ISSN 0028-4793

Iordanous, Y., Seymour, N., Young, A., Johnson, J., Iansavichus, AV., Cuerden, MS., Gill, JS., Poggio, E., Garg, AX. & Donor Nephrectomy Outcomes Research (DONOR) Network. (2009). Recipient outcomes for expanded criteria living kidney donors: the disconnect between current evidence and practice. *Am J Transplant.* Vol. 9, No. 7, pp. 1558-1573, ISSN 1600-6135

Johnson, EM., Remucal, MJ., Gillingham, KJ., Dahms, RA., Najarian, JS. & Matas, AJ. (1997). Complications and risks of living donor nephrectomy. *Transplantation.* Vol. 64, No. 8, pp. 1124-1128, ISSN 0041-1337

Johnson, EM., Anderson, JK., Jacobs, C., Suh, G., Humar, A., Suhr, BD., Kerr, SR., Matas, AJ. & Nevis, IF. (1999). Long-term follow-up of living kidney donors: quality of life after donation. *Transplantation.* Vol. 67, No. 5, pp. 717-721, ISSN 0041-1337

Jones, KW., Peters, TG., Charlton, RK., Lenz, BJ., Walker, GW., Repper, S., Crews, MJ., Antonucci, LE. & Peters, EJ. (1997).Current issues in living donor nephrectomy. *Clin Transplant.* Vol. 11, No. 5 Pt 2, pp. 505-510, ISSN 0902-0063

Kido, R., Shibagaki, Y., Iwadoh, K., Nakajima, I., Fuchinoue, S., Fujita, T. & Teraoka, S. (2009). How do living kidney donors develop end-stage renal disease? *Am J Transplant.* Vol. 9, No. 11, pp. 2514-2519, ISSN 1600-6135

Ladefoged, J. (1992). Renal failure 22 years after kidney donation. *Lancet.* Vol. 339, No. 8785, pp. 124-125, ISSN 0140-6736

Mandelbrot, DA., Pavlakis, M., Danovitch, GM., Johnson, SR., Karp, SJ., Khwaja, K., Hanto, DW. & Rodrigue, JR. (2007). The medical evaluation of living kidney donors: a survey of US transplant centers. *Am J Transplant.* Vol. 7, No. 10, pp. 2333-2343, ISSN 1600-6135

Matas, AJ., Bartlet,t ST., Leichtman, AB. & Delmonico, FL. (2003). Morbidity and mortality after living kidney donation, 1999-2001: survey of United States transplant centers. *Am J Transplant.* Vol. 3, No. 7, pp. 830-834, ISSN 1600-6135

Najarian, JS., Chavers, BM., McHugh, LE. & Matas, AJ. (1992). 20 years or more of follow-up of living kidney donors. *Lancet.* Vol. 340, No. 8823, pp. 807-810, ISSN 0140-6736

Nevis, IF. & Garg, AX. (2009). Donor Nephrectomy Outcomes Research (DONOR) Network. Maternal and fetal outcomes after living kidney donation. *Am J Transplant.* Vol. 9, No. 4, pp. 661-668, ISSN 1600-6135

Okamoto, M., Akioka, K., Nobori, S., Ushigome, H., Kozaki, K., Kaihara, S. & Yoshimura, N. (2009). Short- and long-term donor outcomes after kidney donation: analysis of 601 cases over a 35-year period at Japanese single center. *Transplantation.* Vol. 87, No. 3, pp. 419-423, ISSN 0041-1337

Okamoto, M., Suzuki, T., Fujiki, M., Nobori, S., Ushigome, H., Sakamoto, S. & Yoshimura, N. (2010). The consequences for live kidney donors with preexisting glucose intolerance without diabetic complication: analysis at a single Japanese center. *Transplantation* Vol. 89, No. 11, pp. 1391-1395, ISSN 0041-1337

Pham, PC., Wilkinson, AH. & Pham, PT. (2007). Evaluation of the potential living kidney donor.Am J Kidney Dis. Vol. 50, No. 6, pp. 1043-1051, ISSN 0272-6386

Ramcharan, T. & Matas, AJ. (2002). Long-term (20-37 years) follow-up of living kidney donors. *Am J Transplant.* Vol. 2, No. 10, pp. 959-964, ISSN 1600-6135

Ratner, LE. & Sandoval, PR. (2010). When Disaster Strikes: Death of a Living Organ Donor. *Am J Transplant.* Vol. 10, No. 12, pp. 2577-2581, ISSN 1600-6135

Sansalone, CV., Maione, G., Aseni, P., Rossetti, O., Mangoni, I., Soldano, S., De Roberto, A., Minetti, ME., Perrino, ML. & Civati, G. (2006). Early and late residual renal function and surgical complications in living donors: a 15-year experience at a single institution.*Transplant Proc.* Vol. 38, No. 4, pp. 994-995, ISSN 0041-1345

Schostak, M., Wloch, H., Muller, M., Schrader, M., Offermann, G. & Miller, K. (2004). Optimizing open live-donor nephrectomy - long-term donor outcome. *Clin Transplant.* Vol. 18, No. 3, pp. 301-305, ISSN 0902-0063

Segev, DL., Muzaale, AD., Caffo, BS., Mehta, SH., Singer, AL., Taranto, SE., McBride, MA. & Montgomery, RA. (2010). Perioperative mortality and long-term survival following live kidney donation. *JAMA.* Vol. 303, No. 10, pp. 959-966, ISSN 0098-7484

Shehab, AB., Shaheen, FA., Fallatah, A., Sheikh, IA., Gabal, MS. & Al-Koussi, M. (1994). Residual renal function after living related kidney donation. Is it enough? An early report. *J Egypt Public Health Assoc.* Vol. 69, No. 5-6, pp. 379-395, ISSN 0013-2446

Sickand, M., Cuerden, MS., Klarenbach, SW., Ojo, AO., Parikh, CR., Boudville, N., Garg, AX. & Donor Nephrectomy Outcomes Research Network. (2009). Reimbursing live organ donors for incurred non-medical expenses: a global perspective on policies and programs. *Am J Transplant.* Vol. 9, No. 12, pp. 2825-2836, ISSN 1600-6135

Siebels, M., Theodorakis, J., Schmeller, N., Corvin, S., Mistry-Burchardi, N., Hillebrand, G., Frimberger, D., Reich, O., Land, W. & Hofstetter, A. (2003). Risks and complications in 160 living kidney donors who underwent nephroureterectomy. *Nephrol Dial Transplant.* Vol. 18, No. 127, pp. 2648-2654, ISSN 0931-0509

Textor, SC., Taler, SJ., Driscoll, N., Larson, TS., Gloor, J., Griffin, M., Cosio, F., Schwab, T., Prieto, M., Nyberg, S., Ishitani, M. & Stegall, M. (2004). Blood pressure and renal function after kidney donation from hypertensive living donors. *Transplantation.* Vol. 78, No. 2, pp. 276-282, ISSN 0041-1337

Thiel, GT., Nolte, C. & Tsinalis, D. (2005). The Swiss Organ Living Donor Health Registry (SOL-DHR). *Ther Umsch.* Vol. 62, No. 7, pp. 449-457, ISSN 0040-5930

Ushigome, H., Yasui, H., Okamoto, M., Akioka, K., Nakamura, K., Kadotani, Y., Ohmori, Y., Oka, T. & Yoshimura, N. (2003). Pulmonary embolism in a living-related kidney transplantation donor. *Surg Today.* Vol. 33, No. 5, pp. 399-402, ISSN 0941-1291

Wolters, HH., Heidenreich, S. & Senninger, N. (2003). Living donor kidney transplantation: chance for the recipient--financial risk for the donor? *Transplant Proc.* Vol. 35, No. 6, pp. 2091-2092, ISSN 0041-1345

Young, A., Storsley, L., Garg, AX., Treleaven, D., Nguan, CY., Cuerden, MS. & Karpinski, M. (2008). Health outcomes for living kidney donors with isolated medical abnormalities: a systematic review. *Am J Transplant.* Vol. 8, No. 9, pp. 1878-1897, ISSN 1600-6135

Young, A., Kim, SJ., Gibney, EM., Parikh, CR., Cuerden, MS., Horvat, LD., Hizo-Abes, P., Garg, AX. & Donor Nephrectomy Outcomes Research (DONOR) Network. (2009). Discovering misattributed paternity in living kidney donation: prevalence, preference, and practice. *Transplantation.* Vol. 87, No. 10, pp. 1429-1435, ISSN 0041-1337

Yang, RC., Thiessen-Philbrook, H., Klarenbach, S., Vlaicu, S., Garg, AX. & Donor Nephrectomy Outcomes Research (DONOR) Network. (2007). Insurability of living organ donors: a systematic review. *Am J Transplant.* Vol. 7, No. 6, pp. 1542-1551, ISSN 1600-6135

Yang, RC., Young, A., Nevis, IF., Lee, D., Jain, AK., Dominic, A., Pullenayegum, E., Klarenbach, S., Garg, AX. & Donor Nephrectomy Outcomes Research (DONOR)

Network. (2009). Life insurance for living kidney donors: a Canadian undercover investigation. *Am J Transplant.* Vol. 9, No. 7, pp. 1585-1590, ISSN 1600-6135

12

Perioperative Hydration Policy

Mahmoud M. Othman
Department of Anesthesia,
Urology and Nephrology center,
Faculty of Medicine, Mansoura University,
Mansoura,
Egypt

1. Introduction

The number of Kidney transplants has increased in last decades for many advances in diagnostic and therapeutic reasons. Kidney transplantation results in superior life expectancy and better quality of life if compared to dialysis treatment for patients with end-stage renal failure. The success of graft survival after kidney transplantation is closely associated with early graft function based on intraoperative perfusion characteristics of the allograft and good urine output. Clinicians must carefully adjust intravascular volume and arterial blood pressure to effectively perfuse the graft, and the time course of volume expansion seems important for adequate hydration. The ultimate goal for any renal transplantation patient is to have an optimally functioning graft as early as possible after completion of surgery. Key strategies that are used to achieve this goal involve the optimal management of the intravascular volume and achievement of early urine output. One of the reasons for graft failure after renal transplantation is inadequate graft perfusion caused by mis-management of perioperative hydration policy.

2. Chronic renal failure pathophysiology

Knowledge of the pathophysiologic consequences of chronic renal failure is too important for anesthesiologists, because many of these patients have at least one of these sequences, most commonly hypertension, coronary artery diseases, diabetes mellitus and pulmonary dysfunction. Additionally, disturbance in acid-base, electrolytes and fluid balance are usually related to a marked decline in the glomerular filtration rate (GFR) caused by a variety of systemic diseases such as diabetes mellitus or hypertension, and renal disorders as chronic glomerulonephritis ,cystic kidney disorder ,interstitial nephritis , obstructive uropathy, and lupus nephritis. It is essential to recognize the etiology, because the physician should control the problem and does not rely on the patients' ability to comply with the treatment.

3. Pre-operative Kidney recipient assessment

The practice of anesthesia for kidney transplant requires a thorough understanding of the metabolic and systemic abnormalities in end stage renal disease, familiarity with transplant medicine and expertise in managing and optimizing these patients for the best possible outcome.

Patients undergoing renal transplant surgery possess several risk characteristics like cardiovascular diseases, hypertension, diabetes mellitus, and the problems of dialysis. Therefore a thorough pre-operative assessment is crucial for successful intra- and postoperative management. The preoperative work-up includes Past- medical history, dialysis evaluation (How long? How often? When was the last dialysis?), serum electrolytes (serum potassium), ECG, chest X-ray and cardiac echocardiography. Dialysis is usually indicated within 24-48 hrs before the operation. Overzealous ultra filtration is best avoided. Volume status is roughly estimated by their dry weight. Decline of more than 2-4 kg during dialysis suggests significant intravascular depletion. Therefore it was advisable to restrict fluid removal during preoperative dialysis to a target of 1-2 kg above the formal dry weight. (Schnuelle and Johannes Van der Woude: 2006). Antihypertensive drugs and cardiovascular medications should be continued until the day of surgery.

4. Intra-operative hydration policy

The primary goal of fluid administration is to ensure stable hemodynamics by rapidly restoration the circulating plasma volume. However, excessive fluid accumulation, particularly in the interstitial tissue should be avoided. The intra-operative hydration strategy of both kidney donor and recipient are of paramount important for the insurance the success of kidney transplantation and ensure good function of the graft after surgery.

4.1 Kidney donors hydration policy

Othman and his colleagues (2010) described in their study the hydration regimen of their living kidney donors. The kidney donors, in this study, had received 1500 mls normal saline and 1500 mls Ringer's lactate solution, supplemented by crystalloid titrated to match the urine output from the start of the surgery until the renal vessels were clamped. Kidney donors also received 40 mg furosemide and 150 mL mannitol 10% before nephrectomy.

To maintain good diuresis, fluid administration for kidney donors is usually generous (10-20 ml/kg/hr) using isotonic crystalloids during the intra-operative time (Baxi et al 2009). However, some centers recommend overnight preoperative hydration with intravenous fluids and preloading the patients with colloids just before induction of anesthesia. Good hydration of the donor in addition of good hemodynamic intraoperative stability are essential requirements for the graft to tolerate ischemia time after nephrectomy with less harm till vascular anastomosis being completed.

In our center, the harvested kidney in living kidney donor was usually submerged immediately in iced Ringer's lactate solution, and the renal artery was flushed with 250 to 300 mls cold Ringer's lactate solution (4°C) mixed with papaverine 120 mg, heparin 5000 IU, and verapamil 10 mg until the venous effluent was clear (Othman et al, 2010)..

4.2 Kidney recipient hydration policy

Proper peri-operative fluid management is one of the most important aspects governing hemodynamic function in the surgical patient. Adequate hydration is an integral part of the anesthetic management during renal transplant. Adequate plasma volume is essential in maintaining cardiac output and hence tissue perfusion. The stable hemodynamic status of the recipient during kidney transplant surgery is usually associated with an initial good graft function. To decrease the incidence of postoperative acute tubular necrosis (ATN), a liberal hydration policy is usually employed intra-operatively. The systolic blood pressure is maintained between 130 and 160 mm Hg, and the CVP is maintained between 12 and 14 mm Hg (Ferris et al, 2003). Maintaining adequate CVP is especially important in pediatric recipients because reperfusion of an adult kidney graft after completion of anastomosis may divert a significant amount of cardiac output. Measuring the central venous pressure (CVP) is really an absolute requirement to ensure good plasma volume expansion. The pulmonary artery pressure also can be used to guide fluid therapy in patients with preoperative left ventricular dysfunction (Carlier et al ,1982). Additionally, mean arterial pressure (MAP) less than 100 mmHg and plasma volume below 45 mL/kg at reperfusion of the graft are the usual risk factors for graft failure (Toth et al ,1998). Blood flow to the allograft after reperfusion may predict its immediate function. The early graft function requires adequate perfusion that can be achieved by expansion of the intravascular volume of the recipients.

Recently, a study was designed to examine the time of maximum volume expansion relative to renal ischemia period in living-related recipients and its effect on graft perfusion and early renal function (Othman et al, 2010). The kidney recipients were randomly assigned in this study into to one of two hydration regimens. The hydration regimens that used were either the constant infusion rate (CIR) regimen or the CVP target (CVPT) regimen. The CIR group received normal saline at a constant infusion rate of a range 10 to 12 ml.kg-1.-1h from the start of surgery until the renal vessels were unclamped at the end of anastomosis. Isotonic saline 0.9% was infused using a volumetric infusion pump. The CVPT group received normal saline at two different CVPT phases. The first "pre-ischemia" phase was from the start of surgery until the renal artery in the donor kidney was clamped. During this time, saline was infused slowly to maintain the CVP at target within 5 mmHg. In the second "ischemia" phase, from clamping the donor renal artery until unclamping of the recipient renal artery after vascular anastomosis completion, normal saline was infused to maintain a CVPT of around 15 mm Hg. Systolic, diastolic, mean arterial blood pressure, and CVP values were recorded 30 minutes after induction of anesthesia, at the time of renal artery clamping in the donor (onset of ischemia), at unclamping of the vessels after completion of the vascular anastomosis (end of ischemia), and at the end of surgery. Also renal ischemia time, concurrent saline infusion rate, time of onset of urine production on unclamping of the renal artery, and total urine output from unclamping of the renal vessels to the end of the surgery were recorded. Kidney turgidity was evaluated blindly by the surgical team members on a 3-point scale: score I (soft graft), score II (moderately turgid graft), and score III (highly turgid and firm graft).After surgery, all patients were assessed for the presence of tissue edema, especially in the conjunctiva, eyelids, face, and upper airway. Postoperative graft function was evaluated by estimation of fraction extraction sodium ratio (FENa %) after surgery to assess renal concentrating power: Daily serum creatinine, creatinine clearance, and total urine output were recorded for five days postoperatively. Patients in the CVPT group showed better intraoperative graft turgidity, arterial blood pressure stability, earlier diuresis, and rapid improvement of postoperative graft function. This was achieved in the CVPT group without an overall increase in infused saline volume (ranged 3 liters), vasopressor use, and diuretic doses compared with the CIR. The biphasic hydration regimen applied in the CVPT group with delayed most of the crystalloid administration until shortly before the renal vessels were unclamped (with a calculated range of 45-50 ml/min during ischemia time) had more favorable outcome.

Hypotension may occur after unclamping the renal vessels and reperfusion of the graft. It is important to maintain the blood pressure because renal function is critically dependent on adequate perfusion. The two main factors that may precipitate to immediate revascularization hypotension:

1. Sudden shift of 25% of cardiac output to the renal graft.
2. Release of vasodilator mediators accumulated during renal ischemia period.

It is critical that the patient is adequately hydrated throughout renal transplant surgery in preparation for reperfusion of the graft. Close monitoring of the CVP, and avoidance of deep level of anesthesia during this period can prevent hypotension. The use of vasopressors with α agonist action may comprise blood flow to the transplanted organ. Additional fluid may be required to maintain blood pressure and replace urine output. Furosemide can enhance urine output. Loop diuretics block the Na+/K+ channels in the thin ascending loop of Henle. This prevents reabsorption of electrolytes in this part of the nephron. The high osmolar fluid then prevents reabsorption of water in the distal tubule. A large volume of fluid with high electrolyte content is excreted. Mannitol is freely filtered in the glomerulus, but not reabsorbed. It causes osmotic expansion of urine volume. Loop diuretics and /or mannitol may be used to promote diuresis from the grafted kidney. Mannitol improves renal blood flow, acts as a free radical scavenger and reduces the incidence of impaired renal function immediately after transplant (Kasper et al, 2005).

Another study was previously done for pediatric kidney recepients used average introperative fluids 88 ml/kg with a wide range of 30-90 ml/kg which reflected a large range of preoperative hydration status of recipients. However, younger children received higher volume of fluids per kilogram than older one. Also this study indicated that there was no correlation between the amount of fluid given intraoperatively and the occurrence of postoperative oliguria or acute tubular necrosis. (Coupe et al 2005).However, the intraoperative fluid replacement during kidney transplantation should be carefully titrated to the needs and overload must be avoided to get ride the problems that may developed if the new graft is either delayed to function or failing.

5. The choice of recipient fluid therapy

The choice of a particular solution in a given clinical situation may be guided by an understanding of the solutions' properties, but there is still an ongoing debate on the relative merits of crystalloid and colloid solutions for kidney recipients .The intravenous administration of adequate volumes of fluid is associated with earlier onset of graft function, lower postoperative serum creatinine, higher postoperative creatinine clearance, reduced incidence of delayed graft function, and improved graft survival. Most anesthesiologists avoid potassium-containing fluids during renal transplantation with the belief that it may worsen hyperkalemia in case of impaired graft function. The administration of normal saline and normal saline-based fluids (5% albumin) is the standard of care for fluid management in patients undergoing renal transplant surgery. This policy is primarily based on avoidance of potassium-containing fluids that can contribute to intra-operative hyperkalemia. The recipient's blood is usually typed and screened preoperatively. However, blood loss is usually minimal during uncomplicated kidney transplantation. Also blood transfusion is unlikely practice for kidney recipients except in highly indicated cases because of high possibility of triggering the patient's immune system. The anesthesiologist should attempt to maintain a mean blood pressure range of 60 to 80 mm Hg, central venous pressure (CVP) between 10 to 14 cm H20 and mean pulmonary artery pressure of 18 to 20 mm Hg. The estimated blood loss during the case is usually minimal (< 300 ml). In some cases, greater blood loss may require transfusion of packed red cells. Packed red cells should be cytomegalovirus (CMV) negative.

5.1 Crystalloids

Crystalloids solutions are usually preferred during kidney transplantation to correct fluid and electrolyte imbalance (Table 1). However in certain situation as in severe hypovolemia, colloids may be valuable. A great source of controversy and debate is the choice of intra-operative fluid during kidney transplantation. In a survey conducted in over 90% of renal transplant centers in USA, normal saline was used for hydration during kidney transplantation (O'Malley et al 2002). Many studies have shown that the use of normal saline leads to a major increase in serum potassium compared with Ringer's lactate, most likely due to associated hyperchloremic metabolic acidosis through an extra cellular shift of potassium (O'Malley et al, 2005; Khajavi et al, 2008).

	+Na mMole/l	Cl- mMole/l	K+ mMole/l	Ca++ mMole/l	Mg++ mMole/l	Additives (bicarbonate)
Normal Saline (0.9%)	154	154	-	-	-	-
Lactated Ringer's	130	109	4	1.5	-	Lactate(28)
Acetated Ringer's	130	109	4	1.5	-	Acetate(28)
Plasmalyte	140	98	5	1.5	3	Acetate (27) + Gluconate(23)

Table 1. Commonly used crystalloids and their composition:

Hyperchloremia may have adverse renal effects through vasoconstriction in afferent and efferent arteriolar beds of kidney and may result in a decrease in the urine output (Wilcox, 1983). Consequently, the use of Ringer's lactate is now preferred in renal transplant surgery. It is essential to acknowledge that intravenous fluids are behaved like drugs with indications, contraindications, and side effects. With this in mind, the anesthetist must carefully choose the type of fluid for intra-operative use during kidney transplantation .This choice is based on number of factors. These factors include the physical properties of the solution, the patient's biochemical profile with special reference of serum electrolytes and surgical circumstances.

The principal component of crystalloid fluids is the inorganic salt sodium chloride (NaCl). Sodium is the most abundant solute in the extracellular fluids, and it is distributed uniformly throughout the extracellular space. Because 75 to 80% of the extracellular fluids are located in the extravascular (interstitial) space, a similar proportion of the total body sodium is in the interstitial fluids. Exogenously administered sodium follows the same distribution, so 75 to 80% of the volume of sodium-based intravenous fluids are distributed in the interstitial space.This means that the predominant effect of volume resuscitation with crystalloid fluids is to expand the interstitial volume rather than the plasma volume. An infusion of 1 L of 0.9% sodium chloride (isotonic saline) adds 275 mL to the plasma volume and 825 mL to the interstitial volume. Note that the total volume expansion (1100 mL) is slightly greater than the infused volume. This is the result of a fluid shift from the intracellular to extracellular space, which occurs because isotonic saline is actually hypertonic to the extracellular fluids.

5.1.1 Isotonic (normal)Saline

The prototype crystalloid fluid is 0.9% sodium chloride (NaCl), also called isotonic saline (osmolarity=308 mOsmole/l) or normal saline. The latter term is inappropriate because a one normal (1 N) NaCl solution contains 58 g NaCl per liter (the combined molecular weights of sodium and chloride), whereas isotonic (0.9%) NaCl contains only 9 g NaCl per liter. The pH of isotonic saline (pH=5.7)is also considerably lower than the plasma pH. These differences are rarely of any clinical significance. The chloride content of isotonic saline is particularly high relative to that of plasma (154 mEq/L versus 103 mEq/L, respectively), so hyperchloremic metabolic acidosis is a potential risk with large-volume isotonic saline infusion.

5.1.2 Lactated Ringer's

Ringer's solution was introduced in 1880 by Sydney Ringer, a British physician and research investigator who studied mechanisms of cardiac contraction. The solution was designed to promote the contraction of isolated frog hearts, and contained calcium and potassium in a sodium chloride diluent. In the 1930s, an American pediatrician named Alexis Hartmann proposed the addition of sodium lactate buffer to Ringer's solution for the treatment of metabolic acidoses. The lactated Ringer's solution, also known as Hartmann's solution, gradually gained in popularity and eventually replaced the standard Ringer's solution for routine intravenous therapy.
Lactated Ringer's solution contains potassium and calcium in concentrations that approximate the free (ionic) concentrations in plasma. The addition of these cations requires a reduction in sodium concentration for electrical neutrality, so lactated Ringer's solution has less sodium than isotonic saline. The addition of lactate (28 mEq/L) similarly requires a reduction in chloride concentration and has pH approximate 6.7. The chloride in lactated Ringer's is more closely approximates plasma chloride levels than does isotonic saline. Lactated Ringer's is also not an ideal crystalloid.The calcium in lactated Ringer's can bind to certain drugs and reduce their bioavailability and efficacy.Also,lactated Ringer's is considered a moderately hypotonic (Osmolarity=273 mOsmaole/l) crystalloid solution. So, many studies recommend limited use of lactated Ringer's in patients who at risk of cerebral edema (Feldman et al; 1995).

5.1.3 Acetated Ringer's

Acetated Ringer's isolution is similar in its compostion to lactated ringer's except replacement the lactate with acetate which could converted to bicarbonate in all body cells including muscles(Hahn &Drobin, 2003).

5.1.4 Plasmalyte (Normosl)

Plasmalyte is a balanced salt solution having electrolyte compostion and osmolarity (294 mOsmole/l) similar to that of plasma.The major feature of these solutions is the added buffer capacity, which gives them a pH that is equivalent to that of plasma (pH=7.4). Acetate and gluconate content act as precursors of bicarbonate. This converstion occur predominantly in the liver,although acetate could be converted to bicarbonate in other body tissues resulting in less acidosis.An additional feature is the addition of magnesium, which may provide some benefit in light of the high incidence of magnesium depletion in hospitalized patients .A previous relevant study, which compared different crystalloid solutions on acid-base balance and early kidney functions after kidney transplantation,have concluded that plasmalyte has the best metabolic profile (Hadimioglu et al, 2008).

5.2 Colloids

Natural available colloid as human albumin has been widely applied for the treatment of hypovolemia in critically ill and surgical patients during the last two decades. Albumin is being widely replaced by many synthetic colloids such as dextrans, gelatins, and hetastarch (HES) solutions. Colloids are stayed in the intravascular compartment because of their macromolecules composition. The degree of plasma volume expansion exerted by colloids is determined by their concentration, molecular weight, chemical structure, colloid osmotic pressure, metabolism, and elimination rate. HES solutions have varying effects on coagulation characteristics, which depend on the size of the HES molecules and the degree of hydroxethyl substitution. Impaired platelet function, and impaired coagulation profile as measured by thromboelastography have been reported to arise during the administration of HES. This raises some concern for end stage renal patients undergoing kidney transplantation, because they are prone to bleeding complications because of associated platelet dysfunction (Boccardo et al; 2004). Although it is rare, severe and life-threatening anaphylactic reactions have been reported in association with any of the commonly used semi-synthetic colloids and with albumin. The incidence of severe anaphylactic reactions is probably more frequent for gelatins (0.35%) and for dextrans (0.27%) than for albumin (0.10%) or for starches (0.06%) This required to be considered when weighing the risks/benefits for the use of different plasma volume expanders (Laxenaire et al ;1994). A study with a large series of renal transplants from deceased donors, revealed a statistically significant benefit from the usage of albumin, though mannitol, furosemide, and electrolyte solutions were administered concomitantly (Dawidson et al;1992). Protective properties to the intra-operative administration of mannitol during the vascular phase were attributed to the osmotic diuretic and the antioxidant properties of sugar alcohols substances. Two of the synthetic colloids that have widely replaced albumin in clinical practice - dextrans and gelatins - do not seem on the whole to be preferable to albumin. An old comparative study comparing intra-operative albumin and dextran-40 in renal transplant recipients from a living related donor did not show any significant difference between the two regimens with regards to urine volume output and serial serum creatinine concentrations after transplantation (Dawidson et al; 1987). The clinical value of this study may be limited, because small sample size (17 patients) had no enough statistical power to detect outcome differences. Dextran solutions have been associated with major side-effects, such as coagulation disorders, severe anaphylactic reaction, and acute tubular necrosis .This has led to major limitation for their usage as plasma volume expansion in kidney transplantation (Bergman et al; 1990).

Hetastarch (HES) solutions (table 2) are originally synthesized from natural polymers of amylopectin. The pharmacokinetics of HES solutions depend on their molecular weight and C2/C6 hydroxyethylation ratio which influences their degradation mainly by plasma amylase. Osmotic, nephrosis-like lesions were reported in 80% of transplanted kidneys after the use of routine volumes of HES 200/0.6 in brain-dead donors (Legendre et al ,1993) . The likely mechanism for this action may be swelling and vacuolization of the tubular cells, and tubular obstruction due to hyper-viscous urine. Additionally, the slow degradation of high molecular weight or highly substituted HES may increase plasma osmotic pressure, leading to renal dysfunction and therefore these factors limit their use during kidney transplantation. The latest HES generation, HES 130/0.4, has a total body clearance about 23–31 times faster than that of the first generation hetastarch, and exhibits the best risk/benefit ratio of all available HES (Jungheinrich, and Neff ,2005).

	HES 70/0.5	HES 130/0.4	HES 200/0.5	HES 200/0.5	HES 200/0.62	HES 450/0.7
Concentration (%)	6	6	6	10	6	6
Volume efficacy (%)	100	100	100	130	100	100
Volume effect (hours)	1-2	2-3	3-4	3-4	5-6	5-6
Mean molecular weight (KD)	70	130	200	200	200	450
Molar substitution	0.5	0.4	0.5	0.5	0.62	0.7
C2/C6 ratio	4:1	9:1	6:1	6:1	9:1	4.6:1

Table 2. Characteristics of different available hydroxyethyl starch (HES) solutions.

HES preparations (table 2) are characterized by the following criteria:
(A) Concentration (6%, 10%),
(B) Molecular weight (Mw: the sum of each molecule's weight devided by the total mixture's weight times the weight of the molecule):

- Low-molecular weight [LMW]-HES: 70,000 dalton.
- Medium-molecular weight [MMW]-HES: 130,000 to 260,000 dalton.
- High-molecular weight [HMW]-HES: > 450,000 dalton,

(C) Molar substitution (MS: the molar ratio of the total number of hydroxyethyl groups to the total number of glucose units):

- Low MS: 0.4 and 0.5
- Moderate MS: 0.62
- High MS: 0.7

(D) C2/C6 ratio. The ratio of the C2:C6 hydroxyethylation appears to be key factors for pharmcokinetic behaviour of HES and possibly also for its side effects (e.g. accumulation).
However, there still some debates surrounding the effects of hetastarch solutions on renal function, especially in the field of kidney transplantation.
Over the last few decades, there has been a shift in anesthesia practice from using natural colloids such as blood, albumin and fresh frozen plasma to synthetic colloids .However, the widespread use of synthetic colloids during kidney transplantation is still need more investigations to confirm their safety.
The evidence for Targeted Fluid Administration suggests that administration of colloid provides benefits over crystalloids. However no head-to-head trials of crystalloid versus colloid or colloid versus colloid during kidney transplantation have been performed.

Likewise all the clinical trials of Targeted Fluid Administration used are saline-based fluids. A new controversy surrounds the adequate amount of peri-operative fluid administration. For decades the strategy has been to keep the patient normovolaemic ('well hydrated') in the perioperative period. Early urine production is important in kidney transplantation as a good prognostic factor. It is usually associated with longer graft survival and lower morbidity. Early diuresis is commonly observed in live donor grafts. In dead donor grafts, onset of diuresis is usually delayed due to the variable period of kidney ischemia and their storage at low temperatures in electrolyte solutions until they are implanted. Some measures, such as the administration of large volumes of liquids and diuretics, have been advocated to obtain good diuresis at the end of the surgery. Mannitol induces osmotic diuresis and also has a protective effect on the tubular cells of transplanted kidney from ishaemic injury. The renal protective agents as mannitol used during kidney transplantation seems to be related to its ability to increase renal blood flow. This presumably is due to the result of release of intrarenal vasodilator prostaglandin and atrial naturetic peptide. Also, loop diuretics as furosemide act by blocking the Na+/K+ ATPase channels present in the thin ascending limb of Henle, decreasing tubular oxygen consumption which may offer some protection against ischemic injury(Esson and Schrier;2002).

Hypotension may occur after unclamping the vessels and reperfusion of the graft. It is important that the patient should be well hydrated, as renal function is critically dependent on renal perfusion. It is especially important in paediatric recipients because reperfusion of an adult size graft may divert a significant amount of their own blood volume. A previous study for special fluid strategy in pediatric kidney transplantation, a total mean volume of 18 ml.kg-1.h-1was infused, which divided to include approximately 8 ml.kg-1.h-1 of crystalloid, 7 ml.kg-1.h-1 of fresh frozen plasma, and 2 ml.kg-1.h-1 of washed red blood cells(Yamamoto et al 2003).

Central venous pressure value may decrease around 50% within two hours after revascularization despite aggressive fluid management. This decline is similar in recipients of both cadaveric and living related kidney donor and the cause may be multi-factorial such as redistribution of fluids, changes in vascular permeability or increased nitric oxide levels. The use of vaso-pressors ,with alpha agonist activity, are better to be avoided as they can compromise blood flow to the transplanted kidney. Loop diuretics, and mannitol may be used to enhance urine production. Low dose dopamine was previously used to stimulate dopaminergic receptors (DA1) in the kidney vasculature to induce vasodilatation and increased urine output. However, the utility of this approach is questioned in a denervated kidney, which it may not respond adequately to a low dose of dopamine as normal kidneys do.

6. Monitoring

Standard ASA monitors are adequate, although, patients with more advanced co-morbid conditions require more extensive monitoring such as continuous arterial blood pressure and pulmonary artery monitoring. Routine monitors include noninvasive arterial blood pressure, ECG, core temperature, end-tidal carbon dioxide ($ETco_2$), and arterial oxygen saturation SpO_2. CVP monitoring is required for all patients in order to guide volume management and for postoperative vascular access. .Arterial monitoring is reserved for small children undergoing anastamosis of the allograft to the great vessels. Older children undergoing anastamosis to the iliac vessels do not require arterial monitoring, and in fact it should be avoided in order to preserve sites for future arteriovenous fistulae. Swan-Ganz monitoring of pulmonary artery pressures may be necessary in the infrequent patients with symptomatic hypertensive cardiomyopathy or with symptomatic cardiac dysfunction. All patients have urinary catheters inserted prior to surgery for urine output records. Laboratory investigations every 1-2 hours to follow blood hemoglobin ,Hct, serum K+ and acid-base status. Those with the severe co-morbid conditions, such as symptomatic coronary artery diseases or history of congestive heart failure, should be monitored with a non-invasive transesophageal echocardiography to monitor cardiac functions.

7. Postoperative recipient fluid therapy

Strict monitoring of fluid input and urine output is essential especially in the early postoperative period to guide the function of the new graft. A study showed that recipients of living donor kidneys lost more serum albumin during surgery than their donors, resulting in decreased plasma volume that was associated with reduced post-operative urine output. Therefore, it was recommended that administration of postoperative colloids administration is necessary to replace the additional loss of albumin during transplant surgery (Dawidson et al; 1987). On the first day after successful transplantation, serum creatinine concentration is usually related to mean arterial blood pressure. It is decreased in patients with mean arterial pressure (MAP) above 100 mmHg, whereas it remained stable in patients with MAP of 80–100 mmHg and increased in patients with MAP below 80 mmHg (Toth et al ;1998). Post operative daily graft function was evaluated in another recent study that compared the CVP target regimen(15 mmHg) with constant infusion regimen(10-12 ml.kg-1.hour-1) during transplantation (Othman et al; 2010) .It was based on the renal concentrating ability, as reflected by the fractional excretion of sodium (FENa%) for 6 hours in immediate postoperative time. Also, serum creatinine level, creatinine clearance, and urine output were monitored daily for 5 days after surgery. This study reflected early postoperative faster decrease of serum creatinine with higher creatinine clearance and larger urine output in the CVP target group .This finding could attest to the sustained benefit of the central venous pressure titration approach over the constant infusion approach. .FENa % may be affected by a high diuretic dose that acts by altering the handling of sodium by the kidney. In this study, all patients in the constant infusion regimen group and only 50% of patients in the CVPT group had received variable large doses of furosemide, which might account for the early decrease of FENa %. Therefore, FENa % may be not useful as a renal function test for comparison between the used hydration regimens (Othman et al ; 2010).

Maintenance of crystalloid hydration during postoperative period must be adjusted accordingly to vital signs and urine output. Replace urine output (ml per ml) with crystalloid selected according to graft function and patient serum electrolytes. A rigorous postoperative intravenous hydration protocol in renal transplant recipients may protect against vascular thrombosis. Delayed graft function is mainly defined as the need for dialysis in the first week after transplant. It may result from a collection of various detrimental factors such as recipient's age, tissue match and any surgical complications as vessel thrombosis or bleeding. One-year graft survival of a first transplant is approximately 95%; for recipients of non-identical living-related kidneys, it approximates to 90%; for recipients of cadaver kidneys, it approximates 80%; and for re-transplanted recipients of cadaver kidneys, it is usually less to approximate 70%. Overall, recipient survival of approximately 95% during the first post-transplant year can be expected, although cardiovascular deaths remains a major concern (Flechner ; 1994).

Postoperative fluid management plan for kidney transplantation should be judicious and be modified in favor of maintaining just adequate filling pressures to maintain adequate intravascular volume and baseline hemodynamics .Additional fluids as per need once urine output from the new graft starts to decline guided by CVP and myocardial function and avoid overload that may empress the heart function with the recommendation of dialysis in presence of delayed graft function or acute tubular necrosis.

8. Summary

Graft viability associated with renal transplantation is a product of the proper managing of the kidney donor, the allograft, and the recipient patient. Short- and long-term outcome is influenced by perioperative fluid policy. The function of the transplanted kidney seems to be optimized if graft perfusion is greatly maximized through good hydration policy with CVP target to approximate15 mmHg. A strategy of crystalloid administration to a target central venous pressure resulted in better stability of intraoperative blood pressure, less use of vasopressors and furosemide. This could induce a faster decrease in serum creatinine towards normal vlue. Perioperative close monitoring of recipients and optimization of intravascular fluid volume status to maximize graft perfusion are the usual keys for long-term success of renal transplants. Crystalloids are usually considered as the first choice and some colloids could be used safely as alternatives during the procedure and in early postoperative periods. The ideal crystalloid solution seems resemble the plasma composition with special reference to electrolyte content .Although, lactated and acetated Ringer's solutions are moderately hypo-osmolar, isotonic normal saline has high chloride content that could induce hyperchloermic acidosis. Both lactate and acetate are considered as precursors of bicarbonate where lactate converted to bicarbonate in the liver and acetate converted to bicarbonate in all body tissues resulting in less acidosis. A mixture of normal saline with either lactated or acetated Ringer's solution may be the preferred crystalloid choice of fluid therapy during kidney transplantation. This policy could provide better guidance for perioperative hydration strategy during kidney transplantation until best evidence and multi-center guidelines will be established based upon more research in this field.

9. References

Baxi V, Jain A, Dasgupta D. Anesthesia for renal transplantation: An update. Indian J Anaesth. 2009 Apr;53(2):139-47.

Bergman A, Andreen M, Blomback M. Plasma substitution with 3% dextran-60 in orthopaedic surgery: influence on plasma colloid osmotic pressure, coagulation parameters, immunoglobulines and other plasma constituents. Acta Anaesthesiol Scand 1990; 34 : 21-29.

Boccardo P, Remuzzi G, Galbusera M. Platelet dysfunction in renal failure. Semin Thromb Hemost 2004; 30(5):579-589.

Carlier M, Squiifflet JP, Prison Y, et al. Maximal hydration during anesthesia increase pulmonary arterial pressure and improve early function of human renal transplants. Transplantation 1982;34: 201-204.

Coupe N,O'Brien M, Gibson P et al. Anesthesia for pediatric renal transplantation with and without epidural analgesia- a review of 7 years experience. Paediatr Anaesth 2005;15;220-228.

Dawidson I, Berglin E, Brynger H, Reisch J. Intravascular volumes and colloid dynamics in relation to fluid management in living related kidney donors and recipients. Crit Care Med 1987; 15: 631- 636.

Dawidson IJ, Sandor ZF, Coorpender L, et al. Intraoperative albumin administration affects the outcome of cadaver renal transplantation. Transplantation 1992; 53(4): 774-782.

Esson ML,Schrier RW .Diagnosis and treatment of acute tubular necrosis. Ann Inten Med 2002; 137:744-752.

Feldman Z,Zachari S, Reichementhal E, et al. Brain edema and neurological status with rapid infusion of lactated ringer's or 5%dextrose solution following head trauma. J Neurosurg 1995;83:1060-1066.

Ferris RL, Kittur DS, Wilasrusmee C, et al. Early hemodynamic changes after renal transplantation: determinants of low central venous pressure in the recipients and correlation with acute renal dysfunction. Med Sci Manit 2003; 9(2):CR61-CR66.

Flechner SM: Current status on renal transplantation. Urol Clin North Am 1994; 21: 265–282.

Hadimioglu N, Saadawy I, Saglam T et al. The effect of different crystalloid solutions on acid-base balanca and early kidney function after kidney transplantation. Anesth Analg 2008;107: 264-269.

Hahn RG and Drobin D. Rapid water and slow sodium excretion of acetated Ringer's solution dehydrates cells. Anesth Analg 2003; 97:1590-1594.

Jungheinrich C, Neff TA .Pharmacokinetics of hydroxyethyl starch. Clin Pharmacokinet 2005; 44: 681-699.

Kasper DL, Braunwald E, Fauci AS. Harrison's principles of internal medecine, 16th ed. New York: McGraw-Hill, 2005 ;1645.

Khajavi MR, Etezadi F, Moharari RS. Effects of normal saline vs.lactated Ringer's during renal transplantation. Renal Failure 2008;30 :535-539.

Laxenaire MC, Charpentier C, Feldman L. Anaphylactoid reactions to colloid plasma substitutes: incidence, risk factors, mechanism. A French multicenter prospective study. Ann Fr Anesth Reanim 1994;13: 301-310.

Legendre C, Thervet E, Page B, et al .Hydroxyethylstarch and osmotic-nephrosis-like lesions in kidney transplantation. Lancet 1993; 342: 248-249.

O'Malley CMN, Frument RJ, Bennett EG. Intravenous fluid therapy in renal transplant recipients: results of a US survey. Transplant Proc 2002; 34:3142-3145.

O'Malley CMN, Frumento RJ, Hardy MA, et al. A randomized double blind comparison of lactated Ringer 's solution and 0.9%Nacl during renal transplantation .Anesth Analg 2005;100:1518-24.

Othman MM, Ismael AZ, Hammouda GE.Impact of timing of maximal crystalloid hydration on early graft functions during kidney transplantation. Anesth Analg 2010; 110 (5): 1440-1446.

Schnuelle P and Johannes Van der Woude F. Perioperative fluid management in renal transplantation: a narrative of the literature. Transplant int ,2006 ;19: 947-959.

Toth M, Reti V, Gondos T. Effect of recipients' peri-operative parameters on the outcome of kidney transplantation. Clin Transplant1998; 12: 511–517.

Wicox CS. Regulation of renal blood flow by plasma chloride. J Clin Invest 1983; 71:726-735.

Yamamoto R, Nakai R, Nagasawa M et al. Anesthetic management of pediatric renal transplantation: A review of 15 cases under age of 10 years. Masui. 2003 52(6):631-635.

13

Anaesthesia for Kidney Transplantation

Yasser Haggag and Imran Ahmad
Guy's and St Thomas NHS Foundation Trust
UK

1. Introduction

Kidney transplantation improves the quality of life and the long-term survival of end-stage renal failure (ESRF) patients compared to those on dialysis (1). It has also been shown to be a more economic option than both haemodialysis and peritoneal dialysis (2)
With the increasing incidence of organ failure, the demand for organ transplantation has increased, resulting in longer waiting lists and increased waiting list deaths.
Recently, live organ donation has helped to relieve the shortage of deceased donor grafting. Living donor kidney transplantation offers recipients the best hope for long-term rehabilitation and its advantages are indisputable.
This chapter looks at the anaesthetic principles and management of kidney transplantation, the most frequently performed organ transplantation.

2. Preoperative assessment

Hypertension and diabetes mellitus (DM) are the two most common causes of ESRF
Hypertension should be assessed thoroughly in terms of severity, antihypertensive medications and cardiovascular complications. Hypertension associated with renal failure is usually treated with ACE inhibitors or angiotensin II receptors antagonists. (3)
A target blood pressure of 140/90 or less is usually associated with decreased incidence of left ventricular hypertrophy. (4)
Type 1 DM is usually associated with impaired renal function and can lead to the development of severe nephropathy and ESRF. Diabetic patients have increased cardiovascular risk of peripheral vascular disease. (5)
There are few other medical problems associated with advanced kidney diseases, such as:

- Endocrine abnormalities such as hyperparathyroidism
- increased calcium and phosphate serum levels.
- Dyslipidaemia
- Autoimmune diseases as vasculitis – Systemic Lupus Erythematosus (SLE)

3. Medical history

The preoperative visit plays an important role to alleviate patient's anxiety, especially for patients who have been suffering from a life-long kidney problem and anticipating to undergo a procedure that would change their life style completely.

The importance of such a visit to the anaesthetist cannot be over-emphasised, many of these patients have had general anaesthesia in the past, so useful information may be found from previous anaesthesia charts.
The aetiology of a failing kidney cannot be clearly identified every time, but it is important to be aware of the cause if this has been identified, as this may have other implications to the anaesthetic management. The associated morbidity, whether it is the cause of the renal failure or as a consequence of it, has to be sought very clearly.
The duration of renal failure and the requirement of any renal replacement therapy (RRT), either peritoneal dialysis (PD) or haemodialysis (HD) must also be noted. The longer the duration of renal failure, the more likely there will be implications to the anaesthetic management, for example the patient may have required numerous central venous cannulations in the past, resulting in stenosed or thrombosed central veins or they have had numerous arterio-venous (AV) fistulas which make intravenous access difficult.
It is useful to be aware of the patient's 'dry weight' as this will allow estimation of the preoperative fluid status. The frequency of dialysis per week should be asked and the last dialysis session the patient received must also be noted. Ideally this should be as close to surgery as possible. This will ensure optimised fluid balance (although the patient may be under filled after a session) and electrolyte balance, most importantly the potassium and urea levels. A higher potassium plasma concentration can be accepted in this group of patients, but always try to achieve a normal range.
If the patient is due a dialysis session or has elevated electrolyte levels and appears fluid overloaded, then this patient must undergo haemodialysis prior to general anaesthesia and surgery.
The normal daily fluid intake and daily volume of any native urine output (if present) should also be noted, this will act as a further guided to fluid management intra-operatively.
Prior to anaesthesia, the presence of any AV fistulas should be clearly marked and labelled to avoid cannulation and BP measurements.
A history of previous dialysis line or central line insertions into the internal jugular or subclavian veins should also be sought; this may have implications on the insertion of central lines for monitoring during the kidney transplantation. Long term dialysis lines or numerous central lines can cause stenosis and thrombosis of the central veins.
Exercise tolerance can give an indication of the severity of the condition and its associated problems, it is also a useful guide to the general health of the patient.

4. Examination

Routine examination includes vital signs and the state of hydration. Is the patient dry after recent dialysis or fluid overloaded?
Some patients presenting for renal transplant might have associated rare medical conditions that require thorough examination, conditions like Prune Belly syndrome and VATER association (please see later).
Particular attention should be made to the cardiovascular system, including blood pressure control and clinical signs of left ventricular hypertrophy (LVH).
Assessment of the respiratory system will determine further management of the patients following their surgery, if they have associated respiratory disease then they may require post-operative non-invasive ventilation or prolonged intubation and ventilation.
Airway assessment will determine the management of the patient's airway following induction of anaesthesia, but these patients should always be intubated and ventilated for a

renal transplant. Patients with DM may have associated difficult airways so appropriate equipment and techniques for managing the difficult airway must be available.

5. Investigations

Routine investigations such as full blood count (FBC) and kidney function particularly serum creatinine and blood urea nitrogen (BUN) and creatinine clearance.

Serum potassium should to be within the normal levels; usually less than 5.5 mmol/L. A further cycle on dialysis may be required if raised. Also note the bicarbonate and base excess.

Lots of important information can be obtained from the electrocardiogram (ECG), such as left ventricular hypertrophy, ischaemic heart disease or ECG changes associated with electrolyte imbalances, especially hyperkalaemia.

If the patient has a significant history of cardiovascular disease with associated ECG changes, then further assessment maybe required, such as an echocardiogram, radioactive isotope scan or even angiography. Patients with ESRF as a result of DM, may have undiagnosed cardiovascular disease, so particular care should be taken in these patients.

All patients undergoing renal transplant should at least have blood group and saved, blood should be made available if there is a high risk of bleeding.

6. Anaesthetic technique

Normally patients are not prescribed pre-medications prior to induction of anaesthesia, unless strongly indicated. Temazepam can be given orally 10 - 20 mg the night before and/or the morning of surgery in particularly anxious patients. Rantidine, metoclopramide or sodium citrate orally may also be given if the patient has reflux disease.

Induction of anaesthesia always takes place with the routine monitors ECG, non-invasive blood pressure and oxygen saturation monitoring. In patients with associated cardiovascular disease, invasive blood pressure monitoring should be considered, to ensure close monitoring of the blood pressure.

Haemodynamic stability should be maintained throughout the period of the operation with special attention to depressing the vasopressor response to intubation.

Fluctuations of the blood pressure should be within 20% of the baseline reading, this can be achieved by dampening surgical stimulation with the use of opioids.

Intraoperative opioids can be achieved via repeated boluses of Fentanyl or continuous infusion of Remifentanil, as target controlled infusion (TCI) between 4 to 6 ng/mL.

Atracurium (0.5 mg/Kg) is the muscle relaxant of choice in renal failure, it undergoes Hofmann degradation mainly and ester hydrolysis to a lesser extent.

Other muscle relaxants can be used, including all non-depolarizing muscle relaxants, but care must be taken with large or repeated doses as accumulation may result in a prolonged neuromuscular block.

The only depolarizing muscle relaxant in clinical use (suxamethonium) can be used as long as serum potassium levels are less than 5 mmol/L.

After induction of anaesthesia a central line should be inserted, ideally with ultrasound guidance, this allows monitoring of central venous pressure and the infusion of inotropes if necessary. The preferred site of insertion should be the internal jugular vein, be careful with the subclavian approach, particularly if on the fistula side as the vein may be arterialised and bleed profusely.

Immediately following induction of anaesthesia prophylactic dose of antibiotic should be given, this can vary depending on local protocol, commonly used are:
Amikacin 5 mg/Kg or gentamicin 3 mg/Kg
Co-amoxiclav dose 1.2 g can be given as well
Transplant surgery requires the administration of 'goodies', to reduce the incidence of organ rejection and to help functioning of the transplanted kidney. These are usually administered prior to revascularization and vary from centre to centre. Commonly used drugs are furosemide, mannitol, methylprednisolone (which should given as a slow intravenous infusion over half an hour, if given as a bolus it causes marked vasodilatation and may cause pronounced hypotension).

7. Maintenance of anaesthesia

All inhalational agents can be used safely, with the exception of enflurane (which is hardly being used in clinical practice nowadays)
Total intravenous anaesthesia (TIVA) is successfully being used with propofol and remifentanil to maintain GA.
The use of nitrous oxide is not associated with any ill effects, having said that, there is a trend among anaesthetists to avoid the use of N_2O in patients even with a normal kidney function.
The combination of Desflurane and Remifentanil infusion ensures smooth anaesthesia and a quick response to the challenging heart rate and blood pressure control throughout the procedure. This is in addition to smooth and rapid recovery.
Fentanyl can be given cautiously towards the end of the procedure in multiple small doses of 50 - 100 mcg; the total dose is titrated according to patient's response to pain while recovering from general anaesthesia.

8. Intraoperative monitors

Core Temp should ideally be measured via a nasopharyngeal probe, attention should be paid to keep the patient's temperature within the normal range. Hypothermia delays drug metabolism and is associated with increased incidence of postoperative complications namely chest infection and bleeding diathesis
Central venous pressure (CVP) alone can be a misleading guide to fluid requirements throughout the operation.
Oesophageal Doppler can be used to guide fluid management intraoperatively
Arterial blood gas testing (pH , PaO_2 , $PaCO_2$, bicarbonate, lactate, haemoglobin, potassium, sodium and blood glucose) is helpful if an arterial line has been placed, alternatively a venous sample could be used.
Serum potassium can go either way. Hypokalaemia should not be treated unless K is less than 3.0 mmol/L. Where as hyperkalaemia should be dealt with if K levels is 6.0 mmol/L or more. Calcium gluconate is the drug of choice in this case, as opposed to the traditional dextrose-insulin regimen.
Neuromuscular blockade monitor, an additional dose of muscle relaxants has to be judged carefully. Adequate reversal of the neuro-muscular function is extremely important before planning extubation at the end of the procedure.
Bi-spectral index (BIS) monitor can be used to assess depth of anaesthesia.

9. Fluid management

Transplant procedures are routinely short duration, minimal blood loss and preserved capillary permeability.

Patients undergoing renal transplant operations are usually receiving haemodialysis and their intravascular filling status should be monitored closely. The risk of hypovolaemia and under-filling can impair the perfusion to the transplanted kidney, whereas hypervolaemia from overzealous infusion of intravenous fluids can adversely affect myocardial contractility, especially for patients with pre-existing coronary artery disease (CAD) and impaired left ventricular function.

Even fluid balance and maintenance of the eu-volaemic status is strongly advisable

Type of intravenous fluid is of great importance, as the use of 0.9% sodium chloride is thought to be the standard fluid to be used in transplants patients, but the use of other crystalloid fluids such as Hartmann's solution (Lactated Ringer's) was used safely as long as serum potassium levels are monitored closely. (6)

Colloids could also be used safely in these procedures as long as its use does not exceed 15 mL/Kg.

Careful monitoring of the filling status of the patient is paramount, the use of central venous pressure (CVP) as the sole indicator or in combination with other monitors such as oesophageal doppler is advised. (7)

Immediate urine output can be seen in 90% of live kidney donation and up to 50% of cadaveric donation. Appropriate fluid management is the single most important factor to determine good urine output following the transplant.

It has been clearly demonstrated that it is more important than other pharmacological agents such as dopamine or the use of mannitol and colloids

Blood transfusion is better avoided in transplant procedures as the activation of autoimmune system may induce early rejection of the graft.

Renal failure patients are always anaemic, and it is quite safe to keep their haemoglobin levels as low as 7.0 g/dL in the perioperative period as long as continuous haemoglobin monitoring is available. It is a compromise between a low haemocrit that helps flow to the new kidney and the oxygen carrying capacity and delivery of oxygen to the tissues

10. Low Dose Dopamine (LDD)

Dopamine exerts its effect - at this low dose – mainly via peripheral dopaminergic receptors (renal) rather than its effect via the adrenergic receptors (cardiovascular) (8)

Few studies have shown that dopamine infusion at a rate of up to 2.5 mcg/Kg/min. would increase both urine output and creatinine clearance (9)

Other studies have questioned the value of dopamine infusion following graft of denervated kidney as evidenced by Doppler examination of renal blood flow (10), (11). The rational behind the use of dopamine – in the first 12 hr postoperatively - is mainly to ensure arteriolar vasodilatation and increase the renal perfusion pressure and to prevent acute tubular necrosis (ATN). There is no clear benefit from infusing or withholding dopamine, it is usually left to individual institution guidelines and protocols.

If the patient's blood pressure is thought to be high enough to grant satisfactory renal blood flow and ensure adequate reperfusion of the graft, then here is no need to initiate a dopamine infusion.

It is important to maintain adequate mean arterial pressure and central venous pressure prior to the release of the clamps once the donor kidney has been transplanted. This will ensure good blood flow to the kidney. The target values are dependant on the patient's normal mean arterial pressures.

11. Postoperative management

The postoperative fluid management is an important part of maintaining adequate renal perfusion. Various regimes are available. One commonly used is, crystalloid 50mls/hr plus previous hour's urine output. The urine output should be closely monitored and liase closely with the surgeons, especially if the patient remains anuric.
Local anaesthesia wound infiltration with L-Bupivacaine (2 mg/Kg) by the surgeons at the end of surgery, may help reduce post-operative pain.
Fentanyl patient controlled analgesia (PCA) is the standard pain control method
Bolus dose 10 to 20 mcg with 5 minutes lock out interval and no background infusion, but if high doses of opiates are anticipated or required a background infusions can be established, with careful monitoring.
Morphine can be used for postoperative pain control following transplant procedures; care must be exercised as accumulation of its metabolite morphine-6 glucuronide (M-6-G) may occur (12)

12. Regional anaesthesia

The use of epidural for renal transplant surgery is rare and controversial; the main reason is that uraemic patients tend to have a tendency to develop coagulopathy.
Few recent studies have shown that it is a safe technique to use as long as prothrombin time (PT) is normal and the patient should have heparin-free dialysis sessions before epidural placement.
Epidural can be used as the sole anaesthetic technique or in combination with GA.
Both techniques were found to have similar encouraging results with respect to early graft function. The level of insertion is usually low thoracic to high lumbar (T12 - L1 or L1 - L2). Local anaesthetic infusion of Levo-Bupivacaine or Ropivacaine can be used safely. (13) Facilities to continuously monitor the neurological status of the patient, and to pick early signs of epidural haematoma should be readily available. (14)

13. DVT Prophylaxis

Intraoperatively TEDS elastic stockings and flowtron boots should be routinely used. Un-fractionated Heparin 5000 iu twice daily subcutaneously should be prescribed post-operatively. LMWH are to be avoided, as their metabolic end products are execreted via the kidney and can adversely affect the renal function

14. Conclusion

Kidney transplantation is the only definitive modality of treating ESRF
Patients undergoing transplant procedures present many challenges to the anaesthetist.
Success of transplant is all-dependent on thorough preoperative, close intraoperative monitoring and appropriate fluid management.

The anaesthetic technique plays an important role to ensure the immediate success of the graft. (15)

15. Prune Belly syndrome

This is a congenital abnormality mostly occurring in boys, with an incidence of 1 in 30,000 live births, it is of unknown aetiology and has three characteristic features: underdevelopment of the abdominal muscles, undescended testis and abnormalities of the urinary tract (most commonly hydronephrosis and vesico-ureteric reflux). Mortality is as much as 50% before the age of 2 years, depending on the type and severity of the abnormalities. 25-30% of patients develop chronic renal failure, often requiring renal transplantation. This group of patients has several features which could pose problems for the anaesthetist, so anaesthetic management must focus on airway, pulmonary and renal systems. Micrognathia, pulmonary hypoplasia and urinary tract abnormailities should all be evasluated prior to anaesthesia.

16. VATER association

This arises from abnormalities in mesodermal differentiation and is an acronym for Vertebral abnormality, Anal atresia, Trachoe-oesophageal fistula with oEsophageal atresia and Renal dysplasia. Renal failure is a common, there is also an increased frequency of mental retardation and these patients may also have cardiac anomalies such as ASD, VSD and dextrocardia. Anaesthesia for this group of patients must focus on the cardiovascular, respiratory and renal systems.

17. Anaesthesia for Hand-assisted Laparoscopic Donor Nephrectomy

Hand-Assisted laparoscopic donor nephrectomy (HALDN) is a fairly novel technique to harvest the kidney from a live donor.
It is minimally invasive technique compared to the standard open surgical approach.
The donor is a healthy individual, who is usually related to the recipient. He/she can be either ASA grade 1 or 2 (i.e. with a mild systemic illness that does not affect his physiological reserves).
The conduct of anaesthesia in such cases is not different from any other laparoscopic procedure.
The airway should be secured with a re-enforced endotracheal tube.
Position of the patient is the lateral decubitus, with the operating table broken in the middle
The patient should be securely strapped to the table firmly in order to prevent any change to his position during the operation.
Careful positioning needs extra-padding to protect nerves and bony prominences, the upper arm has to be kept in neutral position on an arm support.

18. References

[1] Wolfe RA, Ashby VB, Milford EL, Ojo AO, Ettenger RE, Agodoa LY et al. Comparison of mortality in all patients on dialysis, patients on dialysis awaiting transplantation, and recipients of a first cadaveric transplant. N Engl J Med 1999; 341:1725-30.

[2] Karlberg I, Nyberg G. Cost-effectiveness studies of renal transplantation. Int J Technol Assess Health Care 1995; 11: 611-622.

[3] Heart Outcomes Prevention Evaluation (HOPE) Study Investigators. Effects of an angiotensin -converting enzyme inhibitor, ramipril, on cardiovascular events in high-risk patients. N Engl J Med 2000; 342: 145–53.

[4] Foley RN, Parfrey PS, Harnett JD, Kent GM, Murray DC, Barre PE. Impact of hypertension on cardiomyopathy, morbidity and mortality in end-stage renal disease. Kidney Int 1996; 49: 1379–85.

[5] Norio K, Makisalo H, Isoniemi H, Groop Ph, Pere P, Lidgren L. Are diabetic patients in danger at renal transplantation? An invasive perioperative study. Eur J Anaesthesiol 2000; 17: 729–36.

[6] Hadimioglu N, Saadawy I, Saglam T, Ertug Z, Dinckan A. The effect of different crystalloid solutions on acid-base bal3ance and early kidney function after kidney transplantation. Anesth Analg 2008;107:264-9.3

[7] De Gasperi A, Narcisi S, Mazza E, Bettinelli L, Pavani M, Perrone L et al. Perioperative fluid management in kidney transplantation: is volume overload still mandatory for graft function? Transplant Proc 2006;38:807-9.

[8] Grundmann R, Kindler J, Meider G, Stowe H, Sieberth HG, Pichlmaier H. Dopamine treatment of human cadaver kidney graft recipients: a prospectively randomized trial. Klin Wochenschr 1982; 60:193-7.

[9] Carmellini M, Romagnoli J, Giulianotti PC, Pietrabissa A, Di Stefano R, Rindi P et al. Dopamine lowers the incidence of delayed graft function in transplanted kidney patients treated with cyclosporine A. Transplant Proc 1994; 26:2626-9.

[10] Kadieva VS, Friedman L, Margolius LP, Jackson SA, Morrell DF. The effect of dopamine on graft function in patients undergoing renal transplantation. Anesth Analg 1993; 76: 362-5.

[11] Sandberg J,Tyden G, Groth CG. Low-dose dopamine infusion following cadaveric renal transplantation: no effect on the incidence of ATN. Transplant Proc 1992; 24:357.

[12] Smith I, Walley G, Bridgman S. Omitting fentanyl reduces nausea and vomiting, without increasing pain, after sevoflurane for day surgery. Eur J Anaesthesiol 2008; 25: 790–913. Hammouda GE, Yahya R, Atallah MM (1996) Plasma bupiva- caine concentrations following epidural administration in kidney transplant recipients. Reg Anesth 21:308–311

[13] Akpek AE, Kayhan Z, Kaya H, Candan S, Haberal M (1999) Epidural anesthesia for renal transplantation: a preliminary report. Transplant Proc 31:3149–3150

[14] Evans M, Pounder D (1988) Anaesthesia and perioperative management for renal transplantation. In: Farman JV (ed) Trans- plant surgery: anesthesia and perioperative care. Elsevier Science, Netherlands, pp 289–318

14

Augmentation Cystoplasty: in Pretransplant Recepients

Ashraf Abou-Elela
Cairo University,
Egypt

1. Introduction

Augmentation cystoplasty is performed to increase bladder capacity and compliance. The primary use of augmentation cystoplasty is to protect renal function, to achieve urinary continence, and often to facilitate urinary tract reconstruction [1]. The most common problems necessitating bladder augmentation are neurogenic bladder dysfunction secondary to myelodysplasia, extrophy of the bladder, and posterior urethral valves. However, many other conditions may require bladder augmentation including tuberculosis, interstitial cystitis, multiple surgeries, chemotherapy and radiation therapy.

Not all patients undergoing augmentation cystoplasty, especially in the pediatric population, can achieve complete emptying of their bladder by spontaneous voiding. It was the success and wide spread acceptance of clean intermittent catheterization (CIC) in the mid-1970s that made augmentation cystoplasty and continent urinary diversion possible especially in children [2].

Conventional enterocystoplasty employs the use of detubularized segments of small or large bowel. Ileum, sigmoid and cecum have all been used; several studies have confirmed the reliability of these segments [3, 4].

Despite the functional success of enterocystoplasty, clinical experience has demonstrated that there are numerous complications that can result from the incorporation of small and large bowel and their heterotropic epithelium into the urinary tract. To avoid some of the deleterious side effects of enterocystoplasty, several procedures have been developed to augment the bladder without the use of the bowel. These include gastrocystoplasty, the use of dilated ureter (either naturally dilated or balloon dilated), autoaugmentation and seromuscular enterocystoplasty [5, 6, 7, 8, 9].

Autoaugmentation involves the excision of the detrusor muscle from the dome of the bladder allowing the epithelium to form a large diverticulum which may or may not be covered with a seromuscular gastric or sigmoid patch as a backing. In addition, recent advances in tissue engineering substrates and biomaterials have enhanced our abilities to possibly regenerate bladder tissue that is clinically useful for augmentation purposes. Generally, three classes of biomaterials have been used for engineering of genitourinary tissues; naturally derived materials, such as collagen and alginate, cellular tissue matrices such as bladder and small intestinal submucosa (SIS) and synthetic polymers such as polyglycolic acid (PGA) and polylactic acid (PLA) [10, 11, 12, 13].

At this time, even so, there are significant potential problems with the use intestinal segments in the lower urinary tract; gastrointestinal (GI) segments remain the gold standard for increasing bladder capacity and improving compliance. These problems include: hyperchloremic metabolic acidosis, hyokalemia, hypocalcemia, ammoniagenic encephalopathy, bone demineralization, vitamin B_{12} deficiency, malabsorption, drug absorption toxicities, growth retardation, mucus secretion, urinary tract infection, urinary calculi and tumor formation. Gastrocystoplasty may be complicated with hypochloremic metabolic alkalosis and hematuria-dysuria syndrome (14).

Therefore augmentation cystoplasty should be offered only after medical intervention such as anticholinergic medications and intermittent catheterization fail to achieve dryness or to improve bladder compliance sufficiently.

The majority of children who undergo augmentation cystoplasty will require intermittent catheterization (1). The commitment and capacity of both child and the family to comply with catheterization must be assessed carefully. All potential complications should be discussed in details with adult patients and with the family of the child.

Conditions that may require bladder augmentation

Neurogenic Bladder
- Myelodysplasia
- Sacral agenesis
- Caudal regression
- Spinal tumors, vascular malformation
- Myelitis
- Idiopathic

Congenital
- Exstrophy (cloacal, classic, epispadias)
- Posterior urethral valves

Cloaca
- Urogenital sinus
- Bilateral single ectopic ureters
- Infantile bladder syndrome
- Ureterocele
- Prune-belly syndrome

Other
- Infection (tuberculosis, viral cystitis, bacterial cystitis)
- Interstitial cystitis
- Iatrogenic (multiple surgeries)
- Chemotherapy
- Radiation therapy
- Tumor (rhabdomyosarcoma, neurofibromatosis)

2. Augmentation cystoplasty using bowel segments (enteroplasty)

2.1 General principles

The initial approach to augmentation cystoplasty is similar regardless of the bowel segments to be used. Cystoscopy should be performed preoperatively to avoid any unsuspected anatomic abnormalities that may affect the surgery. In augmentation cystoplasty, the two critical aspects of the surgery are the preparation of the bladder and the augmentation segment chosen.

2.2 Preparation of the native bladder

In augmentation cystoplasty, the bladder usually is addressed first. Most commonly, a midline incision is used to expose the abdomen & pelvis. If possible, the peritoneum is not entered until the bladder has been prepared for augmentation and other associated procedures such as ureteral reimplantation or bladder neck reconstruction have been performed. This minimizes third space fluid loss. The bladder is then bivalved through a sagittal incision from near the bladder neck anteriorly to near the trigone posteriorly, thus forming a "clam-shell" configuration. This maneuver is extremely important because the bladder must be opened fully to prevent the augmentation segment from acting as a diverticulum with the formation of an "hour-glass" deformity. Such an incision allows a technically easier anastomosis of the bowel segment and leaves the native bladder wings to add to the overall capacity. The bladder wings may also be used for implantation of a continent catheterizable channel (e.g. Mitrofanoff) or ureteral reimplantation.
Supratrigonal cystectomy is generally not recommended. The remaining cuff of the bladder is a relatively small area for anastomosis to the intestinal segment; therefore most of the bowel is approximated to itself which could result in the augmentation segment behaving as a diverticulum (1,15). Nevertheless, other surgeons have recommended that the majority of the "diseased" bladder be excised in preparation for augmentation. A greater circumference for the anastomosis can sometimes be provided by opening the bladder in a stellate fashion with a second transverse incision into the two bladder halves (15).

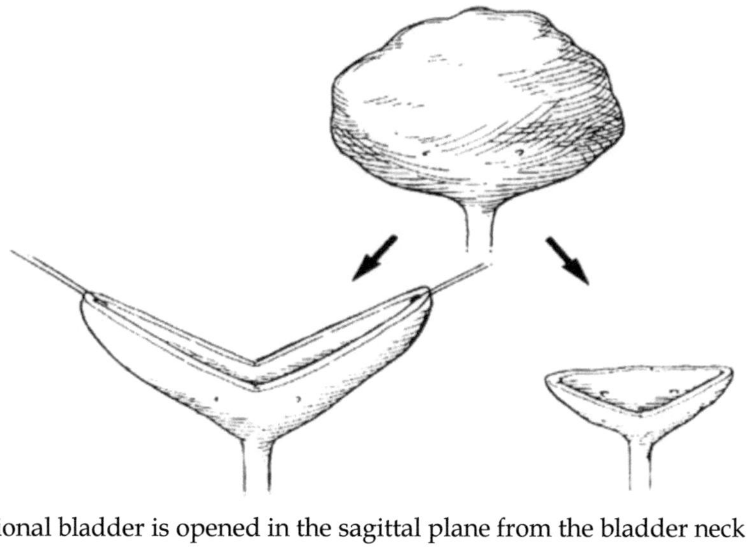

The dysfunctional bladder is opened in the sagittal plane from the bladder neck to the trigone (1).

2.3 Harvesting the augmentation segment

The size and configuration of the augmentation segment are probably more important than the type of bowel used.

Hinman (1988) and Koff (1988) have clearly demonstrated the advantages of opening bowel segments on their antimesenteric border, thereby allowing detubularization and reconfiguration of these segments. Detubularization and reconfiguration maximizes the added surface area to the bladder and thus the benefit of a given segment. Furthermore, the intrinsic innervation is disrupted and peristalsis is decreased significantly (16, 17).

Reconfiguration into a spherical shape provides multiple advantages that improve the overall capacity and compliance. Spherical configuration, by geometry, maximizes the volume achieved for a given bladder wall area. In addition, the spherical configuration also maximizes the radius of curvature, thereby increasing surface tension for a given bladder pressure, which tends to lead to further bladder expansion. This is the relationship of Laplace's law (T = k RP), where T is wall tension, k is a constant dependant on elasticity and wall characteristics, R is the radius of curvature, and P is the luminal pressure.

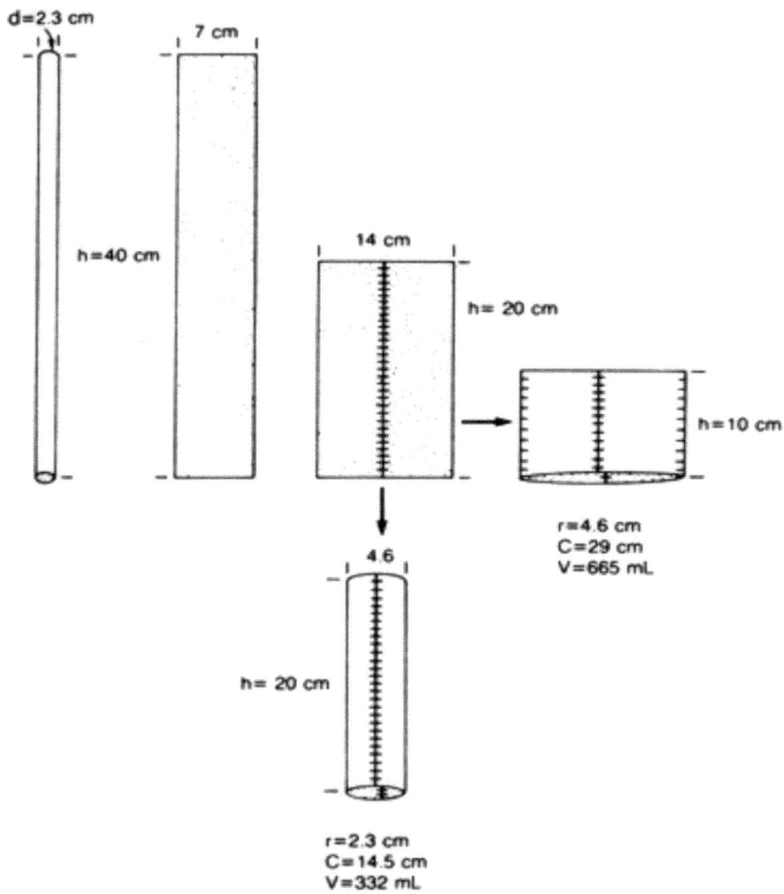

Calculated capacity of 40-cm segment opened and folded twice is 665 mL. C, circumference; d, diameter; h, height; r, radius; V, volume. (From Hinman F Jr. Selection of intestinal segments for bladder substitution: physiological characteristics. *J Urol* 1988;139:521)

The length of the segment used depends on: a) the radius of the bowel used; therefore a larger segment of small bowel usually is required; b) patient's age; c)the size of the pelvis; d) the volume of the native bladder being augmented; if the cystoplasty is being done on a bladder of moderate volume that generates high pressure by uninhibited contractions, less bowel is necessary than for a bladder that is tiny in capacity; e) patient's urinary volumes; patients with upper tract damage, particularly with concentrating ability, may make huge volumes of urine and require a larger capacity.

Depending on the volume needed, 15 to 40 cm of ileum and approximately 20 cm of colon is usually used for cystoplasty. If a segment of stomach is to be used as the augmentation segment, a wedge of at least one-third of the stomach is harvested (19). The gastric wedge requires no reconfiguration as it fits well onto the bivalved bladder. If the ureter is to be used as an augmentation segment, there must be significant dilation and it should likewise be detubularized before being anastomosed to the bladder (20).

The choice of the augmentation segment needs to be tailored individually to each patient. For example, patients with a short ileal mesentery may require the use of the sigmoid to allow for a tension-free anastomosis. Patients with a short gut, renal insufficiency, or a history of pelvic radiation may be better served with a gastrocystoplasty. Patients with myelomeningocele or imperforate anus theoretically could develop diarrhea if the ileocecal valve is taken from their gastrointestinal (GI) tract (21, 22). Other factors to consider include the need for ureteral reimplantation and the need for a continent catheterizable channel. Therefore, it is important to consider each patient individually when selecting the appropriate augmentation segment.

Cystoplasty	Mean	Mean	Mean	Mean Value	First Contraction	Max. Contraction		
	Age (yr)	F/U (mo)	Cap (mL)	At 300 mL cm H_2O	Mean Vol (mL)	Mean P cm H_2O	Mean Vol (mL)	Mean P cm H_2O
Tubular right colon	17.5	9.7	630	18.6	139	37	467	63
Detubularized right colon	28.5	5.1	641	9.4	329	24	596	42
Tubular ileum	66.8	7.0	311	36	110	60	218	81
Detubularized ileum	20.0	5.7	403	14.4	197	22	265	28

From Goldwasser B, et al. Cystometric properties of ileum and right colon after bladder augmentation, substitution or replacement. *J Urol* 1997; 138(2):1007.

Effect of detubularization of colon and ileum on cystoplasty compliance and contraction

3. Types and techniques of enterocystoplasty

3.1 Ileocystoplasty

3.1.1 Technical considerations

Goodwin and colleagues (1959) were among the first to demonstrate the numerous ways of anastomosing a patch of ileum to the native bladder. Virtually all surgeons recognize that ileum should be detubularized and reconfigured to achieve the most spherical shape possible (Q.15).

A segment of ileum at least 15 to 20 cm proximal to the ileocecal valve should be selected. The distal portion of terminal ileum is unique from a physiologic standpoint and should be avoided. The isolated segment should be 15 to 40 cm in length, depending on patient's size, native bladder capacity, type of reconfiguration and desired final capacity. With short ureters, an extra tail of isoperistaltic ileum can be useful to reach the foreshortened ureters. This requires creation of an ileonipple valve to prevent reflux, as in the Kock or hemi-Kock pouch. This type of construction may require up to 60 cm of small intestine.

The segment to be used should have an adequate mesentery to reach the native bladder without tension. After selecting the appropriate segment, the mesentery is cleared from the bowel at either end for a short distance to create a window. The bowel is divided at these ends, and a handsewn ileoileostomy or stapled anastomosis performed. The harvested ileal segment is irrigated clear with 0.25% neomycin solution and opened on its antimesenteric border. The ileum is most commonly folded in a U shape, although longer segments can be folded further into an S or W configuration. The ileum is then anastomosed to itself with running absorbable sutures. The suture line should approximate the full thickness of ileum to ileum while inverting the mucosa. If not opened previously, the bladder is incised in a sagittal plane. The anastomosis of the ileum to the native bivalved bladder is easily done when started posteriorly. The anastomosis may be done in a one-or two-layer fashion, always with absorbable suture. Permanent suture should never be used for any cystoplasty because it may serve as a nidus for stone formation. The mesenteric window at the bowel anastomosis is closed to prevent internal herniation.

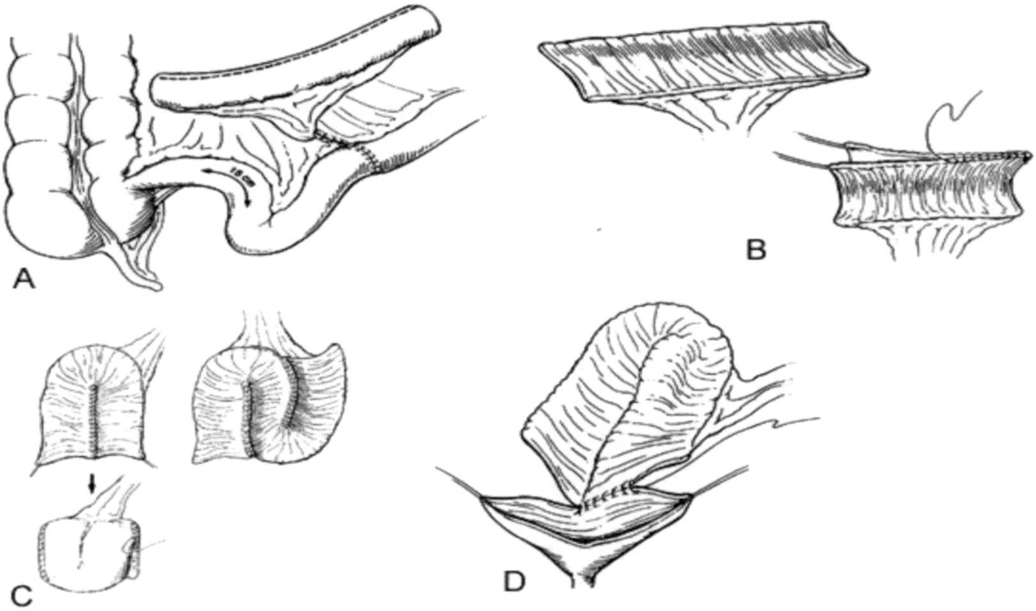

A: 15-40 cm segment of ileum proximal to the ileocecal valve is isolated and an ileoileostomy is performed. **B:** The isolated segment of ileum is opened along the antimesenteric border. The opened segment is then folded and the edges are sutured together. **C:** The opened segment is reconfigured to increase the surface volume. **D:** The reconfigured ileum is anastomosed to the opened bladder beginning at the posterior apex (1).

Ileum does not allow for standard reimplantation of the ureters or the creation of a continent catheterizable channel (i.e., Mitrofanoff), but newer techniques such as the seromuscular trough, as described by Abol-Enein and Ghoneim (22) do allow the use of ileum, should these procedures be required. However, because of its muscle backing, native bladder (or a gastric flap) is still the primary choice for ureteral reimplantation or the construction of a Mitrofanoff valve.

Although the jejunum can be used for urinary reconstruction, yet the high incidence of metabolic complications (hyponatremic, hypochloremic and hyperkalemic acidosis) associated with use of this segment make it less desirable and thus rarely used.

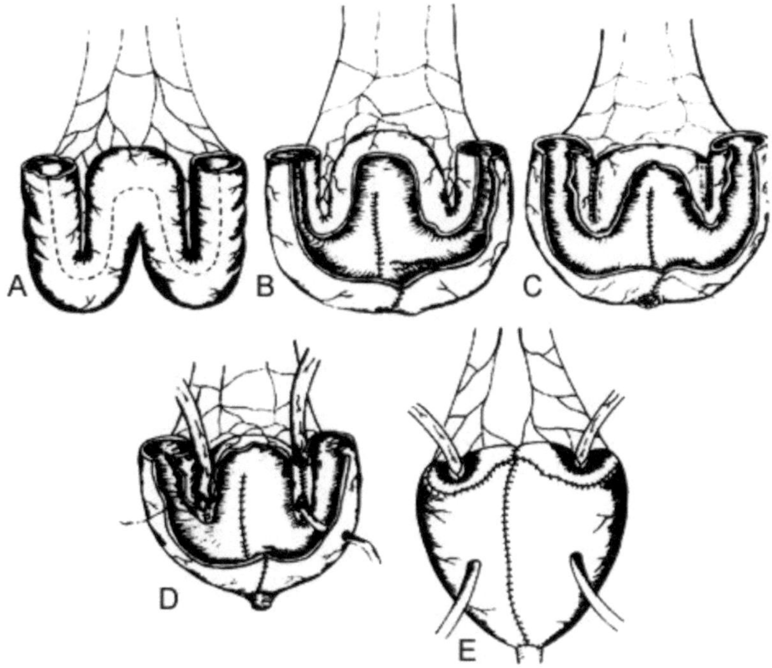

The seromuscular trough formed by anastomosing the edges of the ileum together allows for nonrefluxing ureteral reimplantation into the ileum (22).

3.1.2 Advantages

Ileum is the most commonly used bowel segment for bladder augmentation, as it is:'1) available in large quantity, 2) ease in handling and reconfiguration, 3) has a predictable and abundant blood supply, 4) most compliant segment of bowel, 5) produces moderate mucus compared to colon, 6) causes less severe metabolic complications than colon or stomach, 7) has fewer GI complications than cecum,

3.1.3 Disadvantages

The disadvantages in using ileum include: 1) occasional short mesentery that cannot reach the pelvis, 2) possible development of diarrhea and vitamin B_{12} deficiency, 3) difficulty with creation of submucosal tunnels, 4) hyperchloremic, hypokalemic melabolic acidosis, 5) bowel obstruction, 6) stone formation, 7) mucus production, 8) urinary tract infections, 9) tumor formation which is a risk with large bowel segments as well (14).

3.2 Sigmoid cystoplasty

3.2.1 Technical considerations

Use of the sigmoid colon for augmentation cystoplasty was first reported by Lemoine in 1912 (Q.15) and until nowadays continues to be used commonly.

Because of the strong unit contractions of the sigmoid, it is imperative to detubularize and reconfigure the segment used to provide maximal compliance and disruption of contractions. Fifteen to 20 cm of sigmoid colon is identified and mobilized. Its mesentery is transilluminated to identify the vascular arcade, after which the surgeon must ensure that the segment can reach the bladder without tension. If so, the bowel segment is divided between clamps and a colocolostomy perfomed. Detubularization and reconfiguration is done in a fashion determined by the surgeon's preference. The sigmoid patch is anastomosed to the bivalved bladder.

Sigmoid colon segments are usually reconfigured in one of two ways. Mitchell (1986) suggested closing the two ends and then opening the segment longitudinally opposite its blood supply (23). The segment easily fits on the bivalved bladder. The bowel segment may fit better in either the sagittal or the coronal plane. More radical reconfiguration, and perhaps breakup of unit contractions, may be achieved by folding the sigmoid segment in a U-Shape.

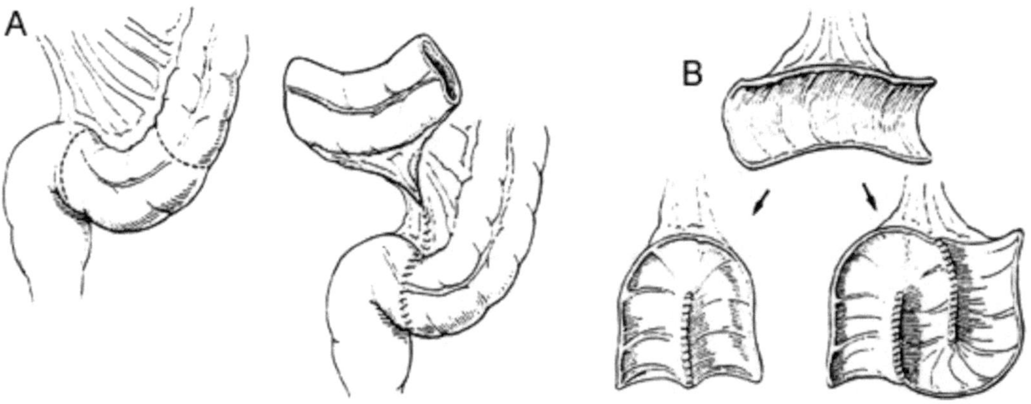

A: A segment of the sigmoid is resected and bowel continuity is reestablished. **B:** The isolated segment of sigmoid is opened on its antimesenteric border and then reconfigured before being anastomosed to the bladder (4).

3.2.2 Advantages

The major advantage of the use of sigmoid colon is the redundancy that is present especially in the spina bifida population. The mobile portion of the sigmoid is so redundant in these children that it often lays in the right lower quadrant. It can be easily opened and reconfigured into a U-shape to increase compliance. The thicker muscle can be used for an antirefluxing ureteral anastomosis as well as for placement of a tunneled continent catheterizable.

3.2.3 Disadvantages

The major disadvantage of the use of the sigmoid colon is the lessened ability to create a large capacity, compliant reservoir. The diameter of the sigmoid may be only similar to the ileum. In certain circumstance, at least a 20 to 30 cm segment of colon is required to create a large enough reservoir. This amount of sigmoid colon can occasionally be difficult to obtain in the non-spina bifida population. In the Indiana series, the highest spontaneous perforation rate occurred among those with sigmoid cystoplasties (19). However, this has not been observed in other large series. Finally hyperchloremic acidosis is more common when the sigmoid colon is employed, compared to other bowel segments. Frequently, these patients will need lifelong alkalinizing agents but this can also be true after ceco or ileocystoplasty as well (24).

3.3 Cecocystoplasty and ileocecocystoplasty

3.3.1 Technical considerations

Couvelair described the use of the cecum for augmentation cystoplasty in 1950 (Q.15). Numerous reports of simple cecocystoplasty have appeared since then. Presently, cecocystoplasty is an uncommon operative procedure; it has largely been replaced by various forms of ileocecocystoplasty.

With the ileocecocystoplasty technique, the cecum is opened, reconfigured, and used to augment the bladder alone, leaving a segment of ileum to reach the ureters or to create a continent abdominal wall stoma based on imbrication of the ileocecal valve and proximal ileum. Conversely, the ileal segment can be opened and used as a patch on the cecal segment before augmentation cystoplasty. Many modifications of the technique exist, but all start with mobilization of the cecum and right colon by incising the peritoneum along the white line of Toldt up to the hepatic flexure. Approximately 15 to 30 cm of the terminal ileum is used. The length of the ileal segment depends on the technique employed. As with all intestinal cystoplasties, before division of the bowel segment, it should be certain that it will reach the bladder without tension.

The isolated ileocecal segment is irrigated clear with neomycin solution and opened on its antimesenteric border through the ileocecal valve for its entire length. In the typical ileocecal augmentation, the ileal and cecal segments are of equivalent length such that the borders of the open segment can be anastomosed and then folded on themselves to form a cup cystoplasty. The anastomosis of the reconfigured segments is done in a one-or two-layer closure with absorbable suture. The opening should be left large enough to provide a wide anastomosis to the bivalved bladder. If more volume is necessary, the ileal segment can be significantly lenghtened, allowing it to be folded before anastomosis to the cecum. The Mainz ileocystoplasty uses an ileal segment twice the length of the cecal segment. The opened edge of the cecal portion is anastomosed to the first portion of the ileal segment. The first and second portions of the ileal segment are next approximated. The compound ileocecal patch is then anastomosed to the bladder.

The ileocecal segment has been used extensively for reconstruction and bladder replacement in the adult population. It has been used less frequently in children because most of the patients undergoing augmentation cystoplasty are doing so because of neurovesical dysfunction. Those patients usually have neuropraxic bowel dysfunction as well. Removal of the ileocecal valve in such children can result in intractable diarrhea (24, 25). Use of the ileocecal valve in such patients should be avoided unless other advantages of the segment outweigh the risk of diarrhea and fecal incontinence.

3.3.2 Advantages

One potential advantage of ileocecocystoplasy is the presence of the appendix. Particularly in children, the appendix is useful in the creation of a reliable continent abdominal wall

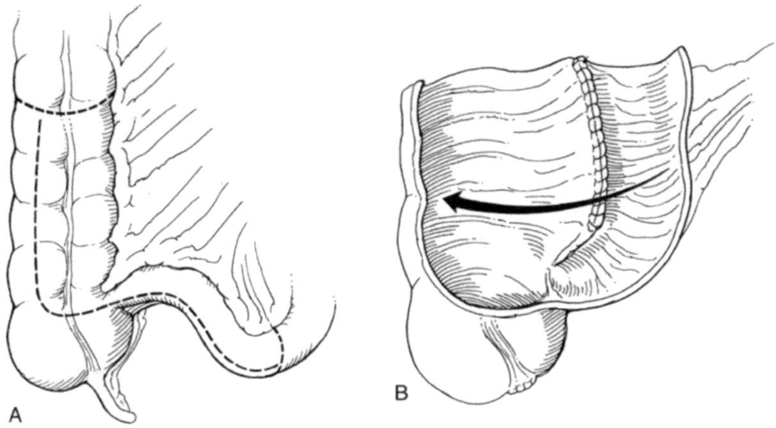

Ileocecocystoplasty. *A)*. An ileocecal segment is selected. The length of segment chosen depends on the technique employed. After removal, it is opened on the antimesenteric border *(dashed lines)*. *B*). The opened ileal and cecal segments are anastomosed to form a cup in the standard ileocecocystoplasty [15].

stoma. The appendix may be removed with a small cuff of cecal wall and tunneled into the native bladder or a tenia of the cecal segment to provide a continent mechanism. Likewise, it may be left in situ and the base safely tunneled by creating a window in the mesoappendix. If the appendix is not to be used, an appendectomy is performed with the standard ileocecocystoplasy.

There are further advantages to the use of the ileocecal segment. Antireflux tunnels can easily be made into the tenia of the cecum when necessary. Again, for the short ureter, a tail of ileum can be left intact to bridge the gap, with the imbricated ileocecal valve used for antireflux. The same imbrication technique can be used to create a continent abdominal wall stoma as with the appendix. Cain and Husmann (1994) and Cain et al (1999) have proposed using the ileocecal segment for augmentation with the plicated ileal segment brought to the abdominal wall as a catheterizable stoma, as in the Indiana pouch [26,27]. Another major advantage of these segments is the use of a portion of bowel that has a large diameter resulting in a capacious and compliant reservoir that often fits the bladder base rather nicely. It also has a well-defined reliable blood supply.

3.3.3 Disadvantages

The major disadvantage to the use of the ileocecal segment is related to the loss of the ilieocecal valve. Patients with neurologic disorders or short gut often have an increased incidence of diarrhea and difficulty with fecal continence. In addition, this segment is not available in the cloacal exstrophy population who has little to no hindgut. The ileocecal segment also reabsorbs urinary wastes which may result in hyperchloremic acidosis. Finally, cecum usually produces more mucus than the ileum which can lead to increased infections and stone formation.

3.3.4 Summary

Through the early 1980s, the cecum and sigmoid colon were more commonly used than ileum for enterocystoplasy. However, because of the shorter mesenteries, increased mucus production, and difficulty with configuration that is associated with large bowel, ileum has come to be the preferred segment of bowel for enterocystopasty for most surgeons. However, detubulairzed large bowel is still used for simple bladder augmentation in select patients (14).

3.4 Gastrocystoplasty

3.4.1 Technical considerations

Two basic techniques exist for the use of stomach in bladder augmentation. Leong and Ong (1972) described the use of the entire gastric antrum with a small rim of body for bladder replacement. With their technique, the left gastroepiploic artery is always used as a vascular pedicle. If the right gastroepiploic artery is dominant and the left vessel ends high on the greater curvature, a strip of body along the greater curvature from the left gastroepiploic artery to the antrum is maintained and provides adequate blood supply. Continuity of the upper gastrointestinal tract is restored by a Billroth I gastroduodenostomy (28).

In the second type of gastrocystoplasly, a gastric wedge based on the midportion of the greater curvature is used (29). The gastric segment used in this technique is made up mainly of body and consequently has a higher concentration of acid-producing cells. The right or left gastroepiploic artery may be used as a vascular pedicle to this segment. The right artery is commonly dominant and therefore is more frequently used. The wedge-shaped segment of stomach includes both anterior and posterior wall. The segment used may be 10 to 20 cm along the greater curvature, depending on patient age and size as well as the needed volume.

The incision into the stomach is stopped just short of the lesser curvature to avoid injury to branches of the vagus nerve that control the gastric outlet. Branches of the left gastric artery just cephalad to the apex of this incision are suture ligated in situ before incision to avoid significant bleeding. Parallel atraumatic bowel clamps are placed on either side of the gastric incisions to avoid excessive bleeding or spillage of gastric contents. Alternatively, the stomach may be incised using a gastrointestinal stapling device that places a double row of staples, on each side of the incision (30). The staple lines, however, must be excised. The native stomach is closed in two layers using permanent sutures on the outer seromuscular layer.

The short gastric branches of the gastroepiploic artery to the antrum on the right or to the high corpus on the left are divided to provide mobilization of the gastroepiploic pedicle leaving the short gastric branches to the augmentation segment intact. In order that the eventual pedicle would be long enough to reach the bladder, the appropriate segment may be higher on the greater curvature if the right vessel is used as a pedicle, or lower if based on the left.

The vascular pedicle, with omentum, should not be free-floating through the abdomen. The segment and pedicle may be passed through windows in the transverse mesocolon and mesentery of the distal ileum and carefully secured to the posterior peritoneum. Despite careful consideration for an adequate pedicle length, on occasion the gastric segment initially does not reach the bladder without tension. Either gastroepiploic artery may be mobilized closer to its origin for further length. The first few branches from the gastroepiploic artery to the isolated gastric segment may also be divided. Because of the rich submucosal arterial plexus in the stomach, devascularization of the isolated segment does not result. Rarely, it may be necessary to approximate some of the isolated gastric segment to itself in one corner. The gastric segment should be approximated to the native bladder with one or two layers of absorbable sutures, taking care to invert the mucosa. Usually the gastric wedge fits well with the bivalved bladder.

Raz and colleagues (1993) have described the use of a much longer, narrower segment of stomach based along the greater curvature. Use of this segment, which includes both body and antrum, somewhat narrows the lumen of the stomach in its entire length except at the fundus and pylorus [(31)] Raz and colleagues (1993) isolated this segment with the use of a gastrointestinal stapler so that the native stomach was never open. Histamine 2 receptor blockers are often given in the early postoperative period to promote healing [(31)].

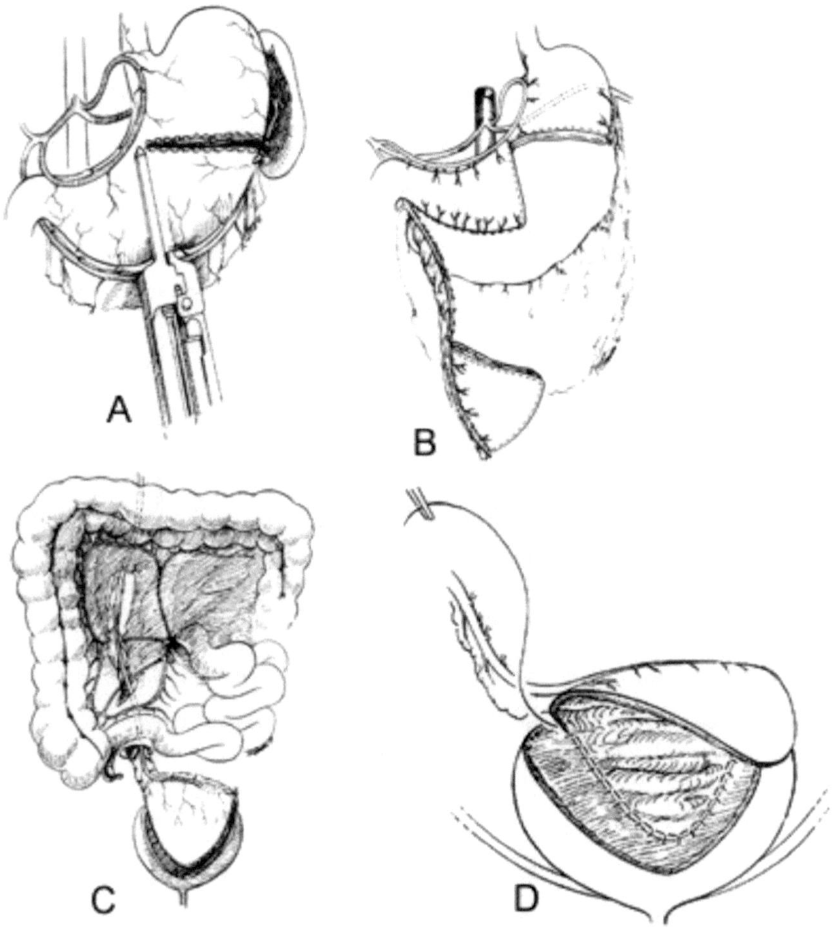

A). A wedge from the body of the stomach is harvested with a stapling device. B). The gastric wedge usually is based on the blood supply from the right gastroepiploic vessel. C). The gastric wedge is brought through the transverse colon and small bowel mesentery to reach the bladder. D). The gastric wedge is sutured to the bladder in two layers [(1)].

3.4.2 Patient selection for gastrocystoplasty

The stomach is unique with special physiologic and metabolic properties. Given the specific advantages and disadvantages that gastric segments exhibit in comparison to intestinal segments, gastrocystoplasty appears to be most appropriate for patients with renal insufficiency and for those with short intestines, as well as in patients with cloacal exstrophy. Also since the development of the hematuria dysuria syndrome is fairly common following gastrocystoplasty, this type of augmentation is most appropriate in patients who have minimal or no perineal and urethral sensation. If gastrocystoplasty is performed in patients that are sensate, it is important to ensure that patients are completely continent. Caution should be exercised when considering gastrocystoplasty in a patient with end stage renal disease in need of transplantation since ulcer formation and perforation of defunctionalized bladders have been reported [(32)]. In general, patients that fulfill the preoperative criteria for conventional enterocystoplasty can also be considered candidates for gastrocystoplasty.

3.4.3 Advantages

Surgically, the stomach is relatively thick and easy to work with. It is readily accessible and has a rich reliable vascular supply. The suppleness of the stomach and the well-defined submucosal plane makes it ideal for reimplantation of ureters and continent catheterizable stomas. Use of stomach for bladder augmentation has clear advantages in patients with renal insufficiency due to its ability to secrete acid. This allows for buffering of systemic acidosis and lessens the need for bicarbonate supplementation. The resultant acid urine also appears to decrease the incidence of bacteriuria.

In comparison to other intestinal segments, there is also decreased mucus production and stone formation. The inherent musculature of the gastric segment may also offer an additional advantage over small and large bowel in more often allowing for spontaneous voiding that can result in more efficient emptying, less residual urine, and decreased need for intermittent catheterization. [(33, 34)]. Lastly both gastrocystoplasty and ileocystoplasty can be accomplished laparoscopically which offers significant advantages in more rapid patient recovery following surgery [(35)].

3.4.4 Disadvantages

The main disadvantage of gastrocystoplasty that currently limits its widespread use in children with a neuropathic bladder is the high incidence of hematuria dysuria syndrome. This is most troublesome in patients that have a sensate urethra and perineum. Caution should be exercised in selecting patients who are sensate and are at risk for incontinence (i.e. bladder exstrophy) when other enteric segments are available.

3.4.5 Results

The urodynamic results of gastrocystoplasty are somewhat variable. Most authors report that it is useful in increasing capacity and compliance similar to large and small bowel [(36)]. In studies that have analyzed both pre- and postoperative urodynamics, gastrocystoplasty has been shown to increase bladder capacity by approximately 150 to 200 percent [(37, 38)]. However it should be noted that there is a wide range of results reported with regard to increased bladder capacity following gastrocystoplasty. In a recent series comparing the urodynamic findings and clinical outcomes following augmentation with stomach versus intestine, it was shown that both stomach and intestine are efficacious in improving compliance but that the use of ileum and colon results in a higher volume reservoir. Intestinal segments appear to expand more readily following augmentation than the stomach [39]. Some of the differences in the literature regarding improvements in capacity and compliance following gastrocystoplasty may be in part explained by variable amounts of stomach that are harvested in individual patients. However, less volume expansion seems inherent to gastric segments compared to ileum and colon.

3.4.6 Summary

Gastrocystoplasty is a useful procedure in the management of children with a neuropathic bladder. However, it has unique properties and potential complications from those seen with conventional enterocystoplasty. From the available experience, it appears that gastrocystoplasty is best suited for patients with renal insufficiency and metabolic acidosis, patients with a small amount of bowel available for augmentation, and patients with an insensate urethra and perineum. Despite some of the metabolic and physiologic advantages of gastrocystoplasty, potential disadvantages still make ileum the preferred intestinal segment for the majority of patients undergoing enterocystoplasty at this time [14].

3.5 Overall results of gastro-intestinal augmentation cystoplasty

The effect of cystoplasty on the patient should be considered in two main categories. First, the effect of removal of a relatively small portion of the gastrointestinal tract for use in urinary reconstruction must be considered. Any more than rare development of gastrointestinal problems would be prohibitive, even if the results were perfect from the standpoint of the urinary bladder. Second the effect of augmentation cystoplasty on the urinary bladder must be reviewed. The primary goal of augmentation is to provide a compliant urinary reservoir. Therefore the main consideration after augmentation is the storage pressure and capacity that are achieved. Any other effect in the urinary bladder is a side effect or complication that exists because bowel is not a perfect physiologic substitute for native bladder.

3.5.1 Bladder compliance after augmentation

An early lesson of past clinical experience with augmentation cystoplasty is the value of detubularization and reconfiguration of the bowel segment [16, 17]. Bowel in its native, tubular form continues to display peristalsis or mass contraction. The tubular form does not maximize the volume achieved for the surface area of bowel used. Hinman (1988) demonstrated with a mathematical model that the maximum volume achieved for a given surface area occurs when a sphere is created. No finished cystoplasty is a perfect sphere but, it should approach that shape as nearly as possible [16].

Many patients who historically underwent augmentation cystoplasty with a tubular segment of bowel have done well, but there have also been numerous failures caused by continued pressure in the bladder from the segment left in its native form. Some surgeons with extensive experience in augmentation cystoplasty and continent diversion have concluded that ileum is superior to other segments in terms of compliance after augmentation [40, 41, 42].Rare reports have suggested superior results with colon compared to ileum. These reports have involved longer colonic segments that were reconfigured in a U shape. Good results have been achieved with all segments in most cases, and it is more important to use a bowel segment well than to choose a particular bowel segment for every patient.

Lytton and Green (1989) demonstrated mass contractions generating pressures of 60 to 110 cm H_2O in right colon reservoirs despite detubularization [44]. Such pressures approach those observed in native cecum [45]. Hedlund and coworkers (1984) reported pressures of only 25 cm H_2O in detubularized cecal segments 1 year after reconstruction [46]. Placement of an ileal patch on a cecal segment can be a more effective mean of decreasing mass contractions than simple reconfiguration [47].

Sidi and associates (1986) demonstrated early peak bladder pressures of 41 cm H2O after cup-patch sigmoid cystoplasty that improved with time [48]. Goldwasser's review of enterocystoplasty using detubularized ileum and colon demonstrated contractions greater than 15 cm H_2O in 42% of patients after ileocystoplasty, compared with, 60% after colocystoplasty[18]. Significant contractions, defined as those greater than 40 cm H_2O at a volume of less than 200 ml, were not noted in any of the ileal augmentations but did persist in 10% of cecal cystoplasties. In continent urinary diversion, ileal reservoirs have been noted to have lower basal pressures and less motor activity [24]. Cecal reservoirs have been noted to generate more pressure per given volume than ileum despite detubularization and to exhibit more obvious uninhibited contractions [49].

Any problems with pressure after augmentation cystoplasty usually occur because of uninhibited contractions, apparently in the bowel segment. It is extremely rare not to achieve an adequate capacity or flat tonus limb unless a technical error has occurred with use of the bowel segment. Occasionally, a small, scarred pelvis prevents adequate expansion of the augmented bladder. When pressure contractions occur in the bladder after augmentation, they are often noted on a rhythmic or sinusoidal pattern, occasionally with increasing amplitude [15].

For most patients, the pressure contractions noted urodynamically are of theoretical interest only and have not affected the clinical result. Contractions that begin at low amplitude later in filling and progress only near capacity may be of no clinical significance at all. Early contractions of higher pressure may occasionally result in persistent incontinence, delayed perforation, hydronephrosis, or vesicoureteral reflux. If patients have such clinical problems after augmentation, repeat urodynamic testing is necessary.

One cannot assume that the bladder is compliant after augmentation. Rhythmic contractions have been noted postoperatively with all bowel segments, although ileum seems the least likely to demonstrate remarkable urodynamic abnormalities, and stomach the most. Rhythmic contractions after cystoplasty have been noted in up to 62% of patients [39, 50]. The segment of stomach initially described for augmentation using the body was much smaller in size than segments of ileum or colon commonly used for cystoplasty. The use of a slightly larger gastric segment that is longer along the greater curvature results in improved urodynamics after augmentation, with less prominent contractions [38, 50]. The antral segment of stomach is less likely to demonstrate such contractions [33].

In perhaps the largest experience with pediatric bladder augmentation, Rink and associates (1995) at Indiana University found that approximately 5% of several hundred patients had significant uninhibited contractions after augmentation cystoplasty causing clinical problems. Rink (1995) found that 6% of more than 300 patients required secondary augmentation of a previously augmented bladder for similar problems in long-term follow-up [51]. These secondary augmentations represent true failures of the primary cystoplasty, not from any side effect or complication but from failure to achieve the objective capacity and compliance. In that series, sigmoid colon, followed by stomach and then ileum, was most likely to require reaugmentation. It should be noted that a colonic segment closed at the ends and not generally reconfigured otherwise was typically used in that experience. Other studies have suggested that stomach is more likely than colon to require secondary intervention [39].

Bowel Segment	Advantages	Disadvantages
Stomach	1. Previous radiation, short gut 2. Prevents systemic acidosis, salt retention 3. Facilitates tunnels for continence and antireflux 4. Reduces infection 5. May potentiate growth in children	1. Acid secretion salt loss, metabolic alkylosis 2. Hematuria-dysuria syndrome 3. More difficult to use
Jejunum	1. Few, not recommended	1. Salt and water loss, metabolic acidosis
Small Bowel	1. Availability 2. Good compliance 3. Less mucus	1. Metabolic acidosis salt resorption 2. Loss of resorption surface in GI tract (B12, folate) 3. Sometimes difficult to work with (no tunnels)
Cecum	1. Availability 2. Good compliance 3. Potential for tunnels and use of IC valve	1. Metabolic acidosis, salt and water resorption 2. Loss of IC valve may cause diarrhea
Sigmoid	1. Most available 2. Good compliance 3. Potential for tunnels	1. Not available in some patients (radiation, constipation) 2. Metabolic acidosis, salt and water resorption 3. Possible increased potential for rupture

GI, gastrointestinal.

Advantages and disadvantages of specific bowel segments [1]

4. Complications of gastrointestinal cystoplasty

4.1 Complications of bowel segment Isolation

4.1.1 Postoperative bowel obstruction

Postoperative bowel obstruction is uncommon after augmentation cystoplasty, occurring in approximately 3% of patients. The rate of obstruction is equivalent to that noted after conduit diversion or continent urinary diversion [51, 52]. Delicate handling of tissues, closure of mesenteric windows, and elimination of sites of internal herniation help to avoid obstruction. The incidence of bowel obstruction is low regardless of the gastrointestinal segment used and should not influence the choice of a particular segment for enterocystoplasty (15).

4.1.2 Malabsorption abnormalities and diarrhea

Loss of the distal ileum may result in fat malabsorption and decrease bile salt and fat soluble vitamin absorption. The distal ileum and ileocecal valve are important for reabsorption and regulation of bowel function. When fecal losses of bile acids exceed production from the liver, fat malabsorption occurs. Steatorrhea then occurs with possible impaired absorption of lipids and fat soluble vitamins (A, D, E & K).

The diarrhea associated with bile acid irritation of the colon can be severe. The secretary diarrhea is secondary to unabsorbed bile salts, causing active secretion of chloride and water in the colon. Reports of chronic diarrhea after bladder augmentation alone have been rare. Diarrhea can occur after removal of large segments of ileum from the gastrointestinal tract even with the preservation of the ileocecal valve (more than 100 cm). Although the length of the segments typically used for augmentation rarely are problematic unless other problems coexist (53, 54). The use of a typical colonic segment for augmentation only rarely results in a change in bowel function and is less of a risk than the use of ileum.

Removal of a segment from the gastrointestinal tract that includes the ileocecal valve is the most likely procedure to cause diarrhea. Patients with neurogenic dysfunction have significant diarrhea after such displacement. Roth et al (1995) reported that 23% of patients in their experience had chronic diarrhea after ileocecal urinary diversion and 11% when ileum alone was used (53). Some children with neurogenic impairment depend on controlled constipation for fecal continence. Removal of the ileocecal valve from the gastrointestinal tract may significantly decrease bowel transit time. Loss of the valve can also allow bacterial backflow into the ileum, and the organisms may interfere with metabolism of fat and vitamin B12.

Oral cholestyramine and a low fat diet can be used to treat the diarrhea. Diarrhea as a result of ileocecal valve resection with decreased transit time can be managed with codeine or lomotil. Some authors reported higher incidence of hypertriglyceridemia and gall stones (54).

4.1.3 Vitamin B12 deficiency

When portions of the alimentary tract are used for urinary reconstruction, nutritional deficiencies can occur. Resection of the terminal ileum can result in vitamin B12 deficiency. Vitamin B 12 (cyanocobalamin) cannot be synthesized by human tissues, so humans must receive their vitamin B12 supply from dietary sources. In the stomach, vitamin B 12 is released from food by hydrochloric acid and digestive enzymes. Intrinsic factor binds to vitamin B12 in the duodenum, and then attaches to receptors in the distal ileum. Vitamin B12 is then stored in the liver and supplies last up to three years.

Deficiency of vitamin B12 causes a megaloblastic anemia and neurologic changes including peripheral neuropathies, optic atrophy, degenerative changes of the spinal cord, and dementia in the late stages (54). Several reports in the literature describe patients in whom the terminal ileum is resected for urinary diversion with a 3.3 to 20 percent incidence of vitamin B12 deficiency (55). Fifty centimeters of ileum appear to be the critical length, with larger resections of small bowel placing the patient at risk for vitamin deficiency (56). Neurological symptoms may occur before serum levels are depressed and without megaloblastic anemia. Pannek and associates recommend starting therapy with 100 mcg of hydroxycobalamin injected intramuscularly monthly one year after surgery for patients losing more than 50cm of terminal ileum [56].

4.2 Metabolic complications of gastrointestinal augmentation cystoplasty

To understand the potential complications of gastrointestinal cystoplasty, one must take into account many factors. These factors include the length and the type of intestinal segment, the general health of the patient, the time urine is in contact with bowel mucosa, and the basic underlying renal and hepatic function.

Serum electrolyte abnormalities are dependent upon the segment of bowel used. Other factors include the constituents of urine in the augmented bladder which depend on many factors including fluid intake, diet and intercurrent illness, gastroenteritis, and dehydration [57].

4.2.1 Hyperchloremic metabolic acidosis

Ileum and colon have similar solute transport properties. Normal urine has higher potassium and hydrogen ion concentration and a lower sodium concentration than normal intestinal contents.

Hydrogen ions in the urine must be excreted with a buffer. As a patient becomes acidotic, the kidneys initially excrete acid buffered with phosphates or sulfates, or titratable acids. As the acidosis becomes chronic however, the kidney generates ammonia (NH3) from the conversion of glutamine to alpha-ketoglutarate. Ammonia buffers the free hydrogen ion and becomes ammonium, NH_4^+. Ileal and colonic mucosa will therefore secrete sodium and bi-carbonate and absorb hydrogen, chloride, and ammonium upon exposure to urine, resulting in the development of a hyperchloremic metabolic acidosis [57]. Patients with good underlying renal function can overcome this acid reabsorption by excreting even more urinary acid.

The majority of the acid load following augmentation cystoplasty is the result of the net ammonium absorption. Ammonia, ionized ammonium and chloride are absorbed when ileum or colon is exposed to urine, and the majority of the acid load is from the absorbed ammonium chloride. Ammonium and hydrogen are then transported with chloride to maintain electric neutrality [58].

In 1987, Mitchell and Piser noted that essentially every patient after augmentation with an intestinal segment had an increase in serum chloride and a decrease in serum bicarbonate level, although full acidosis was rare if renal function was normal [4]. Mild metabolic acidosis is found in 15 percent of patients with ileal conduit diversions. As many as ten percent of patients with ileal conduits require therapy for persistent acidosis. Similarly, 10 to 15 percent of patients with colon conduits develop acidosis. Due to increased urine contact time, metabolic acidosis after bladder replacement with ileum is found in 50 percent of cases. Over 50 percent of colonic reservoirs also have some degree of hyperchloremic metabolic acidosis. Initial reports of ureterosigmoidostomy patients indicate that they have as much as an 80 percent incidence of metabolic acidosis. The risk of acidosis also appears to correlate directly with length of bowel used [54, 59].

The absorptive properties of the intestinal segment may diminish over time. Histological changes occur, including mucosal atrophy and decreased villous height. These histologic findings are believed to cause a reduced absorptive capacity of bowel, however, other studies demonstrate no change in absorptive capacity of the intestinal segment despite histological changes [60]. Most likely, the majority of individuals with metabolic derangement do not develop significant changes in electrolyte transport to protect them from untoward complications.

Patients may present with signs and symptoms of fatigue, diarrhea, weight loss, anorexia, and polydipsia. Laboratory studies demonstrate a significant non-anion gap acidosis with hyperchloremia and azotemia. Arterial blood gases values are more sensitive than serum bicarbonate or chloride levels for detection and early management of acidosis [61].

Acute management includes prompt drainage with treatment of any underlying urinary tract infection and correction of any electrolyte abnormalities. Treatment of mild and chronic forms of metabolic acidosis involves the use of alkalizing agents. Sodium bicarbonate and sodium citrate are useful in restoring acid-base balance. They, however, have untoward side effects, with sodium bicarbonate producing considerable gas and sodium citrate being very distasteful. To neutralize the acid load, supplementation of 1 -2 mEq kg/day of alkali is usually sufficient. In patients with refractory hyperchloremic metabolic acidosis, and those who cannot tolerate or have a contraindication to the alkalizing agents, chlorpromazine has been used successfully in an adult patient with refractory metabolic acidosis. Chlorpromazine and nicotinic acid inhibit cyclic adenosine monophosphate and thereby inhibit chloride transport and absorption in canine models [62]. The usefulness of these agents in humans has not been clinically validated.

4.2.2 Hypokalemia

Hypokalemia can occur in patients with augmentation cysloplasty. The depletion of potassium stores is likely due to the renal wasting of potassium and the chronic metabolic acidosis which causes intracellular potassium depletion. Compared to colon, ileal segments have been shown to have a greater ability to reabsorb potassium when exposed to high concentrations of the ion in urine. Chronic diarrhea may be also a contributing factor for hypokalemia.

The treatment is exogenous potassium replacement. Once the acidosis is corrected, there will be an influx of potassium into the cell because of the extracellular potassium shift. This can lead to profound hypokalemia if not recognized and treated promptly.

4.2.3 Hypocalcemia / Hypomagnesemia

Hypocalcemia and hypomagnesemia are uncommon complication of augmentation cysloplasty. Chronic metabolic acidosis causes loss of calcium from several mechanisms. Symptoms include tetany, tremors and irritability. Treatment consists of calcium replacement either enterally or parenterally depending on the severity. Hypomagnesemia, however uncommon, is due to malabsorption, renal loss, and decreased renal tubular absorption with acidosis. Symptoms are similar to hypocalcemia and the treatment again is exogenous replacement [57].

4.2.4 Ammioniagenic encephalopathy

Urinary ammonium excreted by the kidneys is reabsorbed by the intestinal segment, and then returned to the liver via the portal circulation. The liver metabolizes ammonium to urea via the ornithine cycle. The liver usually adapts to the excess ammonia in the portal circulation without difficulty and rapidly metabolizes it. In the setting of hepatic dysfunction, the hepatic reserve for ammonium metabolism may be exceeded, resulting in the rare complication of ammoniogenic coma. The syndrome also has been described in patients with normal hepatic function (63).

Systemic bacteremia, with endotoxin production, inhibits hepatic function and may precipitate this clinical entity. Urinary tract infections with urea-splitting organisms may also overload the ability of the liver to clear the ammonia. If this syndrome occurs in a patient suspected of having normal hepatic function, systemic bacteremia or obstruction of urinary drainage should be suspected.

Good urinary drainage and treatment of the offending urinary pathogens usually prevents development of the syndrome. Treatment consists of prompt drainage with a Foley catheter. Systemic antibiotics treat the possible underlying infection, and neomycin or lactulose is given to reduce absorption of ammonia in the gastrointestinal tract (54).

4.2.5 Bone disease and retarded growth

A potential long-term complication of intestinal diversion is bone demineralization. This clinical entity was initially found in children developing rickets after ureterosigmoidostomy, but has also been noted in adults with osteomalacia following ureterosigmoi-dostomy, ileal replacement of ureters, and coloplasty (64). In rickets and osteomalacia, bone mineral loss is replaced with osteoid resulting in decreased bone strength. Fortunately, severe defects in bony demineralization are not common.

The cause of bone demineralization appears complex and multi-factorial, with changes in acid-base balance being the major contributing factor. In chronic acidosis, bone serves to buffer the excess acids. Bone minerals released into the circulation, including carbonate and phosphate, buffer the hydrogen ions, decreasing the axial skeleton calcium content. Systemic acidosis also appears to inhibit the conversionof of 25 hydroxycholecalciferol to 1,25 dihydroxycholecalciferol and appears to activate osteoclasts producing further bone resorption. Additionally, patients with urinary diversions have increased excretion of calcium and sulfate. Sulfate has been shown to cause increased excretion of calcium by the kidneys. The effect of sulfate is potentiated by acidosis. Chronic metabolic acidosis therefore results in negative calcium and phosphate balances (65).

Changes in acid-base status may be subtle with patients displaying only a minimal decrease or normal serum calcium and magnesium level and mild depression of serum bicarbonate level. Most patients who present are asymptomatic; however, they may have occult bone mineral defects that place the patient at higher risk for increased orthopedic morbidity.

The diagnosis can be particularly difficult to detect. Parathormone and vitamin D levels are typically normal, and radiologic examination is usually unremarkable. Post-menopausal women and children are at high risk for bone demineralization with several studies showing a reduction in growth potential for children following enterocystoplasty.

Patients presenting with rickets or osteomalacia should have correction of their acid-base disturbance first. Vitamin D and calcium supplements are then used if remineralization does not occur. Administration of vitamin C or oral alkalizing agents to children with urinary diversion may help reinforce normal bone development and prevent bone destruction (66).

4.2.6 Drug absorption toxicities

Absorption of drugs excreted in urine from bowel segments can cause toxicities. One must be aware of the potential toxicities that can result from absorption of active drug such as methotrexate or metabolites in patients with augmentation cystoplasty (54).

4.2.7 Hypochloremic alkalosis

Significant metabolic derangement can occur with gastric diversions. In contrast to ileum or colonic cystoplasty the stomach excretes chloride. This can lead to profound hypochloremic, hypokalemic alkalosis. It has been proposed that the alkalosis results from ongoing chloride loss from the gastric segment in the bladder in the face of decreased oral intake. The decreased ability to excrete bicarbonate from an impaired kidney may compound the problem. Gosalbez and associates (1993) demonstrated persistently increased traditional excretion of chloride despite profound hypochloremia, suggesting that inappropriate gastric secretion is probably the primary problem [39].

Patients may present with lethargy, mental status changes, intractable seizures, and respiratory compromise related to a compensatory respiratory acidosis [39]. Patients are prone to suffer from severe dehydration secondary to a loss of fluid, chloride, and potassium from the gastric segment. A simple viral gastroenteritis illness may trigger severe symptoms of dehydration and alkalosis.

Replacement with normal saline and correction of serum potassium abnormalities usually corrects the metabolic abnormalities. Patients should maintain good oral and normal salt intake. Additional oral salt and potassium supplementation may be needed. Histamine-2 blockers and anticholinergic therapy may also be needed in patients with low-grade alkalosis. Refractory episodes of hypokalemic, hypochloremic metabolic alkalosis may be treated with inhibiting K^+/H^+ exchange with such agents as omeprazole.

4.2.8 Hematuria-dysuria syndrome

Acid secretion by gastric mucosa may result in another unique problem after gastrocystoplasty, the hematuria-dysuria syndrome. Virtually all patients with normal sensation after gastrocystoplasty have occasional hematuria or dysuria with voiding or catheterization beyond that which is expected with other intestinal segments. All patients should be warned of this potential problem, although in most the symptoms are intermittent and mild and do not require treatment. Avoidance of gastrocystoplasty in patients with bladder exstrophy is recommended. The dysuria is certainly not a problem in patients with neurogenic dysfunction.

In the experience of Nguyen and coworkers (1993), 36% of patients developed signs or symptoms of the hematuria-dysuria syndrome after gastrocystoplasty; 14% required treatment with medications, 9% on a regular basis. They believed that patients who are incontinent or have decreased renal function are at increased risk [67]. The symptoms of the hematuria-dysuria syndrome respond well to administration of H_2 blockers and hydrogen ion pump blockers. Bladder irrigation with baking soda may also be effective. It has been demonstrated that urinary pH may decrease remarkably after meals in those who have undergone gastrocystoplasty.

The signs and symptoms of the hematuria-dysuria syndrome are most likely secondary to acid irritation. Acid in urine may cause external irritation and skin excoriation. Recent work has suggested that *Helicobacter pylori* may play a role in this complication, as it may increase acid complications in the native stomach [68]. Such problems are less frequent after antral cystoplasty, where there is a smaller load of parietal cells.

4.2.9 Mucus production

Intestinal segments continue to produce mucus after placement in the urinary tract. The proteinaceous material can potentially impede bladder drainage during voiding or CIC, particularly in pediatric patients who must use small-caliber catheters. Mucus may serve as a nidus for infection or stone formation when it remains in the bladder for long periods. Mucus production often increases after cystoplasty in the presence of cystitis. Colonic segments produce more mucus than ileum and gastric segments produce the least amount. Most patients do not require any routine bladder irrigations for mucus after gastrocystoplasty. Villous atrophy in the ileum has been documented after long-term placement in the urinary tract. It has been suggested that such atrophy may result in decreased mucus production

Hendren and Hendren (1990) noted a decrease in mucus production from colonic segments over years [3], however, others have not been impressed with such changes [51]. Glandular atrophy in colonic mucosa has not been noted histologically. Routine use of daily bladder irrigations to prevent mucus build up may minimize complications of enterocystoplasty such as urinary tract infection and calculi.

4.2.10 Urinary tract infection

Bacteriuria is very common after intestinal cystoplasty, particularly among patients requiring CIC. Recent experience with bowel neobladders has demonstrated that patients who are able to spontaneously void to completion frequently maintain sterile urine. It appears that the use of CIC is a prominent factor in the development of bacteriuria after augmentation cystoplasty; regardless of the segment considered [3, 25].

Bacteriuria has been noted even when patients are maintained on daily oral antibiotics or antibiotic irrigation. Persistent or recurrent bacteriuria occurs in 50% of patients augmented with sigmoid colon, compared with 25% of those undergoing ileocystoplasty. Recurrent episodes of symptomatic cystitis requiring treatment occurred in 23% of patients after cecocystoplasty, 17% after sigmoid cystoplasty, 13% after cecocystoplasty and 8% after gastrocystoplasty. Febrile attacks occurred in 13% [51].

Not every episode of asymptomatic bacteriuria requires treatment in patients performing CIC. Bacteriuria should be treated for significant symptoms such as incontinence or suprapubic pain and perhaps for hematuria, foul-smelling urine, or remarkably increased mucus production. Bacteriuria should be treated if the urine culture demonstrates growth of a urea-splitting organism that may lead to stone formation.

4.2.11 Calculus disease

Patients with augmentation cystoplasty are at risk for upper and lower urinary tract calculus disease. These patients are chronically dehydrated from water loss through the diversion producing concentrated urine which may be a nidus for stone disease. Additionally urinary stasis, mucous production from the intestinal segment and frequent colonization with urea-spitting organisms places the patient at risk [3]. Patients in whom large segments of ileum have been removed may develop enteric hyperoxaluria which places the patient at risk for calcium oxalate stone formation. Hypocitraturia a risk factor for stone disease may be found in patient with chronic metabolic acidosis and malabsorption abnormalities. Hypercalciuria is a result of the acidosis, and can lead to mobilization of calcium from bone and impaired reabsorption from acid renal tubule fluid.

Several series reported calculi in 18% of patients after augmentation cystoplasty [3, 43]. Patients catheterizing through an abdominal wall stoma had the highest risk, probably because of incomplete emptying. Palmer and associates (1993) noted urolithiasis in 52% of patients after augmentation cystoplasty. Rink and colleagues (1995) noted only an 8% rate of bladder stone formation in 231 patients with long-term follow-up after enterocystoplasty (51). The reasons for these remarkable differences are not clear. Stones have been noted after the use of all intestinal segments, with no significant difference noted between small and large intestine. Struvite stones are less likely after gastrocystoplasty probably because of decreased mucus production and acid that minimizes bacteriuria. Uric acid calculi have rarely been noted in the bladder after gastrocystoplasty (37).

Patients should be instructed to keep adequately hydrated. Staples and nonabsorbable sutures should be avoided in the urinary diversion. Infection with urea-splitting organisms should be treated promptly. Patients should be instructed in the importance of regular reservoir catheterizing. Irrigation may be needed if one produces excessive amounts of mucous. Foods high in oxalate should be avoided in patients with enteric hyperoxaluria. Calcium citrate may be given to bind oxalate in the gut reducing its absorption. A low fat diet may reduce calcium saponification and increase the amount of calcium available to bind oxalate.

4.3 Long-term complications

4.3.1 Tumor formation

A well recognized complication of ureterosigmoidostomy has been the development of tumors, primarily adenocarcinoma, at the ureterocolonic anastomotic site. The latency for development of such tumors averaged 26 years and ranged from 3 to 53 years. Adenocarcinomas were the prominent tumors that developed, but benign polyps and other types of carcinoma were also found (15). The exact basis for the increased risk is unknown; however, N-nitroso compounds thought to originate from a mixture of urine and faces may be carcinogenic. These compounds have been noted in the urine of patients with conduit diversion and augmentation (69). Husmann and Spence (1990) suggested that those compounds are more likely enhancing agents rather than a lone cause for tumor development.

It has been proposed that inflammatory reaction at the anastomotic site may induce growth factor production, which, in turn, increases cellular proliferation (68). Filmer and Spencer (1990) identified 14 patients who developed adenocarcinoma in an augmented bladder, and several more have been reported since then. Nine of those tumors occurred after ileocystoplasty and five after colocystoplasty (70).

Experimental work in the rat demonstrated hyperplastic growth in the augmented bladder with all intestinal segments, with no segment showing any particularly increased risk (71). The applicability of such findings to humans is uncertain. The long latency period noted for tumor development after ureterosigmoidostomy suggests that short-term follow-up after augmentation cystoplasty is not adequate to evaluate tumor formation.

Patients undergoing augmentation cystoplasty should be made aware of a potentially increased risk for tumor development. Yearly surveillance of the augmented bladder with endoscopy should eventually be performed; the latency period until such procedures are necessary is not well defined. The earliest reported tumor after augmentation was found only 4 years after cystoplasty (72). Transitional cell carcinoma, hyperplasia, and dysplasia have also been noted near the anastomoses in humans. Urine cytology or flow cystometry may ultimately become useful in surveillance (73).

4.3.2 Delayed spontaneous bladder perforation

Perhaps the most disturbing complication of augmentation cystoplasty is delayed bladder perforation. Patients presenting with spontaneous perforation after augmentation cystoplasty are usually quite ill with abdominal pain, distention and fever. Sepsis has been common. Nausea, decreased urine output, and shoulder pain from diaphragmatic irritation have also been noted. Perforations have been found in the evaluation of virtually asymptomatic pelvic masses Patients with neurogenic dysfunction often have impaired lower abdominal sensation and present later in the course of the illness; severe sepsis and death have occurred. Patients with perforation after gastrocystoplasty often present promptly because of acid irritation.

A high index of suspicion for perforation is necessary. Contrast cystography is diagnostic in most cases. Thorough technique is important to identify as many true-positive cases as possible with cystography. Some reports of perforations have noted a significant false-negative rate on cystography and suggested that ultrasonography and CT improve diagnostic accuracy. They recommended that one of those studies be done in any child with suspected perforation if the initial cystogram is negative (74, 75).

The cause of delayed perforations within a bowel segment is unknown. It has been suggested that perforation might be secondary to traumatic catheterization in some cases. It seems unlikely that catheterization trauma is the lone cause in most patients. The location of the perforations has been variable among patients and even in a single patient with multiple perforations. Perforations have occurred after augmentation in patients who did not catheterize at all. Others have suggested that trauma to the bowel caused by fixed adhesions that result in sheering forces with emptying and filling may result in perforation (15). Chronic, transmural infection of the bladder wall has also been proposed as a cause. Histologic examination of bowel segments adjacent to areas of perforation has revealed necrosis, vascular congestion, hemorrhage, and hemosiderin deposition compatible with chronic bowel wall ischemia. Chronic overdistention of the bladder might result in such ischemia. Chronic ischemia may thus play a significant role in at least some delayed bladder perforations.

Pope and associates (1998) reported perforations occurring in bladders with significant uninhibited contractions after augmentation. High outflow resistance may maintain bladder pressure rather than allowing urinary leakage and venting of the pressure, potentially increasing ischemia. Hyperreflexia alone is unlikely as a solitary cause of perforation, because the complication was essentially never recognized in the era before bowel detubularization and reconfiguration, when persistent pressure contractions were more common after augmentation cystoplasty. Once bowel is reconfigured, however, it may be more prone to ischemia if high pressure does persist.

Once spontaneous perforation has occurred, the chance of recurrence is significant. One third of patients with rupture in one series had a recurrence (74). Consideration must eventually be given to removal of the original segment and replacement by another after repeated perforation.

This problem has been noted with increasing frequency after augmentation cystoplasty and may involve all segments. There may be no particular increased risk of one intestinal segment over another. With the inconsistent differences across multiple large series, it is unlikely that any given enteric segment is at significantly increased risk for perforation and probable that multiple factors influence the risk for the complication (15, 20, 48).

The standard treatment for spontaneous perforation of the augmented bladder is surgical repair, as it is for intraperitoneal rupture of the bladder after trauma. There are reported series of conservative management for suspected perforation consisting of catheter drainage, antibiotics and serial abdominal examinations. It was successful in 87% of patients, although only 2 of 13 patients with suspected rupture had x-ray documentation unequivocally identifying a perforation (74). Even patients who do well with conservative management during the acute episode often require surgical intervention eventually. Such management may be a consideration in a stable patient with sterile urine. The surgeon should certainly have a low threshold for surgical exploration and repair.

Problem	**Stomach**	**Ileum**	**Colon**
Segment loss from GI tract	1. Early satiety 2. Decreased stomach-acid production 3. Increased gastrin production	1. Decreased absorption of B12, folate, and iron 2. Short-gut syndrome	1. Diarrhea 2. Water loss
Acid–base balance	1. Alkalosis 2. Hematuria/dysuria	1. Chronic metabolic acidosis 2. Ammonium and chloride resorption	1. Acidosis 2. Bicarbonate loss 3. Ammonium chloride resorption
Salt balance	1. Sodium and potassium loss	1. Sodium and chloride resorption	1. Sodium and chloride resorption
Mucus	1. More soluble, less apparent	1. Problem with catheter obstruction, irrigation necessary	1. Problem with catheter obstruction, irrigation necessary
Stone formation	1. Rare problem (low pH)	1. Can be a major problem, irrigations recommended	1. Can be a major problem, irrigations recommended
Infection	1. Moderate	1. Common	1. Common
Tumor	1. None documented but too early to tell	1. Reported	1. Significant in ureterosigmoidostomy
Perforation	1. Reported with potential for ulcer formation in anuric or diverted patient	1. Reported, major problem because of potential for infection	1. Reported, major problem because of potential for infection

Metabolic consequences of bladder reconstruction with bowel

5. Alternatives to gastrointestinal cystoplasty

Currently, gastrointestinal segments are commonly used as tissues for bladder replacement or repair. However, gastrointestinal tissues are designed to absorb specific solutes, whereas bladder tissue is designed for the excretion of solutes. As mentioned, when gastrointestinal tissue is in contact with the urinary tract, multiple complications may ensue.
Because of the problems encountered with the use of gastrointestinal segments, numerous investigators have attempted alternative methods, materials, and tissues for bladder replacement or repair. These include autoaugmentation, ureterocystoplasty, methods for tissue expansion, seromuscular grafts, matrices for tissue regeneration and tissue engineering with cell transplantation. Some of these alternatives appear to hold promise, but none has stood the test of time for true comparison to intestinal cystoplasty.
An ideal tissue for increasing capacity and improving compliance would have transitional epithelium so as to be relatively impermeable and avoid metabolic changes. The lining would also prevent mucus production and, probably the increased potential for tumor development. The ability to augment the bladder without violation of the peritoneal cavity would also decrease morbidity. Two such alternative procedures are ureterocystoplasty and autoaugmentation. With ureterocystoplasty, there is good muscle backing of transitional epithelium, whereas collagen eventually backs the transitional mucosa of an autoaugmentation.

5.1 Autoaugmentation

5.1.1 Techniques and results

Cartwright and Snow (1989) described an ingenious method to improve bladder compliance and capacity using native urothelial tissue. In their procedure, known as autoaugmentation they excised detrusor muscle over the dome of the bladder leaving the mucosa intact to protrude as a wide-mouth diverticulum. Initially they made a midline incision through the bladder muscle with the bladder distended with saline so that mucosa bulged from the incision. The muscle was mobilized and excised laterally in each direction. The lateral edges of the detrusor muscle were then secured to the psoas muscle bilaterally to prevent collapse of the diverticulum. Their early experience with a small group of patients resulted in improved compliance in most, with increasing capacity in some [78].
This producer has since been modified by a number of surgeons, particularly in adult patients, each providing a different name for the procedure depending on whether the detrusor muscle was simply incised (vesicomyotomy) or excised (vesicomyomectomy) to create the diverticulum. In an effort to determine whether incision or excision provided superior results, Johnson and colleagues (1994) performed 16 vesicomyotomies and 16 vesicomyomectomies in rabbits after previously reducing the bladder capacity. Functional bladder capacity in the animals increased by 43.5%, and there was no statistical difference between the two techniques. They then performed vesicomyotomies (incision) in 12 patients with neurogenic bladder dysfunction and demonstrated a mean increase in capacity of 40% and a mean decrease in leak point pressure of 33% [78, 80]. They concluded that detrusor excision offered no advantage over incision. All patients demonstrated some increase in capacity (15% to 70%), and no patient in early follow-up clinically deteriorated and required enterocystoplasty.
Detrusorectomy, leaving a small cap of muscle at the dome through which a suprapubic tube can be placed, was proposed by Landa and Moorhead (1994). They have been

concerned that, although these procedures usually improve compliance, the increase in volume is "modest" at best (81).

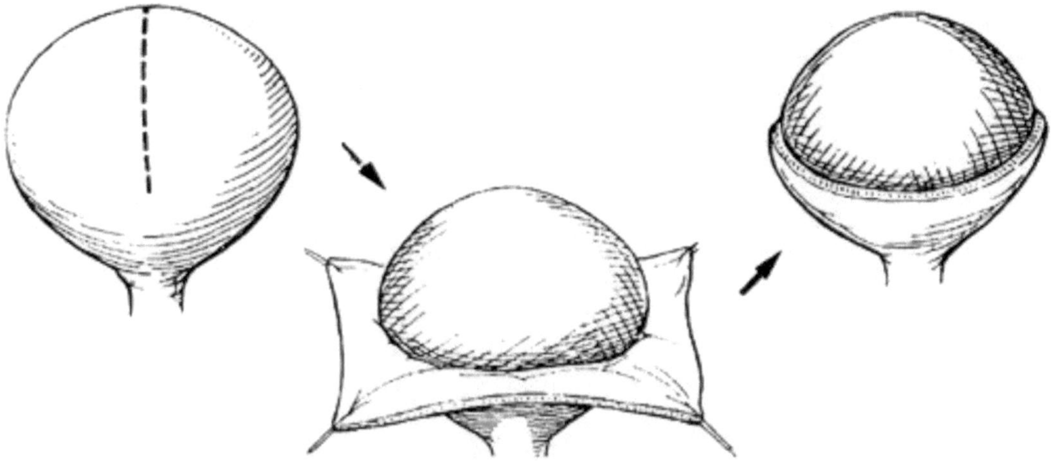

In autoaugmentation, the detrusor is excised leaving the urothelium to act as a diverticulum (1).

The efficacy of autoaugmentation in improving bladder capacity and compliance has been varied. Snow and Cartwright (1999) have follow-up of greater than one year in thirty patients. Nineteen of thirty patients had a neuropathic bladder secondary to spina bifida. All patients had preoperative urodynamic evidence of reduced bladder compliance and detrusor hyperreflexia. While clinical success has been dramatic in some, the overall results have been less impressive. One third of the patients had a significant increase in bladder capacity, an additional third were unchanged, while one third had actual loss of capacity. Evaluation of bladder compliance revealed that 60 percent had an improvement in compliance by greater than 50 percent in comparison to preoperative measurements, 20 percent had a 20 to 50 percent improvement, and the remaining did not change significantly. Overall fourteen patients (47%) had excellent results, showing a significant improvement in compliance, capacity, and dryness. Seven patients (23%) had fair results, described as stability or improvement of the upper tracts without scant improvement in the urodynamic parameters. Nine patients (30%) had poor results, remaining wet or with worsening hydronephrosis (82).

Following autoaugmentation, the majority of patients remained on intermittent catheterization, although 20 percent demonstrated the ability to void spontaneously. Seven patients have required secondary enterocystoplasty following the initial autoaugmentation. Reoperative enterocystoplasty was not hampered by the prior detruserectomy. The urothelial diverticulum at the time of augmentation cystoplasty was noted to be thick and fibrous similar to a leather bag (82).

5.1.2 Advantages

The primary advantage that autoaugmentation has over conventional enterocystoplasty is that it preserves the patient's native urothelium in the augmented segment. This avoids the complications associated with enterocystoplasty related to the presence of heterotopic epithelium in contact with the urine including electrolyte disturbances, mucus, bladder calculi, hematuria dysuria syndrome, and later tumor occurrences. Technically, autoaugmentation is an extraperitoneal procedure that can be performed through a Pfannestiel incision and avoids the complications of bowel surgery including the development of intraperitoneal adhesions and postoperative bowel obstruction. Although autoaugmentation is performed without a formal cystotomy; other bladder procedures such as ureteral reimplantation and appendicovesicostomy can be performed (intravesically or extravesically) at the same time. Lastly, it is important to note that autoaugmentation does not preclude further augmentation procedures if unsuccessful.

5.1.3 Disadvantages

The major drawback of autoaugmentation is that clinical experience has failed thus far to identify the most appropriate patients for this procedure. Mixed results have been obtained clinically with regard to symptomatic and postoperative urodynamic improvement in the autoaugmented bladder. Evaluations of the available data indicate that there is no direct correlation between preoperative urodynamic findings and future success. It works well in some patients while it fails in others. It is of note that many patients have demonstrated clinical improvement after these procedures without a significant change in urodynamics. The exact reasons for the improvement are unknown.

Another drawbacks of autoaugmentation is a limited increase in bladder capacity. Landa and Moorhead (1994) noted that if the maximum capacity and the volume of urine held at 40 cm H_2O are similar, the patient may be better served by immediate intestinal cysloplasty.. The patient and surgeon must be prepared for such an event on occasion. Even if adequate expansion is achieved initially, there is concern that any improvement may not last in the long term. In animals, the surface area of the autoaugmentation site was observed to decrease by approximately 50% at 12 weeks. Progressive thickening and contractor of the site because of collagenous infiltrate was noted. Almost one-half of is adult patients with hyperreflexia who early on had a good result after autoaugmentation failed with longer follow-up (79).

An additional concern with autoaugmentation is the theoretical increased risk of bladder rupture that has been demonstrated in animal studies. Although perforation of the autoaugmented bladder has been reported in one patient, the overall increased risk of bladder rupture as compared to other types of bladder augmentation has yet to be defined (83).

Inadvertent opening of the mucosa during the procedure can make subsequent mobilization more difficult and may promote prolonged postoperative extravasation. Such extravasation usually stops with bladder drainage. Prolonged drainage, however, may lead to compromised results due to collapse of the diverticulum. If concomitant ureteral reimplantation or bladder neck surgery is necessary, various authors have recommended that such procedures should be done first with the bladder then closed before detrusorectomy.

5.1.4 Patient selection for autoaugmentation

Leng and associates (1999), reported good results with the technique among patients with hyperreflexia(85). Adequate preoperative volume may be the most important predictor of success. *Autoaugmentation probably should be considered only in patients who have reasonable capacity but poor compliance due to uninhibited contractions*(82). If a remarkable increase in capacity is needed, autoaugmentation is unlikely to be as definitive as other techniques. However, it should be noted that autoaugmentation has been successful in some patients with a small capacity, poorly compliant bladder.

5.2 Seromuscular grafts and de-epithelialized bowel segments
5.2.1 Technical considerations

Seromuscular grafts and de-epithelialized bowel segments, either alone or over a native urothelium have been attempted [24, 86]. The concept of demucosalizing organs is not new to urologists. More than four decades ago, in 1961, Blandy proposed the removal of submucosa from intestinal segments used for augmentation cystoplasty to ensure that mucosal regrowth would not occur [13].

Hypothetically, this would avoid the complications associated with use of bowel in continuity with the urinary tract. Since Blandy's initial report, 25 years transpired before there was a renewed interest in demucosalizing intestinal segments for urinary reconstruction [87].

Several other investigators have pursued this line of research [24, 86, 88]. These investigative efforts have emphasized the complexity of both the anatomic and cellular interactions present when tissues with different functional parameters are combined. The complexity of these interactions is emphasized by the observation that the use of demucosalized intestinal segments for augmentation cystoplasty is limited by either mucosal regrowth or contraction of the intestinal patch [88].

It has been noted that removal of only the mucosa may lead to mucosal regrowth, whereas removal of the mucosa and submucosa may lead to retraction of the intestinal patch [89].

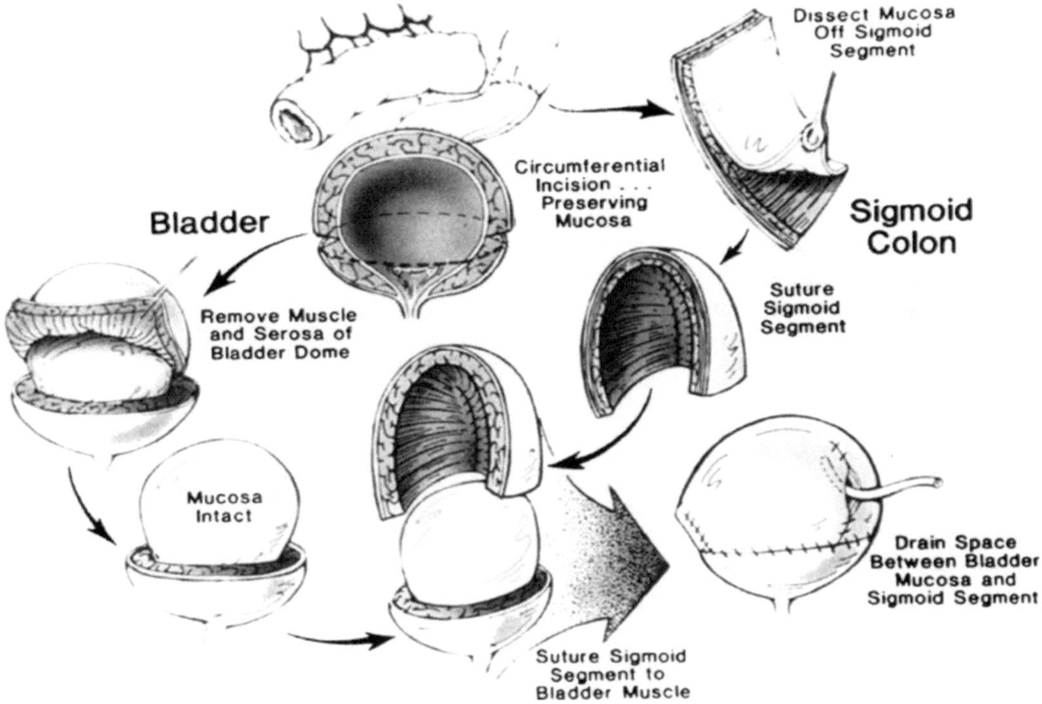

Seromuscular enterocystoplasty using sigmoid colon (SCLU). Detrusor incision is performed similar to autoaugmentation; however, the bulging mucosa is covered with a demucosalized segment of sigmoid colon. (From Buson H, Manivel JC, Dayanc M, et al: Seromuscular colocystoplasty lined with urothelium: Experimental study. Urology 1994;44:745.

Seromuscular enterocystoplasty combines autoaugmentation with a demucosalized flap of colon or stomach. The removal of the gastrointestinal mucosa results in a denuded seromuscular flap that can be placed over the exposed bladder mucosa of an autoaugmented bladder to avoid collagen deposition and contraction. This combination has been done to potentially preserve the advantages of both procedures.

5.2.2 Results

The clinical results of seromuscular enterocystoplasty have been mixed and unpredictable. Initial reports by Dewan and Gonzales in both animal models and humans have been encouraging [24, 86]. In the Gonzales et al series of 16 patients undergoing seromuscular colocystoplasty utilizing sigmoid colon, bladder capacity was increased to almost two and one half times the preoperative volume and end filling-pressures decreased by approximately 50 percent in 14 patients. Two patients failed and required ileocystoplasty their urodynamic data were excluded. Two other patients developed an hourglass deformity [24]. Endoscopic biopsy of the segments was interesting: of 10 biopsies in the series, 1 revealed urothelium with islands of colonic mucosa, and 2 others found only colon mucosa. Removal of all of the enteric mucosa is important when using sigmoid to prevent mucoceles or overgrowth of intestinal mucosa [24].

Dewan and associates (1997) reported on five patients undergoing seromuscular gastrocystoplasty. Four of the five patients have had urodynamic evidence of improved bladder capacity and compliance during the first postoperative year. They believed that preservation of the submucosa eventually promoted regrowth of bowel mucosa. The interaction of the two different tissues will be interesting to follow. The long-term effects on the urothelium by the seromuscular segment and vice versa are unknown. Work has shown that persistent transitional lining will protect from metabolic problems and mucus production [24, 86].

Despite these initial encouraging results, it is important to note that the follow-up in these series has been relatively short and approximately 25 percent of patients have eventually required a secondary operation due to either complication related to the seromuscular flap (contracture) and/or failure to adequately improve bladder capacity and/or compliance [86].

A more recent report of long-term follow-up of 13 patients after seromuscular gastrocystoplasty by Carr et al (1999) describes variable results, at best. The mean follow-up was 50 months. Five patients had a good outcome with regard to objective urodynamic and subjective clinical improvement. Four patients were found to have a "fair" outcome in that they had some objective improvement, while the remaining four patients had a poor result and required re-augmentation [90]. Evaluation of preoperative urodynamic and radiographic data in these patients again demonstrated that it was not possible to predict preoperatively which patients would do well after seromuscular gastrocystoplasty. These procedures are technically more demanding than simple augmentation or autoaugmentation and are associated with more blood loss and a longer operative time [24]. Increased bleeding is particularly likely when using stomach.

These urothelium-lined, seromuscular augmentations are theoretically attractive. Thus far, the failure and reoperation rate after such procedures remains higher than that noted for standard enterocystoplasty [90]. The best results have been reported with the use of colon. Those results may be partially attributed to the learning curve with a new, complex procedure. Longer follow-up and more experience arc necessary to determine whether the complication rate will decrease with experience or increase because of problems with the combination.

In summary, seromuscular enterocystoplasty appears to parallel autoaugmentation that is technically feasible and useful in many patients. However, it has significant shortcomings. It is not possible at this time to define which patients will succeed and which ones will fail. Advantages beyond autoaugmentation appear to be minimal. Further long-term studies are required to determine the true efficacy of this technique. Also, additional studies are needed to determine if there are significant functional differences between seromuscular colocystoplasty and seromuscular gastrocystoplasty.

5.3 Ureterocystoplasty

The use of ureteral tissue for bladder augmentation purposes was first described in 1992 (91). Native ureter is for many reasons the best tissue available for augmentation cystoplasty. It is autologous, lined with urothelium, backed by muscle, distensible, and complaint (92, 93). However, not all patients in need of bladder augmentation have dilated ureteral tissue available for use. Patients that are candidates for ureterocystoplasty should have either i) a nonfunctional renal unit that can be removed making the ureter and renal pelvis available, or ii) a functional renal unit that is associated with a massively dilated, tortuous, and elongated ureter. The lower ureter can then be used for augmentation, while kidney drainage is re-established by reimplantation of the straightened upper ureter into the bladder or by transureteroureterostomy.

An example of an ideal candidate is one with vesicoureteral reflux and dysplasia (VURD) syndrome from posterior urethral valves. In patients with posterior urethral valves, unilateral reflux may behave as a "pop-off" valve to lower intravesical pressures and protect the contralateral upper tract. In many of these patients, the refluxing ureter is massively dilated, draining a poorly functioning or nonfunctioning kidney. It was a logical extension to use this ureteral tissue to augment the bladder. Ureterocystoplasty is also appropriate in patients on dialysis with end-stage renal failure who are awaiting transplantation and are in need of augmentation due to bladder dysfunction.

More recently, the use of ureterocystoplasty has been expanded in an attempt to take advantage of this valuable tissue and make it available to more surgical candidates. Its use has been reported in patients with a duplex system in which either the upper or lower pole is nonfunctioning (96). In patients with a duplex system and a dilated ureter in conjunction with a functioning renal segment, drainage of that segment can be accomplished with an ipsilateral ureteroureterostomy with preservation of the lower portion of the ureter for augmentation. Ahmed et al have also described the "tandem" use of bilateral megaureters for ureterocystoplasty (97).

5.4 Technical considerations

Ureterocystoplasty can be performed through a midline, intraperitoneal incision. This incision provides access to the intestine should mobilization of the ureter be unsatisfactory. Ureterocystoplasty may also be done through two incisions, remaining completely extraperitoneal. The general technique is the same. A standard nephrectomy is performed with great care to preserve the renal pelvic and upper ureteral blood supply. All adventitia and periureteral tissue is swept from the peritoneum toward the ureter during mobilization to protect the ureteral blood supply. Proximally, this blood supply typically arises medially. As the ureter enters the true pelvis, the blood supply arises posteriorly and laterally.

After mobilization of the ureter into the pelvis, the bladder is opened in the sagittal plane. Posteriorly, this incision has typically been carried offcenter directly into and through the ureteral orifice of the ureter used for cystoplasty. The ureter is not detached from the bladder but is opened longitudinally along its entire length, with care taken to avoid its main blood supply. The incision in the bladder and distal ureter should avoid branches of the superior vesical artery, which serves as an important blood supply to the mobilized ureter. The ureter is folded on itself, and the ureter-to-ureter and ureter-to-bladder anastomoses are performed with running absorbable suture.

Alternatively, the bladder incision can be stopped approximately 2 cm from the orifice, with a similar length of distal ureter left in situ and intact without incision. The resulting small loop of intact ureter does not create clinical problems or adversely affect the end volume in a significant manner [20]. This modification of technique is easier and may be safer in that, it avoids potential injury to the blood supply of the mobilized ureter near the ureterovesical junction.

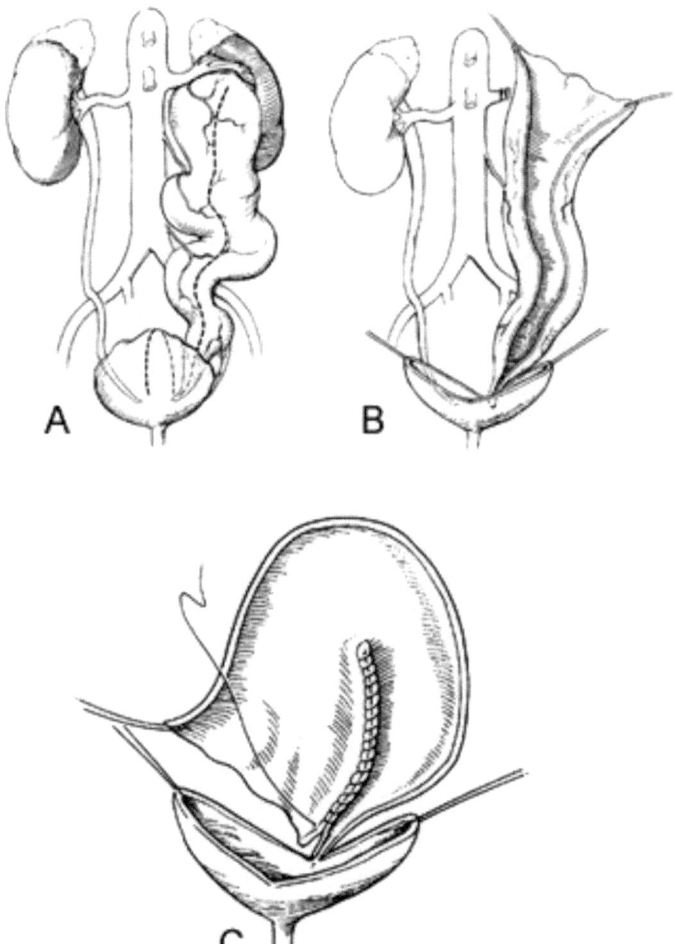

A) A megaureter and poorly functioning kidney are required for ureterocystoplasty.
B) After nephrectomy, the dilated ureter is detubularized, taking care to preserve the blood supply. C) The detubularized ureter is reconfigured before being anastomosed to the bladder [1].

5.4.1 Results

Numerous series have reported good results after augmentation using ureter, some with follow-up as long as 8 years. The upper tracts have remained stable or improved in virtually all patients. Complications have been uncommon, with only a rare early extravasation of urine reported (92).

The largest published series is that of Churchill et al (1993) in which ureterocystoplasty was performed in 16 patients. Thirteen patients had enough urodynamic data available postoperatively for adequate evaluation. Twelve out of thirteen patients had excellent results. As a group, there was a 218 percent increase in bladder capacity, a 284 percent increase in pressure specific bladder capacity, and a 227 percent increase in bladder compliance.

Landau and colleagues (1994), compared age-matched and diagnosis-matched children who underwent ureterocystoplasty or ileocystoplasty. The total mean bladder capacity was 470 ml in the ureterocystoplasty group and 381 ml in the ileocystoplasty group. Bladder volumes at 30 cm H_2O were 413 ml and 380 ml after ureterocystoplasty and ileocystoplasty, respectively. Ureter effectively enhanced both volume and compliance. They reported no significant differences in the postoperative mean increase in bladder capacity and pressure specific bladder volume. Both procedures resulted in excellent functional results (94).

Hitchcock et al (1994) has described similar excellent short-term results in eight patients (95).

5.4.2 Advantages

There are several advantages of using the ureter for augmentation. As is the case with autoaugmentation, the major advantage of ureterocystoplasty is that the native urothelium is preserved, thereby avoiding the specific potential problems associated with the use of bowel. Unlike some cases following autoaugmention, the full thickness opened ureter does not tend to shrink with time, unless the vascular supply is compromised. In patients with end-stage renal disease, the procedure can be performed extraperitoneally, thus, preserving the peritoneum for future peritoneal dialysis. When necessary, concomitant procedures in the bladder may also be performed. It seems likely that the risk of tumor formation will be avoided, and perforation of the augmented bladder may be less probable. However, long-term follow-up will be needed to confirm these notions (92). Lastly, there is increased potential for spontaneous voiding postoperatively in patients who are able to empty their bladders adequately preoperatively.

5.4.3 Disadvantages

The main disadvantage of ureterocystoplasty is that it is only applicable in a minority of patients. Surgical candidates for ureterocystoplasty include patients with either a nonfunctioning renal unit or a megaureter long enough that ipsilateral renal drainage can be re-established following use of the lower ureter for augmentation (92).

6. To the future: Tissue expansion for bladder augmentation

6.1 The experiments

In an attempt to make ureterocystoplasty available to make to patients with non-dilated ureters, some have developed methods of producing a dilated ureter. Lailas et al (1996) have demonstrated in a rabbit model that a temporary cutaneous ureterostomy can be used to perform hydrostatic distention of the ureter with subsequent successful ureterocystoplasty. In this study, the ureteral units were dilated at least 10 fold, as measured by radiography, after daily injection of a saline-antibiotic solution for 1 month. Augmentation cystoplasty was performed with the reconfigured dilated uretral segment. Repeated cystography and cystometry showed an increased bladder capacity ranging from 190 % to 380% (98). In a similar system, a dilating catheter was used to dilate tissue in pigs (99).

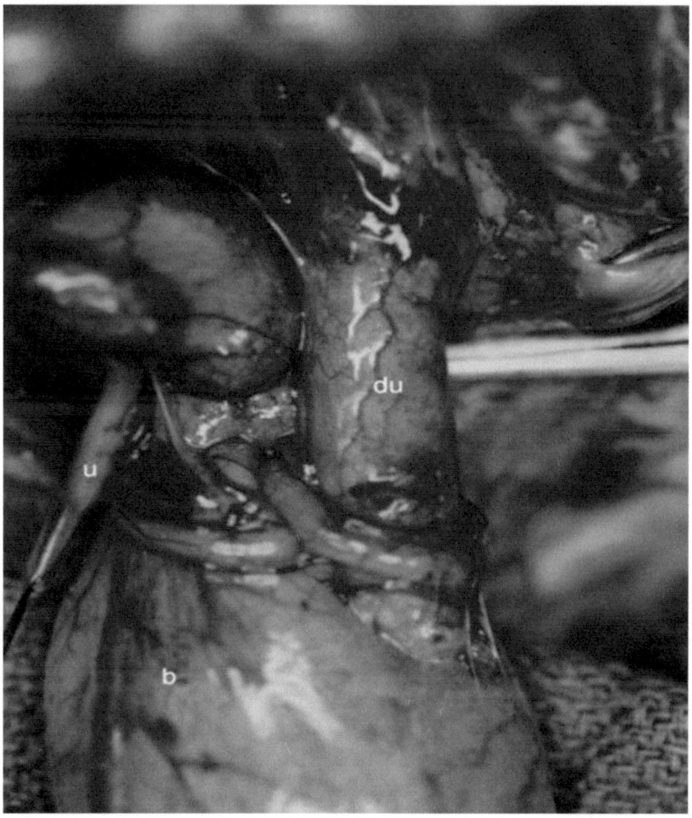

Progressive dilation can be performed in a normal-caliber ureter, which can be subsequently used for ureterocystoplasty. After placement of a ureteral dilation device, comparison is made of progressively dilated ureter (du) and native undilated ureter (u) coming off the bladder (b) (13).

A system for the progressive expansion of native bladder tissue has also been used for augmenting bladder volumes (Satar et al, 1999). Beagle dogs underwent urodynamic studies and the bladders were divided horizontally into two segments: a superior bladder neoreservoir, and an intact smaller bladder inferiorly with both ureters left intact and draining. A silastic catheter was threaded into the newly formed, superiorly located neoreservoir, and connected to an injection port, which was secured subcutaneously. Four weeks after surgery, a saline-antibiotic solution was injected daily into the palpable injection port. Dilating the neoreservoir through the silastic catheter within 30 days after progressive dilation, the neoreservoir volume was expanded at least 10-fold, as measured by radiography and cystometrography. Urodynamic studies of the dilated neoreservoirs showed normal compliance in all animals. Microscopic examination of the expanded neoreservoir tissue showed a normal histology (100).

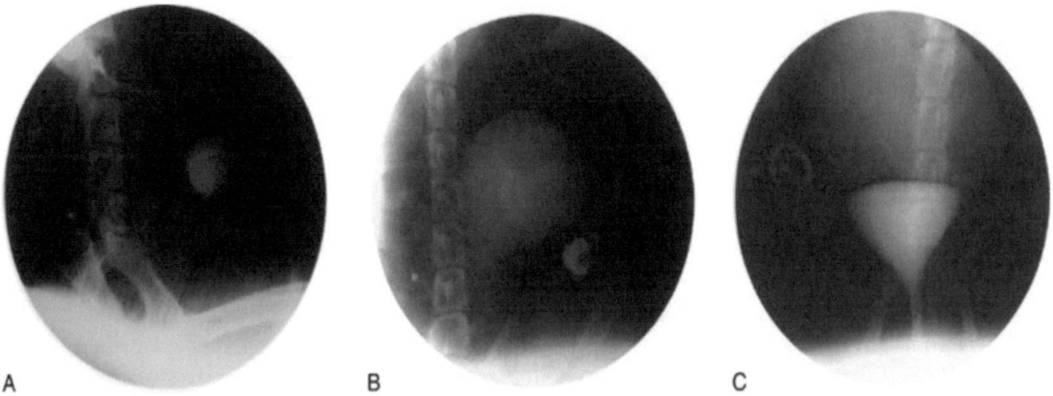

Progressive bladder dilation can be performed with adequate increases in capacity. Cystography of bladder neoreservoir before progressive dilation *(A)* is compared with cystography results after progressive dilation *(B)* and with cystogram showing dilated neoreservoir and intact bladder segment *(C)* (13)

6.2 The expectations

Ideally, bladder tissue expansion could be performed with an indwelling dilation catheter, similar to a Foley catheter with a large balloon. In the future, one could foresee placing a dilating catheter intravesically in a patient who either requires augmentation, in an intermittent fashion (e.g. four times daily) or left indwelling. An expanding balloon within the catheter could then be filled progressively, with either continuous or intermittent filling until the desired bladder volume is achieved. Studies associated with this concept are currently being conducted in the laboratory. Clinical application of these interesting ideas has yet to be undertaken (13).

7. Tissue engineered bladder

The complications that are associated with using various portions of the gastrointestinal tract for genitourinary reconstruction in both adults and children have stimulated the development of tissue engineering techniques for bladder reconstruction through bladder regeneration. Current research efforts are focused on the development of biodegradable materials which are well-characterized with predictable behavior that can be used as alternatives to gastrointestinal segments for bladder reconstruction.

Tissue engineering follows the principles of cell transplantation, materials science, and engineering toward the development of biologic substitutes that can restore and maintain normal function. Bladder reconstruction via tissue engineering and bladder regeneration involve the use of a *biomaterial graft (matrix)*, either permanent or biodegradable, that will function as a suitable scaffold to allow the body's ability of regeneration and growth to occur either naturally (matrices alone unseeded) or with the addition of cultured cells (matrices with cell - seeded) (3, 101).

The ideal graft material is one that would be replaced by the host tissue, provide a low-pressure reservoir, and serve as a scaffold for regeneration of the bladder wall with normal function characteristics. If a suitable graft material can be developed, the need for autogenous tissue and the associated complications of intestinal segments could be eliminated. Currently, there are two types of tissue engineering technologies that have preliminarily been shown to induce bladder regeneration. These are the unseeded and seeded technologies (14).

7.1 Biomaterials

7.1.1 Functions

Biomaterials in genitourinary tissue engineering function as an artificial extracellular matrix (ECM) and elicit biologic and mechanical functions of native ECM found in tissues in the body. Native ECM brings cells together into tissue, controls the tissue structure, and regulates the cell phenotype. Biomaterials facilitate the localization and delivery of cells and/or bioactive factors (e.g. cell adhesion peptides, growth factors) to desired sites in the body; define a three dimensional space for the formation of new tissues with appropriate function. The configuration of the biomaterials can guide the structure of an engineered tissue. The biomaterials provide mechanical support against in-vivo forces of tissue development. The biomaterials can be loaded with bioactive signals, such as cell-adhesion peptides and growth factors, which can regulate cellular function (102).

7.1.2 Design and selection

The design and selection of the biomaterial is critical in the development of engineered genitourinary tissues. The biomaterial must be capable of controlling the structure and function of the engineered tissue in a predesigned manner by interacting with transplanted cells and/or host cells. Generally, the ideal biomaterial should be biocompatible, promote cellular interaction and tissue development, and possess proper mechanical and physical properties.

The selected biomaterial should be biodegradable and bioresorbable to support the reconstruction of a completely normal tissue without inflammation. Such behavior of the biomaterials avoids the risk of inflammatory or foreign body responses that may be associated with the permanent presence of a foreign material in the body. The degradation products should not provoke inflammation or toxicity, and must be removed from the body via metabolic pathways. The degradation rate and the concentration of degradation products in the tissue surrounding the implant must be at a tolerable level (103).

The biomaterials need to be processed into specific configuration. A large ratio of surface area to volume is often desirable to allow the delivery of a high density of cells. A high-porosity, interconnected pore structure, with specific pore sizes promotes tissue ingrowth from the surrounding host tissue. Several techniques have been developed that readily control porosity, pore size, and pore structure (13).

7.1.3 Types of biomaterials

Generally, three classes of biomaterials have been used for engineering of genitourinary tissue: ***synthetic polymers***, such as polyglycolic acid (PGA), polylactic acid (PLA), and poly-lactic-co-glycolic acid) (PLGA), ***naturally derived materials***, such as collagen and alginate; and ***cellular tissue matrices***, such as bladder submucosa and small-intestinal submucosa. These classes of biomaterials have been tested in regard to their biocompatibility with primary human urothelial and bladder muscle cells. Naturally, derived materials and cellular tissue matrices have the potential advantage of biologic recognition. Synthetic polymers can be produced reproducibly on a large scale with controlled properties of strength, degradation rate, and microstructure (105).

7.2 Matrices for bladder regeneration
A. Unseeded matrices (Acellular)

The first technique currently being investigated for bladder regeneration is the unseeded technology. This technology involves placement of matrix graft into the wall of the host-bladder. The body then provides the needed environment for subsequent cell growth and tissue regeneration. This represents an unseeded bladder regenerating process.

Thus far, the major obstacle to unseeded tissue engineering technology has been the inability to develop an optimal biomaterial that will act as a suitable scaffold for the "natural" process of regeneration.

7.2.1 Synthetic non-biodegradable biomaterials

Synthetic non-biodegradable biomaterials such as silicon, Teflon, rubber, polytetrafluoroethylene, and polypropylene have been tried with unsuccessful results because of host foreign body reactions. Most of these attempts have failed because of mechanical, structural, functional, or biocompatibility problems. Usually, permanent synthetic materials used for bladder reconstruction succumb to mechanical failure and urinary stone formation, and use of degradable materials leads to fibroblast deposition, scarring, graft contracture, and a reduced reservoir volume over time.

7.2.2 Synthetic biodegradable biomaterials

As a consequence of these failures with non biodegradable materials, synthetic biodegradable material e.g. collagen and Vicryl (PGA) matrices were developed in the hope that these grafts would allow the host bladder adequate time for regeneration but dissolve prior to sever foreign body reaction. These materials have been used experimentally and have shown less graft encrustation and infectious complications compared to non-biodegradable materials. However, graft shrinkage still limited potential clinical utility of these materials.

Collagen/Vicryl composite membranes were used as a scaffold for tissue ingrowth to repair a full thickness defect in the bladder of rabbits. The collagen membranes were reinforced with meshes of Vicryl, a biodegradable polimer composed of PLGA, to strengthen the collagen membranes, which are too soft to suture reliably. The results of the initial study were not encouraging because of the occurrence of sever infection (Monsour et al, 1987). However, a later study obtained a high success rate when the experiments were repeated using purification and γ irradiation of collagen and postoperative administration of antibiotics. At 3 weeks, a normal urothelium was noted. At 6 weeks, no implanted biomaterial was identified. At 35 weeks, smooth muscle regeneration was evident. During this period, there was no evidence of urinary leakage, infection, or bladder calculi (Scott et al, 1988).

7.2.3 Natural biodegradable materials

Collagen based matrices for tissue regeneration such as placenta, amnion and pericardium have been investigated in dogs and have shown clear evidence of bladder regeneration [(106, 107, 108)]. Functionally, the implanted bladders showed adequate capacity for up to 36 months. Nevertheless, they were observed grossly to undergo graft shrinkage. Histologically, the epithelial layer was present, but the muscular layer was absent.

However, despite initial encouraging results, none of these materials has been found to be suitable for clinical use. The reasons for this are not entirely clear. It can only be speculated from the available literature that long-term experimental results with these biodegradable materials did not recapitulate the initial results and therefore clinical trials were not undertaken.

7.2.4 Acellular Extracellular Matrix (ECM) grafts

Recently there has been the development of new types of biodegradable materials that have shown tremendous potential for the induction of bladder regeneration with unseeded tissue engineering technology. These materials are acellular extracellular matrix (ECM) grafts that are derived from various different organs. The graft is made acellular by a mechanical process that lyses the cells and/or by detergent and enzymatic extraction. These types of ECM grafts may be xenogenic or allogenic and have been derived from full thickness bladder, stomach, and the submucosal layer of small intestine (109).

7.2.5 Xeogenic acellular matrix grafts

Small Intestinal Submucosa (SIS)

The most thoroughly studied collagen based ECM graft for bladder augmentation and urinary reconstruction utilizing unseeded technology is small intestinal submucosa (SIS) (109). SIS is a xenogentic membrane derived from pig small intestine in which the mucosa is mechanically removed from the inner surface and the serosa and muscularies are mechanically removed from the outer surface. This result in a thin, translucent membrane (0.1 mm wall thickness) composed mainly of the submucosal layer of the intestinal wall. Production of SIS is reminiscent of the manufacturing of sausage casing. This unique material has been shown to function well as an arterial or venous graft with rapid replacement by native tissues and evidence of tissue specific regeneration (101).

SIS grafts have been shown to promote full thickness bladder regeneration in both rat and canine animal models. The regenerated bladder tissue is composed of all three layers of the normal bladder wall (urothelium, smooth muscle, and serosa). In addition, the regenerated segment is contractile, compliant, and functionally innervated. Urodynamic studies in a long-term canine augmentation model have demonstrated that the SIS augmented bladder maintains normal bladder capacity and compliance that persist for at least 15 months postoperatively. In vitro muscle strip studies on the regenerated portions of the bladders also demonstrate contractility and compliance that is similar to normal bladder (110).

SIS has been shown to be non-immunogenic with over 1000 cross species transplants and direct challenge testing elucidating no response. In addition, SIS is unique from other biomaterials that have been studied thus far in that it contains a combination of active intrinsic growth factors, cytokines, structural proteins, glyeoproteins, and proteoglycans that may assist in cell migration, cell-to-cell interaction, as well as cell growth and differentiation during the regenerative process. These inherent elements within SIS may prove to be vital to the regenerative process. Further research is needed to identify the functional importance of each of these elements and factors (101).

7.2.6 Allogenic acellular matrix grafts

Bladder Acellular Matrix Grafts (BAMG)

Similar types of cellular ECM grafts to SIS have also been shown to induce bladder regeneration in vivo. Preliminary works have demonstrated that successful morphologic

and functional regeneration of the rat urinary bladder can be accomplished with homologous bladder acellular matrix grafts (BAMG).
The allogeneic acellular bladder matrix has served as a scaffold for the ingrowth of host bladder wall components in rats. The matrix was prepared by mechanically and chemically removing all cellular components from bladder tissue. Partial cystectomy (25% to 50%) was performed, followed by augmentation cystoplasty using acellular bladder matrices. The mucosal lining was complete within 10 days. After 4 weeks, muscular and vascular regeneration was completed. Nerve regeneration continued to improve until week 20. The grafted bladders had significantly better capacity and compliance than the autoregenterated bladders after partial cystectomy alone. The bladders regenerated with acellular matrix grafts exhibited contractile activity to electric and carbachol stimulation. Clinically relevant antigenicity was not evident. However, there was a 26% to 36% incidence of bladder stone formation [111, 112].

B. Seeded matrices

Allogenic Cellular Matrix Grafts

In multiple studies using various materials as acellular grafts for cystoplasty, the urothelial layer was able to regenerate normally, but the muscle layer, although present, was not fully developed [111, 112, 113].
Allogenic bladder submucosa preloaded with cells was used as a biomaterial for bladder augmentation in dogs [113]. The regenerated bladder tissues contained a normal cellular organization consisting of urothelium and smooth muscle and exhibited a normal compliance. Biomaterials preloaded with cells before their implantation showed better tissue regeneration compared with biomaterials implanted with no cells, in which tissue regeneration depended on ingrowth of the surrounding tissue. The bladders showed a significant increase (100%) in capacity when augmented with scaffolds seeded with cells, compared to scaffolds without cells (30%).

7.2.7 Summary

Studies involving acellular matrices that may provide the necessary environment to promote cell migration, growth, and differentiation are being conducted, and demonstrate that bladder regeneration using unseeded tissue engineering technology is feasible without the complications of graft shrinkage, incrustation, and infection. These observations have obvious and significant clinical ramifications. The ability to augment the bladder without the use of bowel or other native host tissue would eliminate many of the complications of conventional enterocystoplasty and would simplify the technical aspects of this operation. Further research into the individual composition of the various biomaterials, the cell-to-cell interaction, and the growth factors that are involved in the bladder regenerative process will be required prior to clinical use of these grafts.

7.3 Bladder tissue engineering with selective cell transplantation (seeded technology)

The second type of tissue engineering technology, the seeded technique, involves the use of *biodegradable materials* that act as cell delivery vehicles for *cultured cells* from the patient. This technique has been applied to the urinary bladder. Initially, this process is begun by harvesting native bladder tissue for the establishment and expansion of primary cultures of

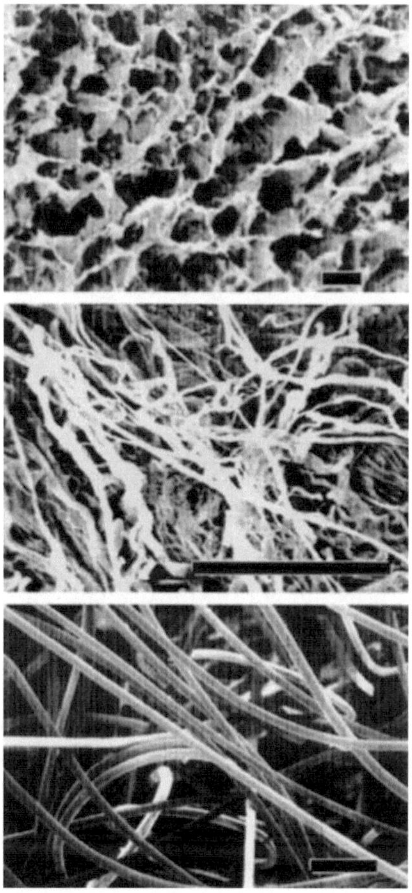

Scanning electron micrographs of biomaterials: collagen sponge *(top)*, acellular matrix prepared from pig bladder submucosa *(center)*, and polyglycolic acid fiber-based matrix *(bottom)*. (Size bars = 100 µm.) (13).

both bladder smooth muscle and epithelial sells. It is possible to expand a bladder epithelial cell culture from a single biopsy specimen such that the cultured cells could cover a surface area of over 400 m within eight weeks (14). Once the cells are grown, they are seeded on a biodegradable membrane in vitro and then transplanted back into the host for continuation of the regenerative process.

In 1992, 1993 Atala and associates demonstrated the successful use of non-woven polyglycolic acid polymers sheets, which allow the in-vitro growth of rabbit and human bladder epithelium and smooth muscle cells (114, 115). Further work demonstrated that these cell-polymer constructs could be implanted into athymic mice with the subequent formation of organized layers of bladder epithelial and smooth muscle cells.

In these studies, urothelial and muscle cells were expanded in-vitro, seeded onto a polymer scaffold (non-wonen polygycolic acid), and allowed to attach and form sheet of cells. The cell-polymer scaffold was then implanted in-vivo. A series of in vivo urologic associated cell-polymer experiments were then performed. Histologic analysis of human urothelial, bladder muscle, and composite urothelial and bladder muscle polymer scaffold, implanted in athymic mice and retrieved at different time points, indicated that viable cells were evident in all three experimental groups (115). Implanted cells oriented themselves spatially along the polymer surfaces. The cell populations appeared to expand from one layer to several layers of thickness with progressive cell organization over extended implantation times. Cell-polymer composite implants of urothelial and muscle cells, retrieved at extended times (50 days), showed extensive formation of multilayered, sheet-like structures and well defined muscle layers. Polymers seeded with cells and manipulated into a tubular configuration showed layers of muscle cells lining the multilayered epithelial sheets. Cell polymers implanted with human bladder muscle cells alone showed almost complete replacement of the polymer with sheets of smooth muscle at 520 days. This experiment demonstrated that composite tissue-engineered structures could be created de novo.

Recently, Yoo et al (1998) and Oberpenning et al (1999), reported on the feasibility of dog bladder augmentation using allogenic bladder submucosa or polyglycolic acid polymers seeded with urothelial and smooth muscle cells (113, 116). Organized bladder histology was noted in the regenerated bladder tissue. More importantly, the regenerated bladder tissue was found to increase bladder capacity and was urodynamically compliant.

In order to determine the effect of implanting engineered tissues in continuity with the urinary tract, Yoo and associates (1998), used an animal model of bladder augmentation. Partial cystectomies, which involved removal of approximately 50% of the native bladder, were performed in 10 dogs. In five, the retrieved bladder tissue was micro dissected and the mucosal and muscular layers separated. The bladder urothelial and muscle cells were cultured. Urothelial and smooth muscle cells were harvested and expanded separately. A collagen-based matrix, derived from allogenic bladder submucosa, was used for cell delivery. This material was chosen for these experiments because of its native elasticity.

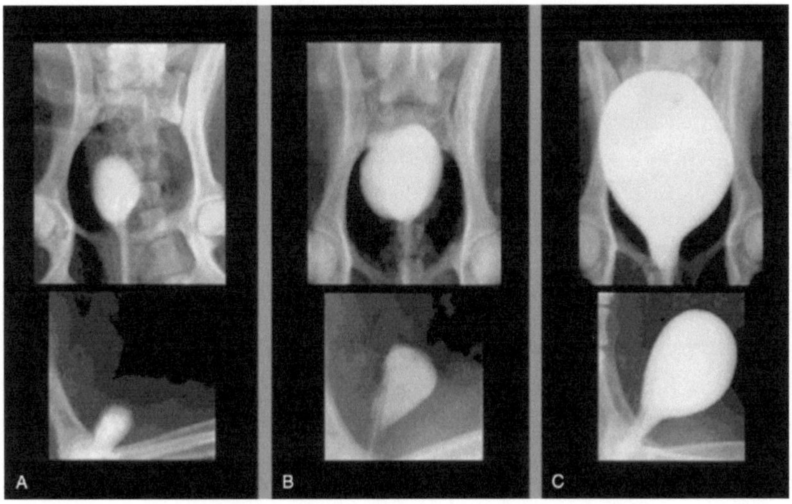

Radiographic cystograms in beagles 11 months after subtotal cystectomy without reconstruction *(A)*; with reconstruction using a polymer without cells *(B)*; and with reconstruction with a polymer and cell-seeded tissue-engineered organ *(C)*. Organs after trigone-sparing cystectomy retained a small-sized reservoir. Tissue-engineered neobladders showed a normal configuration and a larger capacity than the trigones grafted with polymer only (13).

Within 6 weeks, the expanded urothelial cells were collected as a pellet. The cells were seeded on the luminal surface of the allogenic bladder submucosa and incubated for five days. Muscle cells were seeded on the opposite side of the bladder submucosa. Augmentation cystoplasty was performed with the matrix including cells in one group and the matrix without cells in the second group. The augmented bladders were covered with omentum to facilitate angiogenesis to the implant. Bladders augmented with the matrix seeded with cells showed a 99% increase in capacity compared with bladders augmented with the cell-free matrix, which showed only a 30% increase in capacity. Functionally, all animals showed normal bladder compliance as evidenced by urodynamic studies; however, the remaining native bladder tissue may have accounted for these results. Histologically, the retrieved engineered bladders contained a cellular organization consisting of a urothelium-lined lumen surrounded by submucosal tissue and smooth muscle. However, the muscular layer was markedly more prominent in the cell-reconstituted scaffold (113).

7.3.1 Histologic Parameters of Tissue-Engeneered Bladders

It has been well established for decades that the bladder is able to regenerate generously over free grafts. Urothelium is associated with a high reparative capacity. Bladder muscle tissue is less likely to regenerate in a normal fashion. Most of the free grafts (without cells) used for bladder replacement in the past were able to show adequate histology in terms of a well-developed urothelial layer, but they were associated with an abnormal muscular layer that varied in terms of its full development. Because native muscle cells are less likely to regenerate over the free grafts, presence of both urothelial and muscle cells on the matrices used for bladder replacement is important for successful tissue bioengineering.

Both urothelial and muscle ingrowth are believed to be initiated from the edges of the normal bladder toward the region of the free graft. Usually, however, contracture or resorption of the graft has been evident. The inflammatory response toward the matrix may contribute to the resorption of the free graft (89,104).

It was hypothesized that building the three-dimensional structure constructs in vitro, before implantation, would facilitate the eventual terminal differentiation of the cells after implantation in vivo and would minimize the inflammatory response toward the matrix, thus, avoiding graft contractor and shrinkage. The study by Yoo and associates (1998) demonstrated a major difference between matrices used with autologous cells (tissue-engineered matrices) and those used without cells as regards the graft diameter (113). Matrices implanted with cells for bladder augmentation retained most of their implanted diameter, as opposed to matrices implanted without cells for bladder augmentation, in which graft contraction and shrinkage occurs.

7.3.2 Functional parameters of tissue-engeneered bladders

The results of initial studies showed that the creation of artificial bladder may be achieved in vivo; however, it could not be determined whether the functional parameters noted were caused by the augmented segment or by the intact native bladder tissue. To better, address the functional parameters of tissue-engineered bladders; an animal model was designed that required a cystectomy with subsequent replacement organ (116).

A total of 14 dogs underwent a trigone-sparing cystectomy. The animals were randomly assigned to one of three groups. Group A (n= 2) underwent closure of the trigone without a reconstructive procedure. Group B (n= 6) underwent reconstruction with a cell- free bladder

shaped biodegradable polymer. Group C (n=6) underwent reconstruction using a bladder-shaped biodegradation polymer that delivered autologous urothelial cells and smooth muscle cells harvested from autologous bladder biopsy and expanded.
The cystectomy -only controls and polymer-only grafts maintained average capacities of 22% and 46% of preoperative values, respectively. An average bladder capacity of 95% of the original precystectomy volume was achieved in the tissue-engineered bladder replacements.
The subtotal cystectomy reservoirs that were not reconstructed and the polymer-only reconstructed bladder showed a marked decrease in bladder compliance (10% and 42% total compliance). The compliance of tissue-engineered bladders showed almost no difference from preoperative values. Histologically, the polymer-only bladder presented a pattern of normal urothelial cells with a thickened fibrotic submucosa and a thin layer of muscle fibers. The retrieved tissue- engineered bladders showed a normal cellular organization, consisting of a trilayer of urothelium, submucosa, and muscle. The results from this study showed that it is possible to tissue - engineer bladders that are anatomically and functionally normal (116). Clinical trials for the application of this technology are currently being arranged (116).
Progressive bladder dilation can be performed with adequate increases in capacity. Cystography of bladder neoreservoir before progressive dilation *(A)* is compared with cystography results after progressive dilation *(B)* and with cystogram showing dilated neoreservoir and intact bladder segment *(C)*

7.3.3 In summary

It is clear that bladder regeneration is possible utilizing both unseeded and seeded tissue-engineering technologies. Further advances in our current techniques will eventually revolutionize urologic reconstructive surgery, as we know it today. It is important to note that all of the animal studies performed thus far have been in animals with a normal bladder. It is not known whether normal or abnormal bladder regeneration can be achieved with either unseeded or seeded technology in an animal or patient with a neuropathic bladder. Active research is currently investigating this vital question. Additionally, studies are needed to better understand the differences that exist between the unseeded and seeded approaches and the resultant regenerated bladder, so that unseeded and aspect approaches and the resultant regenerated bladder so that the best aspects of each technology may be utilized to achieve a superior result. It is the authors' opinion that future chapters on bladder augmentation will discuss the use of intestinal segments as historical footnote while the major focus will be on the indications and methods for various types of tissue engineering technology.

8. Laparoscopic augmentation cystoplasty

8.1 Laparoscopic enterocystoplasty

8.1.1 Patient selection

Laparoscopy has distinct advantages when compared with open surgical procedures, such as decreased postoperative pain and morbidity, improved cosmoses, a shorter hospital stay, and decreased convalescence. Recent studies have indicated that postoperative intra-abdominal adhesions are reduced significantly after laparoscopic surgery when compared with open surgery (117).

Alternative	Advantages	Disadvantages
Ureter	1. Urinary epithelium, no mucus 2. Good compliance	1. Only applicable if the patient has a dilated ureter 2. Ureter may be scarred (reflux, infection)
Autoaugmentation (bladder myomectomy)	1. Urinary epithelium, no mucus 2. Relatively easy, no bowel resection	1. Inconsistent results can result in bladder scarring 2. Sometimes difficult (bladder scarring or diverticula)
Demucosalized intestinal flap on urothelium (colon, DAWG)	1. Urinary epithelium, decreased mucus 2. More physiologic	1. Difficult procedure 2. Inconsistent results
Bladder regeneration on substrate (SIS)	1. No bowel resection 2. Easily performed	1. Unproven in children 2. Dependent on native bladder potential for regeneration
Tissue engineering	1. Bladder regrowth in laboratory 2. Potentially unlimited capacity, no mucus	1. Unproven in children 2. Dependent on vascular and nerve ingrowth

DAWG, demucosalized augmentation with gastric segment.

Alternatives to intestinocystoplasty

Despite the established role of laparoscopy in diagnostic and ablative urologic surgery, the use of laparoscopic techniques in reconstruction has been limited because of the technical complexity of the procedures involved. The technical steps in performing laparoscopic bladder augmentation are designed to emulate the open surgical counterpart in every aspect, thereby producing similar functional results with an improved recovery.
A relative contraindication specific to laparoscopic bladder augmentation is the presence of extensive intra-abdominal and pelvic adhesions that would preclude laparoscopic dissection. Patients with ventriculo-peritoneal shunts, as noted in cases of myelomeningocele, have increased abdominal adhesions that may preclude a successful laparoscopic approach (117).

8.1.2 Technical considerations

Important elements of the operation include:

- Cystoscopic placement of ureteric catheters (optional).
- Transperitoneal placement of 4 to 5 redially arranged trocars.

- Identification of the cecum and ileocecal junction.
- A 5-mm laparoscope can be introduced through the lower left port to transilluminate the mesentery and identify its vascular pedicle.
- Bowel segment selection and mobilization sufficient for pelvic placement.
- Exteriorizing the bowel loop outside the abdomen through a 2-cm extension of the umbilical port site, preventing twisting of the mesenteric vessels;
- Using traditional open surgical techniques, the bowel segment is isolated, bowel continuity is re-established, mesenteric window is closed, the bowel segment is detubularized along its antimesenteric border and reconfigured (117,118).
- Alternatively, bowel division and side-to-side anastomosis may be done intracorporeally using endoscopic gastrointestinal stapling device with detubularization and freehand intracorporeal suturing to reconfigure the bowel (119).
- Incising the peritoneum, entering the space of Retzius, mobilization of the bladder.
- Vertical incision creating a large cystotomy (bivalving).
- Mobilization of the bowel patch, and fixing it at 6 and 12-o'clock positions.
- Circumferential completion of enterovesical anastomsis in quadrants intracorporeally with running sutures.

8.1.3 Results

Hedican and associates (1999) performed laparoscopic assisted bladder augmentation in eight patients. In addition to using a bowel segment for augmentation, in many of these cases they were also able to laparoscopically mobilize the appendix to perform a Mitrofanoff continent catheterizable stoma. They described using both ileum and cecum as the enteric patch for the bladder. The bladder augmentation was done through a low Pfannenstiel incision. Many of these patients were children and this allowed a rapid recovery with decreased pain as well as a good cosmetic result (120).

Gill and associates (2000) underwent laparoscopic enterocystoplasty for three patients with functionally reduced bladder capacities due to neurogenic causes: ileocystoplasty (n=1), sigmoidocystoplasty (n=1), and cystoplasty with cecum and proximal ascending colon (n=1). In all patients, bowel reanastomosis was performed by exteriorizing the bowel loop outside the abdomen. All three laparoscopic enterovesical anastomoses were water tight without postoperative urinary extravasation. The operative times were 5.3, 8, and 7 hours. The hospital stay was 7, 5, and 4 days (118).

Rackley and associates (2001) performed laparoscopic enterocystoplasty in 12 patients with functionally reduced bladder capacities owing to neurogenic causes. Procedures included ileocystoplasty (2), sigmoidocystoplasty (2), colocystoplasty (1), and cecocolocystoplasty with continent catheterizable ileal stoma (7). Total surgical time ranged from 5.3 to 8 hours (average 7.0 hours). The time of laparoscopic suturing ranged from 1.7 to 3.1 hours (average 2.4 hours). Blood loss was minimal and did not exceed 250 ml during any of the procedures (average 175 ml). The only intra-operative complication was a trocar-induced rectus sheath hematoma. Oral feeding was resumed by 24 hours in 11 of the 12 patients. The average hospital stay was 5.7 days and ranged from 3 to 7 days (117).

Unlike the previously published reports, where portions of the procedure were performed extracorporeally, Elliott and associates (2002) reported their technique of complete laparoscopic ileocystoplasty (119).

8.2 Laparoscopic autoaugmentation

Ehrlich and Gershman (1993), reported the first laparoscopic autoaugmentation in an 8-years-old child with a neurogenic bladder. In this case, the procedure required 70 min, follow-up of the patient at 1 year, documented improvement in his symptoms with rare incontinence (121).

In 1995, McDougall and colleagues described the initial laparoscopic retropubic autoaugmentation of the bladder in an adult (12). In this case, the extraperitoneal approach was used and the incision was made in the detrusor muscle leaving the mucosa intact. There was a significant drop in bladder pressure. At the 6-month follow-up, the bladder capacity increased from 85-350 ml. However, in a second case, while the procedure could be successfully completed, the long-term result was unsatisfactory.

Due to the success of enteric augmentation and the variable results with autoaugmentation, this procedure has largely fallen into disuse (122). Nevertheless, laparoscopic retropubic autoaugmentation allows a brief hospital stay and minor postoperative discomfort. Moreover, the laparoscopic approach should not complicate or preclude subsequent enterocystoplasty if necessary (123).

9. Conclusion

Laparoscopic enterocystoplasty is technically feasible and successfully emulates the established principles of open enterocystoplasty while minimizing operative morbidity. As is true in open surgery, various bowel segments can be fashioned and anastomosed to the bladder laparoscopically. The increased costs associated with laparoscopy and weight minimally invasive surgery in general have been a significant disadvantage; however, a pervious report on the costs of laparoscopic procedures concluded that increased surgical experience reduces the surgical time and length of hospital stay, thereby decreasing costs. Furthermore, the increased use of reusable instruments results in considerable economic benefits. Implementation of appropriate cost-saving strategies ultimately will result in decreased expenses associated with laparoscopy. Although laparoscopic enterocystoplasty is currently a lengthy procedure lasting twice as long as open surgery, further technical modifications and increasing experience will continue to reduce the surgical time involved. For patients with complex co-morbid illness who desire the improved quality of life associated with traditional augmentation cystoplasty, the reduced morbidity observed in the authors' series of patients undergoing a laparoscopic procedure makes this approach an attractive option to consider. The authors' initial experience suggests that laparoscopic enterocystoplasty has the potential to become a viable alternative to open enterocystoplasty.

10. References

[1] Mitchell ME, Plaire JC: Augmentation cystoplasty. In Gillenwater JY, Grayback JT, Howards SS, Mitchell ME (eds): Adult and Pediatric Urology. Philadelphia, Lippincot Williams and Wilkins, 2002, P. 2445.

[2] Lapides J, Diokno Ac, Gould FR, et al. Further observations of self - catheterization. J Urol 1976; 116: 169.

[3] Hendren WH, Hendren RB. Bladder augmentation: experience with 129 children and young adults. J Urol 1990; 144: 445.

[4] Mitchell ME, Piser JA. Intestinocystoplasty and total bladder replacement in children and young adults: follow-up in 129 cases. J Urol 1987; 138: 579.
[5] Nguyen DH, Mitchell ME. Gastric bladder reconstruction. Urol Clin North Am 1991; 18: 649.
[6] Bellinger MF. Urterocystoplasty. Curr Surg Tech Urol 1995; 8: 2.
[7] Cartwright PC, Snow BW. Bladder augmentation: early clinical experience. J Urol 1989; 142: 505.
[8] Cartwright Pc, Snow BW. Bladder augmentation: partial detrusor excision to augment the bladder without use of bowel.l J Urol 1989; 142: 1050.
[9] Dewan PA, Nicholls EA, Goth DW. Ureterocystoplasty: an extraperitoneal urothelial bladder augmentation technique. Eur Urol 1994; 2685.
[10] Ikeguchi HW, Stifelman MD, Hensle TW. Ureteral tissue expansion for bladder augmentation. J Urol 1998; 159: 1665.
[11] Kropp BP, Sawyer BD, Shannon HE, et al. characterization of small intestine submucosa regenerated canine detrusor: assessment of reinnervation in vitro compliance and contractility. J Urol 1996; 156: 599.
[12] Pope JC, Davis MM, Smith ER, et al. ontogeny of canine small intestine submucosa regenerated bladder. J Urol 1997; 158: 105.
[13] Atala A: Tissue Engineering Perspectives for reconstructive surgery. In Walsh PC, Retick AB, Vaughan ED, Jr, Wein AJ (eds); Campbell's Urology. Philadelphia, WB Sauders, 2002, P. 2523.
[14] Colvert JR, Kropp BP, Cheng EY: Bladder augmentation: Current and future techniques. AUA update series 2003: 22 (32) - 250.
[15] DeMarco RT, Koch MO: Metabolic complications of continent urinary diversion AUA update series: 22 (15) - 114.
[16] Hinman F Jr. Selection of intestinal segments for bladder substitution: physical and physiological characteristics. J Urol 1988; 139: 519.
[17] Koff SA. Guidelines to determine the size and shape of intestinal segments used for reconstruction. J Urol 1988; 140: 1150.
[18] Goldwasser B. Barrett DM, Webster GD, et al: Cystometric properties of ileum and right colon after bladder augmentation. Substitution or replacement. J Urol 1987: 138: 1007.
[19] Adams MC, Mitchell ME, Rink RC. Gastrocystoplasty: An alternative solution to the problem of urological reconstruction in the severely compromised patient. J Urol 1988; 140: 1152.
[20] Adams MC, Brock JW, Pope JC, et al. Ureterocystoplasy: is it necessary to detubularize the distal ureter? J Urol 1998; 160: 851.
[21] Gonzalez R, Cabral BHP. Rectal continence after enterocystoplasty. Dialysis Pediatr Urol 1987; 10 (12): 3.
[22] Abol-Enein H, Ghoneim MA: A novel uretero-ileal reimplantation technique: the serous lined extramural tunnel. A preliminary report. J Urol 1994; 151: 1193.
[23] Mitchell ME: Use of Bowel in undiversion. Urol Clin North Am 1986; 13: 349.
[24] Gonzalez R. Buson H. Reid C, Reinbert Y: Sermoucular colocystoplasty lined with urothelium: experience with 16 patients. Urology 1994; 45: 124-129.

[25] King LR: Cystoplasty in children. In King LR, Stone AR, Webster GD (eds): Bladder Reconstruction and Continent Urinary Diversion, 2nd ed. St. Louis, Mosby - Year Book, 1991, 115-125.
[26] Cain MP, Husmann DA: Cecal bladder augmentation with a tapered catheterizable stoma: A modification of the Indiana pouch. Presented at the Urology Section Meeting. American Academy of Pediatrics. Dallas. TX, 1994.
[27] Cain MP, Casale AJ, King SJ, Rink RC: Appendicoversicostomy and newer alternatives for the Mitrofanoff procedure: Results in the last 100 patients at Riley children's Hosptial. J Urol 1999; 54: 909-912.
[28] Leong CH: The use of gastrocystoplasty. Dialog Pediatr Urol 1988; 11: 3-5.
[29] Adams MC, Mitchell ME, Rink PC: Gastrocystoplasty: An alternative solutioni to the problem of urological reconstruction in the severely compromised patient. J Urol 1988; 140: 1152-1156.
[30] Mitchell ME, Rinck RC, Adams MC: Augmentation cystoplasty, implantation of artificial urinary sphincter in men and women, and reconstruction of the dysfunction urinary tract. In Walsh PC, Retik AB. Stamey TZ, Vaughn ED, (eds): Campbell's Urology, 6th ed. Philadelphia. WB Saunders, 1992, pp 2630-2653.
[31] Raz S, Ehrilich RM, Babiarz JW, et al: Gastrocystoplasty without opening the stomach. J Urol 1993; 150: 713-715.
[32] Reinberg Y, Manivel JC, Froemming C, et al: Perforation of the gastric segment of an augmented bladder secondary to peptic ulcer disease. J Urol 1992: 148 (2 pt 1). 369-371.
[33] Sheldon CA, Gibert A, Wacksman J, et al: Gastrocystoplasty: Technical and metabolic characteristics of the post versatile childhood bladder augmentation modality [see comments]. J Pediatr Surg 1995: 30 (2): 283-287: discussion 287-288.
[34] Kajbafzadeh AM, Quinr. FM, Duffy PG, et al: Augmentation cystoplasty in boys with posterior urethral values. J Urol 1995: 154 (2 pt 2): 874-877.
[35] Docimo SG, Moore RG, Adams J, et al: Laparoscopic bladder augmentation using stomach. Urol 1995: 46 (4): 565-569.
[36] Kurzock EA, Baskin LS, Kogaa Ba: Gastocystoplasty: Is there a consensus? World Urol 1998: 16 (4): 242-250
[37] Kurzrock EA, Baskin LS. Kogan BA: Gastrocystoplasty: long–term follow up. J Urol 1998. 160 (6 pt 1): 2182-2166.
[38] Atala A, Bauer SB, Hendren WH, et al: The effect of gastric augmentation on bladder function. J Urol 1993: 149: 1099-1102.
[39] Gosalbez R, Woodard JR, Broecher BH, et al: The use of stomach in pediatric urinary reconstruction. J Urol 1993. 150 (2 pt 1): 438-440.
[40] Goldwasser B, Webster GD: Augmentation and substitution enterocystoplasty. J Urol 1986; 138, 215-224.
[41] Rink RC, Mclaughlin KP: Indication for enterocystoplasty and choice of bowel segment. Probl Urol 1994; 8: 389-403.
[42] Studer UE, Zingg EJ: Ileal orthotopic bladder substitutes: What we have learned from 12 years, experience with 200 patients. Urol Clin North Am 1997; 24: 781-793.
[43] Shekarriz B, Upadhyay J, Demirbilek S, et al: Surgical complications of bladder augmentation: Comparison between various enterocystoplasties in 133 patients. Urology 2000; 55: 123-128.

[44] Lytton B, Green DF: Urodynamic studies in patients undergoing bladder replacement surgery. J Urol 1989; 141: 1984.
[45] Jakobsen H, Steven K, Stigsby B, et al: Pathogensis of nocturnal urinary incontinence after ileocecal bladder replacement: continuous measurement of urethral closure pressure during sleep. Br J Urol 1987; 59: 148-152.
[46] Hedlund H, Lindstrom K, Mansson W: Dynamics of a continent Cecal reservoir for urinary diversion. Br J Urol 1984; 56: 366-372.
[47] Thuroff JW, Alken P, Reidmiller H, et al: 100 cases of Mainz pouch: Continuing Experience and evolution. J Urol 1988: 140: 283.
[48] Sidi AA, Reinberg Y, Gonzalez R: Influence of intestinal segment and configuration on the outcome of augmentation enterocystoplasty. J Urol 1986b; 136: 1201-1204.
[49] Berglund B, Kock NG, Norlen L, Philipson BM: Volume capacity and pressure characteristics of the continent ileal reservoir used for urinary diversion. J Urol 1987; 137: 29.
[50] Adams MC, Bihrle R, Rink RC: The use of stomach in urologic reconstruction. AUA Update Series 1995; 27: 218-223.
[51] Rink RC, Hollensbe D, Adams MC: complications of augmentation in children and comparison of gastrointestinal segments. Americal Urological association Update series 1995: 14: 122-128.
[52] Mitchell ME, Piser JA: Intestinocystoplasty and total bladder replacement in children and young adults: Follow-up in 129 cases. J Urol 1987; 138: 579-584.
[53] Roth S, Semjonow A, Waldner M, Hertle L: Risk of Bowel dysfunction with diarrhea after continent urinary diversion with ileal and ileocecal segments. J Urol 1995; 154: 1696-1699.
[54] Smith RB, Can Cangh P, Skinner DG, et al. Augmentation enterocystoplasty: a critical review. J Urol 1977; 118: 799.
[55] Rogers E, Scardino PT: A simple ileal substitute bladder after cystectomy: Experience with a modification of the Studer pouch. J Urol 1995; 153: 1432-1438
[56] Pannek J, Haupt G, Schulze H, et al: Influence of continent ileal urinary diversion on vitamin B12 absorption. J Urol 1996; 155: 1206-1208.
[57] Mills RD, Studer UE: Metabolic consequences of continent urinary diversion. J Urol 1999; 161: 1057-1066.
[58] Koch MO, McDougal WS, Thomson CO: Mechanisms of solute transport following urinary diversion through intestinal segments: An experimental study with rats. J Urol 1991; 146: 1390-1397.
[59] Poulsen AL, Steven K: Acid – base metabolism following bladder substitution with the ileal urethral Kock reservoir. Brit J Urol 1996; 78: 47-53.
[60] Hall MC, Koch MO, Halter SA, et al: Morphologic and functional alterations of intestinal segments following urinary diversion. J Urol 1993; 149: 664-666.
[61] Stein R. Fisch M, Ermert A, et al: Urinary diversion and orthotopic bladder substitution in children and young adults with neurogenic bladder: A safe option for treatment? J Urol 2000; 163: 568-573.
[62] Kock MO, McDougal WS, Reddy PK, et al: Metabolic alterations following continent urinary diversion through colonic segments. J Urol 1991; 145: 270-273.

[63] Kavaggia FF,Thompson JS, Schaefer EC, et al: Hyperammonemic encephalopathy in urinary diversion with urea-splitting urinary tract infection. Arch intern Med 1990; 150 (11): 2389-2392.
[64] Hessain M: The osteomalaica syndrome after colocystoplasty: A cure with sodium bicarbonate alone. Brit J Urol 1970; 42: 243-245.
[65] Wagstaff KE, Woodhouse CRJ, Rose GA, et al: Blood and urine analysis in patients with intestinal bladders. Brit J URol 1991; 68: 311-316.
[66] Mundy AR, Nurse DE: Calcium balance, growth and skeletal mineralizatin in patients with cystoplasties. Brit J Urol 1992; 69: 257-259.
[67] Palmer LS, Franco I, Koan SJ, et al: Urolithiasis in children following augmentation cystoplasty. J Urol 1993; 150: 726.
[68] Husman DA, Spence HM: Current status of tumor of the bowel following ureterosigmoidostomy: A review. J Urol 1990; 144: 607.
[69] Teriger BFG, Marshall FF: Carcinogenesis and the use of intestinal segments in the urinary tract. Urol Clin North Am 1991; 18: 737.
[70] Filmer RB, Spencer JR: Malignancies in bladder augmentations and intestinal conduits. J Urol 1990: 143: 671.
[71] Little JS, Klee LW, Hoover DM, Rink. RC: long-term histopathologic changes observed in rats subjected to augmentation cystoplasty. J Urol 1994; 152: 720-724.
[72] Carr LK, Herschorn S: Early development of adenocarcinoma in a young woman following augmentation cystoplasty for undiversion. J Urol 1997; 157: 2255-2256.
[73] Barrington JW, Fulford S, Griffiths D, Stephenson TP: Tumors in bladder remnant after augmentation enterocystoplasty. J Urol 1997; 157: 482-486.
[74] Pope JC, 4th, Albers P, Rink RC, Cain MP, et al: Spontaneous rupture of the augmented bladder from silence to chaos. Presented at the European Society of Pediatric Urologists Meeting, Istanbul, Turkey. 1999.
[75] Sheiner JR, Kaplan GW: Spontaneous bladder rupture following enterocystoplasty. J Urol 1988: 140: 1157-1158.
[76] Bauer SB, Hendren WH, Kozakewich H. et al: Perforation of the augmented bladder. J Urol 1992; 148: 699.
[77] Slaton JW, Kropp KA: Conservative management of suspected bladder rupture after augmentation enterocystoplasty. J Urol 1994; 152: 713-715.
[78] Cartwright PC, Snow BW: Bladder augmentation: Partial detrusor excision to augment to bladder without use of bowel. J Urol 1989; 142: 1050.
[79] Johnson HW, Nigro MK, Stothers L, et al: Laboratory variables of autoaugmentation in an animal model. Urology 1994; 44: 260-263.
[80] Stohrer M, Goepel M, Krmaer G, et al: Detrusor myectomy (auto augmentation) in the treatment of hyper-reflexive low compliance bladder. Urology 1999; 38: 30-37.
[81] Landa HM, Moorhead JD: Detrusorectomy. Probl Pediatr Urol 1994; 8: 204-209.
[82] Snow BW, Cartwright P: Why bladder autoaugmentation is a good choice for detrusor instability or bladder hyperreflexia. Contemp Urol 1999:11:96-100.
[83] Ahmed S, Sripathi V, Sen S: Perforation of an autoaugmented bladder autougmentation. New Urol Urdyn 1996 15 (3): 223-233.
[84] Landman J, et al: Laparascopic autoaugmentation of the urinary bladder: Literature review and state of the art. Ped Endo Inno Tech 2000; 4(3): 213-221.

[85] Leng WW, Blalock HJ, Fredriksson WH, et al: Enterocystoplasty or detrusor myectomy? Comparison of indications and outcomes for bladder augmentation. J Urol 1999; 161: 758-763.

[86] Dewan PA: Autoaugmentation demucosalized enterocystoplasty. World J Urol 1998: 16: 255-261.

[87] Salle JL, Fraga JC, Lucib A, et al: Seromuscular enterocystoplasty in dogs. J Urol 1990; 144: 454-456.

[88] Cheng E, Rento R, Grayhack TJ, et al: Reversed seromuscular flaps in the urinary tract in dogs. J Urol 1994; 152: 2252.

[89] Atala A: Commentary on the replacement of urologic associated mucosa. J Urol 1995: 156:338.

[90] Carr MC, Docimo SG, Mitchell ME: Bladder augmentation with urothelial preservation. J Urol (in press) 1999.

[91] Wolf JS Jr, Turzan CW: Augmentation urelerocystoplasty. J Urol 1993: 149(5): 1095-1098.

[92] Churchill BM, Aliabadi H, landau EH, et al: Ureteral bladder augmentation. J Urol 1993. 150 (2 pt 2): 716-720.

[93] Bellinger MF: Urelerocystoplasty update. World J Urol 1998: 16 (4): 251-254.

[94] Landau EH, Jayanthi VR, Khoury AE, et al: Bladder agumentation: Ureterocystoplasty versus ilcocystoplasty. J Urol 1994: 152 (2 pt 2): 716-719.

[95] Hitchcock RJ, Duffy PG, Malone PW: Ureterocystoplasty: The bladder augmentation of choice. Br J Urol 1994: 73(5):575-579.

[96] Ben-Chaim J, Partin AW, Jeffs RD: Ureteral bladder augmentation using the lower pole ureter of a duplicated system. Urol 1996: 47 (1): 135-137.

[97] Ahmed S, Neel KF, Sen S: Tandem Ureterocystoplasty. Aust N Z J Surg 1998: 68(3): 203-205.

[98] Lailas NG, Cilento B, Atala A: Progressive ureteral dilation for subsequent ureterocystoplasty. J Urol 1996: 156 (3): 1151-1153.

[99] Ikeguchi EF, Stifelman MD, Hensle IW: Ureteral tissue expansion for bladder augmentation. J Urol 1998: 159 (5): 1665-1668.

[100] Satar N, Yoo J, Atala A: Progressive bladder dilation for subsequent augmentation cystoplasty. J Urol 1999: 162: 829-831.

[101] Atala A: New methods of bladder augmentation. BJU international (2000), 85, suppl. 3, 24-34.

[102] Kim BS, Mooney DK: Development of biocompatible synthetic extracellular matrices for tissue engineering. Trends Biotechnol 1998: 16:224-230.

[103] Atala A: Future perspectives in reconstructive surgery using tissue engineering. Urol Clin North Am 1999; 26:157-165, ix-x.

[104] Atala A: Autologous cell transplantation for urologic reconstruction. J Urol 1998; 159: 2.

[105] Pariente JL, Kim BS, Atala A: In vitro biocompatibility assessment of naturally derived and synthetic biomaterials using normal human urothelial cells. J Biomed Mater Res 2001: 55: 33-39.

[106] Fishman U, flores En, Scott B, et al: Use of fresh placental membranes for bladder reconstruction. J Urol 1987: 138: 1291.

[107] Kambic H, Kay R, Chen JF, et al: Biodegradable pericardial implants for bladder augmentation: a 2.5 year study in dogs. J Urol 1992; 539-543.
[108] Scott R, Mohammed R, Gorham SD, et al: The evolution of a biodegradable membrane for use in urological surgery: A summary of 109 in vivo experiments. Br J Urol 1988: 62(1): 26-31.
[109] Kropp BP: Small-intestinal submucosa for bladder augmentation. A review of preclinical studies. World J Urol 1998: 16 (4): 262-267.
[110] Kropp BR, Rippy MK, Badylak SF, et al: Regenerative urinary bladder augmentation using small intestinal submucosa: Urodynamic and histopathologic assessment in long-term canine bladder augmentations. J Urol 1996: 155 (6): 2098-2104.
[111] Piechota HJ, Dahms SE, Nunes LS, et al: In vitro functional properties of the rat bladder regenerated by the bladder acellular matrix graft. J Urol 1998: 159(5): 1717-1724.
[112] Probst M, Dahiya R, Garrier S, tanagho EA: Reproduction of functional smooth muscle tissue and partial bladder replacement. Br J Urol 1997; 79: 505-515.
[113] Yoo JJ, Men J, Oberpenning F: A bladder augmentation using allogenic bladder submucosal seeded with cells. Urol 1998: 51(2): 221-225.
[114] Atala A, Vacanti JP, Peters CA, et al: Formation of urothelial structures in vivo from dissociated cells attached to biodegradable polymer scaffolds in vitro. J Urol 1992b; 148:658.
[115] Atala A, Freeman MR, Vacanti JP, et al: Implantation in vivo and retrieval of artificial structures consisting of rabbit and human urothelium and human bladder muscle. J Urol 1993b; 150:608-612.
[116] Oberpenning F. Meng J, Yoo JJ, et al: De novo reconstitution of a functional mammalian urinary bladder by tissue engineering [see comments]. Nat Biotechnol 1999; 17(2): 149-155.
[117] Rackley RR, Abdelmalak JB: Laparoscopic augmentation cystoplasty: surgical technique; Urol Clin Nor Am (2001); 28 (3): 663.
[118] Gill IS, Rackley RR, Merancy AM, et al.: Laparoscopic enterocystoplasty. Urology (2000); 55(2): 178 – 81.
[119] Elliolt SP, Meng MV, Anwar HP, et al.: Complete laparoscopic ileal cystoplasty. Urology (2002); 59(6): 939 – 43.
[120] Hedican SP, Schulam PG, Docimo SG (1999): Laparoscopic assisted reconstructive surgery: J Urol 161(1): 267- 270.
[121] Ehrlich RM, Gershman A (1993): Laparoscopic seromyotomy (auto-augmentation) for non-neurogenic neurogenic bladder in a child: initial case report. Urology 42(2): 175 – 178.
[122] McDougall EM, Clayman RV, Figenshau RS, Pearle MS (1995): Laparoscopic Retropubic autoaugmentation of the bladder. J Urol 153: 123– 126.
[123] Baren V, Bishop MR: Laparosopic bladder autoaugmentation in children. Urol. Clin. N. Am. (1998); 25 (3): 533 – 40.

Part 2

Special Considerations

15

ABO-Incompatible Kidney Transplantation

Mina Hur, Hee-Won Moon and Seog-Woon Kwon
Konkuk University and University of Ulsan
Korea

1. Introduction

ABO antigens are composed of sugar chains and exist not only on red cells but also on many other cells including endothelial cells and epithelial cells of various organs such as kidney, heart, bowel, lung, and pancreas (Marionneau et al., 2001). ABO antibodies, which have been called as isoagglutinins, are preformed antibodies directed against missing A or B antigens. The source of anti-A/B antibodies is thought to be gastrointestinal and environmental bacteria, such as the enterobacteriaceae, which possess ABO-like structures on their lipopolysaccharide coats (Yamamoto, 2004). These preformed ABO antibodies are clinically important in transfusion and organ transplantation medicine because they can cause acute hemolytic transfusion reaction in ABO-incompatible (ABO-I) blood transfusion and hyperacute rejection in ABO-I organ transplantation.

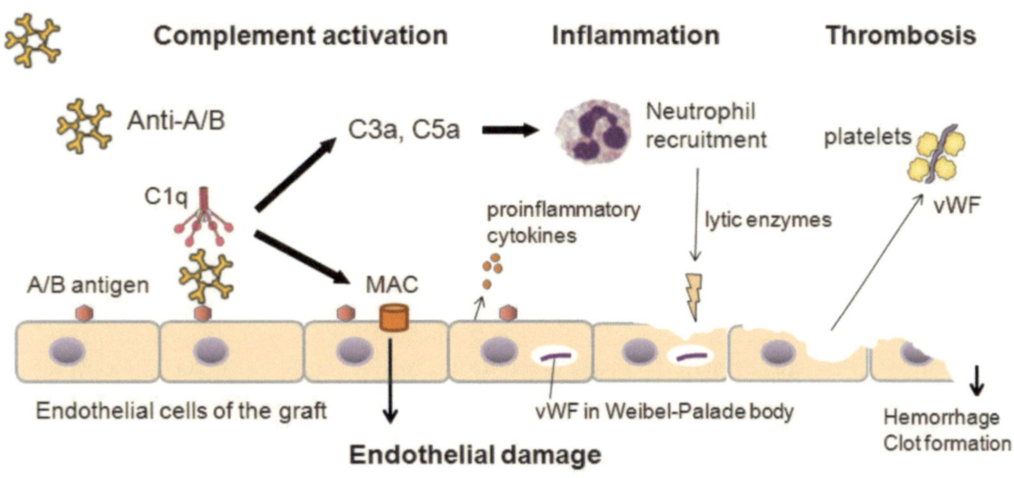

Fig. 1. Proposed mechanism of hyperacute rejection in ABO-incompatible organ transplantion.

Hyperacute rejection is induced by the binding of anti-A/B to antigens expressed on the endothelial cells of the ABO-I graft and activation of complement system (Fig. 1). Subsequently, endothelial damage, inflammation and platelet aggregation can be provoked, leading to vascular thrombosis, occlusion of blood supply and rejection.

ABO-I kidney transplantations were first reported in late 1950s and early 1960s (Hume et al., 1955; Murray et al., 1960; Starzl et al., 1964; Kissmeyer-Nielsen et al., 1966). These early experiences showed that hyperacute rejection could occur, and therefore, crossing the ABO barrier was excluded in the field of kidney transplantation.

In 1981, Slapak et al. first introduced the concept of depleting anti-A/B antibodies when they used modified plasmapheresis and successfully overcame the major donor-recipient blood group incompatibility in kidney transplant patient. Later, the same group reported on pre-transplantation immunoadsorption and plasmapheresis for ABO-I kidney transplantation, showing a high survival rate of 87% (Slapak et al., 1990).

Another group also started a living donor ABO-I kidney transplantation program in 1982, after this group inadvertently experienced an ABO-I cadaver kidney transplantation due to an error in donor ABO typing. In spite of the A_1 to O major ABO-incompatibility, the kidney graft from ABO-I cadaver functioned well with a basic immunusuppressive regimen including a short course of polyclonal antibody with azathioprine, and has been reported to be still functioning 22 years later (Squifflet et al., 2004). In this group, plasmapheresis was chosen to remove antibodies before transplantation and to prevent the occurrence of antibody-mediated hyperacute rejection. In addition, the immunosuppressive regimen was started 3 days prior to transplantation, and splenectomy was performed on the day of transplantation (Alexandre et al., 1985a, 1985b, 1986). Although the transplantation was successful, the return and persistence of anti-donor blood-group antibody was observed in spite of chronic immunosuppression. However, even with the continued presence of these antibodies and the persistence of the target antigen in the kidney, most of the graft continued to function well (Alexandre et al., 1991; Cardella et al., 1987; Reding et al., 1987). It was suggested that ABO blood group incompatibility need not be an absolute barrier to successful kidney transplantation.

2. Accommodation

It has been observed that ABO-I kidney grafts functioned well without rejection in recipients having high titers of anit-A/B antibodies. This phenomenon has been termed accommodation and regarded as an acquired resistance of an organ to immune-mediated damage (Bach et al., 1997; Lynch & Platt, 2008, 2010; Platt et al., 1990). In accommodation state, the graft is not pathologically injured despite the presence of circulating anti-donor antibodies.

The mechanism of accommodation is yet to be elucidated. It was postulated that accommodation might be involved in change in antibodies, change in antigen, modified control of complement, or acquired resistance to injury (Lynch & Platt, 2008). Complement regulation was thought to be essential for the survival of transplants over time and thus for accommodation to be manifested. C4d deposition without signs or symptoms of rejection can be observed in accommodated kidney (Lynch & Platt, 2010). The occurrence of complement activation means that antibody binding is intact in accommodated kidneys, and the lack of lysis means that some regulatory pathways are working for graft survival in the accommodation.

Three possible outcomes of the binding of complement-fixing alloantibody to endothelial cells have been postulated (Colvin & Smith, 2005). Hyperacute or acute rejection can be resulted, if the complement is fully activated. Accommodation can be achieved, if complement activation is completely inhibited. Incomplete inhibition of complement might be sufficient to prevent cell lysis but not to prevent complement activation, leading to endothelial cell activation and chronic antibody-mediated rejection (AMR).

Studies in mice showed that, in the absence of T-cell help, B cells that are exposed to incompatible carbohydrate antigens on allografts differentiate into cells that can produce non-complement-fixing antibody, and these B cells gradually become tolerant after prolonged exposure (Ogawa et al., 2004).

An acquired resistance to injury could reflect accommodation more comprehensively, but does not exclude other mechanisms. Actually, such resistance or protection could be appreciated, if some antibodies bind to graft and some complements are activated. Park et al. (2003) used microarrays, and compared five 1-year protocol ABO-compatible renal graft biopsies to four accommodated ABO-I graft biopsies. They identified significant alterations in gene expression in 440 probe sets, including SMADs, protein tyrosine kinases, TNF-alpha and Mucin 1. They concluded that accommodation is always present in well-functioning, long-surviving ABO-I kidney transplants. Regarding this self-protection against antibody-mediated damage, several novel mechanisms were suggested including the disruption of normal signal transduction, attenuation of cellular adhesion, and the prevention of apoptosis.

Accommodation is regarded as a good response to transplantation. It prevents acute antibody-mediated injury, thus allowing chronic process to ensue over time. Accommodation can be induced when antibodies that would cause rejection of a graft are removed from a recipient and then later return. In addition to this induced type, accommodation can occur spontaneously, without depleting antibodies. In this regard, the prevalence of accommodation would be higher than expected, and spontaneous accommodation may be the most common outcome of clinical organ transplantation (Tang & Platt, 2007). Accommodation still remains an evolving concept, and has a mixed support from experimental and clinical findings. The most important unanswered questions are how often and by which mechanisms accommodation occurs (Lynch & Platt, 2010). Accumulation of clinical evidences and research data would bring progress in understanding the biological implications of accommodation.

3. Current practice

The earlier works in the early 1980s were expanded greatly in Japan, where ABO-I kidney transplantation has been performed in more than 1,000 patients since 1989, and recently accounts for about 18% of all living donor kidney transplants (Takahashi, 2007). Later, a number of centers in USA and Europe have begun ABO-I kidney transplantations using similar protocols (Crew & Ratner, 2010).

The clinical outcome of ABO-I kidney transplantation improved remarkably in the last 10-15 years since the routine use of tacrolimus and mycophenolate. Clinical literatures repeatedly showed that ABO-I kidney transplantation has outcomes comparable to ABO-compatible kidney transplantation (Haidinger et al., 2009; Jeon et al., 2010; Kenmochi et al., 2008; Oettl et al., 2009; Thielke et al., 2007). One-year and five-year survival rates of ABO-I kidney transplants showed little difference from those of ABO-compatible kidney transplants, and their renal functions based on creatinine levels also showed no difference. Recently, the Japanese data on 851 ABO-I kidney transplantations was summarized (Tanabe, 2007a). According to this report, 1-, 3-, 5-, and 10-year patient survivals have been 95%, 92%, 90%, and 85%, respectively, whereas 1-, 3-, 5-, and 10-year graft survivals have been 89%, 85%,

79%, and 61%, respectively. These improved outcomes are attributed to a clearer understanding of the mechanisms underlying accommodation and acute AMR, permitting the development of new therapeutic strategies. There were significant differences in graft survival and the incidence of rejection before and after the introduction of tacrolimus/mycophenolate mofetil.

3.1 Induction therapies

Initial protocols for ABO-I kidney transplantation included splenectomy, which was performed in most recipients until 2004. Recently, a monoclonal antibody directed against CD20 on B cells, rituximab, has replaced splenectomy in most centers (Fig. 2). The use of rituximab eliminated the need for additional surgical intervention, and the outcomes with rituximab infusion alone were equal to those with splenectomy, providing more evidence that splenectomy is unnecessary (Crew & Ratner, 2010; Tanabe et al., 2009).

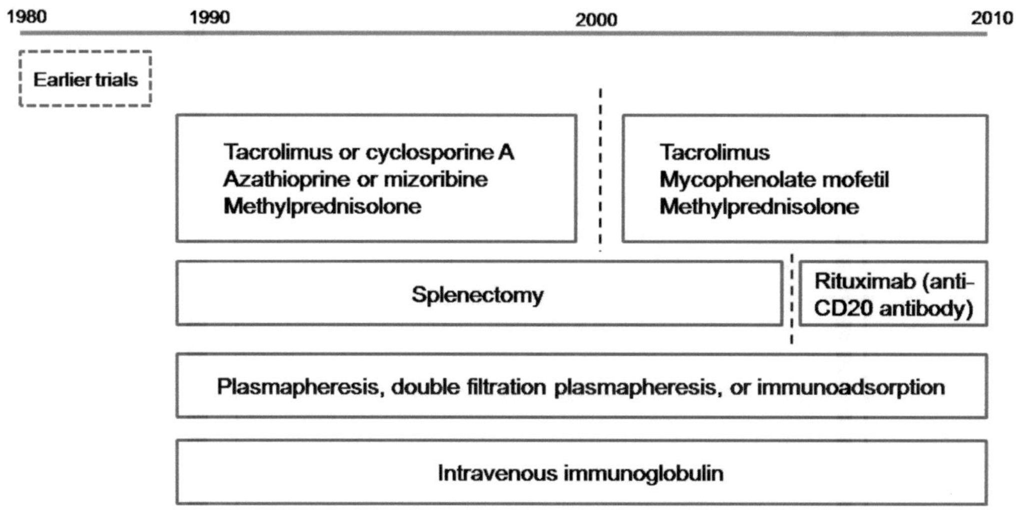

Fig. 2. Changes of preconditioning protocols for ABO-incompatible kidney transplantation. Between 1989 and 1999, a triplicate immunosuppressive regimen consisted of tacrolimus or cyclosporine A plus azathioprine or mizoribine plus methylprednisolone. Since 2000, tacrolimus, mycophenolate mofetil, and methylprednisolone have been used. Splenectomy was performed until 2004, and recently anti-CD20 antibody (rituximab) became an alternative to splenectomy. In most cases, 3-7 sessions of plasmapheresis or immunoadsorption have been performed before transplantation.

Rituximab as an alternative to splenectomy markedly reduced the incidence of AMR and greatly improved the results, becoming a clinically proven effective regimen for a successful ABO-I kidney transplantation. Interestingly, one recent study reported excellent outcomes without splenectomy or rituximab, questioning whether rituximab is indeed necessary (Segev et al., 2005). The authors suggested that rapid allograft accommodation may limit the need for long-term antibody suppression provided by splenectomy or anti-CD20, thereby eliminating the added infectious risk of these modalities and removing another disincentive to ABO-I transplantation.

Before 2000, a triplicate immunosuppressive regimen consisting of tacrolimus or cyclosporine A plus azathioprine or mizoribine plus methylprednisolone was mainly used. Thereafter, tacrolimus, mycophenolate mofetil, and methylprednisolone were used at most institutions. A greater incidence of acute rejection that was observed during the cyclosporine A era was markedly reduced in the tacrolimus era. In particular, the routine use of tacrolimus and mycophenolate mofetil significantly reduced acute rejection rates in patients with high-pretransplant isoagglutinin titers, and improved their outcomes to the levels comparable to those with low titers (Ishida et al., 2007).

3.2 Antibody reduction therapies

In all protocols, plasmapheresis to reduce and control anti-A or –B titers is a central feature. In most cases, ABO-I kidney transplantation recipients underwent 3-7 sessions of plasmapheresis (therapeutic plasma exchange) or double-filtration plasmapheresis before transplantation to reduce isoagglutinin titers. Plasmapheresis effectively removes anti-ABO antibodies, and approximately 20% of reduction is expected in each treatment. Its side effects, which are observed in approximately 5% of patients, are mainly hypocalcemia and pruritus/urticaria, and are usually mild and well tolerated (Tobian et al., 2008, 2009).

Plasmapheresis removes not only ABO antibodies but also the other protective antibodies or clotting factors, potentially increasing the risk of perioperative infection or bleeding. In contrast to plasmapheresis, immunoadsorption method can selectively remove anti-ABO antibodies, unaffecting the levels of the other plasma proteins. The blood type-specific columns can effectively remove anti-A or anti-B antibodies, and approximately 30% of anti-A/B IgM and 20% of anti-A/B IgG levels can be removed after a single treatment (Valli et al., 2009). In spite of its physiologic technique and successful clinical applications, the high cost of immunoadsorption column is a major limiting factor blocking its widespread use. The absence of randomized trials, which compared plasmapheresis and immunoadsorption, makes precise comparison of cost and outcomes impossible at the current point.

Plasmapheresis is a form of therapy to separate plasma from a person's circulating blood, removing pathogenic substances in plasma, and returning the remainder to the patient, usually with replacement fluids. The removal of a pathologic substance is affected by its concentration in circulating blood, the processing volume of blood and the degree of intravascular distribution. For example, IgM or fibrinogen are efficiently removed due to their predominantly intravascular distribution compared to IgG, which is predominantly extravascular. The alteration of immunoglobulin after single-plasma volume exchange was reported as about 63% decrease from baseline (Orlin & Berkman, 1980). An example of the changes of anti-A and anti-B antibody titers and creatinine levels before and after ABO-I kidney transplantation is shown in Fig. 3 (Moon et al., 2009). Efficiency of antibody removal is variable according to the patients. It is important that recipients or potential recipients of ABO-I kidneys should receive plasma that contains no ABO antibody against the graft for transfusion or plasmapheresis.

Plasmapheresis is indicated in various diseases such as thrombotic thrombocytopenic purpura, myasthenia gravis, or hyperviscosity in monoclonal gammopathy. Regarding indication for plasmapheresis, The American Society for Apheresis (ASFA) has published the guidelines and recommendations (Szczepiorkowski et al., 2010). According to this ASFA guideline, ABO-I kidney transplantation is classified as category II, in which plasmapheresis is generally accepted but considered to be supportive or adjunctive to other, more definite treatments, rather than a primary first-line therapy.

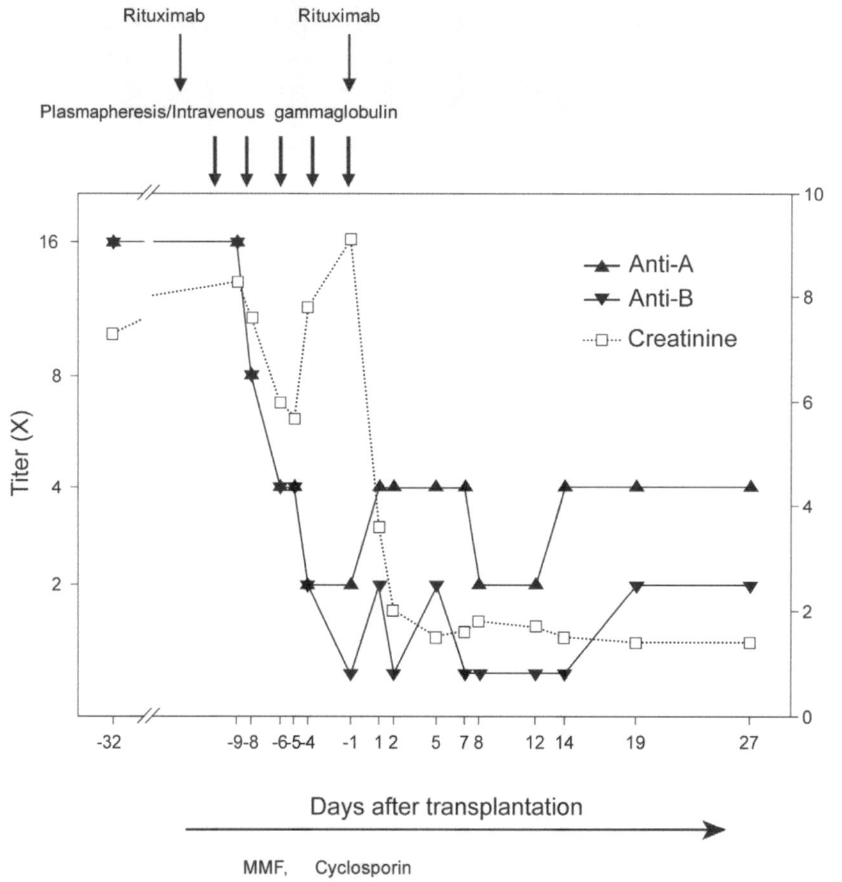

Fig. 3. An example of the changes of anti-A/anti-B antibody titers and creatinine levels before and after ABO-incompatible kidney transplantation. The patient's blood type was O, Rh+ and the donor's blood type was B, Rh+. A combination therapy with plasmapheresis, intravenous gammaglobulin, rituximab and potent immunosuppression was performed. Although the patient's baseline anti-A and anti-B titers were relatively low (1:16 for both anti-A and anti-B), titers were successfully decreased after each plasmapheresis procedure (average 1 fold), finally decreased to 1:1. The kidney transplantation was successful without any sign of hyperacute or acute rejection (modified from the refernece by Moon, et al (2009) with permission of Korean Journal of Laboratory Medicine).

Generally, plasmapheresis is performed using automated instruments. These instruments have specialized devices for blood withdrawal, anticoagulation, separation, return of blood, replacement and discard or collection of separated substances. The separation process is performed by centrifugation or filtration. In centrifugation method, blood components are separated by specific gravity and divided as plasma, platelets, leukocytes and red blood cells. In filtration method, blood is passed through a filter, and blood components are separated by their differences in particle size. Filtration and centrifugation can be combined by using rotating filter.

In conventional plasmapheresis, smaller proteins such as albumin are also removed in addition to pathogenic molecules, antibody or high molecular weight proteins. In general, plasma separated with a plasma separator is discarded and replaced with the same volume of replacement fluid such as fresh frozen plasma or albumin solution. There are several options of plasmapheresis, which separate blood components more selectively.

Double filtration plasmapheresis (DFPP) uses two filters which have different pore sizes. In the first filter, blood is separated as plasma and cell components, and plasma is further separated by the second filter. Large molecular-weight proteins including immunoglobulins such as anti-donor isoagglutinins are removed, while smaller molecular-weight substances such as albumin are returned to the patient's circulation. In this procedure, need of replacement is decreased compared with conventional plasmapheresis, thus adverse effects related to the replacement fluid can be reduced (Fig. 4) (Genberg et al., 2010; Tanabe, 2007b).

In the immunoadsorption, specialized adsorption column selectively adsorbs a specific substance such as immunoglobulin or low-density lipoprotein. This process removes the element of interest specifically and the remaining elements are returned to the patients. Many kinds of immunoadsorption devices for the removal of various types of components are commercially available but generally expensive. For the removal of anti-A and -B antibody, AB antigen-specific carbohydrate columns (Glycosorb AB, Glycorex Transplantation AB, Lund, Sweden) were developed (Tyden et al., 2005) and have been widely used in more than 400 cases of ABO-I kidney transplantation (Genberg et al., 2010; Tyden et al., 2005; Winters et al., 2004). This procedure could decrease the complications associated with plasma exchange such as coagulopathy and transfusion reactions.

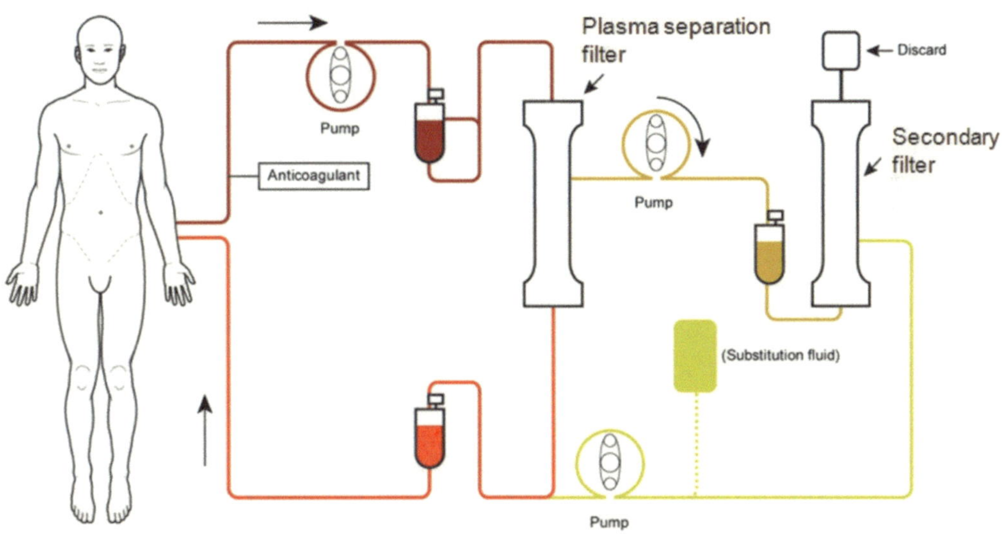

Fig. 4. Schematic presentation of double filtration plasmapheresis (DFPP). In DFPP, plasma separated with a plasma separator (1st filter) passes through the plasma component separator with a small pore size (2nd filter). Molecules that are larger than the pore size such as immunoglobulins are removed, and smaller molecules such as albumin are returned to the patient.

4. Determination of isoagglutinin titer

To reduce isoagglutinin titers prior to ABO-I kidney transplantation, preparative regimens including plasmapheresis, DFPP, or immunoadsorption and immunosuppressive therapy have been used. The clinical significance of isoagglutinin titer in ABO-I kidney transplantation is not entirely clear (Tobian et al., 2011). The goal of isoagglutinin titer to prevent hyperacute rejection is variable across transplantation centers, ranging from ≤ 1:8 to ≤ 1:32 before transplantation (Crew & Ratner, 2010). However, minimal research has been performed to determine the optimal pretransplant titer. The possibility of AMR would decrease as anti-donor antibody titer decreases. In our institution, the titer is lowered to ≤ 1:4 before transplantation. The measurement of isoagglutinin is known to be essential in the assessment of the efficacy of antibody removal, and the prediction of AMR (Kobayashi & Saito, 2006). Although most recipients with AMR had an elevated titer, the positive predictive value of a high titer for AMR was poor (Tobian et al., 2010). Thus, posttransplant titers should be monitored, but must be combined with the other factors assessing AMR.

Accurate measurement of isoagglutinin titer is an important aspect for successful ABO-I kidney transplantation. If the isoagglutinin titer is underestimated compared to the actual titer of patient, we could consider a patient as safe for transplantation and it could lead to rejection or short duration of allograft survival (Crew & Ratner, 2010). IgM antibody mediates complement activation and endothelial damage in AMR, and it is more rapidly removed by plasmapheresis than IgG. However, IgG titers are more emphasized for patient eligibility, rejection risk, and plasmapheresis guidance. Reporting both IgM and IgG titers has been recommended by a working group from US centers (Montgomery et al., 2004). Importantly, measured titers are method-dependent and considerably variable according to assays.

	Tube method	Column agglutination	Flow cytometry
A column ingredient	Not needed	Sephadex gel or glass bead	Not needed
Use of RBC	Yes	Yes	Yes
Antihuman globulin	Yes	Yes	No
Secondary antibody	No	No	Yes
Deletion of IgM	DTT or 2ME	DTT or 2ME	Not needed
Interpretation	Agglutination	Agglutination	Fluorescence detection
Result	Titer	Titer	MFIR or titer
Instrument	Not needed	Not needed	Needed
Cost	Low	Intermediate	Relatively high
Assay time	30 - 60 min	30 - 60 min	1- 2 hours

DTT, dithiothreitol; 2ME, 2-mercaptoethanol; MFIR, mean fluorescence intensity ratio.

Table 1. Various assays for measurement of isoagglutinin titer

There are several options for the measurement of isoagglutinin titers: conventional tube method, gel or bead column agglutination method, and flow cytometry (Krishnan et al., 2008; Stussi et al., 2005). These three methods are summarized in Table 1. In addition, enzyme-linked immunosorbent assay technique (Lindberg et al., 2011; Rieben et al., 1991), surface plasmon resonance (Kimura et al., 2005; Yurugi et al., 2007), and KODE technology (Frame et al., 2007) were developed, although these methods are not routinely available in most institutions.

4.1 Conventional tube method

The conventional tube method has been used in most institutions for the semiquantitative measurement of isoagglutinin titers. IgG and IgM can be measured together, and if dithiothreitol or antiglobulin reagents are used, they can be measured separately. In general, recipient serum is serially diluted and incubated with RBC aliquots of the appropriate blood type in a test tube for about 10 minutes at room temperature. After the mixture is centrifuged, macroscopic agglutinations of RBCs are checked for IgM detection. For IgG detection, additional testing with antihuman globulin is performed to check the agglutination. Titers are determined as the highest dilution that produces 1+ macroscopic agglutination. However, technical variables greatly affect the results, and care should be taken to achieve the most uniform practice (Roback, 2008). Considerable inter-examiner variability may occur, because the titer is determined mainly by visual observation of agglutinated RBCs in tubes. Inter-institutional difference can also occur possibly due to variations in procedures and lack of assay standardizations.

A recent study reported the results of isoagglutinin titers from 26 different labs using sera from six patients of different blood groups (Kobayashi & Saito, 2006). In this report, inter-institutional variation between maximum and minimum value reached as much as 32-fold in IgM and 256-fold in IgG. These variations seemed to be due to different techniques between laboratories, but considerable variation was still noted after standardization of techniques. Another report also showed a large variation of isoagglutinin titers (a median three-fold difference) among three centers performing ABO-I kidney transplants in Germany and Sweden (Kumlien et al., 2007). In this report, gel hemagglutination technique significantly decreased inter-center difference (a median one titer difference) compared with tube methods.

4.2 Gel or bead column agglutination

In gel or bead column agglutination method, a cassette (or card) containing gels or beads is used. Commercially available assays include DiaMed ID Micro Typing system (Bio-Rad, Hercules, CA, USA), BioVue System (Ortho Clinical Diagnosis, Raritan, NJ, USA), or Olympus ID-Micro Typing System (Olympus Co., Tokyo, Japan). In these assays, plasma from the patient is stepwise diluted 1:2 with normal saline or phosphate buffered saline and packed RBCs are used to make a suspension with cell stabilization solution. In each incubation well, recommended cell suspension is mixed with diluted plasma. After incubation and centrifugation, agglutination is observed in card or cassette. In column agglutination method, negative (unagglutinated) test cells pellet to the bottom of the column, and positive (agglutinated) cells are captured at the top of or within the body of column (Fig. 5). The gel or bead particles trap the RBC agglutinates as a filter during centrifugation. The agglutination is graded from 0 to 4 +, and inverted value of the highest plasma dilution that gives a 1+ agglutination reaction is interpreted as the titer (Kumlien et al., 2007).

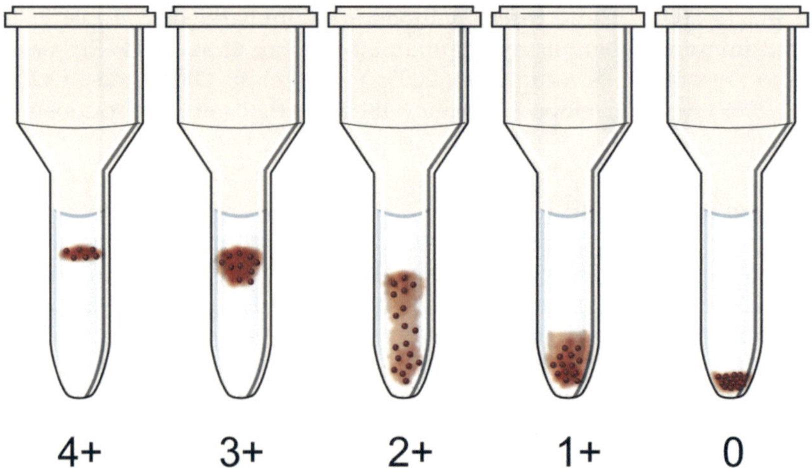

Fig. 5. Interpretation of column agglutination method. The agglutination is graded from 0 to 4+.

4.3 Flow cytometry

In flow cytometry method, quantifications of anti-A/B IgG and IgM are performed using fluorescence conjugated, anti-human IgG and IgM as secondary antibodies. A mixture of RBC suspension and recipient serum is transferred into the test tube and incubated (at 37°C in a CO_2 incubator for IgG antibody; and at room temperature, for IgM antibodies). After washing, fluorescence conjugated, anti-human IgG and IgM secondary antibodies are added in test tube. After incubation and washing steps, binding of anti-A/B antibody is measured by flow cytometry. Human AB serum, which is further depleted by incubation with highly concentrated A and B RBCs, can be used as a negative control, and human serum of blood group O is used as a positive control. Commercially available O RBCs with information of antigen expression are also helpful for the detection of irregular antibodies (Stussi et al., 2005).

Using undiluted serum, quantification of anti-A/B antibody can be determined by calculation of the geometric mean fluorescence intensity ratio (MFIR). This value is calculated by dividing the geometric mean fluorescence intensity of test sera with that of negative control. One study reported that the correlation coefficient between MFIR using flow cytometry and isoagglutinin titer was 0.870 for IgM and 0.783 for IgG (Stussi et al, 2005). For determination of titer using flow cytometry, recipient serum is serially diluted with normal saline solution (2% bovine serum albumin, 0.1% azide). After incubation and washing, secondary antibody is added. After reaction, binding of antibody is determined by flow cytometry. A gated value above assigned cut-off (5% for example) is regarded as positive serum dilution. In a study comparing the reproducibility of the results performed by various assays, flow cytometry showed excellent reproducibility and no measurement deviation was noted, whereas gel column agglutinin assay and tube technique showed two-fold and four-fold differences, respectively (Tanabe, 2007b). However, flow cytometry assay needs the flow cytometry instrument, and the reagents are relatively expensive.

5. Conclusion

The ABO blood group barrier is now being crossed in the field of transplantation, and ABO-I kidney transplantation is becoming more common worldwide. Removing the ABO barrier can expand the donor pool and increase the availability of organs for transplantation. Moreover, it can decrease the time on the organ waiting list, and eventually facilitate the timely transplantation before comorbid conditions develop in the patients. Currently observed long-term results of ABO-I kidney transplantation are similar to those of ABO-compatible kidney transplantation. With the application of adequate antibody reducing strategies, future results would be more promising. To promote accomodation and to prevent acute complement-mediated graft injury, methods for preventing and treating AMR are still needed. Researches for the insights into the mechanism of accomodation will provide us a scientific basis for the development of innovative approaches for the better outcome of ABO-I kidney transplantation.

As the number of ABO-I transplantation increases, there is a need of the optimal methods for ABO isoagglutinin titer for the effective monitoring of ABO-I transplanted patients. Compared with the conventional test tube method, gel card or flow cytometric measurement can provide more accurate and objective results. However, reproducibility, interpretation, and standardization of isoagglutinin titration methods are still unsatisfactory, and further researches should be performed to determine the optimal method for ABO antibody titer assessment. There are also several promising techniques under development, focused on the endothelium, enzymes, or blocking antibodies. Ongoing improvement of promising modalities could make more successful transplantation outcomes in this field.

6. Acknowledgment

The authors appreciate Professor Jin Q Kim, The President of Konkuk University, Korea, for his critical review and valuable comments on this work.

7. References

Alexandre, G.P.J.; De Bruyere, M.; Squifflet, J.P.; Moriau, M.; Latinne, D. & Pirson, Y. (1985). Human ABO-incompatible living donor renal homografts. *The Netherlands Journal of Medicine*, Vol. 28, No. 6, (August 1985), pp. 231-234, ISSN 0300-2977

Alexandre, G.P.J.; Squifflet, J.P.; De Bruyere, M.; Latinne, D.; Moriau, M.; Carlier, M.; Pirson, Y. & Lecomte, C. (1986). ABO-incompatible related and unrelated living donor renal allografts. *Transplantation Proceedings*, Vol. 18, No. 3, (May-June 1986), pp. 452-455, ISSN 0041-1345

Alexandre, G.P.J.; Squifflet, J.P.; De Bruyere, M.; Latinne, D.; Moriau, M. & Ikabu, N. (1985). Splenectomy as a prerequisite for successful human ABO-incompatible renal transplantation. *Transplantation Proceedings*, Vol. 17, No. 1 Pt. I, (January-February 1985), pp. 138-143, ISSN 0041-1345

Alexandre, G.P.J.; Latinne, D.; Gianello, P. & Squifflet, J.P. (1991). Preformed cytotoxic antibodies and ABO-incompatible grafts. *Clinical Transplantation*, Vol. 5, No. 6 Pt. II, (December 1991), pp. 583-594, ISSN 0902-0063

Bach, F.H.; Ferran, C.; Hechenleitner, P.; Mark, W.; Koyamada, N.; Miyatake, T.; Winkler, H.; Badrichani, A.; Candinas, D. & Hancock, W.W. (1997). Accommodation of vascularized xenografts: expression of "protective genes" by donor endothelial cells in a host Th2 cytokine environment. *Nature Medicine*, Vol. 3, No. 2, (February 1997), pp. 196-204, ISSN 1078-8956

Cardella, C.J.; Pei, Y. & Brady, H.R. (1987). ABO blood group incompatible kidney transplantation: a case report and review of the literature. *Clinical Nephrology*, Vol. 28, No. 6, (December 1987), pp. 295-299, ISSN 0301-0430

Colvin R. B. & Smith R.N. (2005). Antibody mediated organ allograft rejection. *Nature Review Immunology*, Vol. 5, No. 10, (October 2005), pp. 807-817, ISSN 1474-1733

Crew, R.J. & Ratner, L.E. (2010). ABO-incompatible kidney transplantation: current practice and the decade ahead. *Current Opinion in Organ Transplantation*, Vol. 15, No. 4, (August 2010), pp. 526-530, ISSN 1531-7013

Frame, T.; Carroll, T.; Korchagina, E.; Bovin, N. & Henry, S. (2007). Synthetic glycolipid modification of red blood cell membranes. *Transfusion*, Vol. 47, No. 5, (May 2007), pp. 876-882, ISSN 0041-1132

Genberg, H.; Kumlien, G.; Wennberg, L. & Tyden, G. (2010). Isoagglutinin adsorption in ABO-incompatible transplantation. *Transfusion and Apheresis Science*, Vol. 43, No. 2, (October 2010) pp. 231-235, ISSN 1473-0502

Haidinger, M.; Schmaldienst, S.; Körmöczi, G.; Regele, H.; Soleiman, A.; Schwartz, D.; Derfler, K.; Steininger, R.; Mühlbacher, F. & Böhmig, G.A. (2009). Vienna experience of ABO-incompatible living-donor kidney transplantation. *Wiener klinische Wochenschrift*, Vol. 121, No. 7-8, (June 2009), pp. 247-255, ISSN 0043-5325

Hume, D.L.; Merrill, J.P.; Miller, B.F. & Thorn, G.W. (1955). Experiences with renal homotransplantation in the human: report of nine cases. *The Journal of Clinical Investigation*, Vol. 34, No. 2, (February 1955), pp. 327-382, ISSN 0021-9738

Ishida, H.; Miyamoto, N.; Shirakawa, H.; Shimizu, T.; Tokumoto, T.; Ishikawa, N.; Shimmura, H.; Setoguchi, K.; Toki, D.; Iida, S.; Teraoka, S.; Takahashi, K.; Toma, H.; Yamaguchi, Y. & Tanabe, K. (2007). Evaluation of immunosuppressive regimens in ABO-incompatible living kidney transplantation--single center analysis. *American Journal of Transplantation*, Vol. 7, No. 4, (April 2007), pp. 825-831, ISSN 1600-6135

Jeon, B.J.; Kim, I.G.; Seong, Y.K. & Han, B.H. (2010). Analysis of the results of ABO-incompatible kidney transplantation: in comparison with ABO-compatible kidney transplantation. *Korean Journal of Urology*, Vol. 51, No. 12, (December 2010), pp. 863-869, ISSN 2005-6745

Kenmochi, T.; Saigo, K.; Maruyama, M.; Akutsu, N.; Iwashita, C.; Otsuki, K.; Ito, T.; Suzuki, A. & Miyazaki, M. (2008). Results of kidney transplantation from ABO-incompatible living donors in a single institution. *Transplantation Proceedings*, Vol. 40, No. 7, (September 2008), pp. 2289-2291, ISSN 0041-1345

Kimura, S.; Yurugi, K.; Segawa, H.; Kuroda, J.; Sato, K.; Nogawa, M.; Yuasa, T.; Egawa, H.; Tanaka, K. & Maekawa, T. (2005). Rapid quantitation of immunoglobulin G antibodies specific for blood group antigens A and B by surface plasmon resonance. *Transfusion*, Vol. 45, No. 1, (January 2005), pp. 56-62, ISSN 0041-1132

Kissmeyer-Nielsen, F.; Olsen, S.; Petersen, V.P. & Fjeldborg, O. (1966). Hyperacute rejection of kidney allografts associated with pre-existing humoral antibodies against donor cells. *Lancet*, Vol. 2, No. 7465, (September 1966), pp. 662-665, ISSN 0140-6736

Kobayashi, T. & Saito, K. (2006). A series of surveys on assay for anti-A/B antibody by Japanese ABO-incompatible Transplantation Committee. *Xenotransplantation*, Vol. 13, No. 2, (March 2006), pp. 136-140, ISSN 0908-665X

Krishnan, N. S.; Fleetwood, P.; Higgins, R. M.; Hathaway, M.; Zehnder, D.; Mitchell, D.; Hamer, R.; Fletcher, S.; Lam, F. T.; Kashi, H.; Tan, L. C.; Imray, C. & Briggs, D. (2008). Application of flow cytometry to monitor antibody levels in ABO incompatible kidney transplantation. *Transplantation*, Vol. 86, No. 3, (August 2008), pp. 474-477, ISSN 0041-1337

Kumlien, G.; Wilpert, J.; Safwenberg, J. & Tyden, G. (2007). Comparing the tube and gel techniques for ABO antibody titration, as performed in three European centers. *Transplantation*, Vol. 84, No. 12 Suppl, (December 2007), pp. S17-S19, ISSN 0041-1337

Lindberg, L.; Johansson, S.M.; Liu, J.; Grufman, P. & Holgersson, J. (2011). Is there a clinical need for a diagnostic test allowing detection of chain type-specific anti-A and anti-B. *Transfusion*, Vol. 51, No. 3, (March 2011), pp. 494-503, ISSN 1537-2995

Lynch, R.J. & Platt, J.L. (2008). Accommodation in organ transplantation. *Current Opinion in Organ Transplantation*, Vol. 13, No. 2, (April 2008), pp. 165-170, ISSN 1531-7013

Lynch, R.J. & Platt, J.L. (2010). Accommodation in renal transplantation: unanswered questions. *Current Opinion in Organ Transplantation*, Vol. 15, No. 4, (August 2010), pp. 481-485, ISSN 1531-7013

Marionneau, S.; Cailleau-Thomas, A.; Rocher, J.; Le Moullac-Vaidye, B.; Ruvoën, N.; Clément, M. & Le Pendu, J. (2001). ABH and Lewis histo-blood group antigens, a model for the meaning of oligosaccharide diversity in the face of a changing world. *Biochimie*, Vol. 83, No. 7, (July 2001), pp. 565-573, ISSN 0300-9084

Montgomery, R.A.; Hardy, M.A.; Jordan, S.C.; Racusen, L.C.; Ratner, L.E.; Tyan, D.B.; Zachary, A.A. & Antibody Working Group on the diagnosis, reporting, and risk assessment for antibody-mediated rejection and desensitization protocols. (2004). Consensus opinion from the antibody working group on the diagnosis, reporting, and risk assessment for antibody-mediated rejection and desensitization protocols. *Transplantation*, Vol. 78, No. 2, (July 2004), pp. 181-185, ISSN 0041-1337

Moon, H.W.; Yun, Y.M.; Hur, M.; Park, J.H.; Lee, H.W.; Chang, S.H. & Yun, I.J. (2009). An experience of ABO-incompatible kidney transplantation using plasmapheresis and anti-CD20 monoclonal antibody. *Korean Journal of Laboratory Medicine*, Vol. 29, No. 6, (December 2009), pp. 585-588, ISSN 1598-6535

Murray, J.E.; Merrill, J.P.; Dammin, G.J.; Dealy, J.B. Jr.; Walter, C.W.; Brooke, M.S. & Wilson, R.E. (1960). Study on transplantation immunity after total body irradiation: clinical and experimental investigation. *Surgery*, Vol. 48, (July 1960), pp. 272-284, ISSN 0039-6060

Oettl, T.; Halter, J.; Bachmann, A.; Guerke, L.; Infanti, L.; Oertli, D.; Mihatsch, M.; Gratwohl, A.; Steiger, J. & Dickenmann, M. (2009). ABO blood group-incompatible living donor kidney transplantation: a prospective, single-centre analysis including serial protocol biopsies. *Nephrology, Dialysis, Transplantation*, Vol. 24, No. 1, (January 2009), pp. 298-303, ISSN 1460-2385

Ogawa, H.; Mohiuddin, M.M.; Yin, D.P.; Shen, J.; Chong, A.S. & Galili, U (2004). Mouse-heart grafts expressing an incompatible carbohydrate antigen. II. Transition from accommodation to tolerance. *Transplantation*, Vol. 77, No. 3, (February 2004), pp. 366–373, ISSN 0041-1337

Orlin, J.B. & Berkman, E.M. (1980). Partial plasma exchange using albumin replacement: removal and recovery of normal plasma constituents. *Blood*, Vol. 56, No.6, (December 1980), pp. 1055-1059, ISSN 0006-4971

Park, W.D.; Grande, J.P.; Ninova, D.; Nath, K.A.; Platt, J.L.; Gloor, J.M. & Stegall, M.D. (2003). Accommodation in ABO-incompatible kidney allografts, a novel mechanism of self-protection against antibody-mediated injury. *American Journal of Transplantation*, Vol. 3, No. 8, (August 2003), pp. 952-960, ISSN 1600-6135

Platt, J.L.; Vercellotti, G.M.; Dalmasso, A.P., Matas, A.J., Bolman R.M., Najarian, J.S. & Bach, F.H. (1990). Transplantation of discordant xenografts: a review of progress. *Immunology Today*, Vol. 11, No. 12, (December 1990), pp. 450-456, ISSN 0167-5699

Reding, R.; Squifflet, J.P.; Latinne, D.; de Bruyere, M.; Pirson, Y. & Alexandre, G.P.J. (1987). Early postoperative monitoring of natural anti-A and anti-B isoantibodies in ABO-incompatible living donor renal allografts. *Transplantation Proceedings*, Vol. 19, No. 1 Pt 3, (Febrary 1987), pp. 1989-1990, ISSN 0041-1345

Rieben, R.; Buchs, J. P.; Fluckiger, E. & Nydegger, U. E. (1991) Antibodies to histo-blood group substances A and B: agglutination titers, Ig class, and IgG subclasses in healthy persons of different age categories. *Transfusion*, Vol. 31, No. 7, (September 1991), pp. 607-615, ISSN 0041-1132

Roback, J. D. (Ed.). (2008). *Technical Manual*. 16th ed. American Association of Blood Banks, ISBN 978-1563952609 (1563952602), Bethesda, USA.

Segev, D.L.; Simpkins, C.E.; Warren, D.S.; King, K.E.; Shirey, R.S.; Maley, W.R.; Melancon, J.K.; Cooper, M.; Kozlowski, T. & Montgomery, R.A. (2005). ABO incompatible high-titer renal transplantation without splenectomy or anti-CD20 treatment. *American Journal of Transplantation*, Vol. 5, No. 10, (October 2005), pp. 2570-2575, ISSN 1600-6135

Squifflet, J.P.; De Meyer, M.; Malaise, J.; Latinne, D.; Pirson, Y. & Alexandre, G.P. (2004). Lessons learned from ABO-incompatible living donor kidney transplantation: 20 years later. *Experimental and Clinical Transplantation*, Vol. 2, No. 1, (June 2004), pp. 208-213, ISSN 1304-0855

Slapak, M.; Naik, R.B. & Lee, H.A. (1981). Renal transplant in a patient with major donor-recipient blood group incompatibility: reversal of acute rejection by the use of modified plasmapheresis. *Transplantation*, Vol. 31, No. 1, (January 1981), pp. 4-7, ISSN 0041-1337

Slapak, M.; Digard, N.; Ahmed, M.; Shell, T. & Thompson, F. (1990). Renal transplantation across the ABO barrier - a 9 year experience. *Transplantation Proceedings*, Vol. 22, No. 4, (August 1990), pp. 1425-1428, ISSN 0041-1345

Starzl, T.E.; Marchioro, T.L.; Holmes, J.H.; Hermann, G.; Brittain, R.S.; Stonington, O.H., Talmage, D.W. & Waddell, W.R. (1964). Renal homografts in patients with major donor-recipient blood group incompatibilities. *Surgery*, Vol. 55, (Febrary 1964), pp. 195-200, ISSN 0039-6060

Stussi, G.; Huggel, K.; Lutz, H.U.; Schanz, U.; Rieben, R. & Seebach, J.D. (2005). Isotype-specific detection of ABO blood group antibodies using a novel flow cytometric method. *British Journal of Haematology*, Vol. 130, No. 6, (September 2005), pp. 954-963, ISSN 0007-1048

Szczepiorkowski, Z.M.; Winters, J.L.; Bandarenko, N.; Kim, H.C.; Linenberger, M.L.; Marques, M.B. ; Sarode, R.; Schwartz, J.; Weinstein, R. & Shaz, B.H. (2010). Guidelines on the use of therapeutic apheresis in clinical practice--evidence-based approach from the Apheresis Applications Committee of the American Society for Apheresis. *Journal of Clinical Apheresis*, Vol. 25, No.3, (June 2010), pp. 83-1217, ISSN 0733-2459

Takahashi, K. (2007). Recent findings in ABO-incompatible kidney transplantation: classification and therapeutic strategy for acute antibody-mediated rejection due to ABO-blood-group-related antigens during the critical period preceding the establishment of accommodation. *Clinical and Experimental Nephrology*, Vol. 11, No. 2, (June 2007), pp. 128-141, ISSN 1342-1751

Tanabe, K. (2007). Japanese experience of ABO-incompatible living kidney transplantation. *Transplantation*, Vol. 84, No. 12 Suppl, (December 2007), pp. S4-S7, ISSN 0041-1337

Tanabe, K. (2007). Interinstitutional variation in the measurement of anti-A/B antibodies: the Japanese ABO-Incompatible Transplantation Committee survey. *Transplantation*, Vol. 84, No. 12 Suppl, (December 2007), pp. S13-S16, ISSN 0041-1337

Tanabe, K.; Ishida, H.; Shimizu, T.; Omoto, K.; Shirakawa, H. & Tokumoto, T. (2009). Evaluation of two different preconditioning regimens for ABO-incompatible living kidney donor transplantation. A comparison of splenectomy vs. rituximab-treated non-splenectomy preconditioning regimens. *Contributions to Nephrology*, Vol. 162, (Febrary 2009), pp. 61-74, ISSN 0302-5144

Tang, A.H. & Platt, J.L. (2007). Accommodation of grafts: implications for health and disease. *Human Immunology*, Vol. 68, No. 8, (August 2007), pp. 645-651, ISSN 0198-8859

Thielke, J.; Kaplan, B. & Benedetti, E. (2007). The role of ABO-incompatible living donors in kidney transplantation: state of the art. *Seminars in Nephrology*, Vol. 27, No. 4, (July 2007), pp. 408-413, ISSN 0270-9295

Tobian, A.A.; Shirey, R.S. & King, K.E. (2011) ABO antibody titer monitoring for incompatible renal transplantation. *Transfusion*, Vol. 51, No. 3, (March 2011), pp. 454-457, ISSN 1537-2995

Tobian, A.A.; Shirey, R.S.; Montgomery, R.A.; Cai, W.; Haas, M.; Ness, P.M. & King, K.E. (2010). ABO antibody titer and risk of antibody-mediated rejection in ABO-incompatible renal transplantation. *American Journal of Transplantation*, Vol. 10, No. 5, (May 2010), pp. 1247-1253, ISSN 1600-6143

Tobian, A.A.; Shirey, R.S.; Montgomery, R.A.; Ness, P.M. & King, K.E. (2008). The critical role of plasmapheresis in ABO-incompatible renal transplantation. *Transfusion*, Vol. 48, No. 11, (November 2008), pp. 2453-2460, ISSN 1537-2995

Tobian, A.A.; Shirey, R.S.; Montgomery, R.A.; Tisch, D.J.; Ness, P.M. & King, K.E. (2009). Therapeutic plasma exchange reduces ABO titers to permit ABO-incompatible renal transplantation. *Transfusion*, Vol. 49, No. 6, (June 2009), pp. 1248-1254, ISSN 1537-2995

Tyden, G.; Kumlien, G.; Genberg, H.; Sandberg, J.; Lundgren, T. & Fehrman, I. (2005). ABO incompatible kidney transplantations without splenectomy, using antigen-specific immunoadsorption and rituximab. *American Journal of Transplantation*, Vol. 5, No.1, (January 2005), pp. 145-148, ISSN 1600-6135

Valli, P.V.; Puga, Y.G.; Fehr, T.; Schulz-Huotari, C.; Kaup, N.; Güngör, T.; Ambühl, P.; Weber, M.; Schanz, U.; Seebach, J.D. & Stussi, G. (2009). Changes of circulating antibody levels induced by ABO antibody adsorption for ABO-incompatible kidney transplantation. *American Journal of Transplantation*, Vol. 9, No. 5, (May 2009), pp. 1072-1080, ISSN 1600-6143

Winters, J.L.; Gloor, J.M.; Pineda, A.A.; Stegall, M.D. & Moore, S.B. (2004). Plasma exchange conditioning for ABO-incompatible renal transplantation. *Journal of Clinical Apheresis*, Vol. 19, No.2, (2004), pp. 79-85, ISSN 0733-2459

Yamamoto F. (2004). Review: ABO blood group system--ABH oligosaccharide antigens, anti-A and anti-B, A and B glycosyltransferases, and ABO genes. *Immunohematology / American Red Cross*, Vol. 20, No. 1, (March 2004), pp. 3-22, ISSN 0894-203X

Yurugi, K.; Kimura, S.; Ashihara, E.; Tsuji, H.; Kawata, A.; Kamitsuji, Y.; Hishida, R.; Takegawa, M.; Egawa, H. & Maekawa, T. (2007). Rapid and accurate measurement of anti-A/B IgG antibody in ABO-unmatched living donor liver transplantation by surface plasmon resonance. *Transfusion Medicine*, Vol. 17, No. 2, (April 2007), pp. 97-106, ISSN 0958-7578

16

Combined Liver and Kidney Transplantation

Cláudia Fagundes and Mónica Guevara*
Liver Unit/Hospital Clinic Barcelona
Spain

1. Introduction

Combined liver and kidney transplant (CLKT) is the procedure of choice for patients with both liver and kidney end-stage-disease. In addition, patients with polycystic liver or kidney disease or with hyperoxaluria, or those with cirrhosis and acute renal failure, including hepatorenal syndrome receiving hemodialysis (HD) for more than two months, may also benefit of CLKT.

The decision to transplant both, the liver and kidney, is more difficult in cases when kidney dysfunction may be temporary. Hepatorenal syndrome is a potentially reversible renal failure caused by advance liver disease. Currently, the treatment of choice of hepatorenal syndrome is liver transplant alone and not a combined liver/kidney transplant.

The model for end-stage liver disease (MELD) replaced the United Network for Organ Sharing status classification for the allocation of liver organs. Due to the heavily weighted serum creatinine value in the calculation of the MELD score, candidates with renal failure have received organs more rapidly. As a result there has been considerable increase in number of combined liver-kidney transplants in the past few years.

The reason to propose both liver and kidney transplant for patients with cirrhosis and renal failure relays on the negative impact that renal failure has on patients submitted to liver transplant alone (LTA). Results of several studies show that renal failure in patients with chronic liver disease is associated with high mortality and morbidity after liver transplant alone. Nevertheless, it's very hard to identify a cut-off point of renal dysfunction that determines those patients who may benefit from combined liver and kidney transplant instead of liver transplant alone.

In this chapter, we will review the main points to be considered when evaluating candidates for combined liver kidney transplant, as well as some concerns that have not been yet clarified.

2.Assessment of renal function and evaluating of CLKT in patients with end stage liver disease

Renal failure in cirrhotic patients is associated with poor prognosis. It is well known that cirrhotic patients with renal failure have decreased survival when compared to patients

* corresponding author. Associate Investigator. IDIBAPS

with normal renal function. This negative effect is also evident when these patients undergo liver transplantation, as shown by reduced graft and patient survival.

Ideally, patients with a high probability of developing end stage renal disease after liver transplantation alone should receive a combination of liver and kidney transplant. However, is still a great challenge to identify these patients who are at higher risk.

The presence and the severity of pretransplant kidney failure are factors independently associated with postoperative sepsis, need for renal replacement therapy and poor graft and patient outcomes.

In addition to the degree of renal dysfunction, duration and cause of renal failure should also be considered when evaluating candidates for liver transplantation alone or combined liver kidney transplantation.

Patients with pretransplant renal dysfunction (defined as pretransplant Scr > 1.5mg/dL) for a period longer than 12 weeks showed higher probability of progression to end-stage renal disease at 3 years post transplant. However in this study the etiology of renal dysfunction was not specified, mainly due to the authors concern of potential bias in classifying renal failure in absence of kidney biopsy.

Renal failure is usually defined by a reduction in glomerular filtration rate (GFR) that can be acute when it occurs in hours to weeks or chronic when it occurs gradually over time.

Currently, serum creatinine remains the most widely used method to assess renal function in cirrhotic patients.

However, patients with liver dysfunction have reduced creatinine production secondary to loss of muscle mass, and therefore, in those patients serum creatinine usually overestimates renal function. As the Cockroft-Gauld and MDRD (Modification of Diet in Renal Disease) formulas are based on serum creatinine concentration, adjusted by race, age, sex and weight, they also overestimate renal function in patients with cirrhosis and should not be used in clinical settings.

In this context, cystatin C has emerged as an option for evaluate renal function since its level is not influenced by muscle mass. Nevertheless, its value has not been well established and is not available as standart test.

More accurate methods, such as determination of inulin clearance or radionuclide markers, represent the gold standard for measuring glomerular filtration rate. Indeed, its use in daily attendance is not feasible, because of its complexity, making repeated measurements that these patients often require difficult. These gold standard methods should be indicated for selected patients when there is a need to accurately assess renal function to decide between performing liver transplantation alone or CKLT. Their routinary use, however, is not mandatory.

Beyond the degree of renal function, the etiology of renal failure should be assessed, as prognosis varies according to the cause of renal failure. In a recent study with a large population of hospitalized patients with cirrhosis, the most common cause of renal failure was due to bacterial infections (46%), followed by hypovolemia (32%), hepatorenal syndrome (13%) and intrinsic nephropathy (9%). Patients with HRS and bacterial infections had lower 3-month survival compare to patients with intrinsic nephropathy. Even though patients with intrinsic nephropathy present better survival among all causes of renal failure in cirrhosis, its chronic form of renal failure has a non-reversible character and are most likely to receive CKLT.

The diagnostic diagram of etiology of renal failure include a complete medical history and physical examination, searching for presence of diabetes and/or hypertension as well as any other evidence of organ damage. Laboratory evaluation should include urinalysis to seek for signs of intrinsic nephropathy, like hematuria, pyuria, cell and granular casts, and 24h urine collection to assess protein excretion.

In addition to urine test, a renal ultrasonography, is useful in evaluating preexisting renal disease. Findings such as alteration of renal echogenicity and reductions in the size of the kidneys indicate the existence of chronic kidney disease.

Finally, a definitive diagnostic may require the realization of a renal biopsy, which may also give prognostic information. In patients with intrinsic nephropathy, marked tubulointerstitial injury is associated with progression to end stage renal disease, even if the primary disease is a glomerulopathy. Among histological findings, the degree of tubular interstitial fibrosis is the most powerful predictor of subsequent progression of renal impairment. There are very limited data on renal biopsies findings in cirrhotic patients. A study evaluated 23 kidney biopsies performed in liver transplant candidates with renal failure of unknown etiology or persisted HRS (> 4 weeks) demonstrated a variety of pathologic findings. These included menbranoproliferative glomerulopathy, IgA nephropathy, diabetes nephropathy and acute tubular necrosis. Of note, 4 patients showed normal histology. In this study CLKT was recommended for 10 of 26 patients with > 40% global glomeruloesclerosis, > 30% of interstitial fibrosis or severe glomerular ischemia/injury. Although these histological criteria have not been evaluated in further studies in patients with cirrhosis, it suggests that renal histopathology changes may alter therapeutic management, including the need for combined liver and kidney transplant.

Therefore according to a recent consensus, a renal biopsy should be performed in patients with an estimated glomerular filtration rate less than 30ml/min with a chronic course .The decision to perform a transjugular or percutaneous renal biopsy should take into account professional experience and patient's clinical conditions, mostly platelet count and coagulation parameters.

Hepatorenal syndrome is a form of kidney failure that is secondary to a severe circulatory disorder in patients with cirrhosis. This particular complication of liver disease can be potentially reversible with the combination of systemic vasoconstrictors and intravenous albumin. Even though the definite treatment of this severe condition remains liver transplantation, the importance of pre-liver transplantation treatment should not be underestimate. Patients with HRS treated with systemic vasoconstrictors and albumin before liver transplantation and pretransplant serum creatinine inferior to 1.5 mg/dL had a three year survival similar to patients transplanted with normal renal function.

Finally, the current criteria to perform CLKT according to the consensus conference is shown in table 1.

1. Evidence of chronic kidney disease and renal biopsy demonstrating more than 30% of glomeruloesclerosis or 30% of interstitial fibrosis.
2. If the biopsy is not possible, the decision is made based on *National Kidney Foundation* criteria for chronic kidney disease, which is an eGFR less than 30ml/min for more than 3 months.
3. Patients with end stage renal disease in renal replacement therapy
4. Patients with hepatorenal syndrome or acute kidney injury with creatinine greater or equal to 2.0 mg/dL and on dialysis for more than 8 weeks.

Table1. Indications for combined liver kidney transplant in patients with end stage liver disease.

3. Evaluation of candidates for CLKT in patients with end stage renal Disease (ESRD)

The benefit of combined liver kidney transplantation is not well established for patients with compensated cirrhosis and ESRD. The decision to perform CLKT or only a liver transplant is matter of debate. In a study of patients with chronic hepatitis C on RRT who underwent kidney transplantation alone, the degree of liver fibrosis correlated with patient and graft survival at 3 years .It is recommended that patients with chronic liver disease and ESRD who are candidates for kidney transplantation should be sought for the presence of significant liver fibrosis and cirrhosis. These patients should be submitted to transjugular liver biopsy with assessment of hepatic venous pressure gradient(HVPG). Patients with cirrhosis and/or clinical significant portal hypertension, determined by an HVPG greater than 10mmHg should be referred to CLKT. The option of kidney transplantation alone should be offered for those patients without these characteristics. Even though most of the data regarding these situations comes from patients with cirrhosis due to hepatitis C, the recommendations are generally applied to all patients irrespective of etiology of cirrhosis.

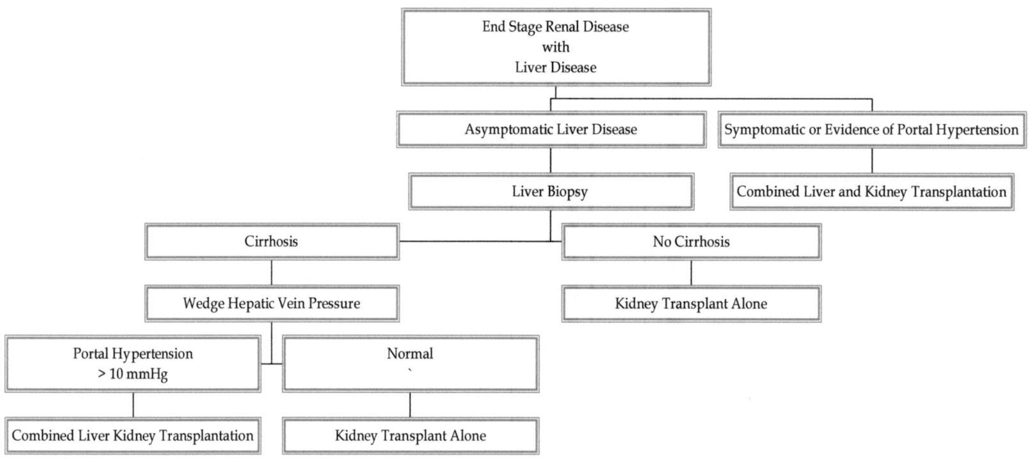

Fig. 1. Diagram for End Stage Renal Disease and Liver Disease (adapted from Consensus Conference on Simultaneous Liver Kidney Transplantation).

4. Outcomes in combined liver and kidney transplantation

Cirrhosis may not be the only indication for CKLT. In a large series of 3520 patients evaluated between 1984-2008, the main indications for combined liver kidney transplantation were: hiperoxaluria type 1 (42.7%), liver cirrhosis and chronic renal failure (23.5%), polycystic liver and kidney disease (15.5%), liver cirrhosis with hepatorenal syndrome (7.1%) and end stage liver disease with renal failure of unknown cause (6%).
Hence, prognosis and outcomes of combined liver kidney transplantation are not well known because most of the data came from series that include patients treated with CLKT

not only with end stage liver disease but also patients with inherited diseases without cirrhosis.

In recent years, MELD score has increasingly been used for liver allocation. Due to the presence of serum creatinine in the formula of MELD score, candidates with renal failure are more likely to receive a liver graft. Although pre transplant renal failure is associated with poor outcomes in liver transplantation settings, this modification on organ allocation system was not followed by changes in survival. The 3-year survival of liver transplant recipients remained almost unchanged when compared pre and pos-MELD era (81% vs. 80%, respectively).

A large case-control study compared the outcomes of patients submitted to liver transplant alone with or without renal failure to combined liver kidney transplants (CKLT) between 1987 and 2006. After adjusting for multiple donor (age, race, cause of death) and recipient (MELD, dialysis status at time of transplant) characteristic's, recipients of CLKT had a similar one-year survival compared to liver transplant alone (82 vs. 81.8%). However, the degree of renal failure in both groups was not described. The only subgroup in which CLKT had benefit on survival was in patients on long-term pre transplant hemodialysis (defined as a period equal to or greater than 12 weeks). In this subgroup, CKLT recipients had a higher survival than those submitted to liver transplantation alone (84.5% vs. 70.8%, P=0.008).

Another study demonstrated that patients on hemodialysis prior to transplantation had a significantly higher 1-year survival for CLKT group when compared to LT alone (79.4% vs. 73.7%, p=0.004). This difference, however, was not observed when only patients with renal failure (defined by serum creatinine ≥ 2.5 mg/dL) not on dialysis where analyzed. In this subgroup, 1-year survival was similar for patients who received CLKT or liver transplant alone (81% vs.78.8%, p= n.s.). An important issue to highlight is that patients receiving CLKT, either on hemodialysis or not, had better liver function at the time of transplant compared to those receiving liver transplantation alone. Mean MELD score of patients receiving LTA or CKLT was 36 vs. 31 for recipients on hemodialysis, and 34 vs. 28 for those with renal failure (serum creatinine >2.5 mg/dl) but not on hemodialysis (p<0.01 for both comparisons).

Most studies of survival in combined liver kidney transplantation analyzed a very heterogeneous population respect to the etiology of liver transplantation. Though, a recent study that only included patients with cirrhosis and chronic kidney disease, showed a 1-year survival lower for patients treated with CKLT compared to liver transplant alone group (80 vs. 97%, p=0.014). The probability of survival at 3 years was also lower in the CLKT group, but the difference between both groups did not reach statistical significance (75% and 88%, respectively). The incidence of complications was also higher for CKLT. Patients with CLKT had a higher incidence of bacterial infections and transfusions requirements compared to LTA group. Nevertheless, the comparison group (liver transplant alone) did not present renal failure at the time of transplant (mean serum creatinine value of 0.96±0.27 mg/dL), because all patients with cirrhosis and advanced chronic kidney disease (defined by a glomerular filtration rate below 30ml/min) were considered candidates for CLKT.

Another important point is the potential reversibility of renal failure after liver transplantation. As mentioned previously, patients with HRS should be treated to reverse the renal failure before liver transplantation. Many of these patients, however, do not respond to treatment and eventually undergo CKLT. Only a few single-center series had described outcomes of patients with hepatorenal syndrome submitted to CLKT. One of them compared the results of patients with HRS on hemodialysis who received CLKT (n=22, median time of pretransplant hemodialysis of 41 days) to those with HRS on hemodialysis who received liver transplant alone (n=80, pretransplant hemodialysis time inferior to 30 days). The one-year survival for patients undergoing CLKT or LTA was similar (72% vs. 66%, respectively, p=0.88). Most of the benefit of performing CKLT was observed in patients on hemodialysis for more than 8 weeks pre transplant. This group had higher survival than those receiving CLKT on hemodialysis for a period inferior than 8 weeks (88% vs.66%, respectively). Among patients receiving liver transplantation alone, recovery of renal function was achieved in 90% of patients at one-month, even though most of them required hemodialysis at post transplant period.

The possible benefit of CLKT on LTA in patients with hepatorenal syndrome was also evaluated in a study comparing patients submitted to CLKT to patients with HRS submitted to LTA. Survival at 5 years was similar for CLKT recipients (48.1%) and patients with HRS receiving LTA (67.1%) (p=ns).

Some recent data on patients who received CLKT (n=75) over a 23 year-period show excellent 1-, 3- and 5- year patients survival (81%, 73% and 67%, respectively). However, short-term mortality (< 90 days) was especially high because of sepsis/infection on postoperative period. In addition, there was no difference in patient survival based on whether or not a recipient was on dialysis pre-transplantion. Nevertheless, the need of post transplant renal replacement therapy was significantly associated with poor prognosis (p=0.0012).

Regarding graft survival, it seems that the liver graft has an immune protective effect on kidney graft when both organs came from the same donor. A study comparing renal allograft outcomes of patients who undergone CLKT to kidney after liver transplantation (KALT) demonstrated a higher incidence of chronic rejection in KALT group than CLKT group (4.6 vs. 1.2%, P < 0.001). One and three-year rejection-free renal graft survival of KALT was lower than CLKT group (77% and 67% KALT vs. 85% and 78% CLKT, respectively; P < 0.001). Renal half-life of KALT allograft was shorter than CLKT group (6.6+/-0.9 vs. 11.7+/-1.3 years, P < 0.001). It has been speculated that this effect is secondary to the secretion of soluble HLA antigens by the liver and to phagocytosis of these reactive antibodies by kupffer cells.

Although many theories have been described to explain the possible hepatic protection on renal graft, some recent findings have questioned this statement. A case report of acute humoral rejection in kidney allograft in an ABO compatible CLKT was described. Even treating, the humoral rejection with plasmapheresis, intravenous immunoglobulin and rituximab, the kidney required 3 months to recovery function and finally progressed to chronic allograft nephropathy.

5. Combined liver and kidney transplantation in special conditions

Polycystic kidney diseases (PKD) compass a group of inherited diseases that causes an irreversible decline in kidney function. Autosomal dominant polycystic kidney disease (ADPKD) is associated with cysts in the kidneys and, in many cases, cysts in the liver and pancreas. The autosomal dominant form (ADPKD) is the most common genetic cause of chronic kidney disease .As survival with dialysis or transplant increase, incidence of liver disease will also increase. When cysts are diffused, fenestration/resection procedures are not successful and LKA offers a good survival option. For combined liver and kidney transplantation one- and two-year patient survival rates were similar to combined transplantation for other indications. For patients with acceptable renal function at time of transplantation, solitary liver transplantation has an excellent outcome.

Primary hyperoxaluria (PHO) is a rare metabolic disorder with autosomal recessive inheritance. PHO is induced by one of two enzymatic defects, both of which result in markedly enhanced conversion of glyoxalate to poorly soluble oxalate which is then excreted in the urine. Combined liver-kidney transplantation is probably the treatment of choice for children with type 1 PHO with progressive renal disease. The liver provides the missing enzyme, thereby lowering oxalate production to the normal range. The outcome may be best if transplantation is performed when the GFR falls to 25 mL/min per 1.73 m2 and prior to marked tissue oxalate deposition. Isolated liver transplantation has been proposed for patients with rapidly progressive disease who still have a glomerular filtration rate above 30 mL/min per 1.73 m^2.

6. Conclusion

Since implementation of MELD score as an organ allocation system, a crescent number of cirrhotic patients with renal failure has been submitted to CLKT. Due to increase shortage of organ donors, is of outstanding importance to define which are the patients who benefit most of this procedure.

The decision to perform orthotopic transplant alone or combined kidney-liver transplantation is still challenging, mainly because there is not enough data on factors that can predict renal function recovery. In patients with possible reversible causes of kidney dysfunction, including those with hepatorenal syndrome and acute renal failure, it is difficult to precise the boundaries between functional and irreversible damage. Therefore, in these cases kidney biopsy should be encouraged in order to evaluate interstitial and glomerular injury.

Combined liver kidney transplantation seems to be an adequate treatment in patients with end stage liver disease and chronic kidney disease on renal replacement therapy, as well as for those with inherited disease. The survival advantage in others subsets of patients is not well established and more studies are needed.

7. Acknowledgment

Supported in part by grants from Fondo de Investigación Sanitaria FIS070443 and 080108. Centro de investigaciones en red de enfermedades hepaticas y digestivas. CIBEREHD is supported by the Instituto de Salud Carlos III. Claudia Fagundes is supported by a grant of Fundación Renal Reina Sofía

8. References

Baccaro, ME. (2010). Combined liver-kidney transplantation in patients with cirrhosis and chronic kidney disease. *Nephrology Dialysis Transplantation,* Vol. 25, No. 7, pp. 2356-63, ISSN 0931-0509

Bahirwani, R. (2008). Transplantation: impact of pretransplant renal insufficiency. *Liver Transplantation,* Vol. 14, No. 5, pp. 665-71, ISSN 1527-6473

Barua M. (2009). Family history of renal disease severity predicts the mutated gene in ADPKD. *Journal of American Society of Nephrology,* Vol. 20, No. 8, pp. 1833-8, ISSN 1533-3450

Brinkert, F. (2009). Transplantation procedures in children with primary hyperoxaluria type 1: outcome and longitudinal growth. *Transplantation,* Vol. 87, No. 9, pp. 1415-21, ISSN 1534-0608

Campbell, MS. (2005).Renal Function after Orthotopic Liver Transplantation is Predicted by Duration of Pretransplantation Creatinine elevation. *Liver Transplantation,* Vol. 11, No. 9,pp. 1048-1055, ISSN 1527-6465

Caregaro, L. (1994). Limitations of serum creatinine level and creatinine clearance as filtration markers in cirrhosis. *Archives of Internal Medicine,* Vol. 154, No. 2, pp. 201-205, ISSN 0003-9926

Cochat, P. (1993). Should liver transplantation be performed before advanced renal insufficiency in primary hyperoxaluria type 1?. *Paediatric Nephrology,* Vol. 7, No. 2, pp. 212-8, ISSN 0931-041X.

Davis, CL. (2007).Simultaneous liver-kidney transplantation: evaluation to de decision making. *American Journal of Transplantation,*Vol.7, No. 7,pp. 1702-9, ISSN 1600-6135

D'Amico, G. (1992).Influence of clinical and histological features on actuarial renal survival in adult patients with idiopathic IgA nephropathy, membranous nephropathy, and membranoproliferative glomerulonephritis: survey of the recent literature. *American Journal of Kidney Disease,* Vol.20, No. 4,pp.315-23, ISSN 0272-6386

D'Amico, G. (2006).Natural history and prognostic indicators of survival in cirrhosis: a systematic review of 118 studies. *Journal of Hepatology,* Vol.44, No. 1,pp.217-231,ISSN 0168-8278

De Eason, JD. (2008). Proceedings of consensus conference on simultaneous liver kidney transplantation (SLK). *American Journal of Transplantation,* Vol.8, No. 11,pp. 2243-51,ISSN 1600-6135

Ginès P, Schrier RW. (2009). Renal failure in cirrhosis. *New England Journal of Medicine,* Vol.13, No. 361, pp.1279-1290, ISSN 0028-4793

Gonwa, TA. (1995). Impact of pretransplant renal function on survival after liver transplantation. *Transplantation,*Vol.59, No. 3,pp.361-365, ISSN 0041-1337

Gonwa, TA. (2006).Continued influence of preoperative renal function on outcome of orthotopic liver transplant (OLTX) in the US: where will MELD lead us? *American Journal of Transplantation,* Vol.6, No. 11,pp.2651-2659,ISSN 1600-6135

Jeyarajah, DR. (1997). Hepatorenal syndrome: combined liver kidney transplants versus isolated liver transplant. *Transplantation,* Vol. 64, No. 12, pp. 1760-5, ISSN 1534-0608.

Jeyarajah, DR. (1997).Hepatorenal syndrome : combined liver kidney transplants versus isolated liver transplant. *Transplantation,*Vol.64, No. 12,pp.1760-1765. ISSN 0041-1337

Locke, JE. (2008). Declining outcomes in simultaneous liver-kidney transplantation in the MELD era: ineffective usage of renal allografts. *Transplantation,* Vol. 85, No. 7, pp.935-42, ISSN 1534-0608

Maluf, DG. (2007). Hepatitis C virus infection and kidney transplantation: predictors of patient and graft survival. *Transplantation,* Vol. 83, No. 7, pp. 853-7, ISSN 1534-0608

Martin-Llahí, M. (2010).Prognostic importance of the cause of renal failure in patients with cirrhosis. *Gastroenterology,*Vol.140, No. 2,pp. 488-496, ISSN 0016-5085

McMillan, RW. (1997). Soluble fraction of class I human histocompatibility leukocyte antigens in the serum of liver transplant recipients. *Clinical Transplantation,* Vol. 11, No. 2, pp. 98-103, ISSN 0902-0063

Mehrabi, A. (2009). A single center experience of combined liver kidney transplantation. *Clinical transplantation,* Vol. 23, Suppl. 21, pp. 102-114, ISSN 0902-0063

Millan MT. (2003). One hundred percent patient and kidney allograft survival with simultaneous liver and kidney transplantation in infants with primary hyperoxaluria: a single-center experience. *Transplantation,.* Vol. 76, No. 10, pp. 1458-63, ISSN 1534-0608.

Nair, S. (2002).Pretransplant renal function predicts survival in patients undergoing orthotopic liver transplantation. *Hepatology* ,Vol.35, No. 5,pp.1179-85, Online ISSN 1527-3350

Nath, KA. (1992).Tubulointerstitial changes as a major determinant in the progression of renal damage. *American Journal of Kidney Disease,* Vol.20, No. 1,pp.1-17. ISSN 0272-6386

Pöge, U. (2006).Calculation of glomerular filtration rate based on cystatin C in cirrhotic patients. *Nephrology Dial Transplan,.*Vol.21, No. 3, pp.660-664, ISSN 0931-0509

Reichmann, TW. (2009). Acute humoral rejection in an ABO compatible combined liver-kidney transplant-the kidney is not always protected, Vol. 9, No. 8, pp1957-60, ISSN 1600-6143

Ruiz, R. (2006). Long-term analysis of combined liver and kidney transplantation at a single center. *Archives of Surgery,* Vol. 141, No. 8, pp. 735-41, ISSN 1435-2451

Ruiz, R. (2010). Indications for combined liver and kidney transplantation: propositions after a 23-yr experience. *Clinical Transplantation,* Vol. 24, No. 6, pp. 807-11, ISSN 0902-0063

Schmitt, TM. (2009). Combined liver-kidney and liver transplantation in patients with renal failure outcomes in the MELD era. *Transplantation International,* Vol. 22, No. 9, pp. 876-83, ISSN 1432-2277

Sherman, DS. (2003). Assessing renal function in cirrhotic patients: problems and pitfalls. *American Journal of Kidney Diseases,* Vol. 41, No.2, pp. 269-78, ISSN 0272-6386.

Skulzacek, PA. (2003). Prediction of GFR in liver transplant candidates. *American Journal of Kidney Diseases,* Vol. 42, No. 6, pp. 1169-76, ISSN 0272-6386.

Simpson, N. (2006). Comparison of renal allograft outcomes in combined liver-kidney transplantation versus subsequent kidney transplantation in liver transplant recipients: Analysis of UNOS Database. , Vol. 82, No. 10, pp. 1298-303, ISSN 1534-0608

Ueno,T. (2006). Liver and kidney transplantation for polycystic liver and kidney-renal function and outcome. *Transplantation*, Vol. 82, No. 4, pp. 501-7, ISSN 1534-0608.

17

Transplantation for the Complex Patient with Hepatitis C and End Stage Renal Disease: A Review

Jorge Ortiz, Jason Andre, Kamran Khanmoradi and Victor Araya
Albert Einstein Medical Center, Philadelphia PA
USA

1. Introduction

Hepatitis C (HCV) and End Stage Renal Disease (ESRD) are two major health issues affecting millions worldwide. The diagnosis of HCV in the dialysis patient has significant prognostic indications and specific interventions are necessary in order to evaluate the extent of liver disease and the feasibility of medical treatment or the need for organ replacement therapy. For the transplant candidate, unique issues with respect to immunosuppressive agents and the appropriate use of HCV positive donors may be particularly vexing. Prior reviews have focused on issues classically limited to nephrology or hepatology, this update will address transplantation issues as well.

2. Epidemiology

The Hepatitis C virus (HCV) is a member of the Flaviviridae family. Approximately 150 million people are infected by this single stranded RNA virus, 5 million of whom live in the United States. It is estimated that 85% of patients will develop chronic infection, which is defined as the presence of HCV RNA for six months after presumed onset. Subsequent spontaneous clearing of the virus is rare. Approximately 10-30% will develop cirrhosis. In the renal dialysis population, the incidence of de novo infection is 3-7% per year. The prevalence ranges from 10-20% and may be underestimated due to cases of low viral load.[1,2,3]

Factors associated with virus acquisition in this patient population include the number of blood units transfused (which has decreased with the advent of erythropoietin alpha and blood bank screening), the length of dialysis therapy and the type of renal replacement therapy. Patients on hemodialysis are at higher risk compared to those on peritoneal dialysis.[4] There are at least six genotypes and many subtypes. HCV accounts for 30-50% of liver transplantation procedures performed and is also associated with many extra hepatic manifestations,[5] (Table 1) most importantly diabetes. The mechanisms underlying the diabetogenicity of HCV likely involve insulin resistance, diminished hepatic glucose uptake and the directly injurious effect of the virus on beta cells of the pancreas.[6] In the kidney, HCV is strongly associated with membranoproliferative glomerulonephritis (MPGN), membranous glomerulonephritis, focal segmental glomerulosclerosis, mesangial proliferative glomerulonephritis[7] and albuminuria.[8] Clinically silent immune complex glomerulonephritis was commonly seen in biopsies of patients with end stage HCV liver disease undergoing liver transplantation.[9]

Antiphospholipid syndrome
Aplastic Anemia
Autoimmune hemolytic anemia
Autoimmune thyroiditis
Chronic fatigue syndrome
Behcet's Syndrome
Carotid atherosclerosis
CRST syndrome
Dermatomyositis
Diabetes
Fibromyalgia
Guillain-Barré syndrome
Hypertrophic cardiomyopathy
Hypocholesterolemia
Idiopathic pulmonary fibrosis
Idiopathic thrombocytopenic purpura
IgA deficiency
Lichen planus
MALToma
Mooren corneal ulcers
Multiple myeloma
Non-Hodgkins lymphoma
Neurocognitive impairment
Pancreatitis Polyarteritis nodosa
Polymyositis Porphyria cutanea tarda
Rheumatoid arthritis
Sialadenitis
Sjogren's syndrome
Systemic lupus erythematosis
Uveitis
Waldenstrom's macroglobuminemia

Table 1. Extrahepatic disease manifestations with HCV infection

3. Evaluation for treatment and kidney transplantation

Evaluation of the potential kidney transplant recipient with HCV involves a careful history and physical examination. Patients with encephalopathy, variceal bleeding, ascites and muscle wasting have significant risk of continued deterioration and should be considered for liver (and kidney) transplantation. The presence of hepatocellular carcinoma within the Milan or UCSF criteria[10] should also be considered an indication for combined liver and kidney transplantation.

False positives (and negatives (0.23%)) are not uncommonly seen with the current generation of ELISA blood tests and therefore a confirmatory PCR should be ordered[11]. The mean time from detection of HCV RNA to the appearance of antibody may be as long as six months[12]. Nevertheless, screening with PCR is not recommended. A negative PCR in a previously positive patient should be repeated because frequent variations in the viral load can be seen. The genotype of the virus may determine its susceptibility to interferon treatment. However, early studies in patients with renal replacement therapy failed to demonstrate that HCV genotype is a factor in interferon responsiveness[13]. Additionally, HCV genotype does not seem to influence survival in renal transplant recipients[14].

4. Biopsy

Liver function tests are not sensitive enough to determine whether there is significant inflammation or even cirrhosis[15]. Liver biopsies are therefore indicated in all HCV positive candidates being considered for kidney transplantation and possible treatment. Studies indicate that advanced fibrosis is a common finding despite normal aminotransferase levels[16]. Histologic features of chronic hepatitis will be seen in 100% of ESRD patients with HCV. 60-80% of patients will have significant fibrosis and 10-12% will have cirrhosis[17]. Established cirrhosis was found to be the most important predictor of death after renal transplantation and is considered a relative contraindication to isolated renal transplantation[18]. If the liver biopsy shows cirrhosis mandatory screening for hepatocellular carcinoma must be instituted[19].

Regarding the biopsy technique, obtaining tissue via the transjugular route may be safer than the percutaneous method especially if the patient has ascites, disorders of the coagulation system or undergoes peritoneal dialysis. An additional advantage of the transjugular approach is the determination of portal pressure gradients which may help to diagnose sub clinical portal hypertension. Radiologic imaging or upper endoscopy (another important screening tool) may demonstrate obvious cirrhosis and varices perhaps obviating the need for this particular intervention. In the absence of cirrhosis, biopsies should be performed at five year intervals. Surrogate serum markers for fibrosis and cirrhosis have been investigated but are not yet the standard of care[20].

5. Hepatocellular carcinoma

The incidence of hepatocellular carcinoma (HCC) is increasing in the general population[21] and is higher in patients with ESRD. The prognosis is also worse for patients with ESRD[22]. Screening is crucial as prognosis after the onset of symptoms is dismal while patients with small expeditiously treated lesions reap a significant survival advantage. The yearly risk of HCC in patients with HCV is highest in those with established cirrhosis (about 2-8% per year). HCV infected patients who do not have cirrhosis have a lower risk of developing HCC. Based on current knowledge all patients with HCV and cirrhosis should undergo surveillance. This should entail a radiologic exam (CT scan, MRI or ultrasound) and alpha fetoprotein monitoring. These screens should be performed (in cirrhotics) at 6-12 month intervals. If HCC is found, metastatic workup includes bone scans and chest CT scans. Surgical resection can be safely performed for patients with ESRD and preserved liver function[23]. For patients with decompensated cirrhosis and small solitary HCC or early multifocal disease (up to three lesions, total tumor burden less than 6.5cm) the best option is liver (and kidney) transplantation[24]. Other modalities used to treat HCC include chemoembolization, alcohol infusion, radiofrequency ablation,Y-90, and acetic acid infusion.

Systemic chemotherapy is not associated with improvements in patient survival. Sorafenib (Nexavar) may be associated with survival improvements in untransplantable patients.

6. Anti viral therapy

Antiviral therapy before transplantation with the objective of eradicating the virus is the current standard of care. Secondary benefits may include the prevention of hepatic decompensation and hepatocellular carcinoma. In dialysis patients, the only recommended treatment is Alpha Interferon monotherapy. The average virological response is 40% and is independent of genotype. Interferon therapy interruption, seen in up to 60% of patients, is due to side effects. The most common of which are flu like symptoms, neurologic symptoms and gastrointestinal symptoms. Sustained viral response (SVR) may be durable (22 months average) post transplantation in those patients successfully treated before surgery. Of the sixteen patients studied in one report, HCV viral counts remained negative in all.[25] Immunosuppressive issues remain troublesome in this complex patient population. Others have also indicated that successfully treated dialysis patients may have an improved graft survival and lower incidence of HCV related kidney disease[26] and new onset post transplant diabetes.

The higher rate of SVR after interferon therapy may result from higher levels of interferon in patients with renal failure. The dose of interferon is 3 million units one to three times a week. Pegylated interferons, although commonly used, are not yet recommended. From a pharmacokinetic standpoint dose adjustments would probably be unnecessary in patients with renal impairment[27]. Absorption may vary with a patient on dialysis[28]. One study reported 87.5% viral clearance in 8 patients after 12 weeks of therapy. All of the 6 patients who completed 48 weeks of therapy achieved a biochemical response[28]. In another report, two of six genotype 1 patients completed a 24 week course of Pegylated Interferon and achieved a SVR[30]. The appropriate dose of Pegylated Interferon Alpha-2 is probably 135 micrograms a week, this gives similar serum levels as 180 micrograms per week in patients with preserved renal function. Pegylated Interferon Alpha-2 should probably be dosed between 0.5-1.0 micrograms/kg (as opposed to 1.0-1.5 ug/kg)[31].

Ribavirin is contraindicated, alone and with interferon, because of the hemolytic anemia associated with it. However, some groups have shown that it can be used in combination with interferon at reduced dosages with plasma monitoring and erythropoietin and iron supplementation[32]. These studies did not prove that ribavirin in low doses, in this population, improved response rates. It is very important to note that if hemolysis results in anemia that necessitates blood transfusion, the patient may be rendered untransplantable because of increased immune reactivity. Amantadine has not proven beneficial.

In kidney transplant recipients, interferon treatment is contraindicated because of the increased risk of acute cellular and antibody meditated rejection[33]. An exception is the patient with fibrosing cholestatic hepatitis (FCH). FCH is characterized by cholestasis with only mild to moderate elevation of transaminases and a rapid deterioration in liver function[34]. Some investigators believe that after combined liver and kidney transplantation, the liver protects the kidney from rejection and interferon can therefore safely be administered.

Ribavirin monotherapy may improve serum aminotransferases and proteinuria, but its effect on liver histology is controversial. Chronic hemolysis may prevent its safe use. Some have recommended that ribavirin be dose adjusted for those renal transplant recipients with HCV who have developed significant proteinuria[35].

7. Prognosis

HCV infection in renal failure patients is usually asymptomatic. The virus seems to have a lower impact on the liver histology of dialysis patients than on the histology of the HCV-positive immunocompetent patients with normal renal function[36]. It would appear that histological progression of liver injury after transplantation is minimal in HCV positive kidney recipients. In fact, fibrosis might regress in some patients[37]. Nevertheless, it is a negative prognostic indicator for survival on dialysis and after kidney transplantation. HCV may intensify oxidative stress in patients with uremia, leading to cardiovascular compromise[38]. Diabetes and cardiovascular disease were statistically significantly associated with patient death (while on dialysis) in one study[39]. Those patients with cirrhosis have a 35% higher death rate than noncirrhotic counterparts.[40,41] In another report, HCC was a statistically significantly more common cause of death in HCV positive dialysis patients[42]. Overall survival in these patients is improved after kidney transplantation compared to remaining on dialysis, despite the theoretical risk of accelerating virus replication with immunosuppression[43], but worse than HCV negative counterparts. This might be related to an increased risk of cardiovascular disease, posttransplant diabetes mellitus, sepsis [44,45,46], and rejection[47]. Thrombotic microangiopathy, MPGN and proteinuria are also associated with HCV infection and may result in lower rates of patient and graft survival[48]. The most common cause of proteinuria post transplant is still chronic allograft nephropathy, and a biopsy is crucial for the diagnosis[49]. All cause hospitalizations are significantly higher in HCV positive kidney recipients compared to HCV negative ones. HCV positive kidney transplant recipients are more likely to be African American, male, older, and have a higher rate of alcohol abuse, experience extended time on dialysis, malnutrition (as measured by serum albumin) and prior transplantation. Those patients with concomitant hepatitis B infection do particularly poorly in terms of patient and graft survival[50]. As do patients with HIV co-infection[51].

8. HCV and Tacrolimus

As stated, HCV infection is associated with pre transplant and de novo post transplant diabetes. This is seen more commonly with Tacrolimus compared to Cyclosporine. Nevertheless, the U.S. FK506 multicenter trial demonstrated higher patient survival in those HCV positive patients who received Tacrolimus compared to Cyclosporine. According to a recent query of the UNOS database (Tables 2-3), 1,3,5 year graft survival for HCV positive recipients of HCV negative organs was 89.7%, 76.7% and 61.6% for those patients treated with cyclosporine. 1,3,5 year graft survival with Tacrolimus immunosuppression was 92.2%, 80.6% and 63.3%. If the donor were HCV positive, 1,3,5 year graft survival for HCV positive recipients was 92.7%, 76% and 56.3% for cyclosporine treated recipients and 89.6%, 74.6% and 52.5% for Tacrolimus treated patients. Patient survival at 1,3, and 5 years for HCV negative donor organs was 94.8%, 88.8% and 80.5% with cyclosporine 95.6%, 89.4% and 79.7% with Tacrolimus. If the donor were HCV positive, patient survival at 1,3 and 5 years was 98%, 91.1% and 82% for cyclosporine and 93.9%, 87% and 75.8% for Tacrolimus.[52] The mechanisms behind diminished graft and patient survival with HCV positive donors and Tacrolimus immunosuppression are not entirely clear.

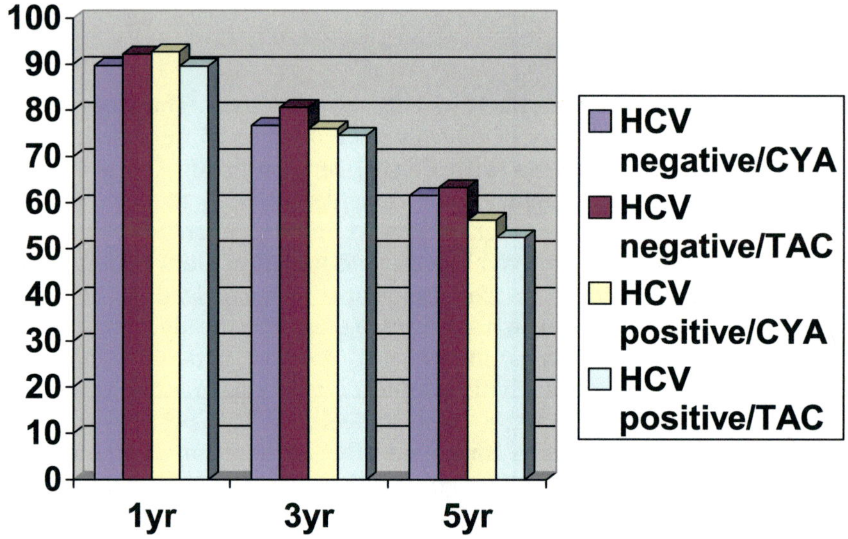

Table 2. Graft Survival by Donor HCV status and Main Maintenance Immunosuppression Agent

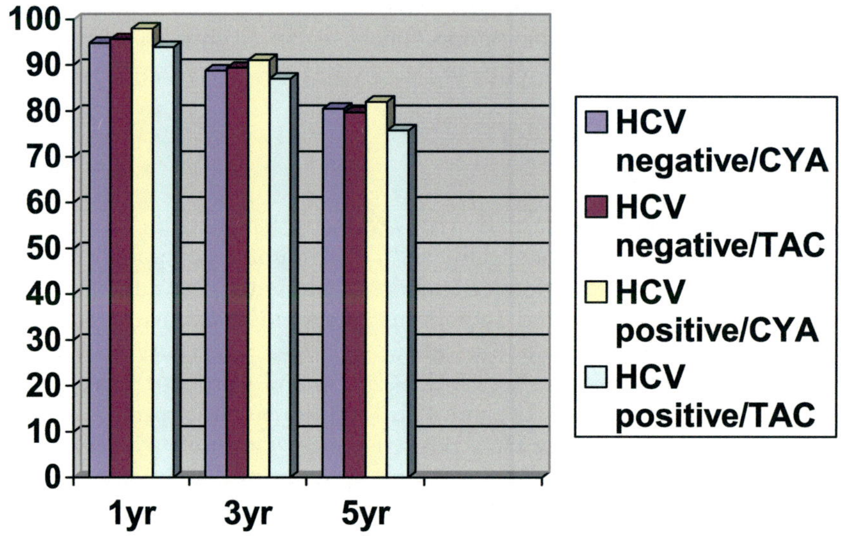

Table 3. Patient Survival By Donor HCV Status and Main Maintenance Immunosuppression Agent

9. Mycophenolate, steroids and induction agents

Another risk factor for diabetes, and a multitude of other complications, is prolonged steroid usage. Early rapid withdrawal has been reported to be safe (at least in the short term) compared with a historic control group[53]. The use of mycophenolate mofetil is associated with improved survival (at least with HCV positive donors) due to fewer infectious deaths[54]. Patients induced with OKT3 or anti-lymphocyte globulin have experienced inferior survivals[54]. The UNOS database was queried for 1,3 and 5 year patient and graft survival for HCV recipients of donor positive and donor negative organs stratified by induction agent (see Table 4). Definitive conclusions pertaining to the best induction agent for the ESRD patient with HCV can not be made until randomized prospective trials are performed.

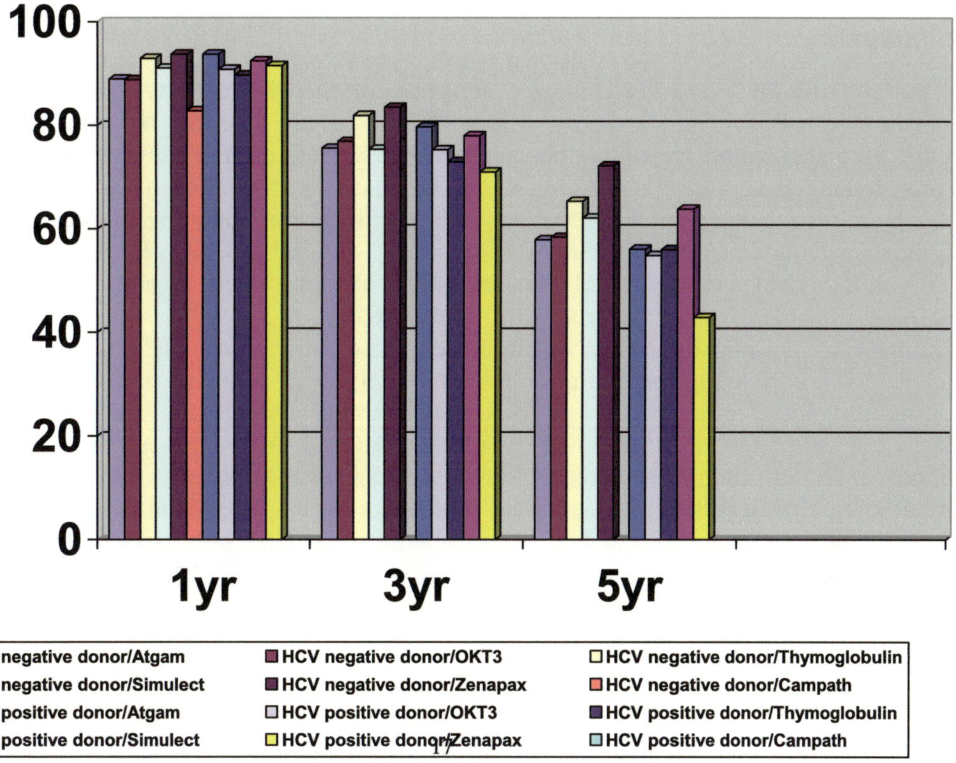

Table 4. Graft Survival by Donor HCV Status and Induction Agent

10. HCV positive donors

The organ donor shortage has compelled centers to transplant kidneys from donors who test positive for HCV. The prevalence and utilization of HCV positive organ donor referrals has increased in the United States. The prevalence of HCV is several fold higher in deceased donors compared to healthy living blood donors. Almost 20% of anti HCV positive donors will be RNA negative[56]. The utilization of HCV positive kidneys for HCV negative recipients is contraindicated[57, 58].

Surprisingly, Bucci et al demonstrated that 34.1% of HCV positive donor kidneys were allocated to HCV negative recipients in the United States in 2000[59]. The use of donor positive kidneys for HCV positive recipients is associated with greater long term mortality compared to virus negative kdneys. Although HCV positive recipients more frequently develop new onset diabetes mellitus (NODM) compared to negative controls, the risk is heightened with HCV positive donors[60]. Nevertheless, in comparison to staying on the waitlist, transplantation with donor virus positive kidneys is associated with increased survival in HCV positive recipients[61]. There is no definitive proof that conversion of genotype after transplantation portends a bad prognosis. Nevertheless, one case reported did implicate a genotypic mismatched kidney transplant in the exacerbation of hepatic dysfunction[62]. Any possible adverse effect of super infection with a different genotype is believed to be outweighed by the beneficial effect of decreased time on dialysis[63].

11. Summary

The patient with HCV and ESRD is very complex. All positive antibody screens should be confirmed with PCR. The standard workup should include a search for clinical signs of hepatic decompensation and a liver biopsy. The biopsy, if it does not show cirrhosis, should be repeated at 5 year intervals. Patients should be treated with interferon if at all possible in order to minimize long term hepatologic complications and to improve outcomes after kidney transplantation. The formulation of interferon and the exact dosing remain a matter of debate. Ribavirin should probably be used only with close follow up and in a setting of a trial. After transplantation, interferon is contraindicated.

Although HCV is a negative prognostic indicator, those patients with HCV are better served transplanted compared to remaining on the waitlist. HCV positive organ donors are also a negative prognostic indicator but nonetheless may confer a significant survival advantage due to the associated decrease in the wait time for a deceased organ. Decompensated cirrhosis is an indication for combined liver and kidney transplantation. At this time well compensated cirrhotics are not considered candidates for single or dual organ transplants, although many centers perform both. Mycophenolate mofetil and steroid freedom have been shown to be safe in this patient population. The results with various calcineurin inhibitors and induction agents have been reviewed. Until randomized perspective trials are performed, the choice of which medication to employ is center specific and experience driven.

12. Conclusion

HCV will remain a major health issue for decades to come. Appropriate communication between disciplines is mandatory in order to ensure excellent patient outcomes. Randomized trials and multi-disciplinary meetings are indicated.

13. References

[1] Hanuka N, Sikueler E, Tovbin D, et al: Hepatitis C virus infection in renal failure patients in the absence of anti-hepatitis C virus antibodies. Journal of Viral hepatitis 2002, 9:141

[2] Lauer GM, Walder BD. Hepatitis C virus infection. N Engl J Med 2001, 345:41

[3] Batty DS Jr, Swanson SJ, Kirk AD, et al. Hepatitis C virus seropositivity at the time of renal transplantation in the United States: associated factors and patient survival. Am J Transplant 2001, 1:179
[4] Pereira BJG. Hepatitis C n organ transplantation: Its significance and influence on transplantation policies. Curr Opin Nephrol Hypertens 1993, 2:912
[5] Agnello V, De Rosa FG. Extrahepatic disease manifestations of HCV infection: some current issues. Journal of Hepatology 2004, 40:341
[6] Masini M, Campani D, Boggi U et al. Hepatitis C virus infection and human pancreatic beta-cell dysfunction. Diabetes care 2005, 28:940
[7] Gopalani A, Ahuja TS. Prevalence of glomerulopathies in autopsies of patients infected with the hepatitis C virus. Am J Med Sci 2001, 322:57
[8] Tsui JI, Vittinghoff E., Shlipak MG, et al., Relationship between Hepatitis C and Chronic Kidney Disease: Results from the Third National Health and Nutrition Examination Survey. J Am Soc Nephrol 2006, 17:1168
[9] McGuire BM, Julian BA, Synon S, et al. Brief Communication: Glomerulonephritis in Patients with Hepatitis C Cirrhosis Undergoing Liver Transplantation. Ann Intern Med 2006, 144:735
[10] Mazzaferro V; Regalia E; Doci R, et al. Liver transplantation for the treatment of small hepatocellular carcinomas in patients with cirrhosis. N Engl J Med 1996, 334(11):693-9
[11] Schneeberger PM, Keur I, Van der Vliet W, et al. Hepatitis C virus infection in dialysis centers in the Netherlands: a national survey by serological and molecular methods. J Clin MIcrobiol 1998, 36:1711
[12] Furusyo N, Hayashi J, Kakuda K, et al. Acute Hepatitis C among Japanese hemodialysis patients: a prospective 9-year study. Am J Gastroenterol 2001, 96:1593
[13] Izopet J, Rostaing L, Moussion F, et al. High rate of hepatitis C virus clearance in hemodialysis patients after interferon-alpha therapy. J Infect Dis 1997; 17:1614
[14] Natov SN, Lau JY, Ruthazaer R, et al. Hepatitis C virus genotype does not affect patient survival among renal transplant candidates. The New England Organ Bank Hepatitis C Study Group. Kidney Int 1999, 56:700
[15] Fabrizi F, Martin P, Dixit V, et al. Acquisition of hepatitis C virus in hemodialysis patients: a prospective study by branched DNA signal amplification assay. Am J Kidney Dis 1998; 31:647
[16] Sterling RK, Sanyal AJ, Luketic VA, et al. Chronic hepatitis C infection in patients with end stage renal disease: characterization of liver histology and viral load in patients awaiting renal transplantation. Am J Gastroenterol 1999, 94:3576
[17] Martin P, Carter D, Fabrizi F, et al. Histopathologic features of hepatitis C in renal transplant candidates. Transplantation 2000, 69:1479
[18] Mathurin P, Mouquet C, Poynard T, et al. Impact of HBV and HCV on kidney transplantation outcome. Hepatology 1999, 29: 257
[19] Llovet JM, Burroughs A, Bruix J. Hepatocellular carcinoma. Lancet 2003; 362:1907-1917
[20] Varaut A, Fontaine H, Serpaggi Je, et al. Diagnostic Accuracy of the Fibrotest in Hemodialysis and Renal Transplant Patients with Chronic Hepatitis C Virsu. Transplantation 2005, 80:1550
[21] El-Serag HB, Mason AC: Rising incidence of hepatocellular carcinoma in the United States. N Engl J Med 1999; 340:745-750

[22] Hayashi H, Ohtake Y, Kashima T, et al: Hepatocellular carcinoma among hemodialysis patients infected with hepatitis C virus-early evolution and rapid prognosis. Clin Nephrol 1999;51:321-323
[23] Cheng S, Wu C Shu K, Ho W et al. Liver Resection for Hepatocellular Carcinoma in Patients With End-Stage Renal Failure. Journal of Surgical Oncology 2001; 78:241-247
[24] Bruix J and Sherman M. Management of Hepatocellular Carcinoma. Hepatology, vol 42, No 5, 2005
[25] Kamar N, Toupance O., Buchler M. Evidence that clearance of hepatitis C virus RNA after alpha-interferon therapy in dialysis patients is sustained after renal transplantation. J Am Soc Nephrol 2003, 14:2092
[26] Cruzado J.M., Casanovas-Taltavull T., Torras J. Pretransplant interferonprevents hepatitis C virus-associated glomerulonephritis in renal allografts by HCV –RNA clearance. Am J Transplant 2003, 3:357
[27] Martin P., Mitra S., Farrington K. Pegylated (40kDa)interferon alfa=2a (Pegasys) is unaffected by renal impairment. Hepatology 2000, 32:370
[28] Barril G., Quiroga J.A. Sanz P. Pegylated interferon alfa 2a kinetics during experimental hemodialysis: impact of permeability and pore size of dialyzers. Aliment Pharmacol Ther 2004, 20:37
[29] Sporea I., Sirli R., Golea O., Peg interferon alfa 2a (40kDA) in patients on chronic hemodialysis with chronic C hepatitis: preliminary results. Rom J Gastroenterol 2004, 20:99
[30] Annichiarico A.E., Siciliano M., Pegylated interferon-alpha 2 monotherapy for hemodialysis patients with chronic hepatitis C. Aliment Pharmacol Ther 2004, 20:123
[31] Fried MW, Shiffman ML, Reddy KR, et al. Peginterferon alfa-2a plus ribavirin for chronic hepatitis C virus infection-a pilot study. N Engl J Med 2002, 347:975
[32] Bruchfeld A, Stahle L, Andersson J, et al. Ribavirin treatment in dialysis patients with chronic hepatitis C virus infection-a pilot study. J Viral Hepat 2001, 8:287
[33] Baid S, Tolkoff-Rubin N, Saidman S, et al. Acute Humoral rejection in hepatitis C-infected renal transplant recipients receiving antiviral therapy. Am J Transplant 2003, 3:74
[34] Toth CM, Pascual M, Chung RT, et al. Hepatitis C virus-associated fibrosing cholestatic hepatitis after renal transplantation. Transplantation 1988, 66:1254
[35] Kamar, N, Ribes D, Izopet J, et al. Treatment of hepatitis C Virus Infection (HCV) After renal Transplantation: Implication for HCV-Positive Dialysis Patients Awaiting a Kidney Transplant. Transplantation 2006, 82:853
[36] Alric L, Di-Martino V, Selves J. et al. Long term impact or renal transplantation on liver fibrosis during hepatitis C virus infection. Gastroenterology 2002; 123(5):1494
[37] Kamar N, Rostaing L, Selves J et al. Natural history of hepatitis C virus-related liver fibrosis after renal transplantation. Am J Transplant 2005, 5:1704
[38] Pawlak K, Pawlak D, Mysliwiec M. Hepatitis intensified oxidative stress, MIP-1 beta and RANTES plasma levels in uraemic patients. Cytoine 2004, 28:197
[39] Bloom RD, Sayer G., Kosuntarty F et al. Outcome of Hepatitis C virus Infected Kidney Transplant Candidates Who Remain on the Waiting List. Am J Transplant 2005, 5:139

[40] Fabrizi F, Poordad FF, et al. Hepatitis C Infection and the Patient with End-Stage renal Disease. Hepatology 2002, 36:3
[41] Marcelli D, Stanhard D, Conte F, et al. ESRD patient mortality with adjustment for comorbid conditions in Lobardy (Italy) versus the United States. Kidney Int 1996: 50:1013
[42] Maisonneuve P., Agodoa L., Geller R. Cancer in patients on dialysis for end-stage renal disease: an international collaborative study. Lancet 1999, 354:93
[43] Knoll GA, Tankerserley MR, Lee JY, et al. The impact of renal transplantation on survival in hepatitis C-positive end stage renal patients. Am J Kidney Dis 1997; 29:608
[44] Yunossi Zzm, Braun WE, Protiva DA et al. Chronic viral hepatitis in renal transplant recipients with allografts functioning for more than 20 years. Transplantation 1999, 67:272
[45] Fabrizi F, Martin P, Dixit V, et al. Post-transplant diabetes mellitus and HCV seropositive status after renal transplantation: Meta analysis of clinical studies. Am J Transplant 2005, 5:2433
[46] Pereira BJ, Wright TL, SchmidCH, Levey AS. The impact of pretransplantation hepatitis C infection on the outcome of renal transplantation. Transplantation 1995, 60:799
[47] Sotsky T, Polyak MR, Riggio R et al. Hepatitis C infection confers increased risk of immunologic failure following renal transplantation. Transplantation 1999; 67 Suppl 1):S577
[48] Baid S, Pascual M, Williams WW, et al. Renal thrombotic microangiopathy associated with anticardiolipin antibodies in hepatitis C-positive renal allograft recipients. J Am Soc Nephrol 1999, 10:146
[49] Nampoory MR, Johny KV, Costandi JN, et al. High incidence of proteinuria in hepatitis C virus infected renal transplant recipients is associated with poor patient and graft outcome. Transplant Proc 2001, 33:3639
[50] Breitenfeldt MK, Rasenack J, Berthold H, et al. Impact of hepatitis B and C on graft loss and mortality of patients after kidney transplantation. Clin Transplant 2002, 16:130
[51] Rostaing L, Izopet J, Cisterne JM, et al: Impact of hepatitis C virus duration and hepatitis C virus genotypes on renal transplant patients: Correlation with clinicopathological features. Transplantation 1998, 65:930
[52] www.UNOS.org OPTN data accessed 12/08/06
[53] Akalin E, Murphy B, Sehgal V, et al. Rapid steroid withdrawal in hepatitis C virus-positive kidney transplant recipients Clin Transplant 2004, 18:384
[54] Abbott KC, Bucci JR, Matsumoto CS, et al. Hepatitis C and renal Transplantation in the Era of Modern Immunosuppression. J Am Soc Nephrol 2003, 14:2908
[55] Gentil MA, Rocha JL, Rodriguez-Algarra G et al. Impaired kidney transplant survival in patients with antibodies to hepatitis C virus. Nephrol Dial Transplant 1999, 14:2908
[56] Pereira B, Milford E, Kirkman R, et al. Prevalence of HCV RNA in organ donors positive for HCV antibody and in the recipients of their organs. N Engl J Med 1992, 327:910
[57] http://www.hdcn.com/symp/03asn/09/per/per.htm
[58] Natov SN, Pereira BJ. Transmission of viral hepatitis by kidney transplantation: donor evaluation and transplant policies (Part 2:hepatitis C virus). Transpl Infect Dis 2002, 4:124

[59] Bucci JR, Matsumoto CS, Swanson SJ, et al. Donor hepatitis C seropositivity: clinical correlates and effect on early graft and patient survival in adult cadaveric kidney transplantation. J Am Soc Nephrol 2002, 13:2974
[60] Abbott KC, Lentine KL, Bucci JR, et al. Impact of diabetes and hepatitis after kidney transplantation on patients who are affected by hepatitis C virus. J Am Soc Nephrol 2004, 15:3166
[61] Abbot KC, Lentine KL, Bucci JR, et al. The Impact of Transplantation with Deceased Donor hepatitis C-Positive Kidneys on Survival in Wait-Listed Long Term Dialysis Patients. Am J. Transplant 2004, 4:2032
[62] Schussler T, Staffield-Coit C., Eason J, et al. Severe Hepatitis C Infection in a Renal Transplant Recipient Following Hepatitis C genotype Mismatch Transplant. Am J Transplant 2004, 4:1375
[63] Gane E, Pilmore H. Management of chronic viral hepatitis before and after renal transplantation. Transplantation 2002, 74:427

18

Combined Kidney-Islet Transplantation

Giuseppe Cavallari, Flavia Neri and Bruno Nardo
Department of General Surgery and Transplantation University of Bologna
Italy

1. Introduction

The possibility to transplant uniquely the endocrine part of the pancreas, islets of Langerhans, with the aim to recovery the endogenous insulin production in diabetic patients has always aroused attention from researches.
The initial experience of this procedure however was unsatisfying especially for what concerns the long term efficacy of the islet transplantation. The exciting results obtained by the Edmonton group in 2000, 100% of insulin independence in seven diabetic patients after 1 year from the islet transplant, encouraged several centers worldwide to approach this technique. Since then several programs of islet transplantation have been launched, and important multicentric clinical trials including an high number of patients were realized.
The Collaborative Islet Transplant Registry (CITR) collects data from 27 North American, 3 European and 2 Australian islet transplant centers and reported that a total of 412 patients underwent an islet transplantation in the time period between 1999-2009.
The global long-term results of CITR demonstrated an insulin independence after islet transplantation in a low percentage of cases but a partial function of the graft, and consequently important advantages for the patients, in the majority of these.
Actually islet transplantation is considered a valid therapeutic option only for selected patients affected by type 1 diabetes mellitus (DMT1). This limitation is a consequence of the benefit/cost ratio between improvement of the glycemic control and the necessity for transplant recipients to be treated with chronic immunosuppressive therapy which has, as well known, important side effects.
These considerations and the availability of new generation basal insulin and sophisticated micro insulin pumps lead the majority of European centers to perform islet transplantation almost exclusively in combination with kidney transplant in DMT1 patients candidate (simultaneous islets-kidney transplant), or just subjected (islet after kidney transplant), to a kidney transplantation for end-stage diabetic nephropathy. These patients therefore would anyway be treated with immunosuppressive drugs.
Even if the combined kidney-pancreas transplantation showed excellent results in DMT1 patients with end-stage diabetic nephropathy, the combined kidney-islet transplantation is considered a valid option in selected cases for this patient category.

2. History of islet transplantation: Past and current era

The history of the islet transplantation is long. The first transplant of fragments of the pancreatic gland in order to cure diabetes dates back even to the 20th December 1893, 28 years before the discovery of the insulin. Two English medical doctors from the Bristol Royal Infirmary Hospital, Dr. Watson-Williams and Dr. Harsant, harvested a pancreas from a deceased sheep and transplanted three pieces of the gland into the subcuticular tissue of a 15-years-old boy with uncontrollable diabetic ketoacidosis. Obviously, despite a temporary improvement of the clinical situation, the xenotransplant failed after three days for acute rejection.

After that first experiment almost one century passed before Paul Lacy and collegues in 1967 developed the technique of islet isolation in rats. Two important innovations made this procedure possible: the injection of digestion enzyme solution in the pancreatic duct and the centrifugation with different density gradients to separate the islets from the discarding tissue.

After few years the improvement of the glycemic control by intraperitoneal transplantation of islets was demonstred in diabetic rats (Younoszai et al., 1970) and subsequently the liver, using the same experimental model, was selected as preferable implantation site (Kemp et al., 1973). Actually the liver, by islets injection through the portal vein, is still the site preferably used for islet transplantation in the clinical setting.

The first clinical series of islet transplantations was reported in the late seventy using azathioprine and steroids as immunosuppressive therapy (Najarian et al., 1977). Although these first cases did not experience any complications the efficacy of the transplant was very limited. Seven patients over seven failed to reach the insulin independence after intraperitoneal or intraportal islet transplantation even though some of them reduced the need of exogenous insulin for a period.

Interestingly the first real clinical success in the field of islet transplantation was reported in one case of combined islet-kidney transplantation performed on a DMT1 uremic patient in Zurich in 1978. This patient reached the insulin independence and maintained it almost one year after the embolization in the spleen of fragments of donor pancreas (Largiader et al., 1979). In 1990 a series of nine islet transplantations was reported by the University of Pittsburgh. The patients underwent multivisceral resections for tumors and sequentially liver, kidney and small bowel transplantation: islets were injected in the portal vein at the liver reperfusion. More than 50% reached and mantained the insulin-indipendence until their death caused by neoplastic relapse (Tzakis et al., 1990). Subsequently other positive experiences were reported (Ricordi et al., 1992) but the global clinical results obtained by the Islet Transplant Registry from the total amount of islets transplantation performed between 1974 and 1999 were very disappointing with an insulin-indipendence presents in only about 10% of cases at one year from the transplant.

In 2000 the group of the University of Edmonton reported 100% of insulin indipendence at 1 year from islet transplantation in a series of 7 patients (Shapiro et al., 2000). Such extraordinary result was possible thanks to the employment of a protocol subsequently called the "Edmonton protocol". The key elements of this protocol were principally two. Firstly the recourse to two or more islets intrahepatic transplants in the same recipients provided an higher total number of transplanted islets (over 11000 IEQ/Kg of the patient body weight). Secondly the use of an immunosuppressive regimen without steroids and their hyperglycemic effect and consisting in interleukin-2 receptor blocking antibody daclizumab (Zenapax®) for induction therapy and sirolimus (Rapamune®) combined with low doses of tacrolimus (Prograf®) for chronic therapy.

Subsequently, with the aim to assess the applicability and reproducibility of the results obtained from the Edmonton group, a multicentric study started using the Edmonton protocol involving 9 transplant centers, 6 of which were American and 3 European.

The data from this study reported in 2006 did not confirm however the Edmonton results, showing an high variability in the outcome of the transplantation according to the isolation centre (Shapiro et al., 2006).
The critical passage in the procedure of islet transplantation is exactly the phase of organ processing in order to isolate the islets of Langerhans. These considerations lead to the development of several networks in which the isolation procedure is performed by few specialized and experienced centers and the islet transplantations are spread to several different centers even at long distance (Kempf et al., 2005).
In 2008 the Collaborative Islet Transplant Registry reported approximately a 30% of insulin independence by 3 years postoperatively over 325 adult recipients which were treated between 1999 and 2007 with an islet alone or a combined kidney-islet transplantations. However more than 75% of the recipients maintained a residual graft functionality detected by the endogenous secretion of C-peptide at 3 years from the transplantation.
This apparently disappointing outcome, showed anyway an important improvement in the quality of life of the patients reducing the episodes of severe hypoglycemia and the development of complications related to the diabetic disease (Alejandro et al., 2008).
In particular some studies have also focused on comparing the outcome of diabetic patients who underwent combined kidney-islet transplantation versus patient operated with kidney transplantation alone.
The group of Milan showed a decreased risk for micro and macroangiopathy, an improvement in the cardiovascular functionality and a reduced neuropathy also in cases of partial islet function after transplantation (Fiorina et al., 2003; Del Carro et al., 2007). Moreover the same authors showed that the improved glycemic control in patients with combined kidney-islet transplantation significantly increased also the kidney graft survival when compared to DMT1 patients with transplantation of the kidney alone (Fiorina et al., 2005).

3. Islets of Langerhans procurement

3.1 Pancreas harvest

The organs used for the islets isolation generally are pancreas previously proposed and not utilized or excluded for the whole pancreas transplantation. This strategy, adopted in order to decrease the competition between the two types of transplantation, allows in the case of pancreas for islets isolation the use of organs from donors with high BMI or >50 years old. Moreover, with the aim to expand the pool of donors, some authors reported positive experience of islet transplantation using donors after cardiac death (Saito et al., 2010).
The harvesting procedure of the gland is similar to the procedure for the whole pancreas transplantation. However, after perfusion with cold preserving solution, the pancreas is collected paying particular attention not to section the pancreatic capsule, event that may impair the enzymatic digestion while, obviously, the accuracy in the isolation and preservation of pancreatic vessels is not important as in case of the pancreas procurement for the transplantation of the whole gland.
The pancreas is harvested en bloc with a portion of duodenum and the spleen. After the pancreas is procured it is kept in cold preservation solution at 4°C. At the moment the pancreas preservation is obtained thanks to a double-layered system: the organ is placed within a superior layer of preservation solution and an inferior layer of perfluorocarbons (PFC) which are constantly oxygenated and help maintaining an high oxygen solubility

coefficient. This method allows the development of a highly oxygenated environment for the pancreas which is of great importance for the protection of the islets (Hering et al., 2002). The gland can be kept in this solution for several hours although it was reported that the best results were achieved when the cold ischemia time was < 16 hours at the beginning of the isolation procedure (Tsujimura et al., 2004).

3.2 Automated method for islets of Langerhans isolation

Before the beginning of the isolation procedure the spleen and the duodenum are removed from the pancreas and an accurate dissection and discard of the peripancretic fat, lymphonodes and vessels is performed (Fig. 1).

The procedure currently used to extract islets from human pancreas is the so called automated method for isolation of the islets of Langerhans, established in 1987 by Ricordi and collegues.

This procedure consists of two phases: digestion and purification phase. The digestion phase includes the digestion of the collagen scaffold of the pancreas releasing the esocrine and endocrine tissues within the gland. It includes a procedure of enzymatic and mechanical digestion. The phase of purification is aimed to obtain only the endocrine part of the gland, islets of Langerhans, separating them from the remain of the gland which is useless (acinar cells, ductal elements, fat tissue, lymph nodes, ganglia, etc).

Digestion phase: after the preparation of the pancreas the gland is devided at the isthmus and the pancreatic duct is cannulated in the proximal part (head and body) and in the distal part (body-tail) with two angiocatheters 18 gauge. The solution containing the digestion enzyme is injected in the Wirsung duct with a pressure of 180 mmHg slowly distending the two parts of the gland. The collagenase at warm temperature (37°C) is activated and starts the enzymatic digestion of the internal scaffold of the pancreas (Fig.2).

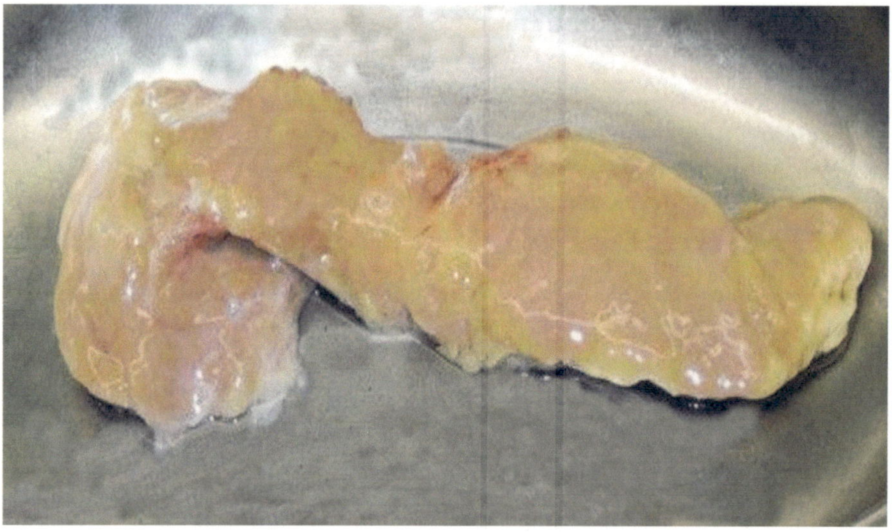

Fig. 1. Pancreas prepared for the isolation procedure.

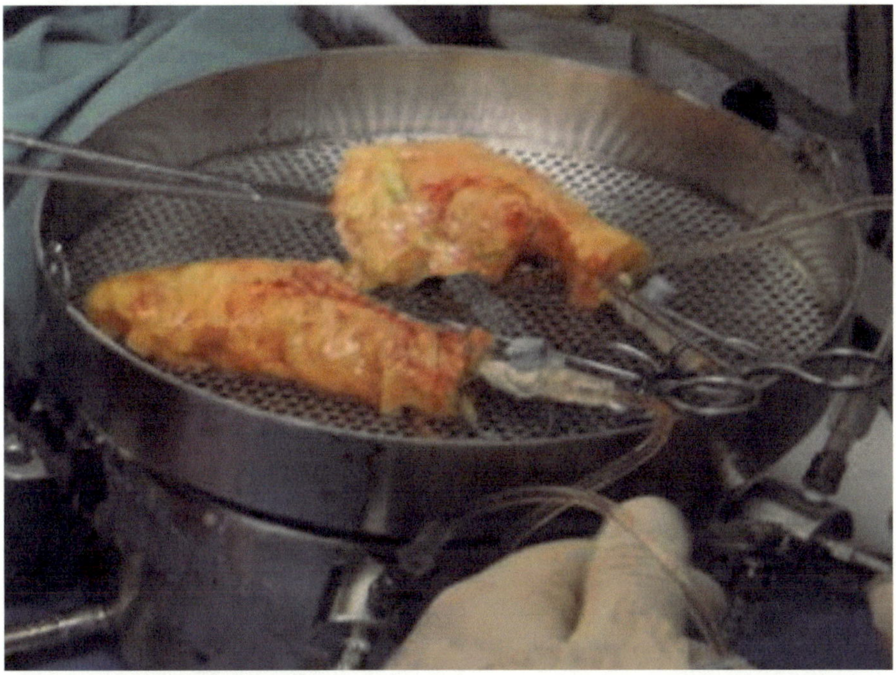

Fig. 2. Cannulation of the pancreatic duct and injection of the collagenase solution.

After some minutes the two portions of the pancreas are divided in smaller pieces and placed in a digestion chamber named "Ricordi chamber" after its inventor. This chamber is composed of a superior and an inferior part divided by a semi-permeable membrane which has holes of about 300 µm. Seven stainless steel balls together with the fragments of the pancreas are put into the inferior part, which is then filled with the digestion solution and closed together with the superior one. The chamber is connected to a mechanical arm with 10 cm excursion which is activated with a sussultory movement (300 oscillation/min) helping the complete mechanical digestion of the pancreas through the steel balls in the chamber. In the meantime a peristaltic pump connected to the system is activated creating a flow of 40 ml/min. The digestion runs in a closed circuit where warm Hank's solution is pumped in the inferior chamber and the tissue released in the solution passes in the superior chamber through the filter. The solution is collected in a cylinder passing in a refrigerator circuit at 4°C; at this temperature the activity of the enzyme and consequently the digestive process is stopped. Samples of the solution are collected from the circuit through a spigot every 2-3 minutes to monitor the progress of the digestion. When free islets are found in the samples the system is converted from closed to open: the solution is collected from the chamber into containers placed on ice. The procedure is stopped when no more islets are detected at samples (Fig 3).

<u>Phase of purification:</u> this includes the separation of the islets from the waste tissue through centrifugation cycles on different Ficoll density gradients. Islets which have a lower specific weight than the other structures, remain in the supernatant, the less dense part of the solution. Nowadays this procedure is generally performed using a COBE® 2991 cell processor system (Fig 4). At the end of the procedure samples of the islets preparation are collected and evaluated through a staining with dithizone (DTZ) which marks zinc in the

insulin granules resulting in a characteristic red stain. Adding few drops of DTZ solution to a sample is possible easily evaluate the morphology and number of the isolated islets through a computerized digital analysis. Specific features of the final volume of islets are required in order to perform the islets transplantation, in particular purity (> 90% of the preparation composed by islets) and adequate number of islets (Fig.5).

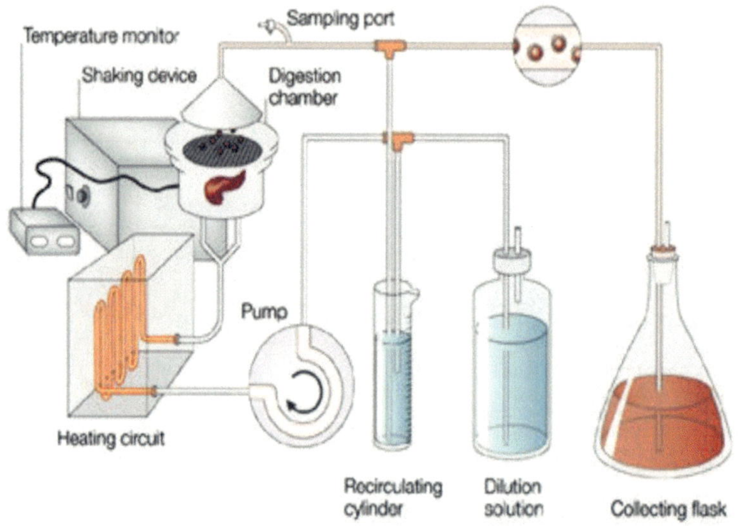

Fig. 3. Schematic representation of the automated method for islets of Langerhans isolation (modified from: Ricordi and Strom, *Nature Reviews Immunology* 2004).

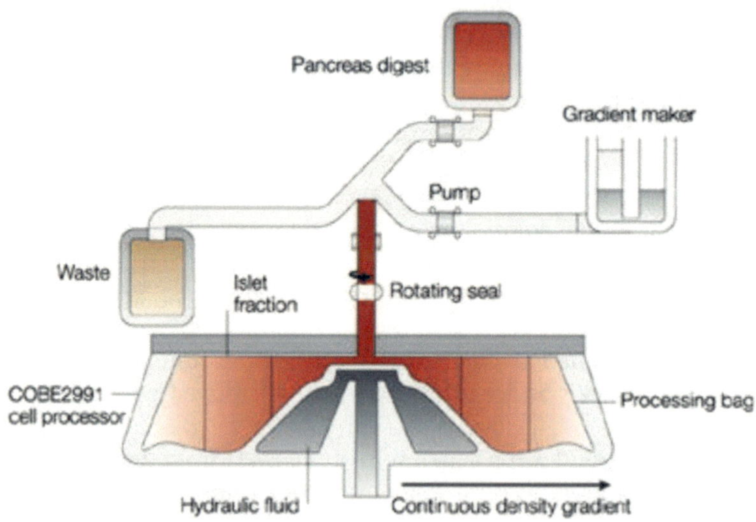

Fig. 4. Islets of Langerhans purification by density gradient separation (modified from: Ricordi and Strom, *Nature Reviews Immunology* 2004).

Although the procedure is quite standardized, only centers with the greatest experience in the field can count on an high percentage of procedures with a satisfactory purity and quantity of islets for the transplantation. Indeed the more the pancreas is manipulated in order to discard the exocrine part, the more islets are lost during this procedure. An additional important variable that reduces the reliability of the isolation process is the different enzyme lot used for the digestion procedure. The adequate amount of islets obtained is calculated with respect to the body weight of the recipient and resuspended immediately before the intrahepatic transplantation in 100 mL of adequate solution (45 mL of HBSS, 0.2 mL od HEPES 1M, 50 mL 20% Human Albumin and 2000 IE of heparin).

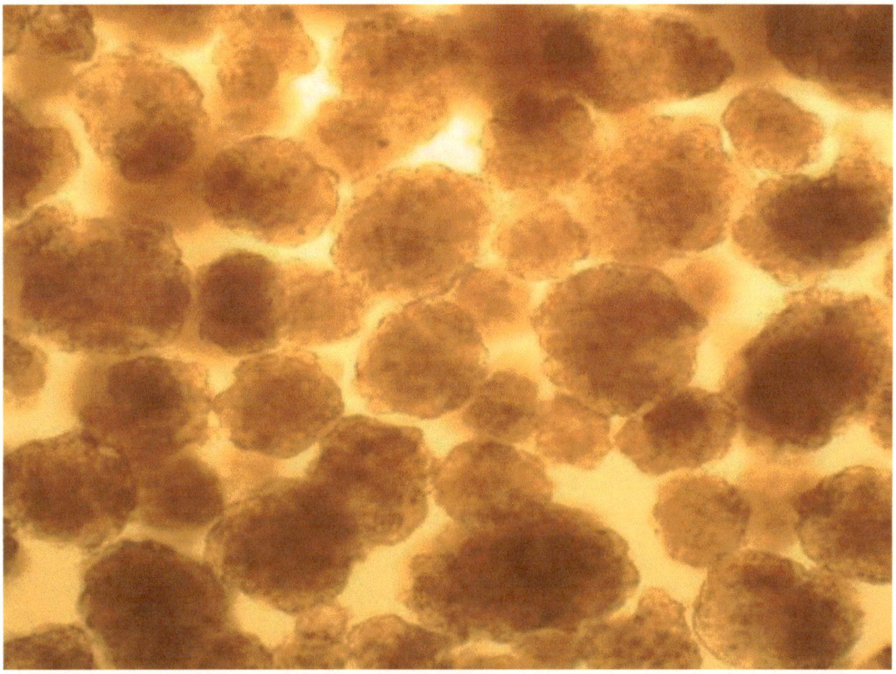

Fig. 5. Highly purified human islets of Langerhans at the end of the isolation procedure.

4. Islet transplantation procedure

The islet transplantation can be performed at the same time as the kidney transplantation (simultaneous islet-kidney transplantation) or in diabetic patients who had previously received a kidney transplant alone (islet after kidney transplantation). In both cases AB0 compatibility and a negative serum cross-match between the pancreas donor and the recipient are required. Obviously when a simultaneous kidney-islets transplantation is performed the pancreas which will undergo the isolation procedure is generally harvested from the same donor of the kidney.

As previously reported in recent years networks have developed connecting several islet transplant centers and single centers dedicated to the procedure of isolation.

The GRAGIL, Swiss-French Multicenter Network of Islet Transplantation, was organized as to send the pancreas to the Genève center for the procedure of isolation; and then distribute the islets obtained to different transplant centers in the south-east area of France.

By this network islet transplantations were performed also in centre at long distance provided that it would be done within 72 hours from the end of the isolation procedure (Langer et al., 2004). This organization allowed a cost decrease and an increase in the experience of the isolation center with a positive rebound on the percentage of successful isolations and consequently on the number of the transplants performed (Kempf et al., 2005). Further similar collaborations were created between north european centers (Nordic Network) and between american centers (Porrett et al., 2007).

In the case of simultaneous kidney-islets transplantation while the pancreas undergoes the procedure of isolation, generally the recipient contemporaneously undergoes kidney transplantation. Once the islets are received, they are infused through a surgical or, radiological procedure.

The implantation site is usually the hepatic parenchyma through the portal system of the recipient. Islets are infused by gravity into the portal circulation and flow with the portal blood to lodge in the hepatic sinusoids (Fig 6).

The surgical procedure is performed after the conclusion of the kidney transplant through injection of the islets in the portal system by opening the peritoneum and catheterization of an ileal vein.

The percutaneous approach is done by a minimally invasive procedure requiring interventional radiology technology. The portal vein is reached by a percutaneous catheter placed under ultrasound or angiographic guidance (Fig. 7).

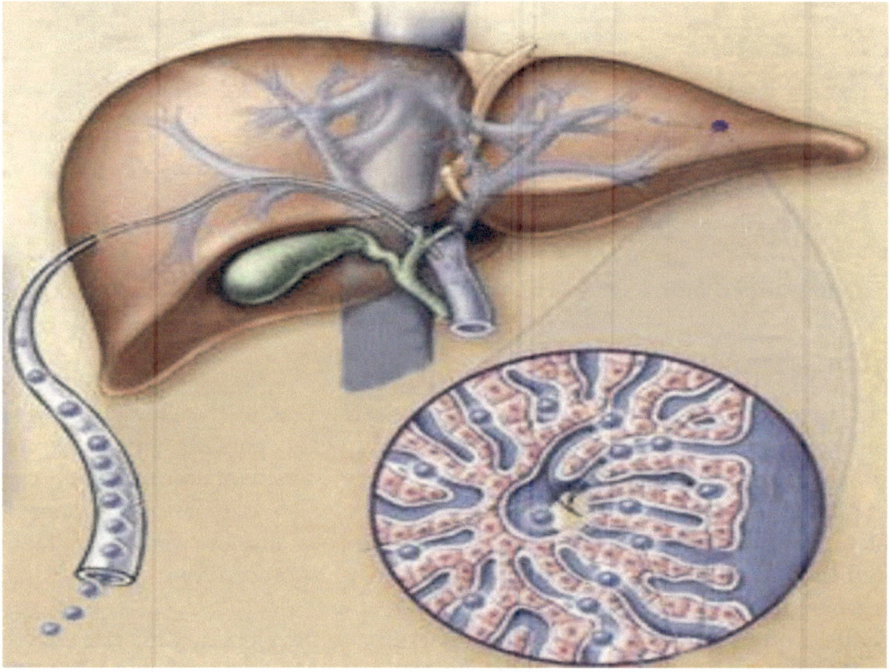

Fig. 6. Islet infusion into the recipient's liver (modified from: Robertson, *New England Journal of Medicine* 2004).

The radiological infusion of the islets can be performed few hours after the end of the kidney transplant or at long time after the operation, as for the islet after kidney transplant or in the case of subsequent islets infusions in patients just transplanted with islets.
Recently other implantation sites have been proposed in the clinical setting , like bone marrow (Cantarelli et al., 2009) or striated muscle (Christoffersson et al., 2010) which probably could show to be valid alternatives in a near future.

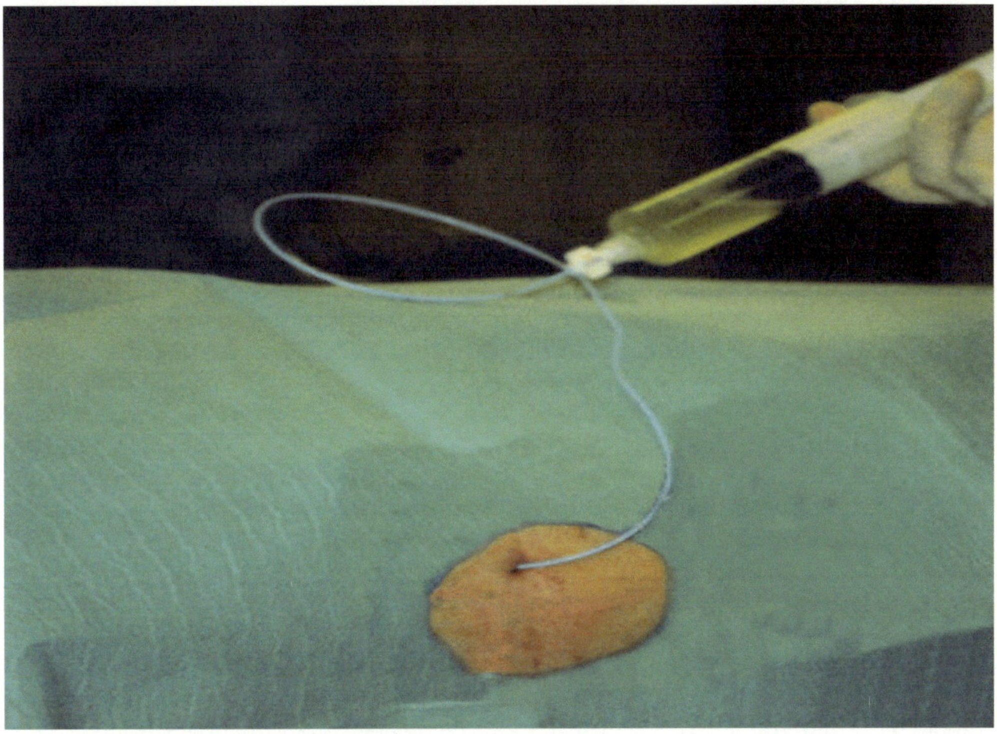

Fig. 7. Islet transplantation through a percutaneous catheter.

5. Complications related to islet transplantation

The procedure of islet transplantation proved to be very safe, especially when compared with the transplant of the whole pancreas. Data from CITR obtained from the analysis of more than 300 recipients showed that no complications occurred in case of injection by surgical approach and less than 10% of complications occurred in case of radiological infusion. Ower and collegues in 2003 showed that the most severe complications occurred in this case were intraperitoneal haemorrhages; anyway these were generally treated conservatively. The exact cause of bleeding in each case is often difficult to determine; however the peri-operative use of heparin to prevent portal thrombosis likely plays a role. The use of fibrin tissue sealant and embolization coils in the hepatic catheter tract seems to be effective in minimizing the bleeding risk.
Another complication related to the intrahepatic islet transplantation procedure is the insurgence of portal hypertension that can occur acutely during the islet infusion especially

in the case of subsequent infusions (Casey et al., 2002). The portal pressure however generally normalizes after the acute phase of the procedure.

Branch portal vein thrombosis was also frequently reported in the past; anyway this complication is generally limited and controlled with appropriate anticoagulation therapy. Actually the use of purer islet preparations, greater expertise in portal vein catheterization and new radiologic devices (catheters medicated for anticoagulation) will constantly reduce the risk of portal vein thrombosis although it will never be completely removed. A complication frequently reported is even the post-transplant elevation of liver enzymes but this is usually temporary and heals without further intervention.

In the past the appearance on magnetic resonance imaging (MRI) of intrahepatic periportal steatosis, occurring in a minority of islet recipients, has raised cautions. This finding is supposed to be due to the local effect of insulin produced by the transplanted islets on the hepatocyte metabolism and is reversible, since the complete resolution of MRI changes was reported in a patient after the graft function failed completely (Markmann et al., 2003). Successively the onset of focal steatosis in patient after islets transplantation was studied by sonogram (Maffi et al., 2005). These authors reported that signs of steatosis were often observed in patients after islet transplantation with total or partial function of the graft and normal liver function anyway was maintained in all of these. It was even proposed to consider the disappearance of this signs as a early marker of graft dysfunction.

6. Combined kidney-islet transplantation: Indications

The American Diabetes Association guidelines (http://www.diabetes.org/) remember that a combined kidney-pancreas transplantation should be always considered in case of uremic patient with DMT1 candidate to kidney transplantation. This recommendation is the result of the beneficial effects observed in terms of quality of life and survival after kidney-pancreas transplantation into patients suffering for DMT1 (Reddy et al., 2003). However since the procedure of pancreas transplantation has an high incidence of mortality and morbidity (Gruessner et al., 2004) it can be proposed only to selected population of patients candidate to kidney transplantation for diabetic nephropathy. In this the European Trial of Immunosuppression in Simultaneous Pancreas Kidney Transplantation (EUROSPK) study group reported that repeated laparotomies in the first 3 months after transplantation were performed in 35% of all the patients. Considering the much lower incidence of complication after islets transplantation several kidney-pancreas centers have also started programs of kidney-islets transplantation basing on the fact that these two procedures are complementary and suitable for patients with different features. Although the success of pancreas transplantation in term of graft survival is higher than islet transplantation with 80% of insulin-independency after 3 years (http://www.iptr.umn.edu/IPTR), some patients can be preferably directed towards a kidney-islet transplantation.

Actually the patient selection for either two therapeutic options is performed after a careful evaluation of possible advantages and disadvantages, with special regard to age and comorbidities. Patients at high risk of intraoperative complications are preferentially assigned to the less invasive procedure of islet transplantation, while younger and healthier patients are generally addressed to pancreas transplantation (Gerber et al., 2008).

In particular kidney-islets transplantation is preferred to kidney-pancreas for patients over 50 years of age or with severe macroangiopathy. Islet transplantation should also be considered for all the patients who underwent kidney-pancreas tranplantation and have functioning pancreatic graft removed for complications as recidivant anastomotic leackage. In this case the possibility to use the removed pancreas for the islets isolation procedure has to be considered. The obtained islets could be then eventually transplanted in the same patient. The esecution of a combined kidney-islet transplantation is also a possibility for uremic patients with DMT1 and a good compliance to insulin therapy with lack motivation to undergo a combined kidney-pancreas transplant. These patients indeed may not accept the elevated peri-operative morbidity associated with kidney-pancreas transplant, which is much higher than with kidney alone transplant. The recipient's weight is also a key factor in the choice between pancreas or islet transplantation. Considering that the volume of islets necessary to obtain success after transplant is calculated with respect to the body weight of the recipient, patients with high weight are generally excluded from the procedure of islets transplantation and treated with a combined kidney-pancreas transplant.

The islet after kidney transplantation should be considered instead of the pancreas after kidney transplantation in patients over 45 years of age or with severe macroangiopathy if the creatinine blood levels are stable below 2 mg/dl at least six months after kidney transplantation and steroids discontinuation (Vantyghem et al., 2009).

Contraindications to the islets transplantion are severe heart diseases (as untreatable coronary artery diseases, severe dilated cardiomyopathy, previous stroke or recurrent transient ischemic attacks) and hepatic diseases as severe steatosis if the recipient liver is used as transplantation site.

In recent years positive experiences have been reported in the field of kidney-pancreas transplant in insulin-dependent patients with type 2 diabetes mellitus (Light et al., 2005). Nath and collegues in 2005 showed that these patients, as well as DMT1 patients, had an higher beneficial effect from a combined kidney-pancreas transplantation than a kidney transplantation alone. On the basis of the high percentage of DMT2 patients with end-stage renal disease and their characteristics, related to macrovascular degeneration, they are generally patients older and in worse clinical conditions than DMT1 patients likely the combined kidney-islet transplantation could be a valid therapeutical option to combined kidney-pancreas transplantation for these patients if they are lean and with low insulin-resistance.

7. Combined kidney-islet transplantation: Aims and results

As previously reported, the global results of the islet transplantations performed in the last decade showed a progressive decline in graft function in the months following the procedure which allows a long-term insulin-independence in a limited number of patients but a residual partial graft function in the majority of them.

In order to extend the period of insulin-independence after transplant several centers have adopted the strategy to perform two or more islet infusions in the same recipient using different pancreas donors. However it was observed that this strategy could increase the risk of sensitization of the patients and therefore jeopardize the possibility of an eventually kidney retransplantation (Campbell et al., 2007). On the basis of these considerations, nowadays the goal of islet in combination with kidney transplantation is not necessarily to arrive at the insulin-indipendence but the achievement of a good glycemic control by a single islet transplantation (Lehmann et al., 2008). A single infusion of functioning islets can reduce long term levels of HbA1c and consequently prevent the occurrence of severe

asymptomatic episodes of hypoglycaemia and delay diabetes-related complications (Alejandro et al., 2008; Cure et al., 2008).
The group of Zurich (Gerber et al., 2008) reported their own experience in the field of combined kidney-islet and kidney-pancreas transplantation. They compared the long-term outcomes of diabetic patients subjected to kidney-islets transplantation and treated with immunosuppression carried out according with the Edmonton protocol versus patients subjected to kidney-pancreas transplant treated with conventional immunosuppression. In particular in the kidney-islet group induction therapy was performed with daclizumab and long-term therapy was carried out through levels of sirolimus and tacrolimus respectively of 7-10 μg/l and 3-6μg/l. In the kidney-pancreas group the induction therapy was performed with basiliximab and chronic immunosuppression was based on tacrolimus, mycophenolate mofetil and prednisone. The study demonstrated a similar kidney function and survival and an improvement of the blood glucose control in both groups.
Actually different protocols of immunosuppression are applied by different transplantation centers to patients trated with a combined kidney-islet transplantation. All of these protocols are steroid free and schedule different combinations beetween daclizumab or etanercept during the induction period plus mycophenolate mofetil or sirolimus and low-dose of tacrolimus or cyclosporine A. Since the number of the islets transplantation performed worldwide is low, a long period of time will be necessary in order to define which immunosuppressive protocol is the most favourable. Nowadays they seem all equally effective as long as steroids free (Alejandro et al., 2008).
As expected the Zurich group study reported a long-term insulin independence much lower in the group transplanted with kidney-islet than in the group transplanted with kidney-pancreas with a global result in line with the findings of the Edmonton trial group and a residual islet graft function sufficient to maintain glycemic control at a near-normal level. Interestingly it was showed that there was only a marginal benefit in terms of glucose control in those patients who received multiple islet infusions compared to patients who received only a single islet infusion. This finding and the not significant difference in glucose control between kidney-islet and kidney-pancreas patients despite much higher C- peptide levels and insulin independence in the latter group showed that even a minor residual beta cell function can significantly improve glycemic control, provided that patients are intensively treated with insulin. This consideration associate to the shortage of organs and the high risk of patient sensitization after multiple islet infusions reinforce the opinion that it preferable to undergo islet transplantation from a single pancreas donor. Moreover the cost is an additional important point in the context of repetitive islet transplantations. The same study reported that the cost of a combined kidney-islet transplantation is lower than the cost for a combined kidney-pancreas transplantation by about 10%, but exceeds in case two or more islet infusions have to be performed (Gerber et al., 2008).

8. Conclusions

The procedure of islet transplantation has made important progresses in the last decade, but the benefit/cost ratio between the improvement of glycemic control and the necessary chronic immunosuppressive therapy makes this option valid only for a restricted category of patients suffering from DMT1.

Actually the most frequent indication to islets transplantation is in combination with the kidney transplant in patients with end-stage diabetic nephropathy; patients therefore who will anyway undergo chronic immunosuppressive therapy.

The islet transplantation allows a long-term insulin independence in a limited number of patients. A residual partial graft function anyway leads to an improvement of the glycemic control, and consequently important advantages, in the majority of treated patients. In consideration of the low incidence of complications and the excellent kidney graft function results using immunosuppressive regimen avoiding steroids the combined kidney-islet transplantation procedure should be considered a valid alternative to kidney-pancreas transplantation for some patients categories.

Patient selection for either one of the two therapeutic options needs to be performed after a careful evaluation of possible advantages and disadvantages, with special regard to age and comorbidities. Patients older than 50 years or considered at higher risk of intraoperative complications were preferentially assigned to the less invasive procedure of kidney-islet transplantation, while younger and healthier patients could be preferentially assigned to kidney-pancreas transplantation.

Endogenous insulin production by transplanted islets combined with optimal insulin therapy is sufficient for maintenance of near-normal glucose levels that allows a delay of all diabetes-related complications and a strong reduction of the episodes of severe hypoglycemic episodes. Actually this should be considered the primary objective of the islet transplantation while the opportunity of increasing the periods of insulin-independence through multiple islets infusions is not commonly acceptable because of the high risk of sensitization to impair the possibility of a kidney retransplant.

In the face of organ shortage and cost procedure-related, these findings may lead to a new paradigm in islet transplantation, where the primary aim is not necessarily to achieve the same insulin-indipendence as in whole-organ transplantation but to improve the glycemic control of the patient through a much less invasive procedure.

Promising fields of research are nowadays focused on increasing the engraftment and survival of the islets after transplantation. If these studies will give positive results it will be possible in future to extend the actual indications of the combined kidney-islet transplantation procedure.

9. References

Alejandro R, Barton FB, Hering BJ et al. (2008). Update from the Collaborative Islet Transplant Registry *Transplantation* 2008 Dec 27;86(12):1783-8.

Campbell PM, Senior PA, Salam A et al. (2007). High risk of sensitization after failed islet transplantation. Am J Transplant 2007; 7: 2311–2317.

Cantarelli E, Melzi R, Mercalli A et al. (2009). Bone marrow as an alternative site for islet transplantation. *Blood* 2009 Nov 12;114(20):4566-74.

Casey JJ, Lakey JR, Ryan EA et al. (2002). Portal venous pressure changes after sequential clinical islet transplantation. *Transplantation* 2002, 74:913-915.

Christoffersson G, Henriksnäs J, Johansson L et al. (2010). Clinical and experimental pancreatic islet transplantation to striated muscle: establishment of a vascular system similar to that in native islets *Diabetes*. 2010 Oct, 59(10):2569-78.

Cure P, Pileggi A, Froud T, et al. (2008) Improved metabolic control and quality of life in seven patients with type 1 diabetes following islet after kidney transplantation. *Transplantation* 2008; 85:801–812

Del Carro U, Fiorina P, Amadio S et al. (2007). Evaluation of polyneuropathy markers in type 1 diabetic kidney transplant patients and effects of islet transplantation: neurophysiological and skin biopsy longitudinal analysis. *Diabetes Care* 2007, 30:3063–3069.

Fiorina P, Folli F, Bertuzzi F et al. (2003) Long-term beneficial effect of islet transplantation on diabetic macro-/microangiopathy in type 1 diabetic kidney transplanted patients. *Diabetes Care* 2003, 26:1129–1136.

Fiorina P, Folli F, Maffi P et al. (2005) Islet transplantation is associated with an improvement of cardiovascular function in type 1 diabetic kidney transplant patients. *Diabetes Care* 2005, 28:1358–1365.

Fiorina P, Venturini M, Folli F et al. (2005). Natural history of kidney graft survival, hypertrophy, and vascular function in end-stage renal disease type 1 diabetic kidney-transplanted patients: beneficial impact of pancreas and successful islet cotransplantation. *Diabetes Care*, 2005, 28: 1303–1310.

Gerber PA, Pavlicek V, Demartines N et al. (2008) Simultaneous islet–kidney vs pancreas–kidney transplantation in type 1 diabetes mellitus: a 5 year single centre follow-up. *Diabetologia*, 2008, 51:110–119.

Gruessner RW, Sutherland DE, Gruessner AC (2004) Mortality assessment for pancreas transplants. *American Journal of Transplantation,* 2004, 4:2018–2026.

Hering BJ, Matsumoto I, Sawada T et al. (2002). Impact of two-layer pancreas preservation on islet isolation and transplantation. *Transplantation,* 2002, 74:1813-1816.

Kaufman DB, Baker MS, Chen X et al. (2002). Sequential kidney/islet transplantation using prednisone-free immunosuppression. *American Journal of Transplantation,* 2002, 2:674-677

Kemp C, Knight M, Sharp D, et al (1973). Effect on transplantation site on the result of pancreatic islets isografts in diabetic rats. *Diabetologia,* 1973, 9:486-491

Kempf MC, Andres A, Morel P et al. (2005) Logistics and transplant coordination activity in the GRAGIL Swiss-French multicenter network of islet transplantation. *Transplantation*. 2005, 79(9):1200-5.

Lacy P, Kostianovsky M (1967) Method for the isolation of intact islets of Langerhans' from the rat pancreas. *Diabetes*, 1967,16:35-39.

Langer RM, Máthé Z, Doros A et al (2004) Successful islet after kidney transplantations in a distance over 1000 kilometres: Preliminary results of the Budapest-Geneva collaboration. *Transplant Proc.* 2004 Dec;36(10):3113-5.

Largiader F, Kolb E, Binswanger U, Illig R (1979). Succesful allotransplantation of an island of Langerhans. *Schweiz Med Wochenschr* 1979,109:1733-1736.

Lehmann R, Spinas GA, Moritz W, Weber M. (2008). Has Time Come for New Goals in Human Islet Transplantation? *American Journal of Transplantation* 2008, 8: 1096–110.

Light JA, Barhyte DY. (2005) Simultaneous pancreas– kidney transplants in type I and type II diabetic patients with end-stage renal disease: similar 10-year outcomes. *Transplant Proc* 2005, 37: 1283

Maffi P, Angeli E, Bertuzzi F et al. (2005). Minimal focal steatosis of liver after islet transplantation in humans: a long-term study. *Cell Transplantation.* 2005;14(10):727-33.

Markmann JF, Deng S, Desai NM et al. (2003). The use of non- heart-beating donors for isolated pancreatic islet transplantation. *Transplantation,* 2003, 75:1423-1429.

Markmann JF, Rosen M, Siegelman ES. (2003). Magnetic resonance-defined periportal steatosis following intraportal islet transplantation: a functional footprint of islet graft survival? *Diabetes* 2003, 52:1591-1594.

Najarian JS, Sutherland RL, Matas AJ, et al. Human islet transplantation: a preliminary report. *Tranplant Proc* 1977, 9:233-236.

Nath DS, Gruessner AC, Kandaswamy R et al. (2005) Outcomes of pancreas transplants for patients with type 2 diabetes mellitus. *Clin Transplant,* 2005, 19: 792.

Owen RJ, Ryan EA, O'Kelly K et al. (2003). Percutaneous transhepatic pancreatic islet cell transplantation in type 1 diabetes mellitus: radiologic aspects. *Radiology* 2003, 229:165-170.

Porrett PM, Yeh H, Frank A et al. (2007). Availability of suitable islet donors in the United States. *Transplantation* 2007, 84:280–282.

Reckard CR, Ziegler MM, Barker CF et al. (1973) Physiological and immunological consequences of transplanting isolated pancreatic islets. *Surgery,* 1973, 74:91-99.

Reddy KS, Stablein D, Taranto S et al (2003). Long-term survival following simultaneous kidney-pancreas transplantation versus kidney transplantation alone in patients with type 1 diabetes mellitus and renal failure. *Am J Kidney Dis.* 2003 Feb;41(2):464-70.

Ricordi C, Lacy P, Finke E et al. (1988) Automated method for isolation of human pancreatic islets. *Diabetes,* 1988, 37(4): 344-354.

Ricordi C, Tzakis AG, Carroll PB et al. (1992). Human islet isolation and allotransplantation in 22 consecutive cases. *Transplantation* 1992, 53:407-414.

Ricordi C and Strom TB (2004) Clinical islet transplantation: advances and immunological challenges. *Nature Reviews Immunology* 2004 April, 4, 259-268.

Robertson RP (2004) Islet transplantation as a treatment for diabetes - a work in progress. *New England Journal of Medicine* 2004 Feb. 12; 350-7:694-705.

Saito T, Gotoh M, Satomi S et al. (2010). Islet transplantation using donors after cardiac death: report of the Japan Islet Transplantation Registry. *Transplantation.* 2010, 90(7): 740-7.

Shapiro AM, Lakey JR, Ryan EA et al. (2000). Islet transplantation in seven patients with type 1 diabetes mellitus using a glucocorticoid-free immunosuppressive regimen. *N Engl J Med,* 2000, 343: 230–238.

Shapiro AM, Ricordi C, Hering BJ et al. (2006) International trial of the Edmonton protocol for islet transplantation. *N Engl J Med* 2006, 355: 1318–1330.

Tsujimura T, Kuroda Y, Avila JG et al. (2004). Influence of Pancreas Preservation on Human Islet Isolation Outcomes: Impact of the Two-Layer Method. *Transplantation,* 2004, 78(1): 96-100.

Tzakis AG, Ricordi C, Alejandro R et al. (1990). Pancreatic islet transplantation after upper abdominal exenteration and liver replacement. *Lancet* 1990, 336:402-405.

Vantyghem MC, Balavoine AS, Kerr-Conte J et al. (2009) Who should benefit from diabetes cell therapy? *Ann Endocrinol*. 2009, 70(6):443-8.

Younoszai R, Sorensen R, Lindall A et al. (1970). Homotransplantation of isolated pancreatic islets. *Diabetes*, 1970, 19:406-407.

19

Kidney-Pancreas Transplantation

Farzad Kakaei[1] and Saman Nikeghbalian[2]
[1]*Tabriz University of Medical Sciences*
[2]*Shiraz University of Medical Sciences*
Iran

1. Introduction

During the past decade, simultaneous pancreas kidney transplantation has been widely accepted as the most effective way to achieve normoglycemia in patients with type 1 diabetes and end-stage renal disease. This procedure was performed for the first time on a human in 1966 but it was in the 1980s, with advances in surgical technique and introduction of cyclosporine for immunosuppression, that the success rates of SPK became acceptable. According to international pancreas transplant (IPTR) report as of December 31, 2004, 23,043 pancreas transplants were performed worldwide. These included more than 17,000 (17,127) performed in the United States (US) and nearly 6,000 (5,916) from outside the US (non-US). In the US, the majority of the cases, 78% (n=11,898), have been simultaneous pancreas-kidney transplants (SPK); 16% (n=2427) are pancreas after kidney (PAK) transplants; 7% (n=1,008) are pancreas transplants alone (PTA).

Indications for pancreas transplantation include the development of diabetic complications such as ESRD, retinopathy or multiple attacks of hypoglycemic unawareness. Unfortunately, pancreas transplantation has been associated with the highest surgical complication rate of all the routinely performed organ transplant procedures (except for small intestinal or multivisceral transplantation) and the risk of pancreas graft loss from surgical complications (technical failures) is higher than from immunological reasons. The overall incidence of surgical complications in PTx is reported to be around 10% to 38%. This high rate of complications leads US centers to preclude PTA in most centers and now over 95% of pancreas transplantations are performed in patients with renal disease or a previous functioning kidney transplant. One year patient, kidney, and pancreas survival rates for recipients of an SPK transplant are 95%, 91%, and 86%, respectively. Compared to patients with diabetes who receive a kidney alone, the addition of a pancreas improves long-term patient and kidney graft survival. Recipients of a pancreas-after-kidney transplant or a pancreas transplant alone have an average 1-year pancreas graft survival rate of 78-83%.

In this chapter we will thoroughly describe many aspects of this complex transplantation procedure including:

- The history of pancreas transplantation
- Indications for pancreas transplantation
- Surgical aspects of pancreas graft procurement from the deceased donor
- Current surgical techniques for pancreas transplantation
- Immunosuppressive regimens

- Postoperative care of pancreas transplant recipients
- Complications of pancreas transplantation
- Long term results of pancreas transplantation

2. History of pancreas transplantation

Experimental transplantation of the pancreas in animals began as early as 1890 with proved success in the treatment of insulin dependent diabetes mellitus (Burke GW , et al, 2004). Grafting 3 pieces of sheep pancreas into the subcutaneous tissue of a diabetic child by Williams in 1893 was another attempt to treat diabetes but the patient died after 3 days because of severe ketoacidosis (Williams PW, 1903). The first clinical attempt to cure type 1 diabetes by vascular pancreas transplantation was done simultaneously with kidney transplantation, at the University of Minnesota in 1966 three years after first successful kidney transplantation (Kelly WD, et al, 1967), but the procedure was not performed with any frequency until many years later. Only 12 cases were done between 1967 till 1973 at the same center but almost all of them rejected before the first year after the operation. Segmental pancreas transplantation from living donors first introduced in 1979. Besides the rejection and vascular problems, dealing with pancreas exocrine secretion was complicated this type of procedure from the early days. By the mid-70s three different techniques were in use: enteric drainage, urinary drainage (into the ureter or directly into the bladder and duct injection. Ureteral drainage was first introduced by Gleidman et al (Gleidman et al , 1973). Bladder drainage first by direct anastomosis of the pancreatic duct to the bladder by Sollinger et al (Sollinger HW, et al, 1984) and then by duodenocystostomy by Nghiem and Corry (Nghiem DD & Corry RJ, 1987) was the most common method for exocrine drainage during the 1980s and 1990s and was still in use in some centers around the world specially for solitary pancreas transplantation. In the early 80's, a dramatic improvement in outcomes happened due to introduction of cyclosporine for immunosuppression (Squifflet JP, et al, 2008). In 1984, Starzl et al (Starzl et al,1984) reintroduced the technique of enteric drainage as originally described by Lillehei which is now is the routine procedure in most pancreas transplant centers.

In 1992, systemic venous drainage which was done through anastomosis of the portal vein to recipient iliac veins was replaced by direct portal drainage by Rosenlof et al (Rosenlof LK, et al, 1992) and also Shokouh-Amiri et al (Shokouh-Amiri MH, et al, 1992) because of its more physiologic pattern of insulin delivery. Now during the modem era of immunosuppression, the whole pancreas transplantation technique with portal - enteric drainage became the gold standard for simultaneous pancreas and kidney transplantation (SPK), and even for pancreas after kidney (PAK) or pancreas transplantation alone (PTA) and as of December 31, 2004, 23,043 pancreas transplants were reported to the international pancreas transplant registry (IPTR) of whom over 60% were performed in the united states.

3. Indications for pancreas transplantation

Patients with type 1 or insulin dependent type 2 diabetes mellitus are eligible for pancreas transplantation when they have any major complications of their disease, but because of complications of this type of surgery and need for lifetime immunosuppression therapy and frequent interventional surveillance (such as protocol biopsies), both the clinicians and the patients should be aware of those conditions that really might benefit from pancreas transplantation. Most common indications are as follows: diabetic nephropathy, retinopathy, neuropathy, disabling or life threatening hypoglycemic unawareness or incapacitating emotional or clinical problems associated with insulin therapy (White et al, 2009). Some of the rare indications (which are not accepted by all transplant surgeons) are diabetic complications after total pancreatectomy, presence of other autoimmune diseases, insulin allergy or resistance to subcutaneous insulin.

Patients should be considered as potential candidate for pancreas transplantation only when their morbidity or mortality risk of the surgical procedure or long term immunosuppressive treatment are lower than the diabetic complications (Meloche RM, 2007). Unfortunately, most patients with chronic diabetes who develop these complications have major comorbidities such as obesity, cardiovascular, cerebrovascular or peripheral vascular diseases, diabetic gastropathy, and vascular or neuropathic diabetic foot. These patients are most suitable for pancreatic islet cell transplantation which is very simpler and has fewer and more minor complications that the relatively complex surgical procedure of whole pancreas transplantation.

Patients with diabetic nephropathy who need concomitant renal transplantation are the most common eligible patients who benefits from simultaneous kidney pancreas transplantation (SPK). Those who previously underwent kidney transplantation are candidate for pancreas after kidney (PAK) transplantation. According to 2004 annual IPTR report (The University of Minnesota, modified on May 28, 2009, available from www.iptr.umn.edu/annual_reports/2004_annual_report/3_txs_cat/home.html) pancreas transplant alone (PTA) now performed in less than 5% of all pancreas transplant recipients because unlike SPK or PAK recipients they don't otherwise need immunosuppression for their renal allograft and surgical complications of this procedure and higher rejection rate of this type of operation outweigh the potential benefits of glycemic control. PTA is best appropriate for those patients with hypoglycemic unawareness, stable renal function, and minimum proteinuria (White et al, 2009), because calcineurin inhibitor immunosuppressive therapy reduces the glomerular filtration rate at least 20% in the first year after pancreas transplantation (Mazur et al, 2004) PAK transplantation is performed mostly in patients who have an appropriate living donor for kidney graft and also are simultaneously candidate for pancreas transplantation. When coordinate logistics available, these operation using kidney graft from the living donor and pancreas graft from a deceased donor may be performed at the same time and at the same center. In some centers partial segmental pancreas transplantation technique is used for SPK when the living donor is suitable for this complex procedure firstly performed by Merkel in 1973 (Merkel et al, 1973).

The contraindications for pancreas transplantation are the same as other types of transplantations (Tiong & Krishnamurthi, 2011): active infections, coronary angiographic evidence of significant non-correctable or untreatable coronary artery disease, recent myocardial infarction, ejection fraction below 30%, history of recent, incompletely treated malignancy (excluding non-melanoma skin cancer), positive HIV serology, positive hepatitis B surface antigen serology, substance abuse, major ongoing psychiatric illness, recent history of noncompliance, inability to provide informed consent, any systemic illness that would severely limit life expectancy or compromise recovery, significant, irreversible hepatic or pulmonary dysfunction. In major pancreas transplant centers like University of Wisconsin, Minnesota, correctable (by stenting, angioplasty or bypass) coronary artery disease is not considered as a contraindication for pancreas transplantation (Sollinger HW, et al, 2009). Most pancreas transplant programs exclude patients older than 45-50 years of age, because higher age is an independent risk factor for predicting poorer surgical outcome, although the rejection rate is significantly lower in this age group (Gruessner AC & Sutherland DE, 2005).

4. Surgical aspects of pancreas graft procurement from the deceased donor

Not all deceased donors are suitable for pancreas graft procurement. Absolute contraindications for pancreas donation are active infection or malignancy, positive serologic evaluation for hepatitis B surface antigen (HBsAg), hepatitis C virus (HCV), human immunodeficiency virus (HIV), and human T cell lymphotropic virus type 1 (HTLV-1), proved diabetes mellitus, pancreatitis (acute/chronic), severe pancreatic steatosis or edema, previous pancreatic surgery and intra-abdominal sepsis. Donor hyperglycemia is common because of stress condition and use of high dose corticosteroids and not a contraindication for use of the pancreas, although it may contribute as a minor risk factor for long-term graft loss (Gores, et al, 1992). Most surgeons only select younger non-obese donors (age 10-50 years, weight 30-100 kg) who are hemodynamically stable without need to high doses of vasopressors. Also a cardiocerebrovascular cause of brain death and massive volume resuscitation are other risk factors for postoperative complications in the recipients (Troppmann C, 2004). Because of these stringent criteria, according to IPTR report, in the United States only 21% of the deceased donor pancreata were used for transplantation during the year 2004. Because pancreas transplantation is not life saving, procurement of other donor organs are more important. If the surgeon considers that the pancreas is not suitable for transplantation it may be used for research or pancreas islet cell transplantation (Shapiro, et al, 2000).

The procedure starts with a long midline incision from suprasternal notch to symphysis pubis area usually by the liver team. All intrathoracic and abdominal organs are evaluated systematically to rule out any suspicious lesion. First, all usual dissections for controlling supraceliac and infrarenal aorta, arc of thoracic aorta and superior or inferior mesenteric vein should be performed, so in case that patient becomes unstable the surgeon can rapidly proceed with cold perfusion of the organs for their safe retrieval. The right colon is completely mobilized from retroperitoneum and then an extended Kocher maneuver is done. All ligaments of the liver are transected and then arterial anatomy of the liver and pancreas is evaluated by palpating the hepatic artery pulsation in the hepatodudenal portion of lesser omentum. The surgeon should have complete knowledge of hepatic artery abnormalities and possibility of existence of a right accessory or right replaced hepatic artery that originate from superior mesenteric artery. In rare cases the entire hepatic artery are originated from superior mesenteric artery. With novel microsurgical techniques none of these anomalies is considered as a contraindication for concomitant liver, pancreas or small intestinal harvesting from a deceased donor. It's better to perform a dissection of the supraduodenal area to reveal the anatomy of common hepatic artery, gastroduodenal and celiac trunk branches specially the origin of the splenic artery. The other dissections may be performed after cold perfusion. The common bile duct is divided and infrarenal aorta and superior or inferior mesenteric vein are cannulated at the next stage. Supraceliac aorta is clamped 3-5 minutes after systemic heparinization and the heart team also clamps the aortic arc and cold perfusion is started.

The most commonly used solutions for cold perfusion are Belzer University of Wisconsin (UW), histidine - tryptophan - ketoglutarate (HTK) and Celsior solution with no significant difference in the results when cold ischemia time is less than 12 hours, but UW is the standard solution in most centers (Fridell et al, 2010).
The donor blood evacuated through the supradiaphragmatic or in some certain cases (such as history of previous thoracic surgery) infrarenal inferior vena cava (IVC). After removing the heart and lungs, liver, pancreas and small intestine usually are procured en bloc and the remaining dissection may be performed in the bench procedure. The duodenal lumen is irrigated by 500 ml of 20% Betadine, 50 mg/ml amphotericin B and metronidazole solution through the nasogastric tube and distal and proximal part are transected by gastrointestinal (GIA) staplers. The portal vein is divided 1 cm to 2 cm above the pancreas border. The gastroduodenal artery is divided and suture ligated and the splenic artery is divided close to its origin and marked by a nonabsorbable 6-0 suture for future identification. The base of mesentery at the inferior border of pancreas is transected by another GIA stapler and the whole pancreas-duodenum-spleen graft removed.
In back table or bench procedure, all excessive fat tissue and spleen should be removed and the origin of mesentery and all small arterial and venous branches in the inferior border of pancreas is reinforced again for future hemostasis. Duodenum is shortened again and reinforced in both distal and proximal side by non-absorbable sutures. Arterial reconstruction is performed by anastomosis of the donor iliac Y-graft, external and internal iliac branches to the graft superior mesenteric and splenic artery, respectively. We also recommend using a small segment of donor left gastric or inferior mesenteric artery for reperfusion of gastroduodenal artery for better circulation of duodenum and head of pancreas to prevent future frequent duodenal ulcers in the graft.

5. Current surgical techniques for pancreas transplantation

Forty five years after the first SPK, controversy continues regarding the site of both venous effluent and exocrine drainage and also many other aspects in this complex surgical procedure. In most centers, SPK is performed separately by two teams. During kidney transplant procedure, the pancreas team prepares the pancreas graft for transplantation. Usually an intraperitoneal approach is used by a long midline incision and the kidney graft is transplanted by standard technique to left iliac fossa (renal artery to internal or external iliac artery and then renal vein to external iliac vein and at last ureter to the bladder or native ureter as described in other chapters of this book). Use of right side for pancreas transplantation is recommended due to more superficial iliac artery position in this side, which makes arterial anastomosis easier. The next step is arterial or venous reconstruction. Except for a few minor changes in arterial reconstruction technique (such as reperfusion of gastroduodenal artery or changing the site of arterial inflow), there is no significant change in the arterial reconstruction technique during these era. There are at least 2 options for venous drainage: systemic or portal drainage. It's better to reconstruct the venous drainage before arterial anastomoses because a short portal vein of the graft may limit the later maneuvers needs for venous anastomosis. In our center we use the recipient superior mesenteric vein at the base of mesentery below the transverse mesocolon for venous outflow(portal drainage) and right common iliac artery for arterial inflow to the donor iliac Y-graft. Those surgeons that prefer to use systemic venous drainage use the right external or common iliac vein as the venous outflow, perfectly as the same manner that they used external iliac artery and vein for kidney transplantation. After completing the arterial and venous anastomoses, the graft is reperfused and complete hemostasis is done. Usually despite every effort for complete hemostasis during back table preparing of the pancreas graft, there is brisk bleeding around the borders of the graft at the time of reperfusion and crystalloid and blood product replacement should be used to prevent hypotension and subsequent damage to the kidney and pancreas grafts. Graft splenectomy is done at this stage by some surgeons. The next step is anastomosis of the graft duodenum to the recipient jejunum (enteric drainage) or bladder (bladder drainage). When portal drainage is chosen, the pancreas head should be directed cephalad and use of bladder drainage is almost impossible and vice versa. In other words, if the surgeon selects bladder drainage for duct management (as is the case for most PTA surgeries), the pancreas head should be directed caudad and use of portal venous drainage won't be possible. Also if portal drainage is used we need a rather longer donor common iliac artery or even an extension graft for arterial reconstruction of the graft.

Drains are inserted at the end of operation around the kidney and pancreas graft separately to monitor for postoperative bleeding and leakages. We prefer to perform the kidney transplant operation retroperitoneally in the left iliac fossa and at the end use the peritoneum to hide the kidney to be able to monitor the kidney graft complications such a urine leakage and lymphocele s1eparately from the pancreas graft.

It is worthwhile to describe briefly about the evolution of these techniques in the leading center of pancreas transplantation in the world, University of Minnesota (Sutherland DE, 2001). For pancreas graft duct management they used many techniques during this long term period: a cutaneous graft duodenostomy, open duct free intraperitoneal drainage, duct occlusion (simple ligation or polymer-injection), enteric drainage (ED) and urinary drainage (bladder and only 4 cases to the ureter). Except for ED and bladder drainage (BD), the other techniques of duct management were used only in the early years of pancreas transplantation evolution in a small portion of their cases because of their recognized complications and now they (along with most other pancreas centers around the world) lose their early enthusiasm to BD technique because of its chronic complications such as hyperchloremic metabolic acidosis, dehydration, chemical cystitis and urethritis, recurrent hematuria, bladder stones, and recurrent graft pancreatitis, recurrent urinary tract infections, urethral stricture and perineal excoriations (Han DJ & Sutherland DE, 2010). They recommended using BD for duct management because they could monitor the graft function by serial measurement of urinary amylase and they had showed that decrease in urinary amylase always preceded hyperglycemia as a manifestation of rejection in pancreas grafts. For SPK bladder drainage transplants, monitoring of urine amylase was less important to detect rejection because a serum creatinine elevation usually preceded a urine amylase decline when the rejection episode affected both organs. In the past, severe complications would lead to conversion of BD to ED in up to 25% of patients within 10 years (Sollinger HW, et al, 1992). Enteric drainage also has many complications (at least risk of enteric contamination) that may be devastating in case of duodenal necrosis and gastrointestinal leakage.

Several options are available for enteric drainage: side-to-side duodenojejunostomy, or duodenojejunostomy with a Roux-en-Y limb and duodenoduodenostomy (Hummel et al, 2008). The site of duodenojejunostomy (distance from the Treitz ligament) and its length are different between authors. Although duodenoduodenostomy complications are more

dangerous but endoscopic biopsy and hemostasis of duodenal ulcers of the transplanted pancreas-duodenum complex will be made feasible by this technique.
Systemic venous drainage is technically less demanding and used with less difficulty and more frequently by those surgeons who are familiar with kidney transplantation technique. In the early days of pancreas transplantation in the University of Minnesota, portal venous drainage was used for the pancreas graft venous effluent only in seven cases. Systemic hyperinsulinemia caused by systemic drainage first was showed by Diem et al (Diem et al, 1990). This concept lead Rosenlof et al (Rosenlof LK, et al, 1992) and Shokouh-Amiri et al (Shokouh-Amiri MH, et al, 1992) to recommend routine use of portal drainage for SPK transplants in 1992 because of its more physiologic pattern of insulinemia, although the carbohydrate metabolism is not different in both groups some authors showed that de-novo hyperinsulinemia predisposes to accelerated atherosclerosis (Fontbonne A, et al, 19991) and increasing the level of low density lipoprotein(LDL) (Hughes TA , et al, 1995) but its relevance to pancreas transplant recipients is not certain.
Some centers now use extra- or retroperitoneal approaches for better accessibility of the pancreas graft for postoperative routine percutaneous biopsies and easier arterial anastomosis and some of them suggest using an en bloc kidney-pancreas transplantation from the same donor. The technique of retroperitoneal pancreas transplantation with portal-enteric drainage was first described by Boggi et al in 2005 (Boggi et al, 2005). This method may be used in patient with severe intraperitoneal adhesions due to multiple previous abdominal surgeries and also for pancreas retransplant. Kahn et al described the same technique by systemic venous drainage (Kahn et al, 2008). They recommend this approach in obese patient with severe iliac artery atherosclerosis because of best exposure of the aorta and inferior vena cava by this method. In the en bloc techniques donor pancreas and left (or right kidney) is harvested en bloc in line with abdominal aorta so that the superior mesenteric, celiac artery and renal artery origins are maintained intact on the aorta and no arterial reconstruction by donor iliac artery would be needed in the back table procedure. Then the aorta could be used as the complex graft inflow conduit. Portal vein and renal vein may be anastomosed separately (Schenker P, et al, 2009) but we recommend to anastomose the graft portal vein to the left renal vein in the bench procedure, and then use the graft renal vein as the venous outflow of the graft. This will reduce the warm ischemia time by reducing the number of vascular dissections and anastomoses.

6. Immunosuppressive regimens

Unlike other solid organ transplantations, pancreas transplantation needs immunosupression for prevention of alloimmune rejection or autoimmune recurrence of diabetes mellitus even in transplant between identical twins (Sutherland DE, et al, 1984). In the early years of pancreas transplantation, only azathioprine and prednisone were used for immunosupression, but such a regimen was not adequate for prevention of rejection in PTA recipients (Sutherland et al, 2001). In the later years Minnesota antilymphocyte globulin added to this regimen for induction and maintenance immunosupression evolved to triple therapy by cyclosporine, azathioprine and prednisone. This change along with better surgical methods and better preservation of the deceased donor pancreas by UW solution resulted in better long term results of pancreas transplantation during the era of late 80's and early 90's. The pancreas rejection rate remained as high as 78% in this era (Stegall MD, et al, 1997). Gradually, cyclosporine and azathioprine were replaced by Tacrolimus

(Prograf™) and Mycophenolate mofetil (MMF, Cellcept™) during the later years and monoclonal anti T cell antibodies such as basiliximab and daclizumab added to induction immunosuppressive regimen of these patients. By use of these new regimens, risk of rejection decreased to less than 8-11% in the modern era of pancreas transplantation (Cantarovich D & Vistoli F, 2009).

The routine immunosupression regimen in most pancreas transplant centers includes a T cell depleting agent such as rabbit antithymocyte globulin (rATG or Thymoglobulin™) with a total dose of 4-12 mg/kg in divided doses, or alemtuzumab (Campath™) or an interleukin-2 receptor antagonist such as basiliximab (Simulect™) or daclizumab (Zenapax™) for induction immunosupression. We add a low dose intravenous methylprednisolone (Solumedrol™) in the day of operation to prevent allergic reactions to these agents. Unfortunately, these induction regimens only reduce the biopsy proven acute rejection (BPAR) episodes, but had no or modest effect on the patient or graft long term survival (Sutherland DE, 2009). Information about use of anti inter leukin-2 receptor antibodies are confounding. For example, Becker *et al.* found no significant differences in patient and graft survival comparing the outcomes of no induction versus daclizumab or basiliximab in 63 SPK transplant recipients receiving tacrolimus, MMF and prednisone. There was, however, a slightly higher rate of deaths due to sepsis in the anti-IL-2R induction group (Becker et al, 2006). Newer data mostly agree with the use of alemtuzumab for induction immunosuppression, without incurring a risk of increased infections or malignancies except for cytomegalovirus. (Sollinger et al, 2011) . A new randomized trial has showed that in the short term follow-up after SPK, alemtuzumab and rATG induction therapies has been similarly safe and effective but alemtuzumab is more cost-effective and has been associated with less BPAR episodes (Farney AC, et al, 2009).

For maintenance immunosupression, perhaps the best current regimen is prednisolone free or rapidly steroid tapering regimens which consist of tacrolimus and MMF combinations. Omitting the steroids from the maintenance regimens results in better wound healing and also prevents from steroid induced insulin resistance. Replacing the MMF with sirolimus has no effect on pancreas rejection rates, but had poorer long term kidney graft survival in the SPK recipients, because sirolimus accentuates the nephrotoxicity of tacrolimus (Gallon LG, et al, 2007). Tacrolimus per se had diabetogenic effects in other solid organ transplant recipients, but such an effect has not been shown in pancreas transplant recipients, may be due to more cautious use of this nephrotoxic drug in SPK recipients or use of healthier donors for pancreas transplantation (Ming CS & Chen ZH, 2007). Because of known nephrotoxicity of calcineurin inhibitors (CNIs) e.g. tacrolimus or cyclosporine, avoidance of these drugs in all pancreas transplant recipients who are potentially at risk of renal damage (SPK or PAK recipients) or future renal failure (PTA recipients) is desirable but all initial attempts with calcineurin inhibitor avoidance or minimization are less promising (Singh RP & Stratta RJ, 2008). Although newer agents such as sirolimus, everolimus, and CTLA-4 Ig are agents known to be either both nonnephrotoxic and nondiabetogenic or less so when compared with CNIs, but their impact on pancreas transplant results are not yet evaluated by randomized trials and their solitary use may be dangerous for the recipients and end up with graft loss (Cantarovich D & Vistoli F, 2009).

7. Postoperative care of pancreas transplant recipients

Perioperative care of pancreas transplant patients has no difference with any other major operation in diabetic patients. Kidney-pancreas recipients should be dilysed briefly for 1-2 hours before the operation to maintain the serum potassium below 5.5 meq/l and also to optimize the platelet function. Complete fluid removal is unnecessary. During the operation all of these patients need routine anesthesiologist monitoring with special attention to hemodynamic stability, tight control of blood sugar (to prevent both hypo- or hyperglycemia) and serum potassium, arterial blood gas and prevention of volume overload by keeping central venous pressure (CVP) around 8-10 mmHg. Ketoacidosis may be occur and should be prevented by intravenous insulin infusion if required. Sterile aseptic techniques are recommended for all venous and arterial line placements.

In kidney-pancreas recipients, usually kidney transplantation is done before the pancreas operation. During the kidney operation the patient is kept mildly volume expanded and before declamping the renal vasculature, the systolic blood pressure should be around 120 mmHg and Mannitol and furosemide should be infused as described in the other chapters of this book. Induction immunosuppressant (methylprednisolone or any types of t-cell receptor or interleukin-2 antibodies) usually started preoperatively and continued throughout the operation. Some surgeons advise to use these agents prior to declamping of vascular anastomoses.

After completion of kidney transplantation, the anesthesiologist should carefully monitor the brisk urine output and maintain it at least around 4 ml/kg/hour with appropriate fluid and electrolyte management throughout the remaining of the operation. Hypovolemia leads to acute tubular necrosis (ATN) of the renal allograft and volume overload will result in bowel and pancreas graft edema and may lead to postoperative abdominal compartment syndrome and graft dysfunction. Anticoagulation is not recommended for general kidney transplant alone recipients unless in the instance of presence of any other indications like mechanical heart valve or history of coagulopathy. But because pancreas is a low blood flow organ, especially when portal drainage is chosen as the preferred method for surgery, before clamping of the inflow veins or arteries, it's better to use systemic heparinization of the patient and we prefer to continue intravenous heparin postoperatively at least for 5 days to maintain the activated partial thromboplastin time (aPTT) around 1.5 times the normal value (between 55 - 85 seconds) to prevent graft vascular thrombosis.

After the operation the patient is transferred to transplant intensive care unit and CVP, vital signs, arterial blood gas, blood pressure, urine output and blood glucose are monitored continuously. Almost all patients are extubated in the operating room and don't need postoperative mechanical ventilation.

Kidney transplant patients usually have large urine outputs (as much as 20 liters/day) that should be replaced according to the patient fluid and electrolyte condition as discussed in the other chapters. Hypotension is usually due to intraabdominal bleeding (even in the absence of drainage from abdominal drains) or gastrointestinal bleeding from duodenal anastomosis and should be treated emergently by reexploration of the patient and fluid management. Hypertension should be avoided and treated appropriately to prevent bleeding and graft malfunction.

Oral immunosuppressive drugs (usually tacrolimus and MMF) are started after the day of operation. Prednisolone replaces intravenous methylprednisolone after 3 days by a dose of 0.5-1 mg/kg/day, but rapidly tapered to near zero during the next 4 weeks-3 months. All patients should receive prophylactic broad spectrum antibiotics for 2-5 days and most centers add antifungal drugs (such as amphotericin B or an azole derivative or caspofungin) and anti cytomegalovirus (CMV) drugs (e.g. gancyclovir) to this regimen. These protocols are different slightly among pancreas transplant centers and its better and mandatory that each physician follow the routines of her/his center to avoid and confusion in the patients and personnel and future evaluations of the center. During the first 24 hours the patient may need small doses of intravenous insulin for maintaining the blood sugar below the 200 mg/dl because of delayed graft function or use of high doses of corticosteroids but after that or in case of any unusual increase in the serum glucose level, prompt assessment of graft vascular status by Duplex ultrasound and appropriate intervention should be done emergently. We routinely monitor the graft vasculature by Duplex ultrasound at least every 12 hours for 5 days after the operation. Many other means are available for continuous monitoring of graft function besides the blood sugar and duplex scanning. Serial measurements of serum amylase and/or lipase, C-peptide, and urine amylase and protocol ultrasonographic or computerized scan (CT) guided biopsies are among them (Han DJ & Sutherland DE, 2010).

Drains should be monitored for unusual leakage or bleeding and removed as soon as possible (usually after 5 days for pancreas drains and 24 after removing the Foley catheter for perirenal drain). Nasogastric tube remains until the return of gastrointestinal function usually for at least 72 hours. A recent study has showed that omission of a nasogastric tube has been associated with earlier return of bowel function, less discomfort, and shorter length of stay (Barth RN, 2008). Ambulation of the patient is desirable in the first 24 hours after the operation to prevent deep vein thrombosis and also other known complications of bedridden patients such as atelectasis or postoperative ileus.

8. Complications of pancreas transplantation

Despite large improvements in immunosuppression and surgical techniques, the history of pancreas transplantation, unlike that of other abdominal organ transplants, has largely been shaped by its associated complications (Troppmann C, 2010). We can discuss about these complications in 3 distinct categories: surgical, infectious, immunologic and other non-immunologic. Infectious complications are not specific for pancreas transplantation and many of their aspects are in common with other solid abdominal organ transplantation and discussion about them is presented in other chapters of this book.

Surgical complications

Surgical complications now decreased to at least 8% in large series reported by experienced pancreas transplant center s around the world and most of them frequently result in graft loss and increase recipient morbidity and mortality significantly and augment transplant cost considerably (Goodman J & Becker YT, 2009). Many of the surgical complications (such as hematuria, duodenocystostomy leakage, reflux pancreatitis, etc) are unique to the bladder drainage as previously discussed. These known complications lead pancreas transplant centers to avoid from bladder drainage and use this technique only for PTA cases. Over 25% of these cases require conversion of BD to ED.

Vascular thrombosis

Vascular thrombosis has remained the most common complication of pancreas transplant procedure with a frequency of 3-10% (Gruessner AC & Sutherland DE, 2009). Other major complications include: intraabdominal bleeding, gastrointestinal bleeding, leakage (from duodenal anastomosis), pancreatitis, pancreatic necrosis, pancreatic fistula, abscess formation and other complications of any other major abdominal surgery such as atelectasis,

pneumonia, deep vein thrombosis, wound infection, dehiscence, and cardiovascular problem which is common in diabetic and chronic renal failure patients.
Graft vascular thrombosis has many factors that most of them are technical because of several vascular anastomoses that needs for pancreas transplantation. Rotation during arterial reconstruction at the time of back table preparing, inadvertent intimal damage to the iliac artery Y-graft during harvesting and over inflation of the arteries during flushing are the known causes of arterial thrombosis. Higher donor age, cardiocerebrovascular cause of brain death and massive fluid resuscitation and hemodynamic instability of the donor and use of HTK as the preservation solution, especially when cold ischemia time is over 12 hours, and recipient hypercoagulable states or use of sirolimus are other important factors (Troppmann C, 2010). Venous thrombosis may be secondary to arterial thrombosis, severe pancreas rejection, and severe graft pancreatitis or may be completely technical or due to use of venous extension graft. There is no difference in the rate of graft thrombosis according to the venous drainage (systemic or portal) technique. Also PAK transplantation has been an independent risk factor for graft vascular thrombosis (Troppmann C, et al, 1996). Most centers use systemic heparinization for prevention of vascular thrombosis and continue this treatment for 5-7 days and after that change this regimen to 325 mg/day acetyl salicylic acid (ASA) or warfarin for selected cases (second transplants or confirmed hypercoagulable state), although some authors hadn't agree with this concept in the past (Sollinger HW, 1996). Usually the first sign of graft thrombosis is increasing the blood sugar level that should be promptly assessed by Duplex ultrasound. The patient may complain from abdominal pain and later abdominal tenderness will be revealed. Venous thrombosis will results in dark hematuric urine if bladder drainage had been used. Except for a few case reports most of these cases needs relaparotomy for graft removal, but if diagnosed early interventional radiologists or reanastomosis may be very rarely salvage the graft.

Leakage

Leakage from duodenojejunostomy or duodenoduodenostomy is a devastating complication of pancreas transplantation that may be associated with high morbidity and mortality, if recognized late. Because of spillage of enteric content, the patients develop signs and symptoms of peritonitis such as abdominal pain and tenderness, fever, high leukocytosis, and bilious content in abdominal drains. Sometimes this leakage is minor and the site of leakage contained by the greater omentum. Using broad spectrum antibiotics and Roux-en-Y reconstruction help more to obscuring the symptoms. In this situation, signs and symptoms may be obscure and only developing ileus, low grade fever, tachycardia and tachypnea, mild hyperglycemia, hyperamylasemia, low platelet count, will lead the surgeon to perform additional imaging studies (mostly abdominal CT scan) to diagnose this problem. The patient should be undergone exploration and in most cases the best option is graft pancreatectomy if peritonitis is diffuse or associated by multiple intraabdominal abscesses, or the patient ids unstable. Leakage from bladder drained pancreas may have milder symptoms and treated by combined bladder decompression and percutaneous drainage or conversion to enteric drainage. In cases of severe sepsis or diffuse infection, graft pancreatectomy is inevitable. Obscure leakages may be revealed as late as 2 weeks after the operation by abdominal abscess or pancreatic fistula that may be treated conservatively by percutaneous drainage, but many times the patient will prefer the graft to be removed because of the associated bothering complications such as skin excoriations by pancreas secretions. Also, pancreas fistula may be a complication of focal necrosis (due to

ischemia, rejection or infection) of the pancreas graft which communicate with the pancreatic duct or a complication of graft pancreatitis.
Many factors is contributed to anastomosis leakage, including technical errors, ischemia of the head of pancreas (due to vascular events, previous atherosclerosis of the donor, edematous duodenum at the time of reconstruction), reexploration for another causes, intraabdominal bleeding or diffuse primary peritonitis, severe acute rejections, and CMV infections. Some surgeons suggest that revascularization of the gastroduodenal artery or even the gastroepiploic artery may prevent ischemia of the head of pancreas and the duodenal C-loop (Nghiem DD, 2008 and Muthusamy ASR et al, 2008). We use this technique in every patient that the gastroduodenal artery is relatively large. This may also protect the duodenum from later ulcers and bleeding.

Pancreatitis

There is no uniformly accepted definition for graft pancreatitis, but all of the available definitions include the signs and symptoms of native pancreatitis with rising lipase and amylase, and maintained endocrine function (Troppmann C, 2010). Unfortunately these serum markers associated poorly with graft pancreatitis and may be prolong elevated after pancreas transplantation. Early pancreatitis is the result of poor graft handling, long ischemia time and preservation and reperfusion injury and may be visible during the operation, by graft edema and diffuse or focal fat necrosis around the graft. Prolonged cold ischemia time over 12 hours, use of HTK as the preservation solution and also poor donor quality are other risk factors (Han DJ & Sutherland DE, 2010). In case of bladder drained pancreas, pancreatitis may be the result of urine reflux. Most of these conditions are self limiting and adding the subcutaneous octreotide (0.1-0.2 mg every 8 hours) for 3-5 days after the operation, bowel rest and temporary total parenteral nutrition is the only treatment that needed. In rare cases it is so severe that the only option for treatment will be graft necrosectomy or pancreatectomy. In BD drained cases, the best treatment for resistant cases is conversion to enteric drainage. Rarely the cause of acute pancreatitis in these patients is CMV or other viral infections that if confirmed should be treated by gancyclovir or other antiviral agents.
Graft pancreatitis may be complicated just like the native pancreatitis with infections, pseudocysts, peripancreatic sterile fluid or pancreatic ascites, pancreatic fistula, and arterial or venous thrombosis or bleeding which should be treated accordingly.

Bleeding

Intraabdominal bleeding is relatively common after this operation. In most cases this is a technical error due to poor hemostasis of the pancreatic graft or the so many vascular anastomoses that used. Sometimes it is due to technical errors in the associated kidney transplant procedure. It may be due to heparin overdose that should be diagnosed by measurement of aPTT and if needs treated by protamine sulfate. Severe graft pancreatitis or pseudoaneurysms of the infected vascular anastomoses are another source of late abdominal bleedings in these patients that may be delayed as long as 2 weeks to several months after the operation. Early postoperative hypertension may cause transient bleeding from vascular anastomoses and through the abdominal drains that will be stopped spontaneously when the hypertension controlled appropriately with any need to reexploration.
Gastrointestinal bleeding is unique complication of enteric drainage. The site of bleeding may be duodenojejunostomy, distal jejunojejunostomy of the Roux-en-Y loop,

duodenoduodenostomy (DD) or mucosal ulcers in the graft duodenal C-loop (Nikeghbalian S, 2009) due to ischemia, rejection or CMV infection. One should rule out other sources of bleeding, such as native small bowel CMV infections, stress native gastric or duodenal ulcers by upper GI endoscopy or enteroscopy and also obscure site of bleeding such as neoplasm or angiodyplasia of the colon. If DD had been used for enteric drainage, endoscopy can be used for diagnosis and treatment. In other cases, angiography, red blood cell isotope scan, or enteroscopy may be used for diagnosis, but in most cases at last the best option is to explore the patient (Orsenigo E, et al, 2005).

Lymphocele and chylous ascites

Because of diverse perivascular dissections (around the aorta, IVC, superior mesenteric vein and iliac arteries and veins) in pancreas transplantation surgery, intraabdominal or perigraft sterile collections due to lymphorrehea are common. These collections may be so much that exit through the abdominal drains and when the patient returns on oral diet being frankly chylous. Perigraft collections are one of the causes of graft dysfunction and should be drains percutaneously. Chylous ascites is usually self-limiting and therapy is only supportive (replacing the fluid and electrolytes and use of oral short chain fatty acids and removing the drains to prevent lymphocyte and protein depletion. The best treatment is prevention by meticulous dissections and ligation of all perivascular lymphatics during the dissections.

Immunologic complications

Acute rejection

Rejection of the pancreas graft is as much as 40 % in the past and pancreas transplant recipients receive the highest level of immunosuppressant drugs among other abdominal organ transplantations. One-year rates of rejection have steadily decreased and are currently in the 10–20% range depending on case mix and immunosuppressive regimen (Singh RP &Strata RJ, 2008). The highest rate of graft loss due to immunologic rejection is seen in PTA recipients and the lowest incidence is in SPK patients, probably due to immunologic protective effect of the renal graft or earlier diagnosis of the rejections with better response to therapy. In the era that BD pancreas transplant was a routine the best indicators of pancreas transplant rejection was decreasing urine amylase and lipase which was preceded by hyperglycemia. In other words, BD experience showed that pancreas exocrine function is affected sooner that its endocrine function and when hyperglycemia presents it would be too late to salvage the pancreas from acute rejection. In the SPK patient, increasing the serum creatinine due to rejection usually preceded the hyperglycemia, and then diagnosis of the renal graft rejection actually means the pancreas rejection as well and both can treated simultaneously by the same antirejection treatment except for rare instances. Nowadays, with increasing experience, protocol percutaneous pancreas biopsies are routine procedure in the armamentarium of any major pancreas transplant unit. By these timely scheduled biopsies, every pancreas rejection could be diagnosed before its clinical and paraclinical symptoms present but until now the controversies continued about the candidates and interval of this time of protocol biopsies for the surveillance of pancreas graft rejection (Gaber LW, 2007).

It's shown that HLA mismatch is a major contributor to pancreas rejection and fully HLA matched recipients has the lowest levels of rejections when on the same immunosuppressive protocol (Burke, et al, 2004). Other series showed that combination immunosuppressive therapy including T-cell depleting antibodies for induction, tacrolimus and MMF could improve the outcome significantly, even in poorly HLA matched PTA recipients (Gruber

SA, et al, 2000). However, in the PTA and PAK categories, HLA matching has remained an important outcome factor (Han DJ & Sutherland DE, 2010).
Signs and symptoms of pancreas rejection are obscure. Only 5-20% of patients developed mild fever, abdominal pain or distension or sometimes ileus or diarrhea (Sutherland DE, et al, 2010). The clinicians should be rely on paraclinical markers and after performing the biopsy the best approach is to treat empirically when a combination of paraclinical changes support existence of an acute rejection episode, if the results of the biopsy prepare with delay. The best treatment for confirmed acute rejection episodes is the use of pulse methylprednisolone therapy plus increasing the dose of oral drugs or adding the sirolimus to the previous drugs. Nephrotoxicity and diabetogenic effect of tacrolimus, and effect of corticosteroids on insulin resistance induction should be in mind. In severe cases use of thymoglobulin or other T-cell depleting antibodies may be required. As previously described many immunosuppressive protocol are under investigation now to better prevent these acute rejection episodes which most of them focused on corticosteroid spring and also use of T-cell depleting antibodies for induction.

Chronic rejection

Previously, chronic rejection does not appear to be as large a problem for pancreas-transplant recipients as it does for renal-transplant recipients (Hopt UT & Drognitz O, 2000). As the number of pancreas transplants surviving beyond the first year increases, chronic rejection is becoming increasingly common (Burke, et al, 2004). The rate of pancreas loss to chronic rejection was 8.8% in 914 pancreas transplants followed for 3 years. Chronic rejection was highest in the PAK (11.6%) and PTA (11.3%) and lowest for SPK (3.7%)(Humar A ,et al, 2003). The most important pathologic changes in chronic rejection are replacing the pancreas tissue with fibrous band with distortion of architecture and loss of acini (Gaber LW, 2007). The severity of chronic rejection is not correlated well to the graft loss, but clinically the patients become hyperglycemic, first with response to oral hypoglycemic agents and then low dose insulin injection an at last completely depend on insulin injection for the rest of their lives. There's no definite treatment for this type of rejection, which may be simply a non-immunologic "physiologic wear and tear "of the organ, but some authors try to use sirolimus in these conditions (Matias P, et al 2008).

Non-immunologic complications

One the known complications of every solid organ transplant is primary nonfunction or delayed graft function. Primary non-function is a definition of inclusion. No other cause of graft nonfunction should be found, e.g. graft vascular thrombosis, graft necrosis, or severe acute rejections or pancreatitis. In this condition the graft is viable and non-inflamed with no need for pancreatectomy, but no insulin secretion is found and the patient needs insulin injection as his/she preoperative situation. Some patients transiently need low doses of insulin for their blood glucose hemostasis, but after a maximum of 1 week this requirement decreased to zero. This condition is named "delayed graft function". In both of this condition no frank anatomic or pathologic changes in the graft is found in the postoperative assessment of the patient. Poor donor quality and poor handling of the graft is the only causes that may contribute to these conditions.
Other non surgical and non-immunologic complications also may be seen in these diabetic patients. Many of these are due to preoperative diabetic complications. Delayed gastric emptying (gastroparesis), constipation or diarrhea, dizziness and lightheadedness (all due to autonomic neuropathy), peripheral neuropathy, poor visual acuity (accelerated

retinopathy)and accelerated cataract are among these complications. Many of these diabetic signs and symptoms are multifactorial and side effects of the immunosuppressant drugs and multiple other antifungals and antivirals that used for these patients plus preoperative poor diabetic control accelerates them. Every effort should be used to diagnose the treatable causes and treat them accordingly. For example for diabetic gastroparesis, use of erythromycin or domeperidone has been moderately successful (Zaman f, et al, 2004). Intractable diarrhea may be due to CMV or other microbial or protozoal infections which should be treated. But when no known cause is found, the best treatment is dividing the dose o MMF to 4 times a day and also use of subcutaneous octreotide. Also every transplant team member should be completely remember the common complications of the immunosuppressive drugs and treat them appropriately or change the drugs if possible.

9. Long term results of pancreas transplantation

Long term results of pancreas transplantation improve day by day with better surgical experience and use of more potent immunosuppressive regimen. Pancreas graft 1 year survival rate improves from 75% in 1998 to 85% at the end of 2003 for SPK cases, and from 55 to 77% for PAK and from 45 to 77% in PTA patients (Gruessner AC & Sutherland DE, 2005). This improvement also is seen in PTA patients that traditionally have the worst outcome, as shows in many studies. For example in a report Stratta et al. by 1 year patient and graft survival has increased to 96% and 86%, respectively (Stratta RJ, et al, 2003). In one the largest recently published studies, the 5-year, 10-year, and 20-year patient survival for SPK recipients was 89, 80, and 58%, respectively (Wai PY & Sollinger HW, 2011).
Now, by decreasing the technical failures, the randomized studies to valuate other effective factors can be performed with better accuracy and less confounding bias. Perhaps the best statistics that show the effect of pancreas transplantation is the statistics about comparing the patient survival in kidney transplant alone recipients with SPK patients. Even in older studies, life expectancy of younger recipients (less than 50 years) of SPK is 10 years longer than diabetic patients who only received a kidney graft from deceased donors (23.4 years *vs* 12.9 years) (Tyden G, et al, 1999, Ojo AO,etal, 2001). When both grafts were procured from deceased donors, SPK transplant recipients has better survival rate than kidney transplant alone (KTA) recipients but this difference is not significant when KTA patients received their grafts from living donors. The presence of a functioning pancreas graft improved survival by 20% at 8 years (Reddy KS, 2003).
Patient survival is not statistically different according to the type of exocrine drainage (BD vs. ED), but quality of life is better and overall complications is less when BD is used (Sollinger HW, et al, 2009). Despite the improved survival, the most common type of death in these patients is death with a functioning graft and cardiovascular morbidity remains a major contributor to patient outcome in these patients (Sollinger HW, et al, 2009).
Comparing with KTA recipients, quality of life in those 95% of patient who survive after SPK transplantation is improved significantly, due to cessation of insulin injections, multiple needling for glucose monitoring and better emotional status (Sutherland De, et al, 2001 & Joseph JT, et al, 2003).

Effect on end organ damage

Pancreas transplantation improves glycemic control in long term follow up, manifested by lower hemoglobin A_{1C} level, improved lipid profile and insulin mediated protein kinetics,

normal hepatic glucose production and counter-regulatory effects of glucagon to hypoglycemia (White SA, et al, 2009).
Sollinger et al suggests that despite numerous reports of improvement in secondary diabetic complications after SPK, retinopathy and cardiac or vascular complications of diabetes are not reversible and show no improvements after SPK, but severe (peripheral and autonomic) neuropathy is an exception to this rule (Sollinger et al, 2009). Diabetic retinopathy will deteriorate after pancreas transplantation in over 30% of patients if it is in an advanced proliferative phase prior to the operation, but after 3 years the pancreas transplantation results in stabilization of retinopathy progression (Chow VC, et al, 1999). Cataract is a known complication of any organ transplantation and is the results of corticosteroids and calcineurin inhibitors and may become evident after pancreas transplantation as well.
Macrovascular effects of diabetes may not improve after pancreas transplantation, especially because of calcineurin inhibitor (CNI) effect on weight gain, dyslipidemia and hypertension, and many other risk factors that are very common in diabetic patients. Also the peripheral vascular disease in diabetics is often far too advanced to reverse. Because, most centers exclude patient with Macrovascular diabetes complications and no conclusive study exists about effect of pancreas transplantation on natural history of macrovascular disease in these patients (Sutherland De, et al, 2001). Deterioration depends on the ongoing risks. Some centers show the benefits of pancreas transplantation on cerebrovascular system, but again the results are inconclusive. Coronary artery disease, diastolic function, left ventricular geometry and cardiac autonomic function may be improved after SPK comparing with KTA recipients after a few years (White SA et al, 2009).
Normoglycemia also improves the diabetic glumerulopathy (but does not reverse it) and decrease the proteinuria. On the other hand, use of CNIs per results in nephropathy and may decrease the creatinine clearance. SPK recipients may not survive enough to benefit from the effects of normoglycemia on their nephropathy. In diabetic KTA recipients, the diabetic nephropathy is progressively leading to lower kidney graft survival and many studies show that PAK transplantation may improves the kidney graft survival by prevention of accelerated diabetic glumerulopathy in these patients.). Some studies shows that PTA (if done early enough) can preserve renal function, but It takes at least 5 years until a pancreas transplant can reverse the lesions of diabetic nephropathy (Sutherland De, et al, 2001).

10. References

[1] Barth RN, Becker YT, Odorico JS, et al. Nasogastric decompression is not necessary after simultaneous pancreas-kidney transplantation. *Ann Surg*. 2008;247:350 -356.

[2] Becker LE, Nogueira VA, Abensur MP, *et al*. No induction versus anti-IL2R induction therapy in simultaneous kidney pancreas transplantation: A comparative analysis. Transplant Proc 2006; 38:1933–1936

[3] Boggi U, Vistoli F, Signori S, et al: A technique for retroperitoneal pancreas transplantation with portal-enteric drainage. *Transplantation* 79:1137, 2005

[4] Burke GW, Ciancio G, Sollinger HW: Advances in pancreas transplantation. *Transplantation*. 2004 May 15;77(9 Suppl):S62-7. Review.

[5] Cantarovich D, Vistoli F: Minimization protocols in pancreas transplantation. *Transpl Int* 2009; 22: 61–68.

[6] Chow VC, Pai RP, Chapman JR, et al: Diabetic retinopathy after combined kidney-pancreas transplantation. *Clin Transplant.* 1999;13:356-362.
[7] Cohn JA, Englesbe MJ, Ads YM, et al. Financial implications of pancreas transplant complications: a business case for quality improvement. *Am J Transplant* 2007; 7:1656–1660.
[8] Diem P, Abid M, Redmon JB, et al. Systemic venous drainage of pancreas allografts as independent cause of hyperinsulinemia in type I diabetic recipients. Diabetes 1990; 39:534 -540.
[9] Farney AC, Doares W, Rogers J, et al: A randomized trial of alemtuzumab versus antithymocyte globulin induction in renal and pancreas transplantation. *Transplantation.* 2009 Sep 27;88(6):810-9.
[10] Fontbonne A, Charles MA, Thibult N, et al. Hyperinsulinaemia as a predictor of coronary heart disease mortality in a healthy population: the Paris Prospective Study, 15-year follow-up. *Diabetologia* 1991 34: 356–61.
[11] Fridell JA, Mangus RS, Powelson JA: Organ preservation solutions for whole organ pancreas transplantation. *Curr Opin Organ Transplant.* 2011; 16(1):116-122
[12] Gaber LW: Pancreas allograft biopsies in the management of pancreas transplant recipients: histopathology review and clinical correlations. (Arch Pathol Lab Med. 2007;131:1192–1199
[13] Gallon LG, Winoto J, Chhabra D, et al: Long-term renal transplant function in recipient of simultaneous kidney and pancreas transplant maintained with two prednisone-free maintenance immunosuppressive combinations: tacrolimus/mycophenolate mofetil versus tacrolimus/sirolimus. *Transplantation* 2007; 83: 1324–29.
[14] Gliedman ML, Gold M, Whittaker J, et al: Clinical segmental pancreatic transplantation with ureter-pancreatic duct anastomosis for exocrine drainage. *Surgery.* 1973;74:171–180
[15] Goodman J, Becker YT: Pancreas surgical complications. Curr Opin Organ Transplant. 2009 Feb;14(1):85-9.
[16] Gores PF, Gillingham KJ, Dunn DL, et al: Donor hyperglycemia as a minor risk factor and immunologic variables as major risk factors for pancreas allograft loss in a multivariate analysis of a single institution's experience. *Ann Surg* 1992; 215: 217–30.
[17] Gruber SA, Katz S, Kaplan B, et al. Initial results of solitary pancreas transplants performed without regard to donor/recipient HLA mismatching. *Transplantation* 2000; 70(2): 388.
[18] Gruessner AC, Sutherland DE. Pancreas transplant outcomes for United States (US) and non-US cases as reported to the United Network for Organ Sharing (UNOS) and the International Pancreas Transplant Registry (IPTR) as of June 2004. *Clin Transplant.* 2005 Aug;19(4):433-55
[19] Han DJ, Sutherland DE: Pancreas transplantation. *Gut Liver.* 2010; 4(4):450-65.
[20] Hopt UT, Drognitz O. Pancreas organ transplantation: short and longterm results in terms of diabetes control. Langenbecks Arch Surg 2000; 385(6): 379.
[21] Hughes TA, Gaber AO, Amiri HS, et al. Kidney-pancreas transplantation. The eff ect of portal versus systemic venous drainage of the pancreas on the lipoprotein composition. *Transplantation* 1995; 60: 1406–1412.

[22] Humar A, Khwaja K, Ramcharan T, et al. Chronic rejection: the next major challenge for pancreas transplant recipients. *Transplantation.* 2003;76:918–923

[23] Hummel R, Langer M, Wolters HH, et al: Exocrine drainage into the duodenum: a novel technique for pancreas transplantation. *Transpl Int* 21:178, 2008

[24] Joseph JT, Baines LS, Morris MC, Jindal RM: Quality of life after kidney and pancreas transplantation: a review. *Am J Kidney Dis.* 2003 Sep; 42(3):431-45

[25] Kahn J, Iberer F, Kniepeiss D, et al: Retroperitoneal pancreas transplantation with systemic-enteric drainage—case report. *Clin Transplant* 22:674, 2008

[26] Kelly WD, Lillehei RC, Merkel FK, Idezuki Y, Goetz FC: Allotransplantation of the pancreas and duodenum along with the kidney in diabetic nephropathy". *Surgery* 1967:61 (6): 827–37

[27] Lillehei RC, Ruiz JO, Aquino C, et al. Transplantation of the pancreas. *Acta Endocrinol (Copenh)* 1976; 83(suppl 205): 303.

[28] Matias P, Araujo MR, Romão JE Jr, Abensur H, Noronha IL.: Conversion to sirolimus in kidney-pancreas and pancreas transplantation. *Transplant Proc.* 2008 Dec;40 (10):3601-5.

[29] Mazur MJ, Rea DJ, Griffi n MD, et al: Decline in native renal function early after bladder-drained pancreas transplantation alone. *Transplantation* 2004; 77: 844–49.

[30] Meloche RM: Transplantation for the treatment of type 1 diabetes. *World J Gastroenterol.* 2007;13(47):6347–6355.

[31] Merkel FK, Ryan WG, Armbruster K, Seim S, Ing TS. Pancreatic transplantation for diabetes mellitus. IMJ Ill Med J 1973;144:477-479 passim.

[32] Ming CS, Chen ZH: Progress in pancreas transplantation and combined pancreas-kidney transplantation. *Hepatobiliary Pancreat Dis Int.* 2007 Feb;6(1):17-23.

[33] Muthusamy ASR, Tzivanakis A, Brockmann JG, et al. Revascularization of the gastroepiploic artery in pancreas transplant. *Transpl Int* 2008; 21:1194– 1195.

[34] Nghiem DD, Corry RJ. Technique of simultaneous renal pancreatoduodenal transplantation with urinary drainage of pancreatic secretion. *Am J Surg* 1987; 153: 405–06.

[35] Nghiem DD. Revascularization of the gastroepiploic artery in pancreas transplant. *Transplant Int* 2008; 21:774–777.

[36] Nikeghbalian S, Bahador A, Salahi H, et al: Non-marginal donor C-loop ulcers as a cause of gastrointestinal bleeding after pancreas transplantation: three case reports. *Transplant Proc.* 2009 Sep;41(7):2930-2.

[37] Ojo AO, Meier-Kriesche HU, Hanson JA, et al: The impact of simultaneous pancreas-kidney transplantation on long-term patient survival. *Transplantation* 2001; 71: 82–90.

[38] Orsenigo E, Fiorina P, Dell'Antonio G, et al: Gastrointestinal bleeding from enterically drained transplanted pancreas. *Transpl Int.* 2005 Mar;18(3):296-302.

[39] Reddy KS, Stablein D, Taranto S, et al: Long-term survival following simultaneous kidney-pancreas transplantation versus kidney transplantation alone in patients with type 1 diabetes mellitus and renal failure. *Am J Kidney Dis* 2003; 41: 464–70.

[40] Rosenlof LK, Earnhardt RC, Pruett TL, et al. Pancreas transplantation. An initial experience with systemic and portal drainage of pancreatic allografts. *Ann Surg.* 1992;215:586–595.

[41] Schenker P, Flecken M, Vonend O, et al: En bloc retroperitoneal pancreas-kidney transplantation with duodenoduodenostomy using pediatric organs. *Transplant Proc*. 2009 Jul-Aug;41(6):2643-5.
[42] Shapiro AJM, Lakey JRT, Ryan EA, et al : Islet transplantation in seven patients with type I diabetes mellitus using a glucocorticoid-free immunosuppressive regimen. *N Engl J Med* 343:230, 2000
[43] Shokouh-Amiri MH, Gaber AO, Gaber LW, et al. Pancreas transplantation with portal venous drainage and enteric exocrine diversion: a new technique. *Transplant Proc*. 1992;24:776–777.
[44] Singh RP, Stratta RJ: Advances in immunosuppression for pancreas transplantation *Curr Opin Organ Transplant* 13:79–84
[45] Singh RP, Stratta RJ: Advances in immunosuppression for pancreas transplantation. *Curr Opin Organ Transplant*. 2008 Feb;13(1):79-84
[46] Sollinger HW: Pancreatic transplantation and vascular graft thrombosis [editorial]. *J Am Coll Surg* 1996; 182:362.
[47] Sollinger HW, Cook K, Kamps D, Glass NR, Belzer FO: Clinical and experimental experience with pancreaticocystostomy for exocrine pancreatic drainage in pancreas transplantation. *Transplant Proc* 1984; 16: 749–51.
[48] Sollinger HW, Odorico JS, Becker YT, et al: Campath vs. basiliximab after simultaneous pancreas–kidney transplantation. *Am J Transplant* (in press).
[49] Sollinger HW, Sasaki TM, D'Alessandro AM, et al: Indications fo enteric conversion after pancreas transplantation with bladder drainage. *Surgery* 1992; 112: 842–45.
[50] Sollinger HW, Odorico JS, Becker YT, et al: One Thousand Simultaneous Pancreas-Kidney Transplants at a Single Center With 22-Year Follow-Up. *Ann Surg* 2009;250: 618–630
[51] Squifflet JP, Gruessner RW, Sutherland DE: The history of pancreas transplantation: past, present and future. *Acta Chir Belg*. 2008 May-Jun;108(3):367-78.
[52] Starzl TE, Iwatsuki S, Shaw BW, Jr, et al. Pancreaticoduodenal transplantation in humans. *Surg Gynecol Obstet*. 1984;159:265–272.
[53] Stegall MD, Simon M, Wachs ME, Chan L, Nolan C, Kam I. Mycophenolate mofetil decreases rejection in simultaneous pancreas-kidney transplantation when combined with tacrolimus or cyclosporine. *Transplantation* 1997; 64: 1695–700.
[54] Stratta RJ, Lo A, Shokouh-Amiri MH, et al. Improving results in solitary pancreas transplantation with portal-enteric drainage, thymoglobin induction, and tacrolimus/mycophenolate mofetil-based immunosuppression. *Transpl Int* 2003; 16(3): 154.
[55] Sutherland DE, Goetz FC, Najarian JS: Living-related donor segmental pancreatectomy for transplantation. *Transplant Proc*. 1980;12:19–25.
[56] Sutherland DE, Gruessner RW, Dunn DL, et al: Lessons learned from more than 1,000 pancreas transplants at a single institution. *Ann Surg*. 2001 Apr;233(4):463-501. Review.
[57] Sutherland DE, Sibley R, Xu XZ, et al. Twin-to-twin pancreas transplantation: reversal and reenactment of the pathogenesis of type I diabetes. *Trans Assoc Am Physicians* 1984; 97: 80–87.
[58] Tiong HY, Krishnamurthi V (2011): Selection and preparation of the pancreas transplant recipient. In: *Kidney and pancreas transplantation, a practical guide.* Srinivas

TR and Shoskesisbn DA, pp. 201-209, Springer science + business media, ISBN: 978-1-60761-641-2, New York

[59] Troppmann C (2004): Surgical complications. In: *Pancreas transplantation.* Gruessner RWG, Sutherland DER, pp. 206–237, Springer, New York.

[60] Troppmann C, Gruessner AC, Benedetti E, et al: Vascular graft thrombosis after pancreatic transplantation: univariate and multivariate operative and nonoperative risk factor analysis. *J Am Coll Surg*. 1996 Apr;182(4):285-316.

[61] Troppmann C: Complications after pancreas transplantation. *Curr Opin Organ Transplant*, 2010;15:112–118

[62] Tyden G, Bolinder J, Solders G, et al:Improved survival in patients with insulin-dependent diabetes mellitus and end-stage diabetic nephropathy 10 years after combined pancreas and kidney transplantation. *Transplantation* 1999; 67: 645–48.

[63] Wai PY, Sollinger HW: Long-term outcomes after simultaneous pancreas-kidney transplant. *Curr Opin Organ Transplant*. 2011; 16(1):128–134.

[64] White SA, Shaw JA, Sutherland DE: Pancreas transplantation. *Lancet*. 2009 May 23; 373(9677):1808-17. Review

[65] Williams PW: Transplantation of Pancreas in Diabetes. *Br Med J* 1903;1:580

[66] Zaman F, Abreo KD, Levine S, Maley W, Zibari GB: Pancreatic Transplantation: Evaluation and Management *J Intensive Care Med* 2004 19: 127

20

Clinical Pharmacokinetics of Triple Immunosuppression Scheme in Kidney Transplant (Tacrolimus, Mycophenolate Mofetil and Corticosteroids)

Robles Piedras Ana Luisa and Monroy Funes Manuel Alejandro
Universidad Autónoma del Estado de Hidalgo
México

1. Introduction

Kidney transplantation is now firmly established as the treatment of choice for most patients with End Stage Renal Disease. The short-term outcomes of renal transplantation have dramatically improved over the past several decades; in a large part, this success is due to improvements in immunosuppression and post transplantation medical care. The goal of immunosuppressive strategies in transplantation is to deliver immunosuppression that result in long-term allograft and patient survival, while minimizing the complications of this immunosuppression. Tacrolimus has been one of the cornerstones of immunosuppressive strategies in clinical transplantation. Currently, regimens that are used for induction and maintenance therapy include the concomitant use of Mycophenolate Mofetil and Corticosteroids. The purpose of this chapter is to provide comprehensive and updated information, about the immunosuppressive drugs tacrolimus, mycophenolate mofetil and corticosteroids, which are used as triple immunosuppression scheme to the control of rejection of the transplanted organ.

2. Tacrolimus

Tacrolimus was isolated from Streptomyces tsukubaensis in 1984 and is a potent immunosuppressant widely used to prevent acute rejection after solid-organ transplantation, it has a macrolide lactone structure (C44H69NO12, 803.5 g/mol) comprising a 23-member carbon ring and a hemiketal masked b-diketoamide function(Scott et al., 2003). In 1984, the compound tacrolimus was discovered in a soil sample taken from the foot of Mount Tsukuba in Tokyo that was found to possess potent in vitro immunosuppressive qualities. Initially called FR000506, tacrolimus was subsequently found to suppress interleukin-2 production associated with T-cell activation, thus inhibiting the differentiation and proliferation of cytotoxic T cells (Fung, 2004). Tacrolimus has a greater effect on the T lymphocyte than does an earlier released calcineurin inhibitor, cyclosporine. In a response to antigenic stimulation, in vitro studies on cultured CD4 helper T lymphocytes have demonstrated that tacrolimus is superior to cyclosporine in selectively inhibiting the secretion of various cytokines, including IL-2 and IL-3. This difference may contribute to the greater effect of tacrolimus than cyclosporine on impairing the expression of alloantigen-stimulated T cells in solid organ transplantation (Vicari-Christensen et al., 2009). The calcineurin inhibitor tacrolimus, has a toxicity profile similar to cyclosporine (Winkler & Christians, 1995). Two types of side effects must be differentiated: (1) those caused by (over)immunosuppression and (2) those caused by drug toxicity. Immunosupression itself results in an increased incidence of infectious complications and malignancies, mainly lymphoma, as well as failure of vaccination. The principal adverse effects associated with tacrolimus treatment include nephrotoxicity, neurotoxicity, disturbances in glucose metabolism, gastrointestinal (GI) disturbance and hypertension. Susceptibility to infection and malignancy is also increased. Many of the adverse effects of tacrolimus are dose-related; nephrotoxicity, neurotoxicity, glucose metabolism disturbances, GI disturbances and infections may occur more frequently or be more severe at higher whole-blood tacrolimus concentrations. Importantly, these adverse events can often be managed by dosage reductions. Concomitant drugs such as corticosteroids may also contribute to some adverse effects (Naesens, 2009¸Plosker, 2000). Because of its variable pharmacokinetics and narrow therapeutic index, monitoring drug concentrations is essential to avoid the risks of over- and under-immunosuppression. For routine clinical practice therapeutic drug monitoring of tacrolimus whole blood concentrations is recommended and target ranges have been defined (Jusko, 1995; Plosker & Foster, 2000). Increased tacrolimus toxicity is observed with increased tacrolimus concentrations. The large variability in the pharmacokinetics of this drug, makes it difficult to predict what drug concentration will be achieved with a particular dose or dosage change (Staatz & Tett, 2004; Venkataramanan, 1995). Therapeutic drug monitoring-guided dosing is an important clinical tool to control Tacrolimus exposure and to improve outcome after transplantation. Therapeutic drug monitoring plays an important role in maintaining effective therapeutic levels and avoiding toxic tacrolimus blood concentrations after systemic administration for the treatment of autoimmune diseases (Christians, 2006). Today, tacrolimus has gained worldwide recognition as the cornerstone of immunosuppressant therapy. It is now commercially available in more than 70 countries and has established a significant role in the field of transplantation. According to statistics issued by the Global Observatory on Donation & Transplantation, an average of 69,300 kidney transplants are performed around the world each year, which constitutes nearly 70% of solid organ transplants performed world-wide (WHO, 2008). There are currently over 100,000 transplant recipients being treated with immunosuppressive drugs, and tacrolimus is being prescribed to patients with new liver and kidney transplant recipients around the world. Studies have also shown that other adjunctive agents can be safely prescribed in combination with tacrolimus.

2.1 Mechanism of action

2.1.1 Immunosuppressive activity

Tacrolimus is a macrolide immunosuppressant that acts by a variety of different mechanisms which include inhibition of calcineurin. The drug inhibits T-lymphocyte activation, this may occur through formation of a complex with FK 506-binding proteins (FKBPs). The complex inhibits calcineurin phosphatase. This is believed to inhibit interleukin-2 (IL-2) gene expression in T-helper lymphocytes. Tacrolimus also binds to the steroid receptor–associated heat-shock protein 56. This ultimately results in inhibition of transcription of proinflammatory cytokines such as granulocyte–macrophage colony-stimulating factor (GM-CSF), interleukin-1 (IL-1), interleukin-3 (IL-3), interleukin-4 (IL-4), interleukin-5 (IL-5), interleukin-6 (IL-6), interleukin-8 (IL-8), and tumor necrosis factor alpha (TNF alpha). The mechanism of action of tacrolimus is largely similar to that of cyclosporin, but tacrolimus is 10 to 100 times more potent. The drugs both inhibit calcineurin but do so via formation of complexes with different immunophilins: Tacrolimus binds to FK-506 binding protein, whereas cyclosporin binds to cyclophilin A. The drugs appear to differ in their effects on patterns of TH2 cell cytokine expression and possibly some aspects of humoral immunity. Furthermore, lymphocyte sensitivity to the drugs may differ between patients. Calcineurin is a protein phosphatase known as protein phosphatase 2B. It is responsible for activating the transcription of interleukin 2 (IL-2), which stimulates the growth and differentiation of a T-cell response. Calcineurin dephosphorylates a nuclear factor of activated T cells, and cytoplasmic component transcription factor can then migrate into the nucleus and activate genes involved in IL-2 synthesis. IL-2 is a powerful inflammatory catalyst implicated in allograft rejection. The allograft rejection process begins when an alloantigen is presented to the T-cell receptor and an increase in the cytoplasmic levels of calcium results. This response activates calcineurin by binding regulatory subunits and calmodulin complexes. Calcineurin induces different transcription factors that are important in the IL-2 genes. IL-2 activates helper T lymphocytes and induces the production of other cytokines. In this way, calcineurin governs the process of rejection. The amount of IL-2 produced by the helper T cells is believed to significantly influence the extent of the immune response (Pascual et al., 2002).

2.1.2 Toxicity

Because cyclosporine has been used for a much longer time, most data in this field pertain to cyclosporine. The effects of tacrolimus are considered to be similar (Naesens et al., 2009). Tacrolimus resembles cyclosporine in that it can result in nephrotoxicity and the hemolytic–uremic syndrome, but it is less likely to cause hyperlipidemia, hypertension, and cosmetic problems and more likely to induce post-transplantation diabetes (Halloran, 2002). Because of its similar mechanism of immunosuppressive activity and its similar clinical toxicity spectrum it is generally assumed that the mechanism involved in tacrolimus toxicity are similar to those for cyclosporine (Christians, 2006). Although the use of cyclosporine and tacrolimus has led to major advances in the field of transplantation, with excellent short-term outcome, the chronic nephrotoxicity of these drugs is the Achilles' heel of current immunosuppressive regimens. Chronic calcineurin inhibitor nephrotoxicity is associated with mostly irreversible histologic damage to all compartments of the kidneys, including glomeruli, arterioles, and tubulo-interstitium, but the nonspecificity of most lesions makes the differential diagnosis with other injurious processes cumbersome. The pathophysiologic mechanisms underlying CNI nephrotoxicity are partly elucidated, although the main question whether nephrotoxicity is secondary to the actions on the calcineurin-nuclear factor of activated t cells pathway remains largely unanswered. It becomes clear that local renal factors are more important for susceptibility to CNI nephrotoxicity than systemic exposure to cyclosporine and tacrolimus. These factors include variability in P-glycoprotein and CYP3A4/5 expression or activity, older kidney age, salt depletion, the use of Non-Steroidal anti-inflammatory drugs, and genetic polymorphism (Hesselink, 2010; Naesens, 2009).

Although the exact mechanism is not clear, calcineurin inhibitors are thought to produce nephrotoxicity through their direct action on the kidney. Long-term use of cyclosporine and tacrolimus can also cause hypertension and diabetes, which could contribute to renal failure. Sirolimus, which is not a calcineurin inhibitor but is structurally related to tacrolimus, has also been linked to nephrotoxicity in patients with focal segmental glomerulosclerosis (Bai, 2010). The long term use of cyclosporine produces diminished renal function associated with macrophage infiltration and interstitial fibrosis in the kidney on biopsy. Cyclosporine exposure is also associated with endothelin expression, which is a regulator of inflammation and fibrosis. Hypertension and renal adverse effects are interrelated, so the mechanisms involved in cyclosporine induced hypertension could also influence its adverse effects on the kidney (Bai, 2010). Tacrolimus has been suspected of inducing more BK-related polyomavirus nephropathy than has cyclosporine in patients who have undergone kidney transplantation, especially when used with mycophenolate mofetil, but renal function may be better with tacrolimus (Halloran, 2002; Meier-Kriesche, 2002).

2.2 Clinical pharmacokinetics

Tacrolimus is usually administered orally in capsules containing the equivalent of 0.5 mg, 1 mg or 5 mg in a solid dispersion in hydroxipropylmethylcellulose, and an injection solution is available in 5 mg/mL, swell as an ointment for the topical treatment of skin lesions during autoimmune diseases (Astellas, 2009).

2.2.1 Absorption

After oral administration absorption of tacrolimus from the gastrointestinal tract after oral administration is incomplete and variable. Generally, bioavailability is about 20 to 25%, but can range from 5% to 93%. The relatively low fraction of tacrolimus absorbed most likely reflects incomplete absorption, the extent of absorption of this drug from the gastrointestinal tract is also influenced by the activity of P-glycoprotein (P-gp) in enterocytes. P-gp is a transmembrane transporter that is closely associated with CYP3A4 and secretes tacrolimus and its metabolites (Undre, 2003). In most subjects, absorption is rapid with peak blood concentrations occurring within approximately 0.5–2 hours of administration (Astellas, 2009; Venkataramanan, 1995). However, in some individuals, drug uptake occurs more slowly, yielding an essentially flat absorption profile, an extended lag time or secondary peaks. Poor aqueous solubility of tacrolimus and altered gut motility in transplant recipients may be partially responsible. Tacrolimus is absorbed rapidily in most subjects, an oral dose of 0.15 mg/kg/12 hours at steady state, the peak concentration (Cmax) averages 45 ng/mL, with a corresponding mean time to peak concentration (Tmax) of 1.5 hours. There is a strong correlation between the area under the concentration-time curve (AUC) and the trough concentration of tacrolimus (Cmin) in whole blood, therefore doses are individualized on the basis of target whole blood trough concentrations (Staatz & Tett, 2004; Undre, 1999). In stable liver transplant recipients, the oral bioavailability of tacrolimus is decreased if it is taken after food containing moderate fat content (Bekersky et al., 2001a, 2001b). However in a study in a study in renal transplant recipients where tacrolimus trough levels were evaluated prospectively during fasting ingestion of tacrolimus and 1 week after nonfasting ingestion, the results observed were statistically and clinically not significantly different (van-Duijnhoven et al., 2002). Data from a study in 7 patients with type 1 diabetes mellitus and 10 nondiabetic patients, all with end-stage renal failure, also showed that the rate of absorption was affected when tacrolimus was taken together with a continental breakfast high in fat content, and food had a greater effect on the absorption of tacrolimus in patients with than without diabetes mellitus (Plosker & Foster, 2000; van-Duijnhoven, 1998).To avoid the possible effect of food on tacrolimus bioavailability, the drug should be given at a constant time in relation to meals. Oral tacrolimus should not be taken with grapefruit juice since this vehicle inhibits CYP3A4 and/or P-gp contained in the GI tract and markedly increases bioavailability (Christians, 2006).

2.2.2 Distribution

In plasma, tacrolimus is highly bound to plasma proteins (99%) mainly to serum albumin and α–1-acid glycoprotein, so the pharmacological activity is considered to be a function of the unbound fraction of tacrolimus. Tacrolimus binds strongly to erythrocytes in the systemic circulation, resulting in a whole blood/plasma concentration distribution range of approximately 4-114 times and whole blood is therefore the medium usually used for assessing therapeutic concentrations (Plosker & Foster, 2000; Undre, 2003). Erythrocyte concentrations vary in transplant patients, especially those who have received hematopoietic stem cell or kidney transplants. α-acid glycoprotein concentrations also vary greatly among patients. Lipophilic drugs such as tacrolimus readily cross membranes and are taken up by adipose tissue. Animal studies indicate that tacrolimus is widely distributed into most tissues, including the lungs, spleen, heart, kidney, pancreas, brain, muscle and liver, tacrolimus crosses the placenta and is detected in breast milk (Staatz & Tett, 2004; Venkataramanan et al., 1995). At steady state, tacrolimus is distributed extensively in the body and at steady state the majority of the drug resides outside the blood compartment; that is, in the tissues. The plasma volume of distribution is greater than 1,000 L and in whole blood is approximately 50 L (Undre, 2003).

2.2.3 Metabolism and elimination

Calcineurin inhibitors like tacrolimus and cyclosporine are metabolized by cytochrome P-450 (CYP) isoenzyme systems 3A4 and 3A5 in the gut lumen before they even reach the portal vein. P-glycoprotein prevents drug absorption from the gut by promoting efflux into the lumen of the intestine, it has also has a role in systemic clearance of drugs by promoting efflux into the bile for excretion (Tsuchiya et al., 2004). After drugs are absorbed, they are subject to first-pass metabolism and systemic metabolism by CYP3A4 and CYP3A5 in the liver. When CYP3A5 is expressed, it accounts for 50% of the total hepatic CYP3A content. After administration, tacrolimus, either injected or absorbed into the body, is excreted from the body after receiving extensive metabolism primarily in the liver and to a lesser extent in the intestinal mucosa, by cytochrome P450(CYP)3A4 isoenzymes, with <0.5% of the parent drug appearing unchanged in urine and feces (Venkataramanan et al., 1995). The specific number of metabolites formed is unclear, but appears to be at least eight metabolites of tacrolimus have been identified, with two of these exhibiting some activity (Op den Buijsch, 2007; Plosker & Foster, 2000). Three mono-demethylated metabolites, three di-demethylated metabolites, one mono-hydroxylated metabolite and one metabolite modifed by reactions have been identified. Three metabolites O-demethylated at the 13-, 31- and 15-methoxy group of tacrolimus, respectively, and one monohydroxylated metabolite at the 12-position. The didemethylated metabolites at the 15- and 31, 13- and 31-, and 13- and 15-methoxy groups of tacrolimus and one metabolite produced after O-demethylation at the 31-methoxy group and formation of a fused 10-membered ring structure through the 19- to 22-carbon of the macrolide ring after oxidation of the 19-methyl group, and of the 36- and 37-vinyl group of tacrolimus (Iwasaki, 2007). Compounds such as tacrolimus that display significant presystemic metabolism and have an intrinsic clearance lower than hepatic blood flow should be sensitive to changes in CYP3A expression. The CYP3A subfamily consists of at least four isoforms: CYP3A4, CYP3A5, CYP3A7 and CYP3A43. As these isoforms have overlapping substrate specificity, it is difficult to segregate their relative contributions to the metabolism of tacrolimus (Staatz & Tett, 2004). While it is known that CYP3A4 is predominantly localized to the liver and intestines, CYP3A5, on the contrary, is predominantly localized to the kidney (Joy et al., 2007). The isoform CYP3A4 is generally the most abundantly expressed CYP in the adult liver, accounting for 30–40% of total CYP content, its expression is highly variable, with 10- to 100-fold interindividual differences (Paine et al., 1997). Althoug there is evidence that cytochrome P4503A is mainly responsible for demethylation of tacrolimus, a minor involvement of cytochrome P450 enzymes other than cytochrome P4503A cannot be excluded (Christians, 2006). The reported elimination half-life ($t_{1/2}$) of tacrolimus is variable, with mean values of approximately 12 hours in liver transplant recipients, 19 hours in renal transplant recipients and 35 hours in healthy volunteers (Meier-Kriesche, 2002). Less than 1% of an intravenous dose of tacrolimus is excreted in the urine as unchanged drug, and total urinary elimination (metabolites and unchanged drug) is just over 2%. Faecal elimination accounts for >90% of an administered dose, and animal data indicate that the main excretory pathway of tacrolimus metabolites is biliary (Plosker & Foster 2000; Venkataramanan et al. 1995).

2.3 Pharmacokinetic variability

2.3.1 Oral bioavailability

Tacrolimus is highly lipophilic and insoluble in water, these physicochemical properties of tracrolimus cause a large amount of intrasubject variability in tacrolimus oral absorption. Tacrolimus is metabolized in the intestine and liver by the cytochrome P450 (CYP) 3A4 and 3A5 oxidative enzymes. It is also substrate for the P-gp drug transporter, a product of the multidrug resistance (*MDR1*) gene. Furthermore, CYP3A isoforms and P-gp are under the transcriptional control of the human pregnane X receptor (PXR). Therefore, the interindividual variability of tacrolimus pharmacokinetics might be explained by heterogeneity in CYP3A4, CYP3A5, P-gp or PXR expressions due to genetic polymorphisms (López-Montenegro Soria, et al., 2010). Extrahepatic metabolism by CYP3A4 in the gastrointestinal epithelium is responsible for presystemic elimination of about half of the absorbed dose, whereas first-pass metabolism by CYP3A4 in the liver accounts for an additional 10% of elimination. The extent of absorption of tacrolimus from the gastrointestinal tract is also influenced by the activity of P-glycoprotein (P-gp) in enterocytes. P-gp is a transmembrane transporter that is closely associated with CYP3A4 and secretes tacrolimus and its metabolites back into the lumen of the gut (Undre et al., 199; Undre, 2003). This extensive presystemic metabolism limits the oral bioavailability of tacrolimus to approximately 25%. The activity of the metabolizing enzyme as well as of the P-gp transporter varies considerably between individuals and between races, and this requires the dosage to be individualized to achieve the desired systemic exposure (Felipe, et al., 2002). Nevertheless, the intra-patient variability in systemic exposure is considered to be low. The low intra-patient variability in the bioavailability of tacrolimus is evidenced by the small number of dose changes required to maintain target whole-blood trough concentrations. While the average oral bioavailability of tacrolimus is 25%, there is a large amount of variation in this parameter among patients (4–89%), small intestine metabolism and/or transport processes contribute greatly (Tuteja et al., 2001). Renal transplant patients may have reduced oral bioavailability for tacrolimus. When given with meals, especially with high fat content food, oral bioavailability of tacrolimus decreases (Venkataramanan et al., 1995). To avoid the possible effect of food on tacrolimus bioavailability, the drug should be given at a constant time in relation to meals. Oral tacrolimus should not be taken with grapefruit juice since this vehicle inhibits CYP3A4 and/or P-glycoprotein contained in the gastrointestinal tract and markedly increases bioavailability. The individual pharmacokinetic response of a renal transplant recipient to immunosuppressive drugs is highly variable. Recent studies have shown that specific genetic variations may alter the pharmacokinetics of these drugs (Rosso Felipe et al., 2009). The metabolic enzyme of tacrolimus is the CYP3A subfamily, including the CYP3A4, CYP3A5, CYP3A7, and CYP3A43 isodynamic enzyme. CYP3A4 and CYP3A5 are the main fractions of these isodynamic enzymes. The mutable site of CYP3A5 is multivariate; the wild type of CYP3A5 is defined as *1, while mutation of 6986A_G is defined as *3. As disclosed by many studies, the CYP3A5 genotype has a great effect on FK506 concentrations. The amount of CYP3A5 in the liver is large among patients with the *1 genotype in contrast to the patients with the *3 genotype, which metabolize tacrolimus faster with lower concentrations in patients with the *1 genotype. Patients with the *3/*3 genotype theoretically have high concentration per dosage ratios (Chen et al., 2002; Rosso Felipe et al., 2009; Tuteja et al., 2001). The presence of the CYP3A5*3 genotype is associated with the absence of protein function. López Montenegro et al., demonstrated that Intestinal absorption and metabolism of tacrolimus is significantly affected by the Single Nucleotide Polymorphisms (SNP) in the CYP3A5 and MDR1 genes. Macphee et al., in 2002 in a study with 180 kidney transplant patients, found that a single nucleotide polymorphism in the CYP3AP1 pseudogene (A/G(44)) that previously has been noted to be more common in African Americans and strongly associated with hepatic CYP3A5 activity correlated well with the tacrolimus dose requirement, and found a weaker association for a polymorphism in the MDR-1 gene, which influences intestinal P-glycoprotein expression. They conclude that the CYP3AP1 genotype is a major factor in determining the dose requirement for tacrolimus, and genotyping may be of value in planning patient-specific drug dosing. As substrates for CYP3A enzymes and P-glycoprotein, drugs that inhibit or induce these mechanisms may increase or decrease blood tacrolimus concentrations, respectively (Van Gelder, 2002). In clinical studies, CYP3A/P-glycoprotein inhibitors and inducers primarily affect the oral bioavailability of tacrolimus rather than clearance, indicating a key role of intestinal P-glycoprotein and CYP3A. Drugs that interact with P-gp may change the distribution of tacrolimus in tissue and modify its toxicity and immunosuppressive activity (Christians et al., 2002). Ketoconazole, an azole antifungal agent, is known to be a potent inhibitor of P-gp and CYP3A4 and have even been used to reduce the dose of tacrolimus and thus save money. If possible, drugs interfering at the level of the CYP system should be avoided. If tacrolimus and either of these drugs are used concomitantly, close monitoring of tacrolimus concentrations should be performed (Van Gelder, 2002).

2.3.2 Ethnicity, pharmacogenetic variability

The importance of interethnic differences in the pharmacokinetics of immunosuppressants has been recognized as having a significant impact on the outcome of transplantation.

Between-patient variability in drug absorption may be the major cause of inferior transplant outcome observed in special populations such as African-Americans, children and diabetic patients. For example, the poorer transplant outcome observed among African-Americans has been attributed mainly to differences in absorption of cyclosporine, tacrolimus and mycophenolate mofetil (Hariharan et al., 1993; Schweitzer et al., 1998; Stein et al., 2001). Also, compared with white recipients, black transplant patients may also require higher doses of sirolimus to achieve comparable acute rejection rates, even without displaying significant differences in drug absorption. Whether this effect is the result of pharmacodynamic differences comparing black and white patients is not known (Felipe et al., 2002). In a retrospective analysis Fitzimmons et al. found that the oral bioavailability of tacrolimus in African American healthy volunteers and kidney transplant patients was significantly lower than in non-African Americans (Fitzsimmons, 1998). There was no statistically significant difference in clearance. These results were confirmed in a healthy volunteer study. The absolute oral bioavailability of tacrolimus in African American and Latin American subjects was significantly lower than in Caucasians. The results suggested that the observed ethnic differences in tacrolimus pharmacokinetics were, instead, related to differences in intestinal P-glycoprotein-mediated efflux and CYP3A-mediated metabolism rather than differences in hepatic elimination (Mancinelli et al., 2001). Other ethnic groups such as the Japanese populations are not different from the Caucasian population because their transplant outcomes were comparable under usual tacrolimus dosages (Ochiai et al., 1995). Drugs metabolized by CYP3A4/5 inhibited tacrolimus metabolism, with ketoconazole being the most potent. Ketoconazole, cyclosporine A, diltiazem, erythromycin, and fluconazole were reported as the drugs that elicit clinically relevant drug interactions with tacrolimus (Christians et al., 2002). These results indicate the potential for metabolic interactions between tacrolimus and co-medicated drugs metabolized by CYP3A4/5. Rifampicin decreased the blood levels of tacrolimus in kidney and liver transplant patients. Rifampicin treatment caused a decrease of tacrolimus blood levels in healthy volunteers when compared to pretreatment levels (Hariharan et al., 1993; Stein et al., 2001). Co-administration of rifampicin significantly increased tacrolimus clearance and decreased tacrolimus bioavailavility. A combination of fluconazole and tacrolimus augments tacrolimus blood levels (Mañez et al., 2002). In kidney transplantation, it was also reported that in a combination of fluconazole at 100 mg to tacrolimus, the dosage of tacrolimus could be reduced by forty percent without changing tacrolimus trough levels (Toda et al., 2002). *CYP3A* proteins are involved in the metabolism of more than 50% of the drugs in use, including tacrolimus. Pharmacogenomic studies have shown that SNP in intron 3 of the *CYP3A5* gene correlate with different expression levels, because of the appearance of a cryptic-splice site resulting in either the presence (*1/*1 and SNP *1/*3) or absence (SNP *3/*3) of the protein (Yu et al., 206; Barrera-Pulido et al.,2008). Interindividual CYP3A expression in the liver varies 10- to 100-fold and up to 30-fold in the small intestine, but there is no significant polymorphism of CYP3A4. Only people with at least one CYP3A45*1 allele express significant amounts of CYP3A45*3and CYP3A45*6 cause alternative splicing and protein truncation that results in the absence of CYP3A5 enzyme (Macphee et al., 2002). Greater than 60% of African Americans compared with less than 10% of the Caucasian population possess the CYP3AP1 G_{-44} allele, which is necessary for CYP3A5 expression. In humans expressing CYP3A5, it represents at least 50% of the total hepatic content of CYP3A. Together with CYP3A4 it is the most abundant CYP enzyme in the small intestine. CYP3A5 is probably the most important genetic contributor to interindividual and interracial differences in CYP3A-dependent drug clearance. As discussed above, another important factor affecting the pharmacokinetics of tacrolimus is the expression of MDR1, the gene encoding the active transporter P-glycoprotein. Homozygous individuals for the T-allele for MDR1, C3435T, have significantly lower intestinal and leukocyte P-glycoprotein expression than C homocygotes ((Macphee et al., 2002; Schaeffeler et al., 2001). MDR1 C3435T is significantly more prevalent in the Caucasian than in the African American population. MacPhee (2002) demonstrated that the dose-normalized tacrolimus blood concentration after renal transplantation was associated with a SNP in the CYP3AP1 gene, probably through linkage with an SNP in the CYP3A5 gene. Individuals with at least one CYP3A5*1 allele synthesize CYP3A5 and CYP3A5*3/*3 homozygotes do not (Paine et al., 1997). In another study MacPhee et al. (2005) showed results with direct typing of the CYP3A5 genotype for a group of 180 kidney-only transplant recipients. South Asian and white patients with at least one CYP3A5*1 allele achieved twofold lower dose-normalized tacrolimus blood concentrations compared with CYP3A5*3/*3 homozygotes, confirming their previous findings for the CYP3AP1 SNP. There was a significant delay in achieving target blood concentrations in those with at least one CYP3A5*1 allele. They conclude that the Determination of the CYP3A5*1/*3 genotype could be used to predict the tacrolimus dose requirement and, given incomplete linkage, would be better than determination of the CYP3AP1 genotype. For renal transplant recipients receiving tacrolimus as an immunosuppressant, practitioners can expect *CYP3A5*1* carriers to have a tacrolimus clearance 25-45% greater than that of *CYP3A5*3* homozygotes, with proportional dosing needs to maintain adequate immunosuppression. Since inadequate immunosuppression is linked to graft rejection, evaluation of CYP3A5 polymorphisms may be helpful in determining an appropriate starting dosage, rapidly achieving adequate immunosuppression, and ultimately improving the outcome of renal transplantation (Utecht et al., 2002).

2.3.3 Sex

Gender-related differences in pharmacokinetics have frequently been considered as potentially important determinants for the clinical effectiveness of drug therapy. The human multidrug-resistance gene 1 (MDR1) gene product P-gp has been identified as a major determinant in the pharmacokinetics of numerous drugs. Additional other drug transporters are also assumed to play a major role in absorption, distribution and/or renal and hepatic excretion of therapeutic agents. Gender differences have been noted in the hepatic expression of MDR1, with women displaying only one-third to one-half of the hepatic P-gp level of men. Low P-glycoprotein activity in the liver is suggested to result in increased hepatic CYP3A metabolism for cosubstrates of CYP3A and P-glycoprotein. Low P-gp activity in the gut wall results in shorter gut wall transit time and, hence, decreased gut wall CYP3A metabolism (Lown et al., 1997; Meibohmet al., 2002). The most important pharmacokinetic parameter influenced by sex differences seems to be oral biovailability (Christians, 2006; Harris et al., 2002). Although no difference in dosing by sex was found in the tacrolimus kidney transplant trials and dosing recommendations for male and female patients are the same, sex differences were found when tacrolimus and ketoconazole were coadministered (Fitzsimmons et al., 1998; Tuteja et al., 2001). Female-specific issues such as pregnancy, menopause, oral contraceptive use and menstruation may also have profound effects on drug metabolism. These effects can often be clinically important (Harris et al., 2001).

2.3.4 Age

As already mentioned, tacrolimus is primarily metabolized by cytochrome P450(CYP)3A enzymes in the gut wall and liver. It is also a substrate for P-gp, which counter-transports diffused tacrolimus out of intestinal cells and back into the gut lumen. Age-associated alterations in CYP3A and P-gp expression and/or activity, along with liver mass and body composition changes, would be expected to affect the pharmacokinetics of tacrolimus in the elderly (Staatz & Tett, 2002). Several changes in hepatic function and structure have been noted in the elderly; among them, two of the most important are an absolute (and relative to bodyweight) decrease in the size of the liver, and reduced regional blood flow to this organ (Hämmerlein et al., 2002). It is likely that inter- and intraindividual pharmacokinetic variability associated with tacrolimus increase in elderly populations. In addition to pharmacokinetic differences, donor organ viability, multiple co-morbidity, polypharmacy and immunological changes need to be considered when using tacrolimus in the elderly. Aging is associated with decreased immune responsiveness, a slower body repair process and increased drug adverse effects. Elderly liver and kidney transplant recipients are more likely to develop new-onset diabetes mellitus than younger patients, elderly transplant recipients exhibit higher mortality from infectious and cardiovascular causes than younger patients, but may be less likely to develop acute rejection, also have a higher potential for chronic allograft nephropathy and a single rejection episode can be more devastating (Staatz & Tett, 2002). Pharmacokinetic parameters observed in adults may not be applicable to children, especially to the younger age groups. In general, patients younger than 5 years of age show higher clearance rates regardless of the organ transplanted or the immunosuppressive drug used (del Mar Fernández De Gatta et al., 2002). Only limited information is available on the pharmacokinetics of tacrolimus in pediatric patients, the rate and extent of tacrolimus absorption after oral administration do not seem to be altered in pediatric patients. The volume of distribution of tacrolimus based on blood concentrations in pediatric patients (2.6 L/kg) is approximately twice the adult value. Blood clearance of tacrolimus is also approximately twice as high in pediatric (0.14 L/h/kg) compared with adult (0.06 L/h/kg) patients. Consequently, $t_{1/2}\beta$ does not appear modified in children, but oral doses need to be generally 2-fold higher than corresponding adult doses to reach similar tacrolimus blood concentrations. More pharmacokinetic studies in pediatric patients are, however, needed to rationalize the use of therapeutic drug monitoring for optimization of tacrolimus therapy in this patient population (Wallemacq & Verbeeck 2001).

2.4 Time after initiation of treatment

It is well established that tacrolimus pharmacokinetics changes with the time after transplantation are the results of a reduced clearance or an increase in oral bioavailability (Staatz & Tett, 2004). Possible reasons include stabilization of the patient with reduction of postsurgical stress, hematocrit, ischemia-reperfusion injury and stabilization of transplant organ function, especially if the latter directly affects tacrolimus pharmacokinetics such as the liver. Also, immunosuppressive drugs affect expression and activity of CYP3A enzymes and P-gp (Christians et al., 2002). There is evidence that induction of CYP3A and P-gp by corticosteroids is responsible for the requirement to reduce tacrolimus doses as corticosteroid doses are tapered (Hesselink et al., 2003; Plosker & Foster 2000; Undre 1998). After cessation of concomitant steroid treatment, tacrolimus exposure increase by 25% (del Mar Fernández De Gattaet al., 2002).

2.5 Drug-Drug interactions

Drug interactions occur when the efficacy or toxicity of a medication is changed by coadministration of another drug (Dresser et al., 2000). The clinical relevance of pharmacokinetic drug interactions depends on a number of considerations, of which the therapeutic index of the drug is the most important. Potential sites of pharmacokinetic drug interactions include the gastrointestinal tract, protein- and tissue-binding sites, drug metabolising enzymes, drug transporter systems, biliary excretion and enterohepatic recirculation as well renal excretion (Van Gelder, 2002). There are several factors involved in absorption of a drug after oral administration, all of which can be the target of drug interactions: delivery to the intestine (pH, gastric emptying and food), absorption from the intestinal lumen (dissolution, lipophilicity, stability, active uptake), intestinal metabolism (phase I or II metabolism), active intestinal drug efflux pumps, and subsequent hepatic first pass extraction (Christians et al., 2002). Drug interactions with tacrolimus fall into two basic categories. The first are agents known to cause nephrotoxicity when administered by themselves, the second category of drug interactions involves inhibition or induction of tacrolimus metabolism. Because tacrolimus is metabolized extensively by CYP3A4 isoenzymes and P-glycoprotein, drugs that are either inhibitors or inducers of this system may increase or decrease serum concentrations of tacrolimus. CYP3A4 inhibitors that increase whole blood concentrations of tacrolimus include antifungal agents (fluconazole, voriconazole, ketoconazole, itraconazole, and clotrimazole), calcium channel blockers (diltiazem, nifedipine, nicardipine, and verapamil), macrolide antibiotics (erythromycin, clarithromycin, and troleandomycin), prokinetic drugs (metoclopramide and cisapride), protease inhibitors (indinavir, saquinavir, ritonavir, nelfinavir, amprenavir, and atazanavir), and grapefruit juice. CYP3A4 inducers that are known to decrease tacrolimus concentrations include anticonvulsants (carbamazepine, phenytoin, and phenobarbital); rifamycins (rifampin and rifabutin), and St John's wort (Vicari-Christensen et al., 2009). Potential pharmacokinetic interactions between tacrolimus and mycophenolate mofetil has been evaluated since these drugs are frequently used in combination (Zucker et al., 2002; Undre at al., 2002; Hübner et al., 1999). Results indicate that mycophenolate mofetil does not significantly affect the pharmacokinetics of tacrolimus in renal and hepatic transplant recipients. However, tacrolimus may have an effect on the pharmacokinetics of mycophenolic acid, the active metabolite of mycophenolate mofetil. In renal transplant recipients who were converted from cyclosporin to tacrolimus therapy (while being maintained on the same dosage of mycophenolate mofetil), plasma trough concentrations of mycophenolic acid were significantly increased (approximately doubled) as were AUC values for mycophenolic acid (increased by about one-third) after conversion from cyclosporin to tacrolimus (although there was no mycophenolate mofetil control group in the study) (Plosker & Foster, 2000). Because of the large number of potentially interacting agents, and the critical nature of the drugs involved in the treatment of transplant patients, complete avoidance of drug interactions with tacrolimus is not possible. Thus, most drug interactions with tacrolimus are managed using appropriate tacrolimus dosage modification with tacrolimus concentration monitoring as a guide.

2.6 Adverse reactions

The calcineurin inhibitors tacrolimusa and cyclosporine, are the mainstay of immunosuppressive therapy in solid organ transplantation. These drugs produce severe adverse effects and tended to occur most frequently in the first few months after transplant and decline thereafter, possibly in ther line with reduction in dosages of the immunosuppressants (Bai et al., 2010). There are several principal adverse effects associated with tacrolimus. Nephrotoxic effects can occur in up to 52% of patients and limit the use of the drug. However, nephrotoxic effects may be difficult to distinguish from other causes of renal failure in kidney transplant recipients. Neurotoxic effects may be manifested by tremors (15%-56%), headache (37%-64%), insomnia (32%-64%), and paresthesias (17%-40%). Post-transplant diabetes mellitus is one of the more serious metabolic disorders associated with calcineurin inhibitors treatment (Scott et al., 2003). Cyclosporine appears to be less diabetogenic than tacrolimus, but both agents may impact directly the transcriptional regulation of insulin gene expression in the pancreatic β cells. Based on an analysis of 3365 kidney recipients, the primary risk factors identified for posttransplantation diabetes included older age, female, increased Body Mass Index, and tacrolimus-based therapy.[24] Other studies have also identified tacrolimus as a risk factor for posttransplantation diabetes in addition to older age (> 40 years), Body Mass Index greater than 25 kg/m^2, positive hepatitis C serology, family history of diabetes, metabolic syndrome, African-American or Hispanic race-ethnicity, and higher mean pretransplantation plasma glucose concentration. The risk factors for posttransplantation diabetes are similar to those for type 2 diabetes (Markell, 2004; González-Posada at al., 2004; Kamar et al., 2007). Hypertension (38-89%) is common, as is drug-induced diabetes (24%), exacerbated by the use of corticosteroids. Gastrointestinal disturbances reported are diarrhea (37%-72%), nausea (32-46%), constipation (23-35%), and anorexia (34%). Malignant neoplasms such as lymphoma and lymphoproliferative disease occur rarely (1.5%). Finally, the risk of bacterial, viral and fungal infections is increased (up to 45%), because of the immunosuppressive effect of tacrolimus..

2.7 Therapeutic drug mpnitoring

Therapeutic drug monitoring has been used as an essential tool to individualize immunosuppressive drug therapy in vascularized organ transplant recipients, allowing a more rational use of drugs with narrow therapeutic index such as cyclosporine, tacrolimus, sirolimus, and mycophenolate acid (Rosso Felipe et al., 2009). Tacrolimus whole-blood through concentrations have been found to correlate well with the area under the concentration-time curve measurements in liver, kidney and bone marrow transplant recipients (r= 0.91-0.99). Thus, through concentrations are a good index of overall drug exposure, and are currently used for routine monitoring as part of patient care posttransplantation (Jusko, 1995; Staatz et al., 2001). This approach offers the opportunity to reduce the pharmacokinetic variability by implementing drug dose adjustments based on plasma/blood concentrations. Drug levels are obtained as predose (12 hours after previous dose) trough concentrations in whole blood (Cattaneo et al., 2009). These trough levels correlate reasonably well with area under the curve, with total area under the curve being an accurate measure of drug exposure (Kapturczak et al., 2004). Therapeutic ranges of tacrolimus after kidney transplantation are reported as a range for various times after transplant: 0-1 month, 15-20 μg/L; 1-3 months, 10-15 μg/L; and more than 3 months, 5-12 μg/L (Scott et al., 2003). Pharmacokinetic therapeutic drug monitoring can only be of clinical relevance when the pharmacodynamics response is correlated to drug exposure. In a retrospective analysis based on adult renal transplant recipients during the first month after transplantation, tacrolimus through blood concentrations measured, were correlated with rejection episodes. The median through blood concentration in patients with rejections (5.6±1.6 ng/mL) were significantly lower than in patients without rejection (9.2±3.5 ng/mL). A rejection rate of 55% was found for patients with median tacrolimus through blood concentrations between 0 and 10 ng/mL, whereas no rejection was observed in patients with median tacrolimus through blood concentrations between 10 and 15 ng/mL (Staatz at al., 2001). Tacrolimus blood concentrations are monitored 3 to 7 days a week for the first 2 weeks, at least three times for the following 2 weeks, and whenever the patient comes for an outpatient visit thereafter (Jusko & Kobayashi, 1993). On the basis of the terminal half-life of tacrolimus, it was suggested to start monitoring tacrolimus blood concentrations 2 to 3 days after initiation of tacrolimus treatment after the drug has reached steady state. However it is important to reach effective drug concentrations early after transplantation to decrease the risk of acute rejection and to avoid excessive early calcineurin inhibitors concentrations that may be severely damaging after reperfusion of the transplanted organ (Shaw et al., 2002). The frequency of therapeutic drug monitoring of tacrolimus should be increased in the case of suspected adverse events or rejection, when liver function is deteriorating, after dose adjustments of the immunosuppressants, change of route of administration, or change of drug formulations, when drugs that are known to interact with CYP3A or P-gP are added or discontinued, or when their doses are changed, in case of severe illness that may affect drug absorption or elimination such as severe immune reactions and sepsis, or if noncompliance is suspected (Christians at al., 2006). Recent advances in molecular biology and genetic information made available through the Human Genome Project has had a great influence in the biomedical and pharmaceutical area. It is well established that large numbers of patients demonstrate great differences in drug bioavailability. Nowadays the advent of the genomic era has brought several new fields of study, including pharmacogenomics, which seek to link drug treatment with the individual's genetic makeup. Pharmacogenomics holds many promises for improved treatment of a large variety of medical conditions, including immunosuppression for organ transplantation (Cattaneo et al., 2004; Danesi et al., 2000). In recent years, extensive studies on pharmacogenetics of immunosuppressive drugs have been focused on the contribution of drug metabolizing enzyme cytochrome P450 (CYP) 3A (CYP3A4 and CYP3A5) and the drug transporter P-gp to the individual administration of cyclosporine and tacrolimus, for they are thought to be the main determinant of the pharmacokinetics of currently used immunosuppressive drugs (Macphee et al., 2002). Those involved in therapeutic drug monitoring are now realizing the potential role of pharmacogenomics in influencing individual patient's exposure to immunosuppressive agents and concomitant therapy. As rapid techniques for assessing genetic polymorphisms become available, they are likely to play a significant part in planning the initial doses of immunosuppressive drugs and tailor maintenance therapy (Cattaneo et al., 2004).

3. Mycophenolate

The search for inhibitors of the *novo* purine synthesis led to the ancient compound mycophenolic acid discovered in 1896. MPA was known to be immunosupresive, to inhibit lymphocyte DNA synthesis, and to inhibit guanine nucleotide synthesis in tumor cells. It was found to block the *novo* purine biosynthesis by inhibit the key enzyme in this pathway, inosine monophosphate dehydrogenase (IMDPH). The principle of the Mycophenolate mofetil arose from de observation that defects in the *novo* purine biosynthesis create immunodeficiency without affecting other tissues. Mycophenolate mofetil (MPM) is the 2-

morpholinoethyl ester of mycophenolic acid (MPA), an immunosuppressive agent IMPDH inhibitor. The chemical name for MMF is 2-morpholinoethyl (E)-6-(1,3-25 dihydro-4-hydroxy-6-methoxy-7-methyl-3-oxo-5-isobenzofuranyl)-4-methyl-4-6 hexenoate. It has an empirical formula of $C_{23}H_{31}NO_7$, a molecular weight of 433.50 (Christians et al., 2006), is a potent, selective, noncompetitive, reversible inhibitor of IMPDH, an essential enzyme in *de novo* synthesis of purines (i.e. guanosine), MPA has potent cytostatic effects on lymphocytes. Inhibits proliferative responses of T and B-cells to both mitogenic and allospecific stimulation and suppresses antibody formation by B-cells. By preventing glycosylation of lymphocyte and monocyte glycoproteins involved in intracellular adhesion to endothelial cells, MPA may inhibit recruitment of leukocytes to sites of inflammation and graft rejection (Pillans et al., 2001; Kiberd, et al., 2004; van Gelder et al., 1999).

3.1 Mechanism of action

The salvage pathway of purine synthesis in lymphocytes is less active than the de novo synthesis of purines. Inosine monophosphate is converted to guanosine monophosphate by inosine monophosphate dehydrogenase. During T-cell activation, the activity of both types I and II inosine monophosphate dehydrogenase enzymes increases by tenfold. Mycophenolate mofetil is converted in the liver by ester hydrolysis to mycophenolic acid, which in turn non-competitively and reversibly inhibits types I and II inosine monophosphate dehydrogenase activity during DNA synthesis in the S phase of the cell cycle. In the salvage pathway, guanine is converted to guanine monophosphate by the enzyme hypoxanthine-guanine phosphoribosyltransferase. MPM is commonly used in transplanted patients; it is a non-competitive reversible inhibitor of 5′-mono phosphate inosine dehydrogenase, which controls the synthesis of guanosine triphosphate; its mechanism of action is by depletion of intracellular levels of guanosine triphosphate (GTP) and deoxyguanosine triphosphate (dGTP), which leads to suppression of DNA synthesis in T and B lymphocytes stimulated with antigens or mitogens. It does not inhibit early events of lymphocytes activation including cytokine production. It also inhibits antibody formation and production of adhesion molecules on the cellular surface. It has been used to prolong transplant survival in animal and human models in 5/6 nephrectomy to reduce cellular infiltration within the tubule and interstitium with decreased renal damage been observed in the remnant kidney (Bullingham, 1996a, 1996b).

3.2 Clinical pharmacokinetics

3.2.1 Onset & plasma concentrations

Peak mycophenolic acid levels occur approximately one hour post dose, with a secondary peak occurring 6 to 8 hours later, due to enterohepatic recirculation of MPA glucuronide (MPAG) and its hydrolysis back to mycophenolic acid in the gastrointestinal tract. The apparent elimination half-life of mycophenolic acid after a single oral dose of MMF is approximately 18 hours. The AUC is found to increase following renal transplantation, stabilising after about a month of therapy. Food reduces the Cmax but has no effect on the AUC. Single dose studies in chronic renal impairment (creatinine clearance < $25mL/min/1.73m^2$) showed that the AUC for mycophenolic acid was 28-75% higher than in individuals with no or milder renal impairment (Christians et al., 2006). A secondary plasma MPA peak is often seen 6 to 12 h after oral administration of MMF, suggesting enterohepatic circulation of the drug. Because of this secondary rise in plasma MPA concentration, the apparent mean terminal half-life of MPA is 17.9 h in healthy subjects. MPA is converted in the liver to the pharmacologically inactive MPAG, which is excreted by the kidney. Plasma MPA is extensively bound to albumin, and a mean protein binding of 97% has been reported in normal plasma (Bullingham, 1996a, 1996b). Renal transplant patients who received oral mycophenolate mofetil 1.5 g twice daily achieved maximal plasma concentrations of 13.5 μg/mL early postransplant (less than 40 days) and 24.1 μg/mL late posttransplant (at least 3 months). The maximum plasma concentrations were achieved at 1.21 hours and 0.9 hours, respectively. Following kidney transplantation, 10 patients who received oral mycophenolate mofetil 1 g twice daily achieved mean maximum plasma concentrations of mycophenolic acid of 11.1 μg/mL, 11.9 μg/mL, and 14.9 μg/mL on days 2, 5, and 28, respectively. The maximum concentration was achieved at 2.18 hours, 1.9 hours, and 1.63 hours (Johnson et al., 1999). Renal transplant patients (n=12) who received oral mycophenolic acid 720 mg twice daily achieved maximal plasma concentrations of 15 μg/mL, 26.2 μg/mL, and 24.1 μg/mL at 2 weeks, 3 months, and 6 months posttransplant, respectively. The maximum plasma concentrations were achieved at 1.8 hours, 2 hours, and 2 hours (Sollinger et al., 1992).

3.2.2 Absorption

MPM is well absorbed orally with a mean bioavailability of 94%. After oral administration, it is rapidly and essentially completely absorbed, and then essentially completely converted to MPA, the active immunosuppressant species. In renal transplant recipients, very low serum levels of mycophenolic acid were achieved after oral mycophenolate mofetil therapy in the early posttransplantation period; serum levels increased significantly after 20 days of treatment, suggesting potentially impaired absorption or altered metabolism of the ester in uremic patients. Following oral and IV administration, MPM undergoes rapid and complete metabolism to MPA, the active metabolite; however, Mycophenolate sodium (MPA 720 mg) and MPM 1 g result in bioequivalent MPA exposure. Food decreases peak plasma concentrations of MPA by 33-40%; no effect on the MPA AUC (Bullingham, et al., 1998).

3.2.3 Distribution

MPA plasma protein binding is ≥ 97-98%, mainly in albumin. Severe renal impairment has been shown to decrease the binding of mycophenolic acid to albumin, thereby elevating the concentration of mycophenolic acid free fraction in serum. In addition, increased levels of the mycophenolic acid glucuronide metabolite in these patients may compete with free mycophenolic acid for binding with albumin. In patients with renal impairment or delayed graft function, protein binding may be decreased (Meier-Kriesche et al., 2000). MPM hydrochloride protein binding is 97%, in albumin principally. MPA half-life is about 8 - 17.9 hours. MPM volume of distribution is approximately 4 L/Kg. The mean volume of distribution for mycophenolic acid was 54 L at steady state and 112 L at elimination phase (Bullingham, et al., 1998).

3.2.4 Metabolism and excretion route

MPM undergoes complete metabolism to MPA; metabolism occurs presystemically following oral administration. MPA is metabolized by glucuronyl transferase to the phenolic glucuronide of MPA. The phenolic glucuronide is converted to MPA via enterohepatic recirculation. MPM is rapidly hydrolysed extensively in the liver to MPA; this metabolite is conjugated to form the pharmacologically inactive mycophenolic acid glucuronide. Approximately 87% of the oral dose is excreted as MPAG in the urine. MPM is excreted in urine (93%) as the phenolic glucuronide of MPA (87%) and in feces (6%). MPS is excreted principally in urine as phenolic glucuronide of MPA (> 60%) and as unchanged MPA (3%). The mean renal clearance of MPA glucuronide was 15.5 mL/min following the administration of delayed release mycophenolic acid to stable renal transplant patients (Christians et al., 2006). Deconjugation of the glucuronide to mycophenolic acid may occur in humans via the action of intestinal or intestinal microflora beta-glucuronidase, with subsequent reabsorption of mycophenolic acid (Mourad et al., 2002; Platzet al., 2002). *In vivo*, mycophenolic acid glucuronide is converted to mycophenolic acid via enterohepatic recirculation. MPM total body clearance is 140 to 193 mL/min. The plasma clearance of MPA is 193 mL/min following oral administration of mycophenolate mofetil. The mean clearance of mycophenolic acid was 140 mL/min following oral administration of the delayed release mycophenolic acid tablet to stable renal transplant patients. The plasma clearance of MPA is 177 (+/- 31) mL/min following IV administration of MPM (Bullingham, et al., 1998; Meier-Kriesche et al., 2000).

3.3 Pharmacokinetic variability

The pharmacokinetics of MMF is complex; some patients achieve a peak in 1 to 2 h and a second peak at 5 to 6 h due to enterohepatic circulation. In some patients, the second peak (Cmax) is as much as 50% of the total peak concentration. A maximum concentration of >10 μg/mL is associated with side effects. There is little correlation with area under the concentration curve (AUC) and dose. The AUC in the first 12 h does correlate with propensity to reject if it is <30 μg.h/mL or toxicity if it is >60 μg.h/mL. The desired exposure is 35 to 60 μg.h/mL (Shaw et al., 2000). Mycophenolic acid AUC is increased by renal dysfunction, which may be clinically relevant early after transplantation or during rejection episodes. Plasma concentrations of MPA glucuronide higher in nontransplant subjects with severe renal impairment than in those with mild impairment or normal renal function. At the same time, plasma concentrations of MPA glucuronide higher in transplant patient with delayed renal graft function than in patients not experiencing delayed graft function. Dialysis does not remove MPA. Plasma concentrations of free (unbound) MPA and total MPA glucuronide have increased in nontransplant individuals with severe chronic renal impairment (GFR < 25mL/minute per 1.73 m^2). Plasma MPA concentrations in patients with delayed graft function similar to values in patients not experiencing delayed graft function. In hereditary deficiency of hypoxanthine-guanine phosphoribosyl-transferase (HGPRT), such as Lesch-Nyhan and Kelley-Seegmiller syndrome, the use of MPM (a inosine monophosphate dehydrogenase inhibitor) is not recommended (Ahsan et al., 1999).

3.3.1 Effect of food consumption, ethnicity and sex

Food delayed MPM absorption, the extent of absorption was not affected by food; however, the maximum concentration of the active metabolite was reduced by 40%. Administration of MPA delayed release tablet with a high fat meal did not affect the extent of absorption of mycophenolic acid, but the maximal plasma concentration was reduced by 33%, and there was a 5 hours delay in the time to reach maximal concentration (Bullingham et al. 1998). A pharmacokinetic study showed that the rate but not the extent of absorption of mycophenolate is affected by food, indicating that mycophenolate may be administered with food (Christians et al., 2010).

Ethnicity and sex do not significantly affect the primary pharmacokinetic parameters of MPA. A study examine MPA pharmacokinetics in 13 African American and 20 Caucasian renal transplant recipients during the first 4 to 90 posttransplant days and found No significant differences in either MPA AUC or free MPA AUC values (Shaw et al., 2000). Another investigation compared MPA pharmacokinetics in 39 African American and 43 Caucasian renal allograft recipients with stable graft function, There were no significant differences in MPA AUC, Cmax and tmax values between the two groups (Pescovitz et al., 2003). MPA pharmacokinetic parameters did not differ significantly in the males versus females in this study. No differences between diabetic and nondiabetic stable renal transplant recipients were found in this study. Limited studies comparing pharmacokinetics parameters between African-American and white renal transplant patients have shown few differences, suggesting that the differences in rejection rates between these two populations are not explained by pharmacokinetic differences alone but are more likely related to differences in innate immunologic response (Ahsan et al., 1999).

3.3.2 Relationship between adult and pediatric patients

There was a considerable inter- and intraindividual variability of pharmacokinetic parameters in both patient groups. Some of this variability appears to be related to the function of the kidney transplant, because in patients with primary transplant dysfunction a bower maximal MPA concentration and a longer time to maximum concentration were observed. This may be due to slower absorption of MMF, most likely as a result of uremic dysmotility of the gastrointestinal tract (Halloran et al., 1997). Because for MMF there is a relationship between the immunosuppressive efficacy in renal transplant recipients and the MPA-AUC, this fact predict that MMF in a dose of 600 mg/m^2 twice a day displays a comparable effectiveness in pediatric transplant recipients, as observed previously in adult patients. This hypothesis is currently being investigated in a large multicenter study. A dose of 600 mg MMF/m2 BSA in children between the ages of 6 and 15 year yielded comparable AUC for MPA and free MPA at 3 weeks after renal transplantation as adults who received 1 g of MMF, the recommended twice daily oral dose in adults (Bullingham, 1996a). Hence, the body surface area (BSA) -adjusted dosing of MMF appears to be appropriate in pediatric renal transplant recipients. MPM pharmacokinetic parameters, including AUC, in children 1 to 18 years of age receiving MPM 600 mg/m^2 (in oral suspension) twice daily following renal transplantation similar to values in adult renal transplant recipients receiving 1 g twice daily. MPS peak plasma concentrations and AUC of MPA in stable pediatric renal transplant patients 5 to 16 years of age receiving a single dose of MPS (MPA 450 mg/m^2) increased (33 and 18% respectively) relative to adults receiving the same dose based on body surface area. Clinical importance is not determined yet (Halloran et al., 1997).

3.4 Effect of time after transplantation on MPA Pharmacokinetics

The dose-interval MPA AUC in renal transplant recipients increases as a function of time. The dose-normalized mean MPA AUC in renal transplant patients is at least 30 to 50% lower in the first few weeks after transplantation than in the later period (1-6 months after transplantation). It has been demonstrated that most of this phenomenon is accounted for in the novo renal transplant patients with impaired renal function. The reason for lower MPA AUC in this patients in the early posttransplant compared with the time when graft function has stabilized (about 1 month after transplant surgery) is most likely the decreased plasma protein binding of MPA leading to an increase clearance of drug by the liver (Shaw et al., 1998). This theory is supported by observations of elevated free MPA fraction values in the early posttransplantation period in patients with impaired renal function that return to normal values by 1 month posttransplantation. A possible additional factor that could contribute to the higher oral clearance of MPA early after transplantation is corticosteroid therapy, which is significantly higher in that period but then is tapered to low dose levels or completely withdrawn. In pediatric patients, as in adult subjects, the median AUC values increase as a function of time after transplantation (from approximately 35 mg.h/L at weeks to approximately 65 mg.h/L at 3 months after transplantation). The intraindividual variability of AUC was high in the immediate posttransplant period, but decline in the stable phase, whereas the wide interindividual variability remained significant (Oellerich et al., 2000).

3.5 Pharmacokinetic Interactions with mycophenolate mofetil

Since mycophenolate mofetil is solely metabolized by glucuronidation, direct pharmacokinetic interactions with drugs metabolised by cytochrome P450 oxidation are not generally expected. Pharmacokinetic interaction with other drugs metabolised by glucuronidation is a theoretical possibility, although a clinically significant interaction is very unlikely. Potential general mechanisms for interactions with mycophenolate mofetil involve either entrohepatic cycling, or renal tubular competition between MPAG and other drugs undergoing transport mediated renal excretion. As regards the former, competitive interaction could occur between MPAG and other drugs at the biliary transporter, although no example has been reported. Once MPAG is excreted into the gut, cholestyramine and other bile acid sequestrants can clearly reduce the plasma mycophenolic acid AUC and hence clinical effectiveness. Deglucuronidation of MPAG in the colon is mediated by the gut flora, and in particular by the Gram-negative anaerobes which contain most of the glucuronidase activity. Antibiotics with activity against such organisms may reduce entrohepatic cycling and hence the mycophenolic acid AUC. With a renal tubular interaction, plasma mycophenolic acid is not affected. No major clinical sequelae appear to follow from raised plasma MPAG concentrations. The clinical significance of any tubular interaction will thus depend on the magnitude and consequence of raised plasma concentrations of the other interacting drug. Being a competitive interaction, high plasma MPAG concentrations are likely to increase the magnitude of the interaction. Renal impairment may thus be the clinical situation where such interactions need special consideration (Bullingham et al. 1998).

3.6 Clinical efficacy

The relationship between MPA pharmacokinetics and clinical outcomes has been reported in at least 1o investigations. The association between MPA AUC and the risk for acute rejection was first noted in a retrospective analysis of pharmacokinetic data obtained during the first 3 weeks after transplantation, in a dose-escalation study of MMF in 41 adult kidney transplant patients (Jeong & Kaplan, 2007; Takahashi et al., 1995). In mid-1990s, three large clinical trials were conducted in kidney transplant recipients to prove clinical efficacy of MMF. These were the largest prospective, randomized, double blind trials ever performed in transplantation, using the incidences of acute rejection as a primary end point. The results demonstrated the superior efficacy of MMF (1.0 or 1.5 g twice daily), combined with cyclosporine and steroids, in reducing the rate of acute rejection during 6 months after kidney transplantation as compared with azathioprine or placebo treatment (Jeong & Kaplan, 2007). Also, they established the safety of MMF in adult renal transplant patients; overall incidence of adverse effects was comparable between groups. The prominent adverse effects of MMF included nausea, vomiting, diarrhea, and hematologic effects, with a high dosage (3 g/d) being associated with increased risk for the adverse effects. Subsequent long-term (1- and 3-years) follow-up studies reported the similar efficacy and safety of MMF. Other maintenance immunosuppressants that have been evaluated in combination with MMF include tacrolimus. A randomized, clinical trial in renal transplant patients who were treated with tacrolimus-based triple regimens (tacrolimus/MMF/steroid) demonstrated a significant reduction in the incidence of rejection compared with the double regimen group when MMF was given at a dosage of 1g twice a day for 1 year after transplantation. However, in the first 6 months of this trial, MMF was discontinued in half of the patients because of gastrointestinal complications or hematologic adverse effects, indicating the need for lower MMF dosages. It was understood later to be because tacrolimus does not inhibit biliary excretion of MPAG, whereas cyclosporine disrupts enterohepatic cycling and intestinal reabsorption of MPA by inhibiting biliary transporters. Subsequent monitoring of MPA levels in renal transplant patients revealed that MPA plasma levels were lower in the cyclosporine-based regimen compared with the tacrolimus combination. In conclusion, MMF is effective in preventing acute rejection and improving graft and patient survival in combination with cyclosporine and tacrolimus. Tacrolimus-based treatment requires a lower dosage of MMF compared with a cyclosporine-based regimen to maintain the similar MPA plasma levels. (Pawinski et al., 2006).

3.7 Therapeutic drug monitoring

The incorporation of MMF into immunosuppressive regimens has been associated with decreased rates of acute rejection and decreased chronic allograft loss. When the drug was introduced into clinical practice, routine therapeutic drug monitoring was not recommended and empiric dosing became the norm of many centers. However, a deeper appreciation for the highly variable pharmacokinetic behavior of MPA and the relationship between concentration of the drug and risk for acute rejection, combined with an increased emphasis on the need for further improvements in clinical outcomes, treatment of patients with greater risk for graft loss than ever before, and the use of strategies for lowering or eliminating concomitant agents such as corticosteroids or CNI, have led to increasing interest in the role of MPA therapeutic drug monitoring in optimizing immunosuppression.
Recent reviews have suggested provisional target therapeutic ranges for MPA AUC and trough concentrations when using MMF in combination with either cyclosporine or tacrolimus. When combined with cyclosporine, the recommended target ranges are 1 to 3.5 mg/L and 30 to 60 mg/h per L for trough concentrations and AUC, respectively. For the combination with tacrolimus, the target ranges of 1.9 to 4.0 mg/L and 30 to 60 mg/h per L for trough and AUC measurements, respectively, have been suggested (Van Gelder et al., 2006). Two ongoing concentration-control *versus* fixed dosage trials in renal transplant patients will hopefully provide the basis for rigorous assessment of these target ranges in the setting of contemporary practice. A proposed schedule for objective assessment of MPA exposure is presented in Table 4. We hope that the ongoing trials will provide more

definitive data on which to base the selection of sample type, test schedule, and the cost-benefit analysis of MPA therapeutic monitoring (Shaw et al., 2007).

4. Corticosteroids

4.1 Mechanism of action

Glucocorticoids exert their effects by binding to a glucocorticoid receptor (GR) localized in the cytoplasm of target cells. There is a single class of GR that binds glucocorticoids, with no evidence for subtypes of differing affinity in different tissues. Recently a splice variant of GR, termed GR-b, has been identified that does not bind glucocorticoids but binds to DNA and may therefore potentially interfere with the action of glucocorticoids (Bamberger et al., 1995).

4.2 Pharmacokinetics

The pharmacokinetic characteristics of the various glucocorticoids depend on their physicochemical properties. Glucocorticoids are lipophilic and are usually administered as prodrugs when given intravenously (Mager & Jusko, 2002).

4.2.1 Absorption and distribution

Glucocorticoids are well absorbed after oral administration and have a bioavailability of 60–100%. They have moderate protein binding and a moderate apparent volume of distribution (Derendorf et al., 1991; Varis et al., 2000). Over 90% of circulating plasma corticosteroids attached to two types of proteins: (1) a non-specific albumin, and (2) a high affinity transcortin, an α-2-globulin important in regulating corticosteroid flowing freely, as allows greater freedom in tissues with an inflammatory response. Transcortin has a high affinity and a low capacity for hydrocortisone and prednisolone, whereas albumin has a low affinity but high capacity. This leads to an increase in the free glucocorticoid fraction once transcortin is saturated at concentrations of about 400 μg/L. Such concentrations are achieved after administration of hydrocortisone or prednisolone doses >20mg (Czock et al., 2005). Protein binding is biologically relevant, because only free drug can reach the biophase (i.e. the site of action) and interact with the receptor. Therefore, pharmacodynamic considerations have to include protein binding. Clinically, decreased protein binding due to low plasma albumin concentrations correlated with glucocorticoid adverse effects in prednisone therapy (Lewis et al., 1971). Generally, however, alterations in protein binding do not have much impact on drug action (Benet et al., 2002; Czock et al., 2005).

4.2.2 Metabolism and excretion

The renal excretion of unchanged glucocorticoids is only 1–20% (Garg & Jusko, 1994). Glucocorticoid metabolism is a two-step process. Firstly, oxygen or hydrogen atoms are added then secondly, conjugation takes place (glucuronidation or sulphation). Subsequently the kidney excretes the resulting hydrophilic inactive metabolites. Intracellular metabolism by 11β-hydroxysteroid dehydrogenase (11β-HSD) controls the availability of glucocorticoids for binding to the glucocorticoid and mineralocorticoid receptors. Type 1 dehydrogenase (11β-HSD1) is widely distributed in glucocorticoid target tissues and has its highest activity in the liver. 11β-HSD1 acts mainly as a reductase, converting the inactive cortisone to the active cortisol (Czock et al., 2005). Type 2 dehydrogenase (11β-HSD2) is found in mineralocorticoid target tissues (kidney, colon, salivary glands, placenta). 11β-HSD2 has a high affinity for endogenous cortisol and by oxidation, converting cortisol to cortisone, it protects the mineralocorticoid receptor from occupation by cortisol. The activity of 11β-HSD2 varies depending on the type of glucocorticoid, which explains to some extent the different mineralocorticoid activities of different glucocorticoids (Diederichet al., 2002).

4.2.3 Prednisolone and prednisone

The pharmacokinetics of prednisolone and prednisone are complicated by dose-dependency due to nonlinear protein binding (Wald et al., 1992). Protein binding of prednisolone decreases nonlinearly from 95% to 60–70%, while the concentration increases from 200 60–70%, while the concentration increases from 200 μg/L to 800 μg/L when protein binding of prednisolone reaches the stationary state (Rose et al., 1981). In consequence, a dose-dependent increase in the volume of distribution (Vd) and drug clearance (CL) is observed at doses over 20mg (Frey et al., 1990; Rohatagi et al., 1997). However, the elimination half-life remains constant and the dose dependencies of Vd and CL disappear when free prednisolone concentrations are measured (Möllmann et al., 1989; Rohatagi 1997). Prednisolone clearance decreases again only at very high doses, which can be explained by saturation of elimination mechanisms. The affinity of prednisone for transcortin is 10-fold lower than that of prednisolone (Czock et al., 2005).

4.2.4 Methylprednisolone

Methylprednisolone (6α-methylprednisolone) has no affinity for transcortin and binds only to albumin (Czock et al., 2005). Accordingly, methylprednisolone pharmacokinetics are linear, with no dose-dependency. The disposition of methylprednisolone is biexponential (Möllmann et al., 1989). A two-compartment model is appropriate for intravenous administration of very high doses. A one compartment model can be used with lower intravenous doses and oral administration (Booker et al., 2002; Lewis et al. 1971).

4.3 Interactions between glucocorticoids and tacrolimus

Corticosteroids are an essential component of most immunosuppressive regimens currently used in renal transplantation because of their efficacy in reducing acute rejection and improving graft survival. The precise mechanism of action of glucocorticoids is not fully understood, although it is apparent that it is multifaceted, involving both direct and indirect mechanisms and affecting proximal and distal events of T cell activation (Almawi et al., 1999). Long-term administration of corticosteroids also is known to be associated with numerous adverse effects that lead to increased patient morbidity and mortality after renal transplantation. The adverse effects of corticosteroids, including new-onset diabetes, hyperlipidemia, hypertension, growth retardation, accelerated bone loss, weight gain, avascular necrosis, cataracts, cosmetic changes, depression, psychotic behavior, and others, have been well documented Hricik et al., 1993; Grotz et al., 1998; Kobashigawa & Kasiske, 1997; Schulak & Hricik, 1994). There also is evidence that they may interfere with the tolerogenic pathways of organ acceptance (Qian et al., 1997; Wang et al., 2001). In addition to affecting the morbidity and the quality of life of renal transplant recipients, corticosteroids increase the long-term cost of their medical. Because glucocorticoids are inducers of the CYP34A4 enzyme involved in tacrolimus metabolism, theoretically glucocorticoid use would be expected to necessitate increased tacrolimus dosing. Indeed, studies in adults have documented increased tacrolimus levels upon steroid withdrawal, but similar data on pediatric patients are not available. In recent years, tacrolimus has been used both steroid based and steroid-free immunosuppressive protocols (van Duijnhoven et al., 2003; Anglicheau et al., 2003). Steroid avoidance or rapid elimination of steroids may have an advantage over steroid withdrawal. Steroid avoidance protocols may avoid the long-term risks of steroid use and the increased risk for rejection when the steroids are withdrawn. Birkeland and Khwaja reported excellent long term graft survival and function (3 and 4 year, respectively) with very low rejection rates. In other studies, a slight increase in acute rejection episodes, especially in the early posttransplantation period, was observed; these were easily reversible, and their impact on long-term graft survival is unclear at this time (Borrows et al., 2004; Cole et al., 2001; Grewal et al., 1998; ter Meulen et al., 2004). Steroids, once thought to be a mandatory component of immunosuppression to preserve graft survival, are gradually being eliminated from current protocols. It has long been recognized that despite the efficacy of maintenance corticosteroids that these medications are far from benign (Jaber et al., 2007). Consequently, corticosteroid-free immunosuppression has become a desirable goal for many in the transplant community. A potential problem of eliminating corticosteroids from an immunosuppressive regimen, however, is an increased risk for acute rejection (Vanrenterghem et al., 2000).

5. References

Ahsan, N., Hricik, D., & Matas, A., Rose, S., Tomlanovich, S., & Wilkinson, A., Ewell, M., McIntosh, M., & Stablein, D., Hodge E. Prednisone withdrawal in kidney transplant recipients on cyclosporine and mycophenolate mofetil--a prospective randomized study. Steroid Withdrawal Study Group. *Transplantation*, Vol. 68, No. 12, (December 1999), pp. 1865-1874, ISSN 1534-0608

Almawi, W.Y., Melemedjian, O.K., & Rieder, M.J. An alternate mechanism of glucocorticoid anti-proliferative effect: Promotion of a Th2 cytokine-secreting profile. *Clinical Transplantation*, Vol. 13, No. 5, (October 1999), pp. 365-374, ISSN 0902-0063

Anglicheau, D., Flamant, M., & Schlageter, M.H., Martinez, F., Cassinat, B., & Beaune, P., Legendre, C., & Thervet, E. Pharmacokinetic interaction between corticosteroids and tacrolimus after renal transplantation. *Nephrology Dialysis Transplantation*, Vol. 18, No. 11, (November 2003), pp. 2409-14, ISSN 1460-6235

Bai, J.P., Lesko, L.J., & Burckart, G.J. Understanding the genetic basis for adverse drug effects: the calcineurin inhibitors. *Pharmacotherapy*, Vol. 30, No. 2, (February 2010), pp. 195-209, ISSN 0277-0008

Bamberger, C.M., Bamberger, A.M., & de Castro, M., Chrousos, G.P. Glucocorticoid receptor beta, a potential endogenous inhibitor of glucocorticoid action in humans. *Journal of Clinical Investigation*, Vol. 95, No. 6, (Jun 1995), pp. 2435-2441, ISSN 0021-9738

Barrera-Pulido, L., Aguilera-García, I., & Docobo-Pérez, F., Alamo-Martínez, J.M., & Pareja-Ciuró, F., Nuñez-Roldán, A., & Gómez-Bravo, M.A., Bernardos-Rodríguez, A. Clinical relevance and prevalence of polymorphisms in CYP3A5 and MDR1 genes that encode tacrolimus biotransformation enzymes in liver transplant recipients. *Transplantation Proceedings*, Vol. 40, No. 9, (November 2008), pp. 2949-2951, ISSN 0041-1345

Bekersky, I., Dressler, D., & Mekki, Q. Effect of time of meal consumption on bioavailability of a single oral 5 mg tacrolimus dose. *Journal of Clinical Pharmacology*, Vol. 41, No. 3, (March 2001), pp. 289-297, ISSN 1552-4604

Bekersky, I., Dressler, D., & Mekki, Q.A. Effect of low- and high-fat meals on tacrolimus absorption following 5 mg single oral doses to healthy human subjects. *Journal of Clinical Pharmacology*, Vol. 41, No. 2, (February 2001), pp. 176-182, ISSN 1552-4604

Benet, L.Z. & Hoener B.A. Changes in plasma protein binding have little clinical relevance. *Clinical Pharmacology and Therapeutics*, Vol. 71, No. 3, (March 2002), pp. 115-121, ISSN 0009-9236

Birkeland, S.A. Steroid-free immunosuppression in renal transplantation: A long-term follow-up of 100 consecutive patients. *Transplantation*, Vol.71 , No. 8, (April 2007), pp. 1089-90, ISSN 1534-0608

Booker, B.M., Magee, M.H., & Blum, R.A., Lates, C.D., Jusko, W.J. Pharmacokinetic and pharmacodynamic interactions between diltiazem and methyl prednisolone in healthy volunteers. *Clinical Pharmacology and Therapeutics*, Vol. , No. , (October 2002), pp. 370-382, ISSN 0009-9236

Borrows, R., Loucaidou, M., & Van Tromp, J., Cairns, T., Griffith, M., & Hakim, N., McLean, A., Palmer, A., & Papalois, V., Taube, D. Steroid sparing with tacrolimus and mycophenolate mofetil in renal transplantation. *American Journal of Transplantation*, Vol. 4, No. 11, (November 2004), pp. 1845-51, ISSN 1600-6143

Bullingham, R., Monroe, S., & Nicholls, A., Hale, M. Pharmacokinetics and bioavailability of mycophenolate mofetil in healthy subjects after single-dose oral and intravenous administration. *Journal of Clinical Pharmacology*, Vol. 36, No. 4, (April 1996b), pp. 315-324, ISSN 1552-4604

Bullingham, R., Nicholls, A., & Hale, M. Pharmacokinetics of mycophenolate mofetil (RS 61443): A short review. *Transplantation Proceedings*, Vol. 28, No. 2, (April 1996a), pp. 925-929, ISSN 0041-1345

Bullingham, R.E., Nicholls, A.J., Kamm, .BR. Clinical pharmacokinetics of mycophenolate mofetil. Clinical Pharmacokinetics, Vol. 34, No. 6, (1998), pp. 429-455, ISSN 0312-5963

Cattaneo, D., Perico, N., & Remuzzi, G. From pharmacokinetics to pharmacogenomics: a new approach to tailor immunosuppressive therapy. *American Journal of Transplantation*, Vol. 4, No. 3, (March 2004), pp. 299-310, ISSN 1600-6143

Chen, J.S., Li, L.S., & Cheng, D.R., Ji, S.M., & Sun, Q.Q., Cheng, Z., & Wen, J.Q., Sha, G.Z., & Liu ZH. . Effect of CYP3A5 genotype on renal allograft recipients treated with tacrolimus. *Transplantation Proceedings*, Vol. 41, No. 5, (June 2002), pp. 1557–6, ISSN 0041-1345

Christians, U., Jacobsen, W., & Benet, L.Z., Lampen, A. Mechanisms of clinically relevant drug interactions associated with tacrolimus. *Clinical Pharmacokinetics*, Vol. 41, No. 11, (2002), pp. 813-51, ISSN 0312-5963

Christians, U., Klawitter, J., & Clavijo, C.F. *Kidney International, Supplement*, No.115, (March 2010), pp. S1-S7, ISSN 0085-2538

Christians, U., Pokaiyavannichkul, T., & Chan, L. (2006). Tacrolimus, In: *Applied Pharmacokinetics and Pharmacodynamics, Principles of Therapeutic Drug Monitoroing*, M.E. Burton, L.M. Shaw, J.J. Schentag, W.E. Evans, (Ed.), pp. 529-562, Lippincott, Williams and Wilkins, ISSN 0-7817-4431-8, Philadelphia, United States of America

Cole, E., Landsberg, D., & Russell, D., Zaltzman, J., & Kiberd, B., Caravaggio, C., and Vasquez, A.R., Halloran, P. A pilot study of steroid-free immunosuppression in the prevention of acute rejection in renal allograft recipients. *Transplantation*, Vol. 72, No. 5, (September 2001), pp. 845-50, ISSN 1534-0608

Czock, D., Keller, F., & Rasche, F.M., Häussler, U. Pharmacokinetics and pharmacodynamics of systemically administered glucocorticoids. *Clinical Pharmacokinetics*, Vol. 44, No. 1, (2005), pp. 61-98, ISSN 0312-5963

Danesi, R., Mosca, M., & Boggi, U., Del Tacca, M. Genetics of drug response to immunosuppressive treatment and prospects for personalized therapy. *Molecular Medicine Today*, Vol. 6, No. 12, (December 2000), pp. 475-482. [Abstract] ISSN 1357-4310

del Mar Fernández De Gatta, M., Santos-Buelga, D., & Domínguez-Gil, A.,García, M.J. Immunosuppressive therapy for paediatric transplant patients: pharmacokinetic considerations. *Clinical Pharmacokinetics*, Vol. 41, No. 2 (2002), pp. 115-135, ISSN 0312-5963

Derendorf, H., Möllmann, H., & Barth, J., Möllmann, C., & Tunn, S., Krieg, M. Pharmacokinetics and oral bioavailability of hydrocortisone. *Journal of Clinical Pharmacology*, Vol. 31, No. 5, (May 1991), pp. 473-476, ISSN 1552-4604

Diederich, .S, Eigendorff, E., & Burkhardt, P., Quinkler, M., & Bumke-Vogt, C., Rochel, M., & Seidelmann, D., Esperling, P., & Oelkers, W., Bähr, V. 11 β-hydroxysteroid dehydrogenase types 1 and 2: an important pharmacokinetic determinant for the activity of synthetic mineralo- and glucocorticoids. *The Journal of Clinical Endocrinology and Metabolism*, Vol. 87, No. 12, (December 2002), pp. 5695- 5701, ISSN 1945-7197

Dresser, G.K., Spence, J.D., & Bailey, D.G. Pharmacokinetic-pharmacodynamic consequences and clinical relevance of cytochrome P450 3A4 inhibition. *Clinical Pharmacokinetics*, Vol. 38, No. 1, (2000), pp. 41-57, ISSN 0312-5963

Felipe, C.R., Silva, H.T., & Machado, P.G., García, R., & da Silva Moreira, S.R., Pestana, J.O. The impact of ethnic miscegenation on tacrolimus clinical pharmacokinetics and therapeutic drug monitoring. *Clinical Transplantation*, Vol. 16, No. 4, (August 2002), pp. 262–272, ISSN 0902-0063

Fitzsimmons, W.E., Bekersky, I., & Dressler, D., Raye, K., & Hodosh, E., Mekki, Q. Demographic considerations in tacrolimus pharmacokinetics. *Transplantation Proceedings*, Vol. 30, No. 4, (June 1998), pp. 1359-1364, ISSN 0041-1345

Frey, B.M. & Frey, F.J. Clinical pharmacokinetics of prednisone and prednisolone. *Clinical Pharmacokinetics*, Vol. 19, No. 2, (1990), pp. 26-46, ISSN 0312-5963

Fung, J.J. Tacrolimus and transplantation: A decade in review. *Transplantation*, Vol. 77, No. 9, (May 2004), pp. S41-S43, ISSN 1534-0608

Garg, V. & Jusko, W.J. Bioavailability and reversible metabolism of prednisone and prednisolone in man. *Biopharmaceutics and Drug Disposition*, Vol. 15, No. 2, (March 1994), pp. 163-172, ISSN 0142-2782

González-Posada, J.M., Hernández, D., & Bayés Genís, B., García Perez, J., & Rivero Sanchez M. Impact of diabetes mellitus on kidney transplant recipients in Spain. *Nephrology Dialysis Transplantation*, Vol. 19, No. S3, (June 2004), pp. iii57–61, ISSN 1460-6235

Grewal, H.P., Thistlethwaite, J.R. Jr., & Loss, GE. Corticosteroid cessation 1 week following renal transplantation using tacrolimus/mycophenolate mofetil based immunosuppression. *Transplantation Proceedings*, Vol. 30, No. 4, (June 1998), pp. 1378-1379, ISSN 0041-1345

Grotz, W.H., Rump, L.C., & Niessen, A., Schmidt-Gayk, H., & Reichelt, A., Kirste, G., & Olschewski, M., Schollmeyer, P.J. Treatment of osteopenia and osteoporosis after kidney transplantation. *Transplantation*, Vol. 66, No. 8, (October 1998), pp. 1004-1008, ISSN 1534-0608

Halloran, P., Mathew, T., & Tomlanovich, S., Groth, C., Hooftman, L., & Barker, C. Mycophenolate mofetil in renal allograft recipients: a pooled efficacy analysis of three randomized, double-blind, clinical studies in prevention of rejection. *Transplantation*, Vol. 63, No. 1, (January 1997), pp. 39-47, ISSN 1534-0608

Halloran, P.F. Immunosuppressive Drugs for Kidney Transplantation. *New England Journal of Medicine*, Vol. 351, No. 26, (December 2002), pp. 2715-2729, ISSN 0028-4793

Hämmerlein, A., Derendorf, H., & Lowenthal, D.T. Pharmacokinetic and pharmacodynamic changes in the elderly. Clinical implications. *Clinical Pharmacokinetics*, Vol. 35, No. 1, (2002), pp. 49-64, ISSN 0312-5963

Hariharan, S., Schroeder, T.J., & First, M.R. Effect of race on renal transplant outcome. *Clinical Transplantation*, Vol. 7, No. 3, (June 1993), pp. 235, ISSN 0902-0063

Harris, R.Z., Benet, L.Z., & Schwartz, J,B. Gender effects in pharmacokinetics and pharmacodynamics. *Drugs*, Vol. 50, No. 2, (2002), pp. 222-239, ISSN 0012-6667

Hebert, M.F., Fisher, R.M., & Marsh, C.L., Dressler, D., & Bekersky, I. Effects of rifampin on tacrolimus pharmacokinetics in healthy volunteers. *Journal of Clinical Pharmacology*, Vol. 39, No. 1, (February 1999), pp. 91-96, ISSN 1552-4604

Hesselink, D.A., Bouamar, R., & van Gelder, T. The pharmacogenetics of calcineurin inhibitor-related nephrotoxicity. *Therapeutic Drug Monitoring*, Vol. 32, No. 4, (August 2010), pp. 387-393, ISSN 0163-4356

Hesselink, D.A., Ngyuen, H., & Wabbijn, M., Gregoor, P.J., Steyerberg, E.W., & van Riemsdijk, I.C., Weimar, W., & van Gelder T. Tacrolimus dose requirement in renal transplant recipients is significantly higher when used in combination with corticosteroids. *British Journal of Clinical Pharmacology*, Vol. 56, No. 3, (September 2003), pp. 327-30, ISSN 1552-4604

Hricik, D.E., O'Toole, M.A., & Schulak, J.A., Herson, J. Steroid-free immunosuppression in cyclosporine treated renal transplant recipients: a meta-analysis. *Journal of the American Society of Nephrology*, Vol. 4, No. 6, (December 1993), pp. 1300-1005, ISSN 1046-6673

Hübner, G.I., Eismann, R., & Sziegoleit, W. Drug interaction between Mycophenolate mofetil and tacrolimus detectable within therapeutic mycophenolic acid monitoring in renal transplant recipients. *Therapeutic Drug Monitoring*, Vol. 21, No. 5, (October 199), pp. 536-539, ISSN 0163-4356

Iwasaki, K. Metabolism of Tacrolimus (FK506) and Recent Topics in Clinical Pharmacokinetics. *Drug Metabolism and Pharmacokinetics*, Vol. 22, No. 5, (October 2007), pp. 328–335, ISSN 1347-4367

Jaber, J.J., Feustel, P.J., & Elbahloul, O., Conti, A.D., & Gallichio, M.H., Conti, D.J. Early steroid withdrawal therapy in renal transplant recipients: a steroid-free sirolimus and CellCept-based calcineurin inhibitor-minimization protocol. *Clinical Transplantation*, Vol. 21, No. 1, (January-February 2007), pp. 101-109, ISSN 0902-0063

Jeong, H. & Kaplan, B. Therapeutic monitoring of mycophenolate mofetil. *Clinical Journal of the American Society of Nephrology*, Vol. 2, No. 1, (January 2007), pp. 184-191, ISSN 1555-9041

Johnson, A.G., Rigby, R.J., & Taylor, P.J., Jones, C.E., Allen, J., & Franzen, K., Falk, M,C., & Nicol, D. The kinetics of mycophenolic acid and its glucuronide metabolite in adult kidney transplant recipients. *Clinical Pharmacology and Therapeutics*, Vol. 66, No. , (November 1999), pp. 492-500, ISSN 0009-9236

Joy, M.S., Hogan, S.L., & Thompson, B.D., William, F., & Finn, W.F., Nickeleit, V. Cytochrome P450 3A5 expression in the kidneys of patients with calcineurin inhibitor nephrotoxicity. *Nephrology Dialysis Transplantation*, Vol. 22, No. 7, (July 2007), pp. 1963–1968, ISSN 1460-6235

Jusko, W.J. Analysis of tacrolimus (FK 506) in relation to therapeutic drug monitoring. *Therapeutic Drug Monitoring*, Vol. 17, No. 6, (December 1995), pp. 596-601, ISSN 0163-4356

Jusko, W.J. & Kobayashi, M. Therapeutic monitoring of tacrolimus (FK 506). *Therapeutic Drug Monitoring*, Vol. 15, No. 4, (August 1993), pp. 349, ISSN

Jusko, W.J., Thomson, A.W., & Fung, J., McMaster, P., & Wong, S.H., Zylber-Katz E. Consensus document: therapeutic monitoring of tacrolimus (FK506). *Therapeutic Drug Monitoring*, Vol. 17, No. 6, (December 1995), pp. 606-614, ISSN 0163-4356

Kamar, N., Mariat, C., & Delahousse, M., Dantal, J., Al Najjar, A., & Cassuto, E., Lefrançois, N., Cointault, O., & Touchard, G., Villemain, F., & Di Giambattista, F., Benhamou, P.Y. Diabetes mellitus after kidney transplantation: a French multicentre observational study. *Nephrology Dialysis Transplantation*, Vol. 22, No. 7, (July 2007), pp. 1986-1993, ISSN 1460-6235

Kaplan, B., Meier-Kriesche, H.U., & Friedman, G., Mulgaonkar, S., Gruber, S., & Korecka, M., Brayman, K.L., Shaw, L.M. Pharmacokinetics of mycophenolic acid in renal transplant patients whit delayed graft function. *Journal of Clinical Pharmacology*. 1998;39(7):715-20

Kapturczak, M.H., Meier-Kriesche, H.U., & Kaplan, B. Pharmacology of calcineurin antagonists. *Transplantation Proceedings*, Vol. 36, No. 2S, (March 2004), pp. 25S-32S, ISSN 0041-1345

Khwaja, K., Asolati, M., & Harmon, J., Melancon, J.K., & Dunn, T., Gillingham, K., & Kandaswamy, R., Humar, A., & Gruessner, R., Payne, W., & Najarian, J., Dunn, D., & Sutherland, D., Matas AJ. Outcome at 3 years with a prednisone-free maintenance regimen: A single-center experience with 349 kidney transplant recipients. *American Journal of Transplantation*, Vol. 4, No. 6, (June 2004), pp. 980-987, ISSN 1600-6143

Kiberd, B.A., Lawen, J., & Fraser, A.D., Keough-Ryan, T., & Belitsky, P. Early adequate mycophenolic acid exposure is associated with less rejection in kidney transplantation. *American Journal of Transplantation*, Vol. 4, No. 7, (July 2004), pp. 1079–1083, ISSN 1600-6143

Kobashigawa, J.A. & Kasiske, B.L. Hyperlipidemia in solid organ transplantation. *Transplantation*, Vol. 63, No. 3, (February 1997), pp. 331-338, ISSN 1534-0608

Lewis, G.P., Jusko, W.J., & Graves, L., ND Burke, C.W. Prednisone side-effects and serum-protein levels: a collaborative study. *The Lancet*, Vol. 2, No. 7728, (October 1971), pp. 778-780, ISSN 0140-6736

López-Montenegro Soria, M.A., Kanter Berga, J., & Beltrán Catalán, S., Milara Payá, J., & Pallardó Mateu, LM., Jiménez Torres, N.V. Genetic Polymorphisms and Individualized Tacrolimus Dosing. *Transplantation Proceedings*, Vol. 42, No. 8, (October 2010), pp. 3031–3033, ISSN 0041-1345

Lown, K.S., Mayo, R.R., & Leichtman, A.B., Hsiao, H.L., & Turgeon, D.K., Schmiedlin-Ren, & P., Brown, M.B., Guo, W., & Rossi, S.J., Benet, L.Z., & Watkins, P.B. Role of intestinal P-glycoprotein (MDR1) in interpatient variation in the oral bioavailability of cyclosporine. *Clinical Pharmacology and Therapeutics*. Vol. 62, No.3 , (September 1997), pp. 248-260, ISSN 0009-9236

Macphee, I.A., Fredericks, S., & Mohamed, M., Moreton, M., & Carter, N.D., Johnston, A., & Goldberg, L., Holt, D.W. Tacrolimus pharmacogenetics: the CYP3A5*1 allele predicts low dose-normalized tacrolimus blood concentrations in whites and South Asians. *Transplantation*, Vol. 79 , No. 4, (February 2002), pp. 499-502, ISSN 1534-0608

Macphee, I.A., Fredericks, S., & Tai, T., Syrris, P., & Carter, N.D., Johnston, A., & Goldberg, L., Holt, D.W. Tacrolimus pharmacogenetics: polymorphisms associated with expression of cytochrome p4503A5 and P-glycoprotein correlate with dose requirement. *Transplantation*, Vol. 74, No. 11, (December 2002), pp. 1486-1489, ISSN 1534-0608

Mager, D.E. & Jusko W.J. Quantitative structure-pharmacokinetic/pharmacodynamic relationships of corticosteroids in man. *Journal of Pharmaceutical Sciences*, Vol. 91, No. 11, (November 2002), pp. 2441-2451, ISSN 0022-3549

Mancinelli, L.M., Frassetto, L., & Floren, L.C., Dressler, D., & Carrier, S., Bekersky, I., & Benet, L.Z., Christians, U. The pharmacokinetics and metabolic disposition of tacrolimus: a comparison across ethnic groups. *Clinical Pharmacology and Therapeutics*, Vol. 69, No. 1, (January 2001), pp. 24-31, ISSN 0009-9236

Mañez, R., Martin, M., & Raman, D., Silverman, D., & Jain, A., Warty, V., & Gonzalez-Pinto, I., Kusne, S., & Starzl, T.E. Fluconazole therapy in transplant recipients receiving FK506. *Transplantation*. Vol. 57, No. 10, (May 2002), pp.1521-1523 , ISSN 1534-0608

Markell M. New-onset diabetes mellitus in transplant patients: pathogenesis, complications, and management. *American Journal of Kidney Disease*, Vol. 43, No. 6, (June 2004), pp. 953-965, ISSN 0272-6386

Meibohm, B., Beierle, I., & Derendorf, H. How important are gender differences in pharmacokinetics? *Clinical Pharmacokinetics*, Vol. 41, No. 5, (2002), pp. 329-342, ISSN 0312-5963

Meier-Kriesche, H.U. & Kaplan, B. Cyclosporine microemulsion and tacrolimus are associated with decreased chronic allograft failure and improved long-term graft survival as compared with Sandimmune. *American Journal of Transplantation*, Vol. 2, No. 1, (January 2002), pp. 100-104, ISSN 1600-6143

Meier-Kriesche, H.U., Shaw, L.M., & Korecka, M., Kaplan, B. Pharmacokinetics of mycophenolic acid in renal insufficiency. *Therapeutic Drug Monitoring*, Vol. 22, No. 1, (February 2000), pp. 27-30, ISSN 0163-4356

Möllmann, H., Rohdewald, P., & Barth, J., Verho, M., Derendorf H. Pharmacokinetics and dose linearity testing of methylprednisolone phosphate. *Biopharmaceutics and Drug Disposition*, Vol. 10, No. 5, (September-October 1989), pp. 453-64, ISSN 0142-2872

Mourad, M., Wallemacq, P., & König, J., de Frahan, E.H., & Eddour, D.C., De Meye,r M., & Malaise, J., Squifflet, J.P. Therapeutic monitoring of mycophenolate mofetil in organ transplant recipients. Is it necessary? *Clinical Pharmacokinetics*, Vol. 41, No. 3, (2002), pp. 319-327, ISSN 0312-5963

Naesens, M., Kuypers, D.R., & Sarwal, M. Calcineurin Inhibitor Nephrotoxicity. Clinical *Journal of the American Society of Nephrology*, Vol. 4, No. 2, (February 2009), pp. 481–508, 1555-9041

Ochiai, T., Fukao, K., & Takahashi, K., Endo, T., & Oshima, S., Uchida, K., & Yokoyama, I., Ishibashi, M., & Takahara, S., Iwasaki, Y. Phase III study of FK 506 in kidney transplantation. *Transplantation Proceedings*, Vol. 27, No. 1, (February 1995), pp. 829-833, ISSN 0041-1345

Oellerich, M., Shipkova, M., & Schütz E., Wieland, E., Weber, L., & Tönshoff, B., Armstrong, V.W. Pharmacokinetic and metabolic investigations of mycophenolic acid in pediatric patients after renal transplantation: implications for therapeutic drug monitoring. *Therapeutic Drug Monitoring*, Vol. 22 No. 1, (February 2000), pp. 20-26, ISSN 0163-4356

Op den Buijsch, R.A., Christiaans, M.H., & Stolk, L.M., de Vries J.E., & Cheung, C.Y., Undre, N.A., & van Hooff, J.P., van Dieijen-Visser, & M.P., Bekers, O. Tacrolimus pharmacokinetics: infuence of adenosine triphosphate-binding cassette B1 (ABCB1) and cytochrome (CYP) 3A polymorphisms. *Fundamental & Clinical Pharmacology*, Vol. 21, No. 4, (August 2007), pp. 427-35, ISSN 0767-3891

Paine, M.F., Khalighi, M., & Fisher, J.M., Shen, D.D., & Kunze, K.L., Marsh, C.L., & Perkins, J.D., Thummel, KE. Characterization of interintestinal and intraintestinal variations in human CYP3A dependant metabolism. *The Journal of Pharmacology and Experimental Therapeutic*, Vol. 283, No. 3, (December 1997), pp. 1552-1562, ISSN 0022-3565

Pascual, M., Theruvath, T., & Kawai, T., Tolkoff-Rubin, N., & Cosimi, A.B. Strategies to improve long-term outcomes after renal transplantation. *New England Journal of Medicine*, Vol. 346, No. 8, (February 2002), pp. 580-590, ISSN 0028-4793

Pawinski, T., Durlik, M., & Szlaska, I., Urbanowicz, A., & Majchrnak, J., Gralak, B. Comparison of mycophenolic acid pharmacokinetic parameters in kidney transplant patients within the first 3 months post-transplant. *Journal of Clinical Pharmacy and Therapeutics*, Vol. 31, No. 1, (February 2006), pp.27-34, ISSN 0009-9236

Pescovitz, M.D., Guasch, A., & Gaston, R., Rajagopalan, P., & Tomlanovich, S., Weinstein, S., & Bumgardner, G.L., Melton, L., & Ducray, P,S., Banken, L., & Hall, J., Boutouyrie, B.X. Equivalent pharmacokinetics of mycophenolate mofetil in African-American and Caucasian male and female stable renal allograft recipients. *American Journal of Transplantation*, Vol. 3, No. 12, (December 2003), pp.1581-1586, ISSN 16006143

Pillans, P.I., Rigby, R.J., & Kubler, P., Willis, C., & Salm, P., Tett, S.E., & Taylor, P.J. A retrospective analysis of mycophenolic acid and ciclosporin concentrations with acute rejection in renal transplant recipients. *Clinical Biochemistry*, Vol. 34, No. 1, (February 2001), pp. 77-81, ISSN 0009-9120

Platz, K.P., Eckhoff, D.E., & Hullett, D.A., Sollinger, H.W. RS-61443 studies: review and proposal. *Transplantation Proceedings*, Vol. 23, No. 2S2, (April 2002), pp. 33-35, ISSN 0041-1345

Plosker, G.L., & Foster, R.H. Tacrolimus: a further update of its pharmacology and therapeutic use in the management of organ transplantation. *Drugs*, Vol. 59, No. 2, (2000), pp. 323-89, ISSN 0012-6667

Prograf Product Monograph Astellas Pharma Canada, Inc. Revision 2009.

Qian, S., Lu, L., & Fu, F., Li, Y., & Li, W., Starzl, T.E., & Fung, J.J., Thomson, A.W. Apoptosis within spontaneously accepted mouse liver allografts: evidence for deletion of cytotoxic T cells and implications for tolerance induction. *Journal of Immunology*, Vol. 158, No. 10, (May 1997), pp. 4654-4661, ISSN 1550- 6606

Rohatagi, S., Barth, J., & Möllmann, H., Hochhaus, G., & Soldner, A., Möllmann, C., & Derendorf H. Pharmacokinetics of methylprednisolone and prednisolone after single and multiple oral administration. *Journal of Clinical Pharmacology*, Vol. 37, No. 10, (October 1997), pp. 916-925, ISSN 1552-4604

Rose, J.Q., Yurchak, A.M., & Jusko, W.J. Dose dependent pharmaco kinetics of prednisone and prednisolone in man. *Journal of Pharmacokinetics and Biopharmaceutics*, Vol. 20, No. 6, (August 1981), pp. 389-417, ISSN 0090-466X

Rosso Felipe, C., de Sandes, T.V., & Sampaio, E.L., Park, S.I., & Silva, H.T. Jr., Medina, and Pestana, .JO. Clinical impact of polymorphisms of transport proteins and enzymes involved in the metabolism of immunosuppressive drugs. *Transplantation Proceedings*, Vol. 41, No. 5, (June 2009), pp. 1441-1455, ISSN 0041-1345

Salvadori, M., Holzer, H., & de Mattos, A., Sollinger, H., & Arns, W., Oppenheimer, F., & Maca, J., Hall, M. Enteric-coated mycophenolate sodium is therapeutically equivalent to mycophenolate mofetil in de novo renal transplant patients. *American Journal of Transplantation*, Vol. 4, No. 2, (February 2004), pp. 231-236, ISSN 1600-6143

Schaeffeler, E., Eichelbaum, M., & Brinkmann, U. Frequency of C3435T polymorphism of MDR1 gene in African people. *The Lancet*, Vol. 358, No. 9279, (August 2001), pp. 383-384, ISSN 0140-6736

Schulak, J.A., & Hricik DE. Steroid withdrawal after renal transplantation. *Clinical Transplantation*, Vol. 8, No. 2 Pt 2, (April 1994), pp. 211-216, ISSN 0902-0063

Schweitzer, E.J., Yoon, S., & Fink, J., Wiland, A., & Anderson, L., Kuo, P.C., & Lim, J.W., Johnson, L.B., & Farney, A.C., Weir, M.R., & Bartlett, S.T. Mycophenolate mofetil reduces the risk of acute rejection less in African-American than in Caucasian kidney recipients. *Transplantation*, Vol. 65, No. 2, (January 1998), pp. 242-248, ISSN 1534-0608

Scott, L.J., McKeage, K., & Keam, S.J., Plosker, G.L. Tacrolimus: a further update of its use in the management of organ transplantation. *Drugs*, Vol. 63, No. 12, (2003), pp. 1247-97, ISSN 0012-6667

Shaw, L.M., Figurski, M., & Milone, M.C., Trofe, J., & Bloom, R.D. Therapeutic drug monitoring of mycophenolic acid. *Clinical Journal of the American Society of Nephrology*, No. 2, Vol. 5, (September 2007), pp. 1062-1072, ISSN 1555-9041

Shaw, L.M., Holt, D.W., & Keown, P., Venkataramanan, R., & Yatscoff, R.W. Current opinions on therapeutic drug monitoring of immunosuppressive drugs. *Clinical Therapeutics*, Vol. 21, No. 10, (October 2002), pp. 1632-1652, ISSN 0149-2918

Shaw, L.M., Holt, D.W., & Oellerich, M., Meiser, B., & van Gelder, T., Shaw, L.M., & Holt DW, Oellerich M. Current issues in therapeutic drug monitoring of mycophenolic acid: report of a roundtable discussion. *Therapeutic Drug Monitoring*, No. 23, Vol. 4, (August 2001), pp. 305-315, ISSN 0163-4356

Shaw, L.M., Korecka, M., & Aradhye, S., Grossman, R., & Bayer, L., Innes, C., & Cucciara, A., Barker, C., & Naji, A., Nicholls, A., & Brayman, K. Mycophenolic acid area under the curve values in African American and Caucasian renal transplant patients are comparable. *Journal of Clinical Pharmacology*, Vol. 40, No. 6, (June 2000), pp. 624-633, ISSN 1552-4604

Shaw, L.M., Mick, R., & Nowak, I., Korecka, M., & Brayman, K.L. Pharmacokinetics of mycophenolic acid in renal transplant patients with delayed graft function. *Journal of Clinical Pharmacology*, Vol. 38, No. 3, (March 1998), pp. 268-275, ISSN 1552-4604

Sollinger,. H.W., Belzer, F.O., & Deierhoi, M.H., Diethelm, A.G., & Gonwa, T.A., Kauffman, R.S., & Klintmalm, G.B., McDiarmid, S.V., & Roberts, J., Rosenthal, J.T. RS-61443 (mycophenolate mofetil). A multicenter study for refractory kidney transplant rejection. *Annals of Surgery*, Vol. 216, No. 4, (October 1992), pp. 513-518, ISSN 1528-1140

Staatz, C., Taylor, P., & Tett, S. Low tacrolimus concentrations and increased risk of early acute rejection in adult renal transplantation. *Nephrology Dialysis Transplantation*, Vol. 16, No. 9, (September 2001), pp. 1905-1909, ISSN 1460-6235

Staatz, C.E., & Tett, S.E. Clinical pharmacokinetics and pharmacodynamics of tacrolimus in solid organ transplantation. *Clinical Pharmacokinetics*, Vol. 43, No. 10, (2004), pp. 623-53, ISSN 0312-5963

Staatz, C.E., & Tett, S.E. Pharmacokinetic Considerations Relating to Tacrolimus Dosing in the Elderly. *Drugs Aging*, Vol. 22, No. 7, (2002), pp. 541-557, ISSN 1170-229X

Stein, C.M., Sadeque, A.J., & Murray, J.J., Wandel, C., & Kim, R.B., Wood, A.J. Cyclosporine pharmacokinetics and pharmacodynamics in African American and white subjects. *Clinical Pharmacology and Therapeutics*, Vol. 69, No. 5, (May 2001), pp. 317-323, ISSN 0009-9236

Takahashi, K., Ochiai, T., & Uchida, K., Yasumura, T., & Ishibashi, M., Suzuki, S., & Otsubo, O., Isono, K., & Takagi, H., Oka, T. Pilot study of mycophenolate mofetil (RS-61443) in the prevention of acute rejection following renal transplantation in Japanese patients. *Transplantation Proceedings*, No. 27, Vol. 1, (February 1995), pp. 1421-1424, ISSN 0041-1345

ter Meulen, C.G., van Riemsdijk, I., & Hené, R.J., Christiaans, M.H., & Borm, G.F., van Gelder, T., & Hilbrands, L.B., Weimar, W., & Hoitsma, A.J. Steroid-withdrawal at 3 days after renal transplantation with anti-IL-2 receptor alpha therapy: A prospective,randomized, multicenter study. *American Journal of Transplantation*, Vol. 4, No. 5, (May 2004), pp. 803-10, ISSN 1600-6143

Toda, F., Tanabe, K., & Ito, S., Shinmura, H., Tokumoto, T., & Ishida, H., Toma, H. Tacrolimus trough level adjustment after administration of fluconazole to kidney recipients. *Transplantation Proceedings*, Vol. 34, No. 5, (August 2002), pp. 1733-1735, ISSN 0041-1345

Tsuchiya, N., Satoh, S., & Tada, H., Li, Z., & Ohyama, C., Sato, K., & Suzuki, T., Habuchi, T., & Kato, T. Influence of CYP3A5 and MDR1 (ABCB1) polymorphisms on the pharmacokinetics of tacrolimus in renal transplant recipients. *Transplantation*, Vol. 78, No. 4, (October 2004), pp. 1182-1187, ISSN 1434-0608

Tuteja, S., Alloway, R., & Johnson, J., Gaber, O. The effect of gut metabolism on tacrolimus bioavailability in renal transplant recipients. *Transplantation*, Vol. 71, No. 9, (April 2001), pp. 1303–1307, ISSN 1534-0608

Undre, N.A., & Schäfer, A. Factors affecting the pharmacokinetics of tacrolimus in the first year after renal transplantation. *Transplantation Proceedings*, Vol. 30, No. 4, (June 1998), pp. 1261-1263, ISSN 0041-1345

Undre, N.A. Pharmacokinetics of tacrolimus-based combination therapies. Nephrology Dialysis Transplantation, Vol. 18, No. S1, (May 2003), pp. i12-i15, ISSN 1460-6235

Undre, N.A., Stevenson, P., & Schäfer, A. Pharmacokinetics of Tacrolimus: Clinically Relevant Aspects. *Transplantation Proceedings*, Vol. 31, No. S7A, (November 1999), pp. 21S–24S, ISSN 0041-1345

Undre, N.A., van Hooff, J., & Christiaans, M., Vanrenterghem, Y., & Donck, J., Heeman, U., & Kohnle, M., Zanker, B., & Land, W., Morales, J.M., & Andrés, A., Schäfer, A., & Stevenson, P. Pharmacokinetics of FK 506 and mycophenolic acid after the administration of a FK 506-based regimen in combination with mycophenolate mofetil in kidney transplantation. *Transplantation Proceedings*, Vol. 30, No. 4, (June 2002), pp. 1299-1302, ISSN 0041-1345

Utecht, K.N., Hiles, J.J., & Kolesar, J. Effects of Genetic Polymorphisms on the Pharmacokinetics of Calcineurin Inhibitors. *American Journal of Health-System Pharmacy*, Vol. 63, No. 23, (December 2002), pp. 2340-2348, ISSN 1079-2082

van Duijnhoven, E.M., Boots, J.M., & Christiaans, M.H., Stolk, L.M., & Undre, N.A., van Hooff, J.P. Increase in tacrolimus trough levels after steroid withdrawal. *Transplant International*, Vol. 16, No. 10, (October 2003), pp. 721-725, ISSN 0934-0874

Van Gelder T. Drug interactions with tacrolimus. *Drug Safety*, Vol. 25, No. 10, (2002), pp. 707-12, ISSN 0114-5916

van Gelder, T., Hilbrands, L.B., & Vanrenterghem, Y., Weimar, W., & de Fijter, J.W., Squifflet, J.P., & Hené, R.J., Verpooten, G.A., & Navarro, M.T., Hale, M.D., Nicholls, A.J. A randomized double-blind, multicenter plasma concentration controlled study of the safety and efficacy of oral mycophenolate mofetil for the prevention of acute rejection after kidney transplantation. *Transplantation*, Vol. 68, No. 2, (July 1999), pp. 261-266, ISSN 1534-0608

Van Gelder, T., Le Meur, Y., & Shaw, L.M., Oellerich, M., & DeNofrio, D., Holt, C., & Kaplan, B., Kuypers, D., & Meiser, B., Toenshoff, B., & Mamelok, R.D. Therapeutic drug monitoring of mycophenolate mofetil in transplantation. *Therapeutic Drug Monitoring*, Vol. 28 No. 2, (April 2006), pp. 145-154, ISSN 0163-4356

van-Duijnhoven, E.M, Christiaans, M., & Undre, N., Stevenson, P., &van Hooff, J. The effect of breakfast on the oral bioavailability of tacrolimus in diabetic and nondiabetic patients before transplantation. *Transplantation Proceedings*, Vol. 30, No. 4, (June 1998), pp. 1268-1270, ISSN 0041-1345

van-Duijnhoven, E.M., Christiaans, M.H., & Boots, J.M., van Hooff, J.P. Evidence That Fasting Does Not Significantly Affect Trough Levels of Tacrolimus in Stable Renal Transplant Recipients. *Transplantation Proceedings*, Vol. 34, No. 5, (August 2002), pp. 1723-1725, ISSN 0041-1345

Vanrenterghem, Y., Lebranchu, Y., & Hené, R., Oppenheimer, F., & Ekberg, H. Double-blind comparison of two corticosteroid regimens plus mycophenolate mofetil and cyclosporine for prevention of acute renal allograft rejection. *Transplantation*, Vol. 70, No. 9, (November 2000), pp. 1352-1359, ISSN 1534-0608

Varis, T., Kivistö, K.T., & Backman, J.T., Neuvonen, P.J. The cytochrome P450 3A4 inhibitor itraconazole markedly increases the plasma concentrations of dexamethasone and enhances its adrenal-suppressant effect. *Clinical Pharmacology and Therapeutics*, Vol. 68, No. 5, (November 2000), pp. 487-494, ISSN 0009-9236

Venkataramanan, R., Swaminathan, A., & Prasad, T., Prasad, T., & Jain, A., Zuckerman, S. Clinical pharmacokinetics of tacrolimus. *Clinical Pharmacokinetics*, Vol. 29, No. 6, (December 1995), pp. 404-430, ISSN 0312-5963

Vicari-Christensen, M., Repper, S., & Basile, S., Young, D. Tacrolimus: review of pharmacokinetics, pharmacodynamics, and pharmacogenetics to facilitate practitioners understanding and offer strategies for educating patients and promoting adherence. *Progress in Transplantation*, Vol. 19, No. 3, (September 2009), pp. 277-842, ISSN 1526-9248

Wald, J.A., Law, R.M., & Ludwig, E.A., Sloan, R.R., & Middleton, E. Jr., Jusko, W.J. Evaluation of dose-related pharmacokinetics and pharmacodynamics of prednisolone in man. *Journal of Pharmacokinetics and Biopharmaceutics*, Vol. 20, No. 6, (December 1992), pp. 567-589, ISSN 0090-466X

Wallemacq, P.E., & Verbeeck, R.K. Comparative Clinical Pharmacokinetics of Tacrolimus in Paediatric and Adult Patients. *Clinical Pharmacokinetics*, Vol. 40, No. 4, (2001), pp. 283-295, ISSN 0312-5963

Wang, C., Sun, J., & Sheil, A.G., McCaughan, G.W., & Bishop, G.A. A short course of methylprednisolone immunosuppression inhibits both rejection and spontaneous acceptance of rat liver allografts. *Transplantation*, Vol. 72, No. 1, (July 2001), pp. 44-51, ISSN 1534-0608

Winkler, M., & Christians, U. A risk-benefit assessment of tacrolimus in transplantation. *Drug Safety*, No. 12 Vol. 5, (May 1995), pp. 348-57, ISSN 0114-5916

World Health Organization (WHO). Global Activity in Organ Transplantation. Estimates 2008.

Yu, S., Wu, L., & Jin, J., Yan, S., & Jiang, G., Xie, H., & Zheng, S. Influence of CYP3A5 gene polymorphisms of donor rather than recipient to tacrolimus individual dose requirement in liver transplantation. *Transplantation*, Vol. 81, No. 1, (January 2006), pp. 46-51, ISSN 1534-0608

Zucker, K., Rosen, A., & Tsaroucha, A., de Faria, L., & Roth, D., Ciancio, G., & Esquenazi, V., Burke, G., & Tzakis, A., Miller, J. Augmentation of mycophenolate mofetil pharmacokinetics in renal transplant patients receiving Prograf and CellCept in combination therapy. *Transplantation Proceedings*, Vol. 29, No. 1, (February-March 2002), pp.334-336, ISSN 0041-1345

21

Desensitization and Induction Immunosuppressive Therapy in Highly HLA-Sensitized Patients Receiving Cadaveric Renal Allograft

Juana Margarita Rufino Hernández[1], José Manuel González-Posada Delgado[1] and Domingo Hernández Marrero[2]
[1]Nephrology Section. Hospital Universitario de Canarias, Tenerife
[2]Nephrology Section. Hospital Universitario Carlos Haya, Málaga
Spain

1. Introduction

Approximately 15-20% of patients on the waiting list for cadaveric renal transplant are highly HLA-sensitized. It is well known that the presence of alloantibodies against human class I (A, B, C) and class II (DR, DQ) HLA antigens in transplant recipients waiting for a renal transplant has a significant increase in acute and chronic rejection rates and a poor graft outcome. There are interesting options for minimizing these immunological problems such as national paired kidney exchange program or acceptable mismatch program similar to the one developed by Eurotransplant program. However, despite these efforts, these patients can wait up to 5 years for a kidney graft and just get it finally only 30% of them. It is therefore vital to develop strategies to reduce waiting time and decrease the risk of transplant rejection, through the elimination or reduction of circulating lymphocytotoxic antibodies.

There have been several retrospective and prospective studies that have used immunoabsorption or plasmapheresis together with immunosuppressants and intravenous immune globulins with highly variable success rates that, while not providing a high level of evidence, constitutes a promising therapeutic alternative for these patients.

In addition, the use of rituximab in living donor transplantation ABO incompatible, hypersensitive patients with positive crossmatch, acute rejection resistant to standard treatments and pretransplant desensitization are running with very interesting results. Moreover, newer approaches for treating acute humoral rejection such as the proteosome inhibitor (bortezomib) or eculizumab (an anticomplement monoclonal antibody), are emerging as successful therapeutic options (Gloor J& Stegall, 2010).

Long-term follow- up of these patients and the application on a wider scale of these treatments, will provide the definitive answers about their real efficacy (Nocera, 2009). Nevertheless, acute antibody-mediated rejection (AMR), occurring in 20-50% of patients, and subclinical AMR even in the absence of allograft dysfunction, may decrease allograft survival by chronic histological abnormalities.

The aim of this chapter is to review the current data about approach therapy in highly HLA-sensitized patients receiving deceased renal allograft.

2. Definition of highly HLA-sensitized patients

Patients with PRA (panel reactive antibodies) permanently > 75%, plus HLA-polyspecific reactivity by complement dependent cytotoxicity (CDC) or flow cytometry and multiple previous positive crossmatch, should be considered highly HLA-sensitized patients. HLA antibodies, are present in hyperimmunized patients as a result of pregnancies, blood transfusions and previous failed grafts, and make up an important barrier to renal transplantation.

There are different assays that can be used to determine the PRA, but it is necessary to ensure efficiency and reliability of these tests, so that that each laboratory must continuously monitor its processes and results (Ercilla MG, 2010). Monitoring is guaranteed by the accreditation of processes as well as quality control of results, evaluated by external organisations of experts on histocompatibility (for example, the accreditation programme of the European Federation for Immunogenetics and the American Society for Histocompatibility and Immunogenetics).

2.1 The complement dependent cytotoxicity (CDC) assay

A complement-mediated cytotoxicity reaction occurs when an IgM or IgG reacts against an antigen present on the cell surface of specific tissues. After this reaction, the complement system activation leads to cell membrane damage and, secondarily, cell lysis. In addition, the cells covered by the antibody (opsonized) are susceptible to be ingested by the monocyte-macrophage system, as it reduces the ionic charge of the cell surface directly through immune adherence or by binding to C3.

The complement dependent cytotoxicity (CDC) assay estimates PRA by adding potential recipient serum to microtiter plates that contain a pool of lymphocytes with defined HLA antigens. Rabbit complement is added and the plates are viewed after addition of a vital stain. The PRA can then be determined based upon the number of cytotoxic reactions that are observed. The classic assay CDC crossmatch has a high positive predictive value for graft loss in the first 48 hours if positive, which therefore contraindicates transplantation. Alloantibody testing should be performed every three months in all candidate patients for renal transplantation and 15 days after each sensitising event (transfusion, graft loss and pregnancy). This sequential study helps to reveal antibodies that may have been identified in the past but that may not have been detected at the time of transplantation. If the crossmatch is positive by CDC, the process is repeated with the addition of Dithiothreitol (DTT). This step reduces the disulfide bonds present when the antibody is IgM.

A test that is CDC positive/DTT negative (presence of an IgM antibody only) should not preclude transplantation: in this case, the determination of solid-phase anti-HLA alloantibody screening (by immunoabsorption ELISA or flow cytometry, Luminex) is negative in serum that was CDC-PRA positive. By comparison, the presence of a CDC positive/DTT positive test is an indication of IgG anti-donor antibody and is a contraindication to transplantation without the use of a desensitization procedure, especially if a donor specific antibody has been defined. (Klein, 2010; Ercilla MG, 2010)

2.2 The enzyme-linked immunoabsorption (ELISA)

This assay uses microtest trays containing known HLA antigens to which potential recipient serum is added. This test is faster than the CDC assay and the HLA antigens used for screening can be adjusted as necessary to reflect the presumed potential donor pool. As in the cytotoxicity technique, the mix of antigens should be representative of the general population. In case of anti-HLA antibodies, a colorimetric reaction enzyme occurs. This reaction is quantified by spectrophotometer.

By ELISA assay, we detect all anti-HLA antibodies, including complement fixing and non-fixers. Once it has detected the presence of anti-HLA antibodies (class I or II), specificity against which these antibodies are directed can also be determined by a high definition ELISA plates or unique antigens with the same methodology. Solid-phase anti-HLA alloantibody screening is useful when autoantibodies are suspected and there is a need to rule out them in a patient with positive CDC-PRA. This indicates presence or absence of type IgG anti-HLA antibodies against anti-HLA-I and anti-HLA-II and, in some kits, anti-MICA. By using purified HLA antigens, non-anti-HLA antibodies are not identified. If anti-HLA antibodies are not revealed by cytotoxicity but are detected by solid phase, it is highly recommended that more sensitive crossmatch techniques should be used, such as flow cytometry or virtual crossmatch (VCM) in order to better define the risk for these patients. (Klein, 2010; Ercilla MG, 2010).

2.3 Flow cytometry. Single-antigen bead flow cytometry (SAB-FC)

Flow cytometry measures the fluorescence after patient serum has been added to a defined set of HLA antigen flow beads. A positive test is determined by the mean channel shift in intensity, that is, mean intensity of fluorescence (MFI). This assay allows to identify specific HLA antigens to which the patients are sensitized and constitutes what we know as "virtual lymphocyte crosssmatch (VCM)." VCM is indicated in patients who are candidates for retransplantation, women who have previously been multiple pregnant and those with positive results in the solid-phase screening but negative for CDC as well as also is recommended for all living-donor transplants.

In the event that the only positive result is that of the positive VCM, this will indicate a 55% probability of an antibody-mediated rejection episode in the first year versus a 5% probability in the case of a negative VCM and the graft survival at one year is slightly lower. However, a positive VCM, by itself, does not imply that a transplant is necessarily contraindicated, but a careful monitoring and immunosuppression aimed to controlling alloantibody production are needed for a thorough treatment.

A positive B-cell negative T-cell crossmatch usually occurs in presence of anti-HLA-II antibodies, presence of low-titre anti-HLA-I antibodies detectable only in B lymphocytes and presence of specific B lymphocytes autoantibodies. In these cases, the decision for transplantation must be individualised. In others words, T cell negative/B cell positive reactions may be secondary to either class I or class II antibodies, while a T cell positive/B cell negative reaction most likely results from a non-HLA antibody, as class I antigen is expressed on both T and B cells. For living donor recipients, perform a monocyte crossmatch should be useful as may help to detect anti-endothelial antibodies.

Clearly identifying the reactivity of antibodies with the donor (DSAs) is logistically difficult because it requires donor cells which may be stored frozen in liquid nitrogen, or determined of the living donor who has to be present for each determination. Therefore, is in these cases, when the crossmatch cannot be performed due to lack of donor cells, where this assay plays an important role as it allows identify specific HLA antigens to which the patient is sensitized (virtual lymphocyte crosssmatch).

Singh N et al showed the impact that produces pre-Tx DSAs detected by SAB-FC on early clinical outcomes. They tested pre-Tx sera from all consecutive deceased-donor kidney transplants performed between January 2005 and July 2006 (n=237), 66% had a high-immunologic risk. MFI more than or equal to 100 for class I and more than or equal to 200 for class II were the lowest DSA thresholds associated with inferior antibody-mediated rejection-free graft survival (Singh N et al., as cited in Ercilla MG, 2010). The presence of class I-anti-HLA antibodies post-transplant precedes, even by years, the development of glomerulopathy. In addition, the presence of anti-class II antibodies is strongly associated with chronic rejection in living-donor kidney recipients, but it appears that the worst prognosis is associated with the simultaneous detection of anti-HLA-I and anti-HLA-II antibodies.

There is evidence that it is possible to reduce pre-existing circulating alloantibodies in some patients to levels where the antibodies are unable to trigger hyperacute rejections. This does not imply that there are no B lymphocytes with the capacity to restart alloantibody production, but the short-term survival of grafts transplanted in some centres under these conditions is acceptable. (Klein, 2010; Ercilla MG, 2010).

Compared with the cell-based method, the fluorometric bead system is not as susceptible to drug interference, such as antithymocyte globulin, intravenously administered immunoglobulin (IVIG), and rituximab. IVIG may interfere with the bead assay for a few days after administration. Nonetheless, these new techniques allow for greater identification of HLA antibody specificities and a more accurate interpretation of cross-match results. Patients with high DSA and donor-specific cross matches SFI units are considered at high risk for AMR and warranted more frequent antibody-level monitoring posttransplantation, may need desensitization treatments, or plan biopsies, in order to reduce DSA levels or detect early AMR respectively; sometimes, increase in DSA imply retreatment as can result in reduction in DSA, levels to $\leq 10^5$ SFI units is usually associated with a low risk of AMR.

3. Immunosuppressive therapy in high immunologic risk patients receiving cadaveric renal allograft

3.1 Immunosuppressive agents

3.1.1 Anti-lymphocyte antibodies

Thymoglobulin is a polyclonal immunosuppressive agent that is generated in rabbits, containing antibodies to a wide variety of human T-cell surface antigens, including the major histocompatibility complex (MHC) antigens. These antibodies have the ability to block a number of adhesion molecules, cytokines, chemokines, among others. Anti-lymphocyte antibodies have long been an integral part of induction regimens and, nowdays, continue to be used in the management of patients at risk of early rejection. They are used in combination with steroids, mycophenolate and calcineurin inhibitors or, less frequently, proliferation signal inhibitors and are treatment of choice for acute graft rejection grade II and III of Banff or unresponsive to steroid boluses. Among the available polyclonal globulin, thymoglobulin, has shown a great efficacy and typically requires between 7 and 10 doses.

The reaction of these globulins with some lymphocyte antigens can trigger activation of these cells to release cytokines, which may present with chills, fever and systemic symptoms, mainly with the first dose. Steroids, antihistamines and antipyretics intravenous infusion may prevent these early reactions; polyclonal antibodies will be made through a central venous catheter in at least 6 hours.

Side effects in the medium and long term are related to its immunosuppressive effect. Polyclonal antibodies can increase the risk of infection (herpes simplex virus, varicella-

zoster virus, cytomegalovirus or Epstein-Barr virus) and patients may benefit from prophylactic antiviral strategies. Other opportunistic infections may be due to pneumocystis jiroveci and aspergillus, but are related to immunosuppression accumulated by the patient rather than the administration of polyclonal antibodies. Treatment with antilymphocyte globulin and a serum test for Epstein-Barr virus receptor are associated with the risk of lymphoproliferative disorders in renal transplant population. (Gaber ,AO et al., 2010; Oppenheimer, F et al., 2010) .
Currently almost 70% of renal transplant patients in the United States receive antibody induction, either antithymocyte globulin (Thymoglobulin) or inhibitors of IL-2. Brennan, D et al. (Brennan, C et al., 2006) compared the efficacy and safety of randomized use of basiliximab versus thymoglobulin in patients at high risk of rejection (retransplantation, PRA greater than 20% black, one or more HLA incompatibilities) or delayed graft function who received a cadaveric renal transplantation. After 12 months of follow-up, incidence of biopsy proven acute rejection was 15.6% for Thymoglobulin, and 25.2% for basiliximab ($p = 0.02$) and the antibody-treated acute rejection was lower in patients with thymoglobulin (1.4% vs 8.0%, $p = 0,005$). The overall rate of adverse events was 99.3% to 98.5%, was similar between boths induction treatment. The overall incidence of infection was 85.8% to 75.2% with thymoglobulin and basiliximab ($p = 0.03$). This difference appears to be attributable to a higher frequency of urinary tract infection and no CMV viral infections. CMV infection was lower with Thymoglobulin (7.8% vs 17.5%, $p = 0.02$), probably due that a prophylactic antibiotics were used less in patients with thymoglobulin (18.9% vs 30.9%, $p = 0.03$).

3.1.2 Alemtuzumab

Alemtuzumab is a humanized IgG1 kappa monoclonal antibody, genetically engineered, specific for a surface glycoprotein of lymphocytes, 21-28 kD (CD52) present on T and B lymphocytes, natural killer cells and to a lesser extent on monocytes and macrophages. It is indicated for the treatment of patients with chronic lymphocytic leukemia who have been treated with alkylating agents and who have not achieved a complete or partial response. Alemtuzumab causes lysis of lymphocytes by binding to CD52, the antibody mediates lysis of lymphocytes by complement fixation and cell-mediated cytotoxicity, antibody-dependent. The antigen has been detected in a small percentage (<5%) of granulocytes, but not detected in erythrocytes or platelets. Alemtuzumab does not appear to damage the hematopoietic stem cells or progenitor cells. Side effects include first-dose reactions, less severe than those due to OKT3, as well as anemia, leukopenia and pancytopenia. Further long-term controlled studies are needed to establish the potential benefit in terms of efficacy and safety after kidney transplantation.

3.1.3 OKT3

OKT3 is a murine monoclonal antibody against the T3 antigen of human lymphocytes which acts as an immunosuppressant by blocking a molecule (CD3) located in the membrane of human T cells. This molecule appears to be associated with the structure of antigen recognition of T cells. It is indicated to treat acute rejection reaction in renal transplant patients. It must be only used in intravenous form and the dose of other immunosuppressive agents used concomitantly with OKT3 should be decreased to minimal levels and restarted about three days before the end of treatment with OKT3. It produces a rapid and concomitant decrease in the number of circulating T cells (CD3, CD4 and CD8) after the administration. After discontinuation of treatment, CD3 cells reappear rapidly and reach pretreatment levels within a week. OKT3 should not be used in patients with hypersensitivity to this or any other product of murine origin and in patients with fluid overload or with a history of seizures or a predisposition to allergies. After the first dose of OKT3 patients may experience fever, chills, malaise, encephalopathy, aseptic meningitis, dysnea and with minor frequency, fatal severe pulmonary edema. The most common infections were cytomegalovirus (19%) and herpes simplex (27%). To summarize, OKT3 was the first monoclonal antibody against CD3 used but adverse effect profile makes little used today.

3.1.4 Intravenous immunoglobulin (IVIG)

Intravenous immunoglobulin (IVIG) products: are derived from pooled human plasma and have been used for the treatment of primary immunodeficiency disorders, autoimmune and inflammatory disorders and recently in the treatment of sensitized patients. Mechanism of action: neutralization of circulating antibodies through idiotype-idiotype interactions to inhibit the binding of Ac antiHLA to their target cells in a dose-dependent form; inhibition of secretion of cytokines and other soluble mediators; stimulation of cytokine receptor antagonists; interaction with antigen-presenting cells by blocking T cell activation through the Fc receptor; inhibition of binding of the fractions of complement to target cells because they have a high affinity for activated complement components C3b and C4b resulting in decreased formation of the potent anaphylatoxin C5a and the C5b-C9 membrane attack complex, inhibition of proliferation of T and B cells and "down regulation" of the synthesis of antibodies and others.
Plasmapheresis, in combination with intravenous immunoglobulin, produces durable, donor-specific antibody suppression as effect of plasmapheresis is short-lived, and a rebound occurs usually when plasmapheresis is discontinued and half-life of IVIg is about 3 weeks; therefore, in most protocols its administration is repeated every 4 weeks. In adition, IVIG are useful in the treatment and prevention of posttransplant infectious complications including cytomegalovirus, parvovirus B19 and polyoma BK virus. Adverse effects are minor: headaches, fever, fatigue, myalgia, hypotension, sweating, dizziness, chills, chest tightness, wheezing. They all probably are secondary to increased levels of inflammatory cytokines and vasoactive substances and with high velocity perfusion. Anaphylactic reaction and shock can occur in patients with total or partial deficiency of IgA. In these cases, epinephrine, and diazepam for muscle spasms are indicated. Another adverse effect is renal dysfunction, because of the content of sucrose or sorbitol which can cause osmotic nephrosis in the proximal tubule. This can be avoided by reducing the osmolarity of immunoglobulin products containing sucrose, using restorative with sterile water instead of saline and lowers the concentration of Igs and sucrose to <9%. Other life-threatening side effects are thrombotic events. Very slow infusion using IVIG at a concentration of 5%, with low or no sodium content and low osmolarity, and using molecular weight heparin reduces the incidence.

3.1.5 Rituximab

It is a chimeric antibody mouse / human directed against the CD20 antigen on B lymphocytes (expressed in mature B lymphocytes and prelinfocito B). Directly inhibits B cell proliferation, induces apoptosis and reduces the production of antibodies. It has been used for the treatment of non-Hodgkin's lymphoma B cells, rheumatoid arthritis, autoimmune diseases such lupus, idiopatic thrombopenic purpure, cryoglobulinemia and organ transplantation. It produces rapid reduction of B cells with subsequent recovery at 12 months. Recent clinical data suggest that the beneficial effects of rituximab may be due to depriving T cells of antigen-presenting cell activity provided by antigen-specific B cells, thus altering effect or functions and inducing a regulatory profile. These data suggest that the beneficial effects of rituximab on autoimmune disease are more likely related to modification of dysfunctional cellular immunity rather than simply a reduction in antibody. A single dose of 375 mg/m2 in renal transplantation produces depletion of CD19 and CD20 cells for long periods in peripheral blood and tissue level.

Rituximab can be administered in a peripheral vein and, although rare, can cause anaphylactic reactions, which suggests his administration under close monitoring. The use of rituximab, which is directed against the CD20 antigen, would seem to be a logical strategy, since reduction or elimination of B cells that express CD20 and make anti-HLA antibodies, should have a beneficial effect. However, there are problems with this concept. First, anti-CD20 activity has no effect on plasma cells, which are the primary source of acute antibody production and second, rituximab has no immediate effect on circulating antibody levels. These problems might limit the benefit of rituximab if were used as the sole treatment, however, it appears that the use of rituximab in combination with other treatments, e.g., plasmapheresis which eliminates circulating antibodies, and intravenous immune globulin, that acts neutralizing circulating antibodies through idiotype-idiotype interactions to inhibit the binding of Ac antiHLA, or both, might constitute an improved approach for the management of allosensitization.

There are concerns regarding the use of rituximab, because it has been reported to induce reactivation of polyomavirus JC virus, resulting in progressive multifocal leukoencephalopathy. Optimal treatment of AMR probably requires a combination of rituximab with PP and low-dose IVIG or with high-dose IVIG (1–2 gm/kg) due to the inability of rituximab to deplete CD20-negative plasma cells that continue to produce DSA and mediate graft injury.

3.1.6 Calcineurin-inhibitors

Cyclosporine A binds to an intracellular receptor (cyclophilin) and form an active complex that binds and inhibits the phosphatase activity of calcineurin. Calcineurin participates in the transcriptional control of ribonucleic acid for the synthesis of cytokines (IL-2, IFN-γ, IL-4 and TNF-α). Thus, inhibits the proliferation of T cells preventing clonal expansion of helper and cytotoxic T cells; suppressor T cells are not affected.

Tacrolimus is a macrolide that forms a complex intracytoplasmic with a specific immunophilin (FKBP) capable of blocking the phosphatase activity of calcineurin, and thereby inhibit transcription of different genes (IL-2 and others). It inhibits the activation and proliferation of T cells and the synthesis of cytotoxic T lymphocytes. It also slows the growth and differentiation of B cells by interfering with the expression of IL-4 receptor and IL-5 synthesis. Unlike cyclosporin, tacrolimus does not interact with the receptor of transforming growth factor beta (TGF-β) type 2, which would provide more efficacy in preventing chronic graft rejection. Tacrolimus is used to prevent acute graft rejection and for treatment of corticosteroids-resistant acute rejection. It is administered in combination with steroids and derivatives of mycophenolic acid and mTOR inhibitors.

Adverse effects with greater clinical significance are nephrotoxicity, similar to that produced by cyclosporine A, carbohydrate intolerance and diabetes mellitus, neurological disorders: tremor, headache, dizziness, and severe neurological (seizures, encephalopathy, etc.) and also increased susceptibility to development of infections and malignancies. (Oppenheimer, F et al., 2010).

3.1.7 Derivatives of mycophenolic acid, mycophenolate mofetil or enteric-coated mycophenolic acid

Mycophenolate is an ethyl ester of mycophenolic acid that selectively inhibits de novo synthesis of purines, the proliferation of T and B lymphocytes, the expression of adhesion molecules and proliferation of smooth muscle cells of the vascular wall. The enteric-coated mycophenolic acid sodium salt is designed to try to improve gastrointestinal tolerance. The efficacy and safety of both drugs are similar. Its main indication is the prevention of acute graft rejection and may play an important role in preventing chronic rejection. Commonly used with cyclosporine A or tacrolimus to prevent acute graft rejection and have also been proposed for the treatment of corticosteroid-resistant acute rejection or refractory to treatment. May appear blood disorders (anemia, leukopenia and thrombocytopenia), which are not severe. Viral infections, especially citomegalolvirus are more frequent than when used in place of mTOR inhibitors. (Oppenheimer, F et al., 2010)

3.1.8 mTOR inhibitors, sirolimus and everolimus

Anti-mTOR drugs, sirolimus and everolimus are potent immunosuppressants with antiproliferative and anti-migratory capacity that act by blocking the intracellular signalling that regulates the growth and proliferation of T2 cells. mTOR inhibitors are macrolide acting in a late stage cell proliferation by inhibiting cytokine-specific signals. To act it requires form a complex with an immunophilin, but unlike the tacrolimus, do not inhibit calcineurin. Everolimus is a derivative of sirolimus with a shorter elimination half-life and greater oral bioavailability.

In primary immunosuppression, associated with cyclosporine A, have a synergistic immunosuppressive effect, and the incidence of acute rejection varies between 10 and 20%. While competing for the same tacrolimus cyclophilin, the association of mTOR inhibitor-tacrolimus is, at least, as effective as tacrolimus, mycophenolic acid association. Its main advantage is a reduction in the appearance of de novo tumours and the absence of nephrotoxicity, although significant proteinuria has been reported, especially after late use in grafts with impaired function. In cases of nephrotoxicity may be useful in association with mycophenolate, after discontinuation of calcineurin. An additional advantage is the lower rate of cytomegalovirus infection. Its side effects are: hypercholesterolemia, hypertriglyceridemia and thrombocytopenia, which are related to the administered dose. These side effects may offset their benefits in the longer term in highly renal transplant considering that are patients with high immunological risk whose should remain on full-dose triple therapy.

3.1.9 Proteosome inhibitor (bortezomib)

Bortezomib, a proteasome inhibitor approved for the treatment of multiple myeloma, induces plasma cell apoptosis. Its role in desensitization protocols and treatment of humoral rejection may offer promise results in transplant recipients. The pharmacokinetics of bortezomib can be characterized by rapid and wide distribution, a prolonged elimination half life, and hepatic cytochrome P-450 (CYP) isoenzyme metabolism. Side effects more frequent are a low-grade gastrointestinal side effect, mild to moderate anemia, neutropenia, and thrombocytopenia, and primarily mild cases of peripheral neuropathy. Despite the mild decrease in PRA levels, bortezomib therapy led to more than 50% decrease in the levels of anti-HLA antibodies triggering C4d deposition on single antigen Luminex beads as measured in MFI with single-antigen bead flow cytometry.

Results in desensitization of patients with this agent before transplantation are less consistent. Wahrmann et al. could not observe a significant decrease of circulating HLA antibodies in two highly sensitized dialysis patients who were treated with two cycles of bortezomib, indicating that this agent is not able to eliminate long-lived plasma cells. Furthermore, in vitro studies indicate that contact with alloantigen enhances the susceptibility of plasma cells to proteasome inhibition-mediated apoptosis, which might also serve as an explanation for the observed differences in the effectivity of bortezomib in the pre- and posttransplant phases.

In the study by Walsh et al., two patients undergoing acute AMR with high DSA and positive C4d staining on biopsy two weeks after kidney transplantation were treated with a multiday regimen consisting of plasmapheresis, methylprednisolone and bortezomib along with a single dose of rituximab. By nearly 14 days after treatment, DSA levels had dropped significantly as well as repeat biopsy showed faint peritubular capillary C4d labeling and decreased glomerular C4d deposition.

Trivedi et al. (Trivedi et al., 2009, 2010) reported thirteen living donor renal transplant patients treated with bortezomib one to two cycles and plasmapheresis to remove HLA antibodies posttransplant. All patients treated with bortezomib/plasmapheresis resulted in a primary DSA reduction of more than 50% measured by means of single antigen bead on Luminex. In 10 of 13 patients, complete DSA removal, below than 1000 mean fluorescent intensity occurred. At 1 year posttreatment, antibody intensity remains significantly depressed in the group as a whole, despite tetanus toxoid and measles IgG levels remained unchanged and above the level of protection. These data suggest that proteasome inhibitors plus plasmapheresis results in prolonged reduction of HLA antibodies while leaving protective immunity intact. Some patients had reappearance of anti-HLA antibodies despite initial effective reduction, and the authors suggested that certain patients may need more than one cycle of treatment to decrease DSA levels.

3.1.10 Eculizumab (anti-C5, anticomplement monoclonal antibody)

The monoclonal antibody eculizumab, which binds to complement factor C5 and prevents formation of the membrane attack complex C5b-9, is currently in clinical use for the treatment of paroxysmal nocturnal hemoglobinuria and being tested for the treatment of atypical hemolytic uremic syndrome. Its use combined with plasmapheresis or IVIg decrease C5b-C9 complex deposition in the kidney. It is very important to be immunized against meningitis (Neisseria meningitidis) to all patients two weeks before the administration of eculizumab as due to its mechanism of action, the use of this drug increases the patient's sensitivity to meningococcal infection.

Eculizumab selectively inhibits the human complement protein C5, preventing its division into C5a and C5b, thus annulling the formation of C5b-9 terminal complement, which is behind the formation of transmembrane channels that cause cell lysis. The adverse reactions most frequently reported are headache, nasopharyngitis, nausea, pyrexia, myalgia, fatigue and herpes simplex, observed in at least 5 of every 100 patients. The most serious side effect was meningococcal septicemia.

Complement activation plays a critical role in mediating AMR after kidney transplantation. As eculizumab has the ability to inhibit C5b-C9 MAC and C5a generation, it should act as a strong accommodation promoter and prevent AMR. Fortunately, recent data presented by Stegall et al. (Stegall et al.,2010, as cited in Jordan, S, 2010) supports this contention. These investigators treated ten patients who underwent desensitization with plasmapheresis + IVIG with eculizumab after transplantation. After nearly 12 months of follow-up for all patients, none developed AMR. Several protocol biopsies showed C4d deposits but no evidence of AMR. This finding is suggestive of incomplete complement activation, which is permissive for accommodation. This author says, that a combination of high-dose IVIG with eculizumab maybe act to modify elements of cellular immunity, humoral immunity, and complement effectors. Confirmation of these ideas awaits clinical trials.

3.1.11 Receptor antagonists interleukin-2 (I1-2R): Basiliximab

This anti-CD25 monoclonal antibody, one chimeric (basiliximab) are widely used in renal transplantation patients with low-moderate immunological risk during the induction phase. Usually, induction therapy with basiliximab is used in combination with calcineurin-inhibitors, derivatives of mycophenolic acid and prednisone This antibody is directed against a chain of IL-2 receptor, whose expression on the cell surface requires activation of the T cell. Basiliximab is used in two doses of 20 mg each, for intravenous injection at time of transplantation and on the fourth day after transplantation, respectively. The first dose should be administered before reperfusion of the organ. Hypersensitivity reactions, including anaphylaxis, have been reported in isolation with the use of these antibodies, which, moreover, are considered safe and an adverse event profile similar to those reported with placebo.

3.1.12 Therapeutic apheresis

Plasmapheresis is a plasma exchange procedure to removal from blood plasma molecules with specific antigen recognition like antibodies or autoantibodies, molecules that alter the physical properties of plasma, immune complexes, toxic molecules and others. The therapeutic goal of plasma is to reduce circulating levels of these molecules to mitigate the underlying disease process. The vast majority of disorders successfully treated by plasmapheresis treatment involving the removal of IgG, as it has a longer half life and low rate of synthesis. Other factors removed as complement, coagulation proteins or inflammatory mediators contribute to a lesser extent the therapeutic benefit of plasmapheresis by its short half-life and high rate of synthesis.

Therapeutic plasma exchange has been used successfully in the treatment of many hematological, neurological, renal, and metabolic disorders, rheumatic and acute humoral rejection. This last is a condition that requires early diagnosis and intervention. Many groups have developed protocols for immunosuppression and immunomodulation that often include therapeutic plasma exchange.

Plasmapheresis therapy is successfully used in the treatment or prevention of rejection in solid organ transplantation. Although the cellular immune response is responsible for mediating most of the rejections of allografts, acute humoral rejection of the transplanted organ refers to a severe dysfunction associated with the presence of antibodies directed against the donor organ. This type of rejection is generally resistant to immunosuppressive and immunomodulatory therapies, occurs more frequently in patients with preexisting antibodies to the ABO system antigens or HLA expressed by the graft and is associated with a poor prognosis for graft survival. Numerous studies showed evidence of HLA antibodies decreased with plasmapheresis; in addition, patients with refractory acute rejection, the use of plasma exchange schemes and IVIG results in a better renal graft survival. The number of plasmapheresis sessions is greater the higher the antibody titer donor-specific. In addition, as soon as plasmapheresis stops, there is a rebound in the title antibody. Therefore, plasmapheresis is considered an additional technical assistance to other therapeutic procedures, particularly treatment with IVIG.

Extracorporeal immunoadsorption is other technique for the elimination of pathogenic antibodies and circulating immune complexes. Immunoadsorption is capable to eliminate huge amounts of immunoglobulins from the patient's circulation with a minimum of side effects (associated with the substitution of fresh frozen plasma or albumin or removal of other plasmatic factors to above 50%).

Most evidences about immunoadsorption are based on uncontrolled case series and individual observations. Indications for extracorporeal immunoadsorption are presently limited to HLA-pre-sensitised kidney recipients, rapidly progressive glomerulonephritis, haemolytic uraemic syndrome, life-threatening autoimmune diseases among others. Immunoadsorption devices can be subdivided into non-selective, semi-selective and highly selective adsorbers. In patients with acute vascular rejection after renal transplantation, immunoadsorption can be used to remove anti-HLA antibodies in combination with conventional anti-rejection therapy. It seems feasible to apply immunoadsorption instead of plasmapheresis for acute, vascular rejection although a controlled trial should demonstrate whether one or the other is more effective and associated with less adverse effects.

Immunoadsorption could also be successfully used for the reduction of anti-HLA antibody titre before transplantation for obtaining a negative cross match in highly sensitised patients. A median of plasma processed during the pre-transplant immunoadsorption session could be high and may not be achieved with the use of plasmapheresis due to a high likelihood of adverse reactions attributable to the administration of fresh frozen plasma or albumin. By contrast to plasmapheresis, immunoadsorption allows the treatment of higher plasma volumes with a greater reduction of immunoglobulins (immunoadsorption is capable of removing >85% of IgG during one session). In the future, immunoadsorption may replace plasmapheresis in the treatment of some but not all diseases, however, the high costs associated with immunoadsorption therapy must be taken into account. (Schwenger,& Morath,C, 2010).

3.1.13 Others agents in Phase I, II or III clinical trials

ISA247 (voclosporine), a cyclosporine analogue, has the advantage of inducing less postransplantation diabetes and reduced nephrotoxicity (Phase III study).

CP-690550, a specific inhibitor of the JAK3 protein kinase, has an effect comparable to tacrolimus on the acute rejection rate and kidney function. Orally is administered with basiliximab, mycophenolate and steroids. Initial results suggest that co-administration with mycophenolate involves excessive immunosuppression, with increased BK virus infection and cytomegalovirus.

Belatacept, is a humanized antibody that blocks the costimulatory signal by binding to CD80 and CD86 antigen presenting cells, thereby promoting anergy and apoptosis of T cells. Its efficacy is similar to that of cyclosporin A, but with a more favorable toxicity profile. The

need for intravenous injection and a slight increase in the development of lymphoproliferative disease in liver transplantation recipients with negative serology to Epstein-Barr virus could partially limit its use (Multiple Phase II and III trials).
Alefacept and Efaluzimab are humanized antibodies that inhibit T-cell adhesion and are in Phase I and II clinical trials.

3.2 Clinical evidences on desensitization therapy strategies in high immunological risk patients

In this section, we review the most relevant publications related to therapies in high immunologic risk patients, making emphasis on aspects such as incidence of acute rejection, long-term allograft survival and function, mortality and others. Highly sensitized transplant recipients, regardless of the desensitization protocol used, are at increased risk for AMR. Both desensitization and AMR are managed with the similar therapeutic arsenal; however protocols are center-specific and there are no consensus guidelines. The two desensitization protocols more frequently used are high-dose IVIG or low-dose IVIG with either plasmapheresis or immunoadsorption. Additionally, some transplant centers may add intravenous steroids, rabbit antithymocyte globulin, or rituximab. For variant of AMR where over 30% of infiltrating cells are mature plasma cells, which do not express CD20, several transplant centers have utilized bortezomib instead of rituximab.
Yuan XP et al (Yuan XP et al., 2010) evaluated the efficacy of plasmapheresis plus low-dose intravenous immunoglobulin in highly sensitized patients waiting for a deceased-donor renal transplant. In 25 patients (group 1), a positive T- and/or B-cell cytotoxicity crossmatch was rendered negative by plasmapheresis plus low-dose intravenous immunoglobulin treatment. During the same time, 32 highly sensitized patients (group 2), without desensitization, had a negative crossmatch and received deceased-donor renal transplants. Group 1 showed a numerically higher rate of acute rejection and antibody-mediated rejection, but the difference was not statistically significant. No differences in Kaplan-Meier graft survival were found between group 1 and group 2 after long-term follow-up. They conclude that desensitization with plasmapheresis, plus low-dose intravenous immunoglobulin enables successful deceased-donor renal transplant in highly sensitized patients with a positive crossmatch and achieve results similar to highly sensitized patients with negative crossmatch. Moreover, antibody-mediated rejection occurred predominantly in recipients with donor-specific antibodies of high titers. They used anti-thymocyte globulin for induction in both groups.
Loupy A, (Loupy A et al., 2010), combined posttransplant prophylactic intravenous immunoglobulin, rituximab and plasmapheresis in kidney recipients with preformed donor-specific antibodies. All patients had a concomitant evaluation of glomerular filtration rate, protocol biopsies, and DSA mean intensity of fluorescence (MFI) at 3 month and 1 year posttransplant. The first strategy combined posttransplant quadritherapy and intravenous immunoglobulin (group 1, n=36) and the second added to the above protocol rituximab and plasmapheresis (group 2, n=18). Peak and day-0 class-I or II DSA max-MFI were similar in both groups. The rate of acute antibody-mediated rejection (AMR) was similar in both groups (about 19.6% vs. 16.6%, respectively). At 1 year posttransplant, group 2 was characterized significantly by lower score microcirculation inflammation lesions, a lower rate of transplant glomerulopathy and a lower rate of chronic AMR. The decline in DSA-MFI from day 0 to 1 year was about 44% in group 1 compared with 80% in group 2 and the 1-year glomerular filtration rate was about 43 vs. 54 ml/min/1.73 m2, respectively. The

study raises the possibility that a more prophylactic immunosuppressive strategy at day 0 combining intravenous immunoglobulin/anti-CD20/plasmapheresis in high-risk population, is associated with significant differences in long-term function and chronic AMR rate, although similar rates of early acute clinical humoral rejection may be observed.

Vo A, et al (Vo AA et al., 2010, 2008) used high-dose intravenous immune globulin (2 g/kg x2 doses) and rituximab (2 doses) for desensitization of highly HLA-sensitized patients awaiting kidney transplantation. All patients received intravenous ganciclovir while staying at the hospital and valganciclovir for 6 months as outpatients, with dose adjustments for renal function. Both fungal and bacterial infection prophylaxis, including Pneumocystis carinii, was performed in all patients according to standard clinical practice. From July 2006 to February 2009, seventy-six treated patients (31 living donors, 45 deceased donors) were transplanted. For living donors (LD) and deceased donors (DD) recipients, significant reductions were seen in T-cell flow cytometry crossmatch from pretreatment to time of transplant. Patients received their kidney transplants when the complement-dependent cytotoxicity (CDC) T-cell crossmatch was negative at a 1:2 dilution of serum or the mean flow-channel shift in the T-cell flow-cytometric crossmatch was below 250. Time on wait list for DD recipients was reduced from a mean of 95 to 4.2 months after treatment; 37% experienced acute rejection but patient and graft survival up to 24 months was 95% and 84%, respectively. The mean serum creatinine, at 12 and 24 months were about 1.5 and 1.3 mg/dl, respectively. They concluded that IVIG and rituximab seems to offer significant benefits in reduction of anti-HLA antibodies allowing improved rates of transplantation for highly sensitized patients, especially those awaiting DD, with acceptable antibody-mediated rejection and survival rates at 24 months. All patients had reduced numbers of CD19+ cells after rituximab infusion. No patients developed neurologic symptoms suggestive of progressive multifocal leukoencephalopathy or required further hospitalization, and the rate of urinary tract infection was not greater than that among transplant recipients who were not highly sensitized. No other important infectious complications were noted.

Although 13 of 16 patients who received a kidney transplant had a persisting positive crossmatch at the time of transplantation (below the threshold given above), no hyperacute rejection episodes were noted. The same group developed an in vitro test system to predict whether intravenous immune globulin might reduce PRA or crossmatch positivity in individual patients. For patients who did not respond well in this test system or who had high antibody titers before desensitization, intravenous immune globulin and rituximab were considered not to be sufficient alone, and the patients received in addition plasmapheresis.

Vo AA, Jordan SC, et al (Vo AA; Jordan, SC. et al., 2008, 2009), analyzed the use of subcutaneous alemtuzumab induction therapy with intravenous immune globulin and rituximab in an uncontrolled study in 54 highly HLA-sensitized patients from 3/05 to 4/07. No patient developed acute injection-related reactions after alemtuzumab, however, bone marrow suppression was occasionally seen requiring reduction or elimination of mycophenolate mofetil approximately 1-2 months posttransplant. Patient and graft survival at 12 month was 98%/96%, respectively. Acute rejection episodes occurred in 35% with 20% being C4d+ acute rejection. Mean serum creatinine at 12 month was about 1.4 mg/dl. Infections occurred in eight patients (five with polyoma BK viremia, one CMV/PBK and two with CMV viremia). They concluded that induction therapy with alemtuzumab appears feasible and indeed promising, but awaits more definitive study.

Scemla A et al (Scemla A et al., 2010), revised the incidence of infectious complications in 38 highly sensitized renal transplant recipients treated by rituximab. They compared this population with 26 highly sensitized renal transplant recipients who received comparable

treatment but without rituximab. Mean posttransplant follow-up was 25.5±11.5 and 34.6±16.4 months in the rituximab and control groups, respectively. A total of 84 severe infectious episodes occurred in 39 patients (rituximab 55.3% vs. controls 69.2%, ns). Two patients died in each group. Three of these four deaths were related to infectious complications. Specifically, rituximab was not associated with an increased risk of infection.
Kamar N et al (Kamar N et al., 2010), revised the occurrence of infectious disease and its outcome after rituximab therapy (375 mg/m^2, 2-8 courses) in 77 kidney-transplant patients between April 2004 and August 2008. Their results were compared with a control group (n=902) who had received no rituximab. After a median follow-up of 16.5 months for rituximab patients and 60.9 months for control patients, the incidence of infectious disease was 45.45% and 53.9% (ns), respectively. The incidence of bacterial infection was similar between the two groups, whereas the viral-infection rate was significantly lower, and the rate of fungal infection was significantly higher in the rituximab group. Nine out of 77 patients died after rituximab therapy, of which seven deaths were related to an infectious disease, compared to 1.55% in the controls (p=0.0007). They concluded that in the whole population, the independent predictive factors for infection-induced death were the combined use of rituximab and antithymocyte-globulin given for induction or anti-rejection therapy, recipient age, and bacterial and fungal infections.
Flechner SM et al (Flechner SM et al., 2010), revised the role of proteasome inhibition with bortezomib in the treatment of antibody-mediated rejection in 20 patients. AMR was diagnosed about 19.8 months posttransplant. De novo class I DSA was detected in 55% and class II DSA in 90% recipients. Patients received intravenous corticosteroids followed by a 2-week cycle on days 1, 4, 8 and 11 of plasmapheresis and 1.3 mg/m^2 bortezomib; then 0.5 mg/kg intravenous immunoglobulin four times. Their results were a significantly decrement in peak-nadir dominant DSA. Patient survival was 100%, and graft survival 85% with a mean follow-up of 9.8 months. The treatment was generally well tolerated but caused fatigue, gastrointestinal complaints, fluid retention, and thrombocytopenia in a number of patients. The last follow-up estimated glomerular filtration rate was 41.9±16.8 ml/min, however, only 25% returned to their baseline renal function. They concluded that the bortezomib-containing regimen demonstrated activity in AMR but seems to be most effective before the onset of significant renal dysfunction or proteinuria and the use of bortezomib to treat AMR should be evaluated in controlled trials using dosing strategies that include longer courses or retreatment schedules.
Something similar was found by Raghavan R et al (Raghavan R et al, 2010), this author revised the use of bortezomib in kidney transplantation and said that the use of this biological agent in the field of transplantation may seem to show promise in the realm of transplant recipients desensitization and treatment of AMR, and will be defined better as more clinical data and trials become available.
Lonze BE et al (Lonze BE et al., 2010) review a 43-year-old patient with end-stage renal disease and 100% panel reactive antibody who was treated with desensitization protocol using two cycles of bortezomib undertaken after anti-CD20 and intravenous inmunoglobulins. A flow-positive, cytotoxic-negative cross-match live-donor kidney at the end of an eight-way multi-institution domino chain became available. The patient received three pretransplant plasmapheresis treatments. Intraoperatively, the superior mesenteric vein was the only identifiable patent target for venous drainage. Eculizumab was administered postoperatively in the setting of antibody-mediated rejection and an inability to perform additional plasmapheresis. Creatinine remains normal at 6 months

posttransplant and flow cross-match remained negative. In this report, they described the combined use of new agents (bortezomib and eculizumab) and modalities (nontraditional vascular access, splanchnic drainage of graft and domino paired donation) in a patient who would have died without transplantation.

Wahrmann M et al, (Wahrmann M et al., 2010), analized two sensitized hemodialysis patients that were selected to receive two subsequent bortezomib cycles (1.3 mg/m^2 on days 1, 4, 8, and 11). Dexamethasone was added to the second cycle to enhance treatment efficiency. During a half-year follow-up period, cytotoxic panel reactive antibody decreased from 87% to 80% (patient 1) and 37% to 13% (patient 2). Patient 1 showed a 40% reduction in binding intensities of identified Luminex HLA single antigen reactivities and, in parallel, slight reductions in ABO blood group antibody and total immunoglobulin levels. In patient 2, bortezomib did not affect circulating antibody levels in a meaningful way. Both patients showed a more than 50% reduction in the levels of anti-HLA antibody-triggered C4d deposition to Luminex beads. They concluded that, without additional immunosuppressive measures, bortezomib has modest effects on circulating antibodies against HLA or blood group antigens. Hovewer, the reduced levels of antibody-triggered complement fixation, imply potential clinical relevance of proteasome inhibition for recipient desensitization.

Sberro-Soussan R (Sberro-Soussan R, et al., 2010), evaluated the in vivo efficacy of one cycle of bortezomib (1.3 mg/m^2 x 4 doses), used as the sole desensitization therapy, in four renal transplant recipients experiencing subacute antibody-mediated rejection with persisting DSA (>2000 Mean Fluorescence Intensity, MFI). Bortezomib treatment did not significantly decrease DSA MFI within the 150-day posttreatment period in any patient. In addition, antivirus (HBV, VZV and HSV) antibody levels remained stable following treatment suggesting a lack of efficacy on long-lived plasma cells. They concluded that one cycle of bortezomib alone does not decrease DSA levels in sensitized kidney transplant recipients in the time period studied and need to evaluate this new desensitization agent properly in prospective, randomized and well-controlled studies.

Locke JE et al, (Locke JE et al., 2009) present a single case in which eculizumab was used combined with plasmapheresis e inmunoglobulins to salvage a kidney undergoing severe AMR. They showed a marked decrease in C5b-C9 (MAC) complex deposition in the kidney after the administration of eculizumab.

Stegall et al. recently reported on their results obtained in a first series of patients in whom the use of eculizumab was tested for the prevention of AMR in crossmatch-positive kidney transplantation. Sixteen crossmatch-positive kidney transplantations realized under the usage of eculizumab were compared to a historical control group of 51 transplantations where desensitization had been performed without eculizumab. Acute humoral rejection was found in only 6% of patients desensitized with eculizumab as compared to a 40% rate in the historical control group. However, 4 of 16 patients in the eculizumab group with persistent levels of high DSA after transplantation showed signs of chronic allograft injury, including endothelial cell activation and transplant glomerulopathy (Stegall,2010, as cited in C. Siisal & Morath C, 2011).

Thielke et al. reported that a negative crossmatch was successfully achieved in 51 of 57 positive-crossmatch patients treated with antithymocyte and anti-CD20 antibody induction therapy in addition to plasma exchange and low-dose intravenous immunoglobulin. The rate of allograft survival was 93% at 1 year and 81% at 2 years.

Glotz et al (Glotz et al., 2002) reported 15 patients with either a panel reactive antibody (PRA) of >50 percent or with a positive crossmatch to their potential living donor who were given 2 g/kg of IVIG monthly for three months. Thirteen of the 15 showed evidence of desensitization (reduction of PRA by at least 50 percent or a repeat negative crossmatch to the living donor) and underwent renal transplantation. The mean decrease in PRA for recipients was 80 percent and a post-IVIG administration NIH cytotoxicity crossmatch was negative prior to transplantation. The IVIG was repeated at the same dose on post-transplant day zero and one. Thymoglobulin was used for induction and maintenance immunosuppression consisted of mycophenolate, corticosteroids and tacrolimus. The IVIG was again repeated at post-transplant day 20 or 21 and 40 or 41. One graft was lost secondary to thrombosis and one graft was lost secondary to rejection. No other episodes of rejection were reported in the remaining allografts during follow-up of over one year.

Kaposztas et al. reported 2-year outcomes in their recent retrospective study looking at 54 patients treated for AMR. Group A had 26 patients who underwent treatment with plasmapheresis and rituximab, and group B had 28 patients who received plasmapheresis without rituximab. Patients who had low serum IgG levels also received IVIG. Two-year graft survival was significantly better in the group that received rituximab (90% vs 60%), with the difference attributed to rituximab. A trend toward improved graft survival was also seen in those who received IVIG. This retrospective study has one of the largest cohorts reported to date and supports the use of rituximab for treating AMR, with good short-term allograft survival; however, many patient variables were not consistent between the groups (Kaposztas et al, 2009, as cited in Jordan, S, 2010).

Gloor et al, (Gloor et al., 2003) described 14 patients with a positive cytotoxicity crossmatch to a potential living donor. Patients underwent plasmapheresis on days four, three, and one pretransplant, on the day of transplantation, and on day one and three post-transplantation. Intravenous immunoglobulin 100 mg/kg was administered after each plasmapheresis session. Rituximab at a dose of 375 mg/m^2 was given on post-transplant day four. Splenectomy was performed at the time of transplantation in those with an intact spleen (two had previously been splenectomized). Thymoglobulin was used for induction and tacrolimus, mycophenolate and corticosteroids were used for maintenance therapy. Patient survival at a mean follow-up of 15 months was 86 percent. Histologic evidence of AMR occurred in 43 percent. The risk of AMR was related to the baseline anti-HLA antibody titer. All four subclinical episodes responded to treatment and follow-up protocol biopsies showed no histologic evidence of rejection. Both episodes of rejection defined as clinically significant AMR demonstrated evidence of chronic allograft nephropathy on subsequent biopsies.

Stegall et al (Stegall et al, 2006, as cited in C. Siisal & Morath C, 2011) deigned one study to compare high dose IVIG (13 patients) with plasmapheresis/low dose IVIG protocols (32 patients) in renal transplant recipients with high DSA levels. Plasmapheresis plus low dose intravenous inmunoglobulins (IVIG) received also anti-CD20 antibody (32 patients), and 19 of the 32 patients in this group also underwent splenectomy; post-transplant plasmapheresis and low dose IVIG were continued on post-surgery days one to three for a total of two to three sessions. High single dose IVIG (13 patients), which is the high dose IVIG group. Plasmapheresis plus low dose IVIG plus anti-CD20 antibody plus pretransplant Thymoglobulin combined with post-transplant DSA monitoring (16 patients), was the plasmapheresis/monitoring group. Achieving a negative crossmatch was significantly more likely with both plasmapheresis protocols versus high dose IVIG (84, 88, and 38 percent respectively). Significantly lower humoral rejection rates were also reported with the plasmapheresis protocols (37, 29, and 80 percent, respectively), although none of the patients in the high single dose IVIG group received rituximab or post-transplant administration of

IVIG. Patients with low baseline antibody titers responding to high dose IVIG may do equally as well with further optimization of therapy. However, whether or not the administration of rituximab or the routine post-transplant administration of IVIG would be of benefit in reducing the incidence of acute rejection in a high dose IVIG protocol is unclear at this time as this study not included randomization and only participated a low numbers of patients.

4. Remarks and conclusions

The main goal of monitoring circulating antibodies is to measure PRA and identify specific antibodies in order to evaluate the patient's immunological risk and interpret a crossmatch. The introduction of HLA antibody characterization based on interactions between recipient serum and purified HLA antigens bound to solid-phase substrates has improved detection and quantification of donor-specific antibodies (DSAs).

Currently, few kidney transplant options exist for hypersensitive patients on the waiting list if they do not undergo previously to desensitising treatments or strong induction therapy. In this respect, high doses of intravenous immunoglobulins may reduce the level of circulating antibodies, but, many patients only respond partially, and the efficacy varies among patients. Plasmapheresis can decrease circulating antibodies, but there is normally a significant increase in their titre levels once the sessions have been completed. Therefore, this technique is now considered a complement to the use of immunoglobulins for decreasing antibody levels. Likewise, rituximab has also been shown to have a beneficial effect when combined with immunoglobulins and plasmapheresis to reduce anti-HLA antibodies rate and to treat antibody-mediated rejection. On the other hand, newer interventions aimed at the prevention of DSA-mediated allograft injury using complement blockade, or the inhibition of DSA synthesis using proteasome inhibitor-mediated plasma cell depletion are promising.

In any case, the best therapeutic strategy may be of combining these drugs, particularly when there is early detection of acute antibody-mediated rejection through histological or serological techniques. Whether long-term beneficial outcomes are achived with these drugs without life-threatening side-effects, remains to be elucidate.

According to our previous results, we tentatively propose the following desensitization and induction protocol:

Recipients with positive cytotoxicity crossmatch or retransplantation recipients with positive cytometry crossmatch and negative cytotoxicity crossmatch are potential candidates for pre-transplant desensitisation. For first transplant recipients with positive cytometry crossmatch but with negative cytotoxicity crossmatch, desensitisation may not be necessary. For patients who are only positive for virtual lymphocyte crosssmatch, with negative cytotoxicity and cytometry crossmatches, there are currently insufficient data that support the appropriateness of desensitisation. Patients on the waiting list more than 12 months and at least three studies quarterly permanently with PRA> 50-75% polyspecific, multiple previous positive crossmatch, and multiple HLA-antigens positive reactivity that makes transplantation highly unlikely, if they have absence of IgA deficiency and antibodies antiIgA, they could receive high dose of immunoglobulins, plus plasmapheresis and one or two doses of rituximab.

Requirements for performing kidney transplantation in these patients would be:

a. Pre-transplant negative cytotoxicity crossmatch, and
b. Negative virtual crossmatch test prior to the kidney transplant, i.e., abscense of all class I or II HLA antigens in the donor that have produced an alloresponse in the recipient at any time.

c. Induction therapy with thymoglobulin tacrolimus, mycophenolate, methylprednisolone.
d. Desensitisation treatment would consist in rituximab, various plasmapheresis sessions with IV immunoglobulin infusion following each session.
e. Monitorization of CD19+/CD20+ lymphocyte populations and checking for any appearance of opportunistic infections using a PCR assay for CMV, Epstein-Barr viral serology, B-19 parvovirus and polyomavirus BK are necessary.
f. Cytomegalovirus infection prophylaxis with gancyclovir/valgancyclovir 6 months, pneumocistis jirovecii prophylaxis with trimethoprim sulfamethoxazole and fungal infection prophylaxis with nystatin or oral fluconazole must be considered.
g. Monitoring PRA title every 15 days the first 3 months and then monthly during first year and before or after any deterioration of renal function. A rising DSA titter may suggests the need for intensification of therapy with potential modification of maintenance immunosuppression or initiating intensive therapy using IVIG and/or plasmapheresis.
h. Monitoring of neurological symptoms: progressive multifocal leukoencephalopathy, reactivation of polyoma JC virus also is very important.
i. In the case of immunoligal-mediated renal dysfunction, it is important perform a graft biopsy and C4d staining. Treatment for apparent AMR is essentially by combining metilprednisolone, plasmapheresis (or immunoadsorption) and IVIG, with a duration that will be dependent upon an improvement in renal function, decrease in the titter of DSA or improvement of biopsy findings. If there is no good response to treatment, individual assess whether repeated rescue therapies, such as rituximab or eculizumab. In the case of appearance of plasma cells in the renal graft biopsy, it should be assessed individually using bortezomib as salvage therapy. Subclinical rejection (as defined by positive C4d staining associated with histologic evidence of antibody mediated rejection) on protocol biopsies may be associated with future AMR or subsequent evidence of chronic allograft injury. Whether or not treatment of subclinical rejection in this setting has a benefit on long-term graft survival is unknown, however, given the high risk of acute rejection, most physicians would favor restarting plasmapheresis/IVIG or other treatment.
j. An additional critical issue is antibody development against allogeneic antigen systems on graft other than HLA that are not necessarily detected in routine antibody testing, like anti-major histocompatibility complex class I related A (anti-MICA), antiendothelial antibodies, antibody binding to angiotensin type-1 receptor and others. These antibodies have found a strong association with antibody-mediated rejection in recipients whose sera did not contain antibody to donor HLA, indicating that antibodies directed against non-HLA antigens also have a certain impact. These issues are not reasons for this chapter and may be addressed in future. More studies are required in this field to determine the frequency and magnitude of damage caused by non-HLA immunity.

5. References

Brennan,C.; Daller, JA.; Lake, KD.; Cibrik, D. & Del Castillo, D. (2006). Thymoglobulin Induction Study Group. Rabbit antithymocyte globulin versus basiliximab in renal transplantation. *N Engl J Med* Vol.355 No.9, (Nov 2010), pp. 1967-1977, ISSN 0028-4793

Ercilla, MG. & Martorell, J. (2010). Immunologic study of the donor-receptor couple. *Nefrologia,* Vol.30, suppl. 30, (Nov 2010), pp. 60-70, ISSN 2013-7575.

Everly, MJ.; Terasaki, PI.; Hopfield, J.; Trivedi, HL & Kaneku, H. (2010). Protective immunity remains intact after antibody removal by means of proteasome inhibition. *Transplantation,* Vol.90, No. 12, (Dec 2010), pp. 1493-1498, ISSN 1534-0608.

Flechner, SM.; Fatica, R.; Askar, M.; Stephany, BR.; Poggio, E.; Koo, A.; Banning, S.; Chiesa-Vottero, A. & Srinivas, T. (2010). The role of proteasome inhibition with bortezomib in the treatment of antibody-mediated rejection after kidney-only or kidney-combined organ transplantation. *Transplantation,* Vol 27. No 12, (Dec 2010), pp. 1486-1492, ISSN.

Gaber, AO.; Knight, RJ.; Patel, S. & Gaber, LW. (2010). A review of the evidence for use of thymoglobulin induction in renal transplantation. *Transplant Proc,* Vol.42, No. 5, (Jun 2010), pp. 1395-1400, ISSN 0041-1345

Gloor, JM.; DeGoey, SR.; Pineda, AA.; Moore, SB.; Prieto, M.; Nyberg, SL.; Larson, TS.; Griffin, MD.; Textor, SC.; Velosa, JA.; Schwab, TR.; Fix, LA. & Stegall, MD. Overcoming a positive crossmatch in living-donor kidney transplantation. *Am J Transplant,* Vol 3. No 8, (Aug 2003), pp. 1017-1023, ISSN 1600-6143.

Gloor, J. & Stegall, M. (2010). Sensitized renal transplant recipients: current protocols and future directions. *Nat. Rev. Nephrol,* Vol 6. (March 2010), pp. 297-306, ISSN 1759-5061,1759-507X.

Glotz, D.; Antoine, C.; Julia, P.; Suberbielle-Boissel, C.; Boudjeltia, S.; Fraoui, R.; Hacen, C.; Duboust, A. & Bariety J. (2002). Desensitization and subsequent kidney transplantation of patients using intravenous immunoglobulins (IVIg). *Am J Transplant,* Vol 2. No 8, (Sep 2002), pp. 758-760, ISSN 1600-6143.

Jordan, SC.; Peng, A. &Vo, AA. (2009). Therapeutic strategies in management of the highly HLA-sensitized and ABO-incompatible transplant recipients. *Contrib Nephrol,* Vol 162. (2009), pp. 13-26, ISSN 0302-5144 .

Jordan S, Reinsmoen, N,; Peng,A.; Lai, C.; Cao, K.; Villicana, R.; Toyoda,M.; Kahwaji, J & Ashley A. (2010). Advances in diagnosing and managing antibody-mediated rejection. *Pediatr Nephrol,* Vol.25, No.10, (Oct 2010), pp. 2035-2048, ISSN 0931-041X

Jordan, SC.; Toyoda, M.; Kahwaji, J. &Vo, AA. (2011). Clinical aspects of intravenous immunoglobulin use in solid organ transplant recipients. *Am J Transplant,* Vol 11. No 2, (Feb 2011), pp. 196-202, ISSN 1600-6143.

Kamar, N.; Milioto, O.; Puissant-Lubrano, B.; Esposito, L.; Pierre, MC.; Mohamed, AO.; Lavayssière, L.; Cointault, O.; Ribes, D.; Cardeau, I.; Nogier, MB.; Durand, D.; Abbal, M.; Blancher, A. & Rostaing, L. (2010). Incidence and predictive factors for infectious disease after rituximab therapy in kidney-transplant patients. *Am J Transplant,* Vol 10. No 1, (Jan 2010), pp. 89-98, ISSN 1600-6143.

Klein,C, Brennan,D (Sep2010). HLA and ABO sensitization and desensitization in renal transplantation, In: *Up to Date,* 9.2010, Avalaible from http://learn.uptodate.com/index.

Locke, JE.; Magro, CM.; Singer, AL.; Segev, DL.; Haas, M.; Hillel, AT.; King, KE.; Kraus, E.; Lees, LM.; Melancon, JK.; Stewart, ZA.; Warren, DS.; Zachary, AA. & Montgomery, RA. (2009). The use of antibody to complement protein C5 for salvage treatment of severe antibody-mediated rejection. *Am J Transplant,* Vol 9. No 1, (Jan 2009), pp. 231-235, ISSN 1600-6143.

Lonze, BE.; Dagher, NN.; Simpkins, CE.; Locke, JE.; Singer, AL.; Segev, DL.; Zachary, AA. & Montgomery, RA. (2010). Eculizumab, bortezomib and kidney paired donation facilitate transplantation of a highly sensitized patient without vascular access. *Am J Transplant,* Vol 10. No 9, (Sep 2010), pp. 2154-2160, ISSN 1600-6143.

Loupy, A.; Suberbielle-Boissel, C.; Zuber, J.; Anglicheau, D.; Timsit, MO.; Martinez, F.; Thervet, E.; Bruneval, P.; Charron, D.; Hill, GS,; Nochy, D, & Legendre, C. (2010). Combined posttransplant prophylactic IVIg/anti-CD 20/plasmapheresis in kidney recipients with preformed donor-specific antibodies: a pilot study. *Transplantation,* Vol. 15, No. 89, (Jun 2010), pp.1403-1410, ISSN 1534-0608

Nocera, A. (2009). Desensitization protocols in immunized living donor kidney transplant recipients. *G Ital Nefrol* , Vol. 26, No. 4,(Jul-Aug 2009), pp. 499-515, ISSN.Oppenheimer, F.; Pascual, J. & Pallardo.L. (2010). Inmunosuppression in renal transplant, In: *Nefrología al día,* V. Lorenzo Sellares, J.M. López Gómez, ALM, de Francisco Hernandez & D. Hernandez Marrero, (Ed.), 731-747, Grupo Editorial Nefrología de la Sociedad Española de Nefrología, ISBN 978-84-96727-97-7, Barcelona, Spain.

Raghavan, R.; Jeroudi, A.; Achkar, K.; Gaber, AO.; Patel, SJ. & Abdellatif, A. (2010). Bortezomib in kidney transplantation. *J Transplant,* Vol 2010. (Sep 2010), pp. 1-6, ISSN.

Sberro-Soussan, R.; Zuber, J.; Suberbielle-Boissel, C.; Candon, S.; Martinez, F.; Snanoudj, R.; Rabant, M.; Pallet, N.; Nochy, D.; Anglicheau, D.; Leruez, M.; Loupy, A.; Thervet, E.; Hermine, O. & Legendre, C. (2010). Bortezomib as the sole post-renal transplantation desensitization agent does not decrease donor-specific anti-HLA antibodies. *Am J Transplant,* Vol 10. No 3, (Mar 2010), pp. 681-686, ISSN 1600-6143.

Scemla, A.; Loupy, A.; Candon, S.; Mamzer, MF.; Martinez, F.; Zuber, J.; Sberro, R.; Legendre, C. & Thervet, E. (2010). Incidence of infectious complications in highly sensitized renal transplant recipients treated by rituximab: a case-controlled study. *Transplantation,* Vol 90. No 11, (Dec 2010), pp. 1180-1184, ISSN 1534-0608.

Schwenger V & Morath,C. (2010). Immunoadsorption in nephrology and kidney transplantation. *Nephrol Dial. Transplant* Vol. 25, No 8, (May 2010) pp. 2407-2413. Online ISSN 1460-2385 - Print ISSN 0931-0509

Siisal, C & Morath, C. (2011). Current approaches to the management of highly sensitized kidney transplant patients. *Tissue Antigens,* Vol 77. No 3, (Mar 2011), pp. 177-186, ISSN 1399-0039.

Stegall, MD.; Gloor, J.; Winters, JL.; Moore, SB. & Degoey, S. (2006). A comparison of plasmapheresis versus high-dose IVIG desensitization in renal allograft recipients with high levels of donor specific alloantibody. *Am J Transplant* Vol 6. No 2, (Feb 2006), pp. 146-351, ISSN 1600-6143

Trivedi, HL.; Terasaki, PI.; Feroz, A.; Everly, MJ.; Vanikar, AV.; Shankar, V.; Trivedi, VB.; Kaneku, H.; Idica, AK.; Modi, PR.; Khemchandani, SI & Dave SD. (2009)Abrogation of anti-HLA antibodies via proteasome inhibition. *Transplantation,* Vol.87, No. 10, (May 2009), pp. 1555-1561, ISSN 1534-0608.

Vo, AA.; Wechsler, EA.; Wang, J.; Peng, A.; Toyoda, M.; Lukovsky, M.; Reinsmoen, & N, Jordan SC. (2008). Analysis of subcutaneous (SQ) alemtuzumab induction therapy in highly sensitized patients desensitized with IVIG and rituximab. *Am J Transplant,* Vol 8. No 1, (Jan 2008), pp. 144-149, ISSN 1600-6143.

Wahrmann, M.; Haidinger, M.; Körmöczi, GF.; Weichhart, T.; Säemann, MD.; Geyeregger, R.; Kikić, Z.; Prikoszovich, T.; Drach, J. & Böhmig, GA. (2010). Effect of the proteasome inhibitor bortezomib on humoral immunity in two presensitized renal transplant candidates. *Transplantation,* Vol 89. No 11, (Jun 2010), pp. 1385-1390, ISSN 1534-0608.

Yuan, XP; Wang, CX.; Gao, W. & Fu Q, He XS. (2010). Kidney transplant in highly sensitized patients after desensitization with plasmapheresis and low-dose intravenous immunoglobulin. *Exp Clin Transplant,* Vol. 2, No. 2, (Jun 2010), pp. 130-135, ISSN 1304-0855.

Part 3

Surgical Approaches and Complications

22

The Transplantation Operation and Its Surgical Complications

Junjie Zhao, Zhenli Gao and Ke Wang
Yantai YuHuangDing Hospital
China

1. Introduction

Over the past decades, the outcomes of kidney transplantation have improved markedly due to advancements in prevention and treatment of acute rejection episodes, management of posttransplant complications and better knowledge of immunosuppressive drugs. As a result, transplantation has become the mainstay and preferred treatment for patients of all ages with end-stage renal disease. However, the surgical technique for renal transplantation has changed little from the original pelvic operation described in 1951 by Küss et al. It seems the operation has been standardized and there is little need for further discussions over the topic. In fact, the argumentation on surgical technique has never ceased since its birth, for optimization of the surgical outcomes, many aspects of operative techniques have been modified and novel techniques have been invented. In modern immunosuppressive era, the pattern of surgical complications has evolved and gains some fresh features. In this chapter, we will review the standard operative procedures performed today and introduce the updated surgical techniques as well. Meanwhile, the characteristics of major surgical complications and the evolvement of their diagnosis and treatment will be expatiated on. After all, the surgical operation is invariably the key of a successful transplantation; surgical techniques are constantly related to the morbidity and mortality of the patients.

2. Standard surgical technique on kidney transplantation

The standard kidney transplant procedure is the pelvic operation originally used by French surgeons Küss, Dubost, and Servelle and their associates in 1951 and refined subsequently by Murray and Harrison for the first successful kidney transplantation in human history. The heterotopic pelvic approach has been widely accepted for its multiple advantages and considered a standard access. The classical surgical techniques of revascularization and urinary tract reconstruction have also been broadly used to this day. Each renal transplantation operation is a review of original historic work both in urological and vascular discipline.

2.1 Site

The operative site for standard kidney transplantation is pelvic fossa, however, there is always a disagreement on the criteria to select the appropriate side to accommodate the transplant. Initially, it is recommended that placing the donor kidney in the recipient's contralateral side to ensure the renal pelvis and ureter are anterior in case those future surgeries are required (John, 2002). Afterward, it is stated that the more important consideration is to avoid sites of previous transplants, other operations, or peritoneal dialysis catheters though the dissection on the right is slightly easier (James, 2004). Subsequently, suggestion from scholars is presented that each side of the recipient's pelvis is acceptable, however the right external iliac vessels are longer and more horizontal compared to the left side, which facilitates the vascular anastomoses (Stuart, 2008). With progresses of surgical technique and accumulation of clinical experience the concept of selecting the right pelvic fossa as the preferred site for the first transplantation has been universally accepted. However, the ipsilateral severe atherosclerotic vascular disease, venous disorders such as previous deep venous thromboses and femoral dialysis catheters should be routinely excluded. The peritoneal dialysis catheters and previous minor abdominal operation such as appendectomy, conventional herniorrhaphy are not absolute contraindications according to our experiences. It also elicits one issue for nephrologists that the initial peritoneal dialysis catheter or femoral dialysis catheter is properly intubated on the left side for the potential renal recipients. The standard Gibson incision can avoid most stoma of peritoneal dialysis catheters. On the other hand, the minor transperitoneal surgeries or small operations on abdominal wall usually yield limited adhesion at the place to accomplish the transplantation. But, the transplantation is strongly not recommended at the side where has a history of herniorrhaphy with propylene mesh or ipsilateral open operation of ureter and bladder. Because the propylene mesh results in inflammatory response and connective tissue proliferation conducing to fibrosis formation and a thick scar plate on the inner surface of lower abdominal wall, which make the dissection of bladder a formidable task. Previous ipsilateral pelvic surgeries generally preclude the sequent transplantation due to local inordinate anatomical features and severe perivesical tissue conglutination. Massively enlarged polycystic kidneys are challenges for urologists; one would choose the side of the smaller kidney. However, bilateral extremely enlarged polycystic kidneys would make the transplant surgery very difficult or impossible. In that occasion, right or bilateral native nephrectomy might be considered. Sequential and simultaneous laparoscopic bilateral native nephrectomies have all been testified safe and effective. For the second transplantation patients the kidney is implanted on the contralateral side, usually left side.

2.2 Incision and exposure

The kidney transplant operation can be performed via many different routes, however two important issues must be considered when deciding the incision for a renal transplant: a good access to the iliac fossa and bladder and a minimal rate of wound related morbidity. Historically, three classic incisions have been recommended for kidney transplant surgery: pelvic Gibson incision, the hockey stick incision and oblique incision. Curvilinear incision made in lower quadrant of the abdomen, known as the "pelvic Gibson incision", which affords relatively atraumatic and convenient access to the iliac fossa and bladder is mainly used for renal transplantation. Oblique incision and inverted J-shaped incision, known as the "hockey stick incision" are the other two frequently used incisions in some centers. Nanni and colleagues compared the two incisions with regard to the incidence of long-term complications, they concludes that the oblique surgical incision was better than the hockey-stick incision for lower incidence of hernia and abdominal wall relaxation and the more favorable cosmetic results (Nanni et al. 2005). Paramedian, midline incision and even transverse incision are lately introduced to the practice of living kidney transplantation for better cosmetic appearance, but these incisions are of same inherent drawback of difficult exposure of operative bed, which can be possible alternatives for special candidates.(Filocamo et al., 2007; Park et al., 2008).

When a Gibson incision is made, the external oblique muscle and fascia are divided in the line of the incision and split to the lateral extent of the wound. The internal oblique and transverse muscles are divided with cautery in the line of the incision, or in a more beneficial way to divide the two layers of muscles on the confluence of the oblique muscles and the rectus sheath, which avoids division of the internal oblique and transversus muscles. The latter method, most frequently used in our institute, has two major advantages both for patients and surgeons. Firstly it markedly reduces the blood loss resulting from capillary hemorrhage of muscle wound surface during the transplantation, which is usually underestimated by surgeons. Uraemic patients often have a bleeding diathesis at the time of surgery due to malfunctioned platelet, especially when being heparinized during pretransplant hematodialysis. In addition, the muscle fibers could disrupt during closure because of high tension of the wound covering the graft, particularly, if there is a large kidney for a small recipient. The pararectus division of muscles and aponeurosis facilitates the process of wound closure and diminishes the incidence of muscles collapse and wound complications.

The inferior epigastric vessels are ligated and divided, but if there are multiple renal arteries, the inferior epigastric vessels should be preserved in the beginning in case the inferior epigastric artery is required for anastomosis to a lower polar renal artery. Division of the spermatic cord has not been advocated during past decades for its drawback of inducing secondary testicular complications, but freed laterally and retracted medially. The round ligament can be divided for adequate exposure.

The exposure of iliac vessels seems to be an effortless process, but bearish expansion of the extraperitoneal space might cause the peritoneum injury and subsequent enterocele, a rare but potentially fetal surgical complication, described as "renal paratransplant hernia" in recent year. We have encountered three cases of the rare surgical complication in early years. In our opinion, in most, if not all cases, paratransplant hernia is an iatrogenic surgical complication as a result of an unnoticed defect of the peritoneum due to improper maneuvers during the transplantation. Meticulous dissection may help avoid this complication. And if a peritoneal defect is found, it should be closed immediately, regardless of its size to avoid the occurrence of a postoperative paratransplant hernia.

A self-retaining retractor is usually inserted to obtain optimal exposure, which allows the assistant to free both hands to assist the anastomoses. However, the position of the retractor should be checked carefully before fixing it because the inadvertent retractor injury was one of the causes to femoral neuropathy, an unusual complication after kidney transplantation, with major clinical features of reversible muscle weakness or paralysis of hip flexion. The lymphatics that course along and over the vessels must be ligated with a nonabsorbable suture and divided, rather than cauterized, to prevent the later occurrence of a lymphocele. The surgeon must be cautious not to mistake the genitofemoral nerve for a lymph vessel. The former lies on the medial edge of the psoas muscle, and a branch may cross the distal external iliac artery.

2.3 Vascular reconstruction

In general, it is preferable to do the end-to-side venous anastomosis first, and then the end-to-side arterial anastomosis. Some scholars argued that the arterial anastomosis should be done first if the renal artery is to be anastomosed to the internal iliac artery. Although end-to-side anstomosis to the external iliac vein and end-to-end anstomosis to the internal iliac artery is once the classical vascular anastomosis pattern, and also practiced in some centers now, many facts have revealed that the internal iliac artery is not a preferred option for the arterial anastomosis compared with external iliac artery. Firstly, dissection of the internal iliac artery is not as straightforward as that of the external iliac artery. Meanwhile, a mobilization of a length of the external and common iliac arteries is also needed when the internal iliac artery is considered as the candidate of arterial anastomosis because of the application of vascular clamps and prevention of kinking of artery when being rotated laterally for anastomosis, which increases the operative time and risk of surgical complications. Furthermore, it is an intractable problem to handle if the concomitant internal iliac vein is inadvertently damaged during the dissection. Moreover, the risk of anastomosis site stenosis and erectile dysfunction is much higher than that of external iliac artery following the transplantation. Lastly, the short internal iliac artery and variation are common. Therefore, the routine end-to-end anstomosis to the internal iliac artery is not recommended.

Since Carrel described a 3-point anastomosis technique for an end-to-end allograft arterial anastomosis in 1902, transplant surgeons have invented different techniques for arterial and venous anastomoses. Most efforts have been made to decrease ischemic time and promote the quality of anastomosis. The classical and universally used technique is the 2-point anastomosis, with initial sutures placed at either end of the venotomy or arteriotomy. Sometimes, an anchor suture is placed at the midpoint of the lateral wall to prevent posterior or anterior wall being caught up in the suture line. Another running anastomoses fashion, so called "1-suture, 1-knot technique", which does not need to turn the kidney medial and lateral, has showed some advantages especially in obese patients and recipients with deep iliac fossa. Mital and associates, in 1996, performed arterial and venous anastomoses using 4-stay sutures and several vascular clips for each anastomosis, without a continuous vascular suture. (Mital et al, 1996). Afterwards, sutureless vascular anastomosis technique using vascular clips or titanium ring pin staplers have been described and suggested safe and time-saving in small series (Jones, 1998; Ye, 2006). However, these sutureless techniques seem not to be popularized, and their long-time outcomes need further observation.

2.3.1 Venous anastomosis

The renal vein is anastomosed end-to-side, usually to the external iliac vein using a continuous 5-0 monofilament vascular suture following an appropriate venotomy performed in the external iliac vein. In rare conditions such as thrombosis or hypoplasia of both iliac veins, the renal vein has to be anastomosed to other site. Anastomosis to the inferior vena cava is the most common alternative, usually associated with a native nephrectomy. The usage of infra-renal inferior vena cava or infra-hepatic inferior vena cava has been described in the literature. Otherwise, portal venous drainage system, inferior mesenteric vein, superior mesenteric vein, even venous collaterals with large caliber secondary to thrombosis of the inferior vena cava and iliac veins such as a presacral collateral vein and the left ovarian vein have been utilized for renal transplantation with satisfactory results (Wong et al, 2008).

Short right renal vein, particularly from living donors, represent a technical challenge to the transplant surgeon. Usually, the satisfactory anastomosis can be achieved by thorough mobilization of the recipient common and external iliac veins. Sometimes, the techniques of donor vein elongation are needed especially in obese recipients. Right renal vein extension using the inferior vena cava is an excellent option and frequently used in deceased kidney transplantation, but is not suitable to living donors. A variety of techniques have been developed to elongate the short live donor vein, and extension techniques using saphenous, gonadal vein or superficial femoral vein grafts or a polytetrafluoroethylene graft have demonstrated nice results. Extensively elongation of renal vein should be avoided either in live or deceased transplantation for prophylaxis of occurrence of renal vein thrombosis.

2.3.2 Arterial anastomosis

The end-to-side arterial anastomosis is generally placed more proximally than the vein, usually performed using an appropriately trimmed cuff of aorta attached to the renal artery with a continuous 5-0 or 6-0 monofilament vascular suture after a suitable arteriotomy placed in the external iliac artery. The arterial clamps should be applied with great care to avoid the disruption of vascular calcified plaque. Endarterectomy is usually unnecessary. An opening of proper caliber created with artery puncher in the external iliac artery may facilitate the anastomosis of renal arteries from live donors in the absence of "Carrel patch". Careful suture performance is absolutely crucial for the allograft to maintain normal arterial blood flow and function. Appropriate full-thickness suture of arterial wall must be achieved in each stitch, particularly in patients with arteriosclerosis.

Kidney with multiple arteries is a challenge before artery anastomosis. There are various anastomosis patterns for this situation. How best to manage multiple arteries depending on the characteristics of multiple arteries and individual transplant surgeon's preference. Anastomosis of two arteries close together on an aortic patch of a left-sided deceased donor kidney is comparatively straightforward. If they are more than 2 cm apart, consideration could be given to perform two separate anastomoses. Dual arteries to a right-sided kidney often make positioning of the kidney difficult without kinking one or the other artery, sometimes the arteries have to be shortened to fulfill two separate anastomoses. Most complicated cases are encountered in live transplant setting, cuff of aorta is impossible, multiple and short arteries are common with the increasing popularity of laparoscopic living donor nephrectomy. For double arteries, two separate anastomoses are recommended in most occasions. Double parallel anastomoses to the external iliac artery are most common pattern. Sometimes the lower hilar artery or lower polar artery can anastomose to internal iliac artery or inferior epigastric artery in an end-to-end manner. Very small accessory renal arteries, particularly at the upper pole, can be ligated without problems. Arteries reconstruction on the back table operation before revascularization is an effective way suggested by many authors. The advantages of ex vivo reconstruction techniques are that they preserve the small accessory renal arteries by an end-to-side or conjoined anastomosis to renal artery stem and reduce the operative time by simplifying the anastomosis. Multiple short arteries or arteries with other vascular anomalies can also be salvaged. Theoretically, the incidence of vascular complications may be higher using complicated reconstruction techniques on back table. It is necessary to consult the vascular surgeons to achieve the difficult reconstruction under magnification.

2.4 Urinary tract reconstruction

Reconstruction of urinary tract begins following a successful revascularization. The type of urinary tract reconstruction is various. The standard and usual form of urinary tract reconstruction is ureteroneocystostomy. But the classical status of ureteroneocystostomy has been challenged recently. Pyeloureterostomy and ureteroureterostomy conventionally is considered salvage procedures when the transplant ureter's blood supply seems to be compromised or the urinary bladder is difficult to identify. Nie and associates recently compared the overall incidence of urological complications between ureteroureterostomy and ureteroneocystostomy in kidney transplantation, no difference was found, moreover, ureteroureterostomy decreased the incidence of urine leakage and therefore was advocated a good first option for urinary tract reconstruction with a greater possibility of resolving a ureteral stenosis with endourology and no risk of reflux (Nie et al, 2010). Timsi and collages compared results in 151 consecutive kidney transplantations with routine pyeloureterostomy and that in 129 procedures with extravesical anti-reflux ureteroneocystostomy, the outcomes from routine pyeloureterostomy group were even better and also had the similar advantages as the ureteroureterostomy's (Timsit et al, 2010). However, ureteroneocystostomy is still the preferred selection of urinary tract reconstruction for most surgeons because of its various advantages. ureteroneocystostomy is a familiar technique we often applied in general urological surgeries. Deep dissection of native ureter and native nephrectomy are unnecessary. It can be performed regardless of the quality or presence of the native ureter and retains the possibility of conversion to an ureteroureterostomy or pyeloureterostomy if the implant fails. The location of ureteroneocystostomy is usually several centimeters away from the vascular anastomoses, which facilitate the examination and correction of a possible urinary complication during the reinterventions.

2.4.1 Ureteroneocystostomy

There are a variety of techniques for ureteroneocystostomy, which in general can be categorized into transvesical or extravesical and antireflux or non-antireflux. The Leadbetter-Politano (LP) technique is the classic transvesical ureteroneocystostomy described by Murray et al in 1954 for the first successful renal transplant. This technique utilizes one cystostomy to access the interior of the bladder and another cystostomy to recreate a new ureteric orifice in a normal anatomic position. The ureter is tunneled in the submucosal space to prevent reflux. The extravesical ureteroneocystostomy was first described by Witzel in 1896, then again by Gregoir in April 1961, and soon thereafter by Lich et al, who published the technique in November 1961. The Lich-Gregoir (LG) technique was designed to avoid a second cystostomy, yet retain an antireflux mechanism. It creates a 2-3 cm submucosal tunnel with muscle backing of the ureter to provide a valve effect. In addition to the avoidance of a separate cystostomy, other comparative advantages were less bladder dissection, a shorter ureteral length, and no interference with native ureteral function. Additionally, the LG was noted to be rapid and technically easier to perform than the LP technique. Several variations of the LG implantation have been described, such as the use of running instead of interrupted sutures to create the ureteral mucosal anastomosis, performance of a tunnel by submucosal blunt dissection instead of muscular imbrication, placement of a single horizontal Halsted stitch at the proximal apex of the bladder incision to the ureter to prevent tension at the acute angle of the anastomosis, placement of an anchor stitch on the distal ureteral tip to the full thickness of the bladder, folding back the tip of the ureter to make a terminal cuff, incorporation of the muscular layer with the mucosal layer of the bladder in the anastomosis and the parallel-incision technique with a submucosal tunnel created between the two parallel incisions in the lateral bladder. All of

these so-called modified Lich ureteroneocystostomies include extravesicular access, the formation of an antireflux tunnel, and an urothelial anastomosis (Kayler et al, 2010).
Another extravesical approach to ureteroneocystostomy that also includes an antireflux tunnel but lacks an urothelial anastomosis, called the U-stitch technique. By elimination of the urothelial anastomosis, this technique was demonstrated to shorten operative times even further than that of the LG technique. But this technique is associated with an increased risk of a urinary complication and abandoned at our center, and being against by many other institutions.
The techniques without an antireflux mechanism are least often described. Althrougt early comparative analyses have failed to show significant differences between reflux and antireflux techniques, but most non-antireflux techniques have been marginalized and abandoned.
The management of double ureters is something like management of dual arteries to some extent. If there is a common part, a straightforward ureteroneocystostomy can be done as a single ureter. Two separate ureteroneocystostomy using L-G technique is preferred in our center when two ureters are not in one common sheath. The dual ureters can also be reconstructed on back table conjoining them into one common stem to anastomose with bladder or native ureter

2.4.2 Other alternatives

There are some unusual forms of urinary tract reconstruction technique using in special conditions, such as pyelopyelostomy in orthotopic renal transplantation, ureteroenterostomy into an intestinal conduit or an intestinal pouch and pyelovesicostomy when the native ureter and the renal transplant ureter are unsuitable for urinary tract reconstruction. No matter what method is used, a tension-free and watertight anastomosis is most important.

2.5 Closure

There are three aspects should be taken into consideration before closing the wound: Haemostasis, reexamination and placement of drains. Careful haemostasis is necessary for every surgery especially for a uremic patient. The special attention should be paid to the vascular anastomosis site and renal pedicle area in case there is active bleeding from an unrecognized leak or an unligated vessel, which is a cause of emergent reoperation during the very early postoperative period even before leaving the operating room. The significance of reexamination is to find if there are some grave technique faults and correct them before the closure. Vessels are always the emphasis for checking, besides the bleeding the strength of renal artery pulsation and the vascular tension of renal vein should be sensed gently using fingers, adjusting the position of graft if there is a kinking or compression of long vessels. In the mean time, the ureter should be tension free and burden free from adjacent structures after the graft is properly placed. No urine leak is permitted. Drain placement is a very important step that can not be ignored, the related issues we will discuss soon.
The value of obtaining a baseline biopsy specimen before closure remains controversial, but it is the fact that it incurs some unnecessary biopsy-induced vascular complications for some grafts with perfect function. A capsulotomy of the transplanted kidney before closure basically has been abandoned in adult transplantation because it is of no use on the whole.
The process of closure is not as easy as incision making. Muscular tension often higher either from an additional graft or descending effect of muscle relaxant. A running #1 polydioxanone

suture (PDS) provide a convenient choice for closure, some centers routinely close muscles and aponeurosis with single-layer PDS suture (Nanni et al. 2005), which reduce the closing time but is also a risk factor of wound complications. Our experience is to close the wound with two-layer PDS suture plus five to six interrupted anchor stitches in muscle layers with nonabsorbable sutures, which has been proved an appropriate method. Otherwise, attention should also be paid to avoid injuring the peritoneum when closing the incision, for one careless stitch can tear the peritoneum leading to a defect and the paratransplant hernia especially in patients with obesity and ascites. The vaulted transplanted ureter under the muscle layer should not be involved by suture when closing. Furthermore, excessive tension on the suture may lead to compression of the kidney or lead to defects resulting in wound complications, a mesh could be used to achieve a tension free closure.

2.6 Stent, catheter and drains

The debate about the three types of tube has never stopped. The viewpoints varies too much, some of disputes are swordplay. Double J stent is an object full of controversy since its introduction to urology. Its function in renal transplants to significantly reduce ureteric complications is broadly accepted. One meta-analysis has addressed the prophylactic routine stenting in renal transplants is cost-effective (Mangus et al, 2004). The minor flaw such as an increased risk of urinary tract infection, an additional cystoscopy and patient discomfort from bladder spasm is relatively unimportant and controllable, can not counteract its contribution to a markedly lowered incidence of ureteric complications, which sometimes can be a cause of graft loss. The optimal duration of prophylactic stenting has also not been determined. Based on local center preference, it is usually 2 to 6 weeks. In our center, stent is removed during an office visit 4 weeks after tranplantation, accompanying with a routine general checkup.

A dwelling catheter is necessary for every kidney transplantation patients, it is important to maintain the catheter in an unobstructed condition during the early postoperative period. The reported duration time usually is 5 to 7 days, our experience is 7 days. Seven-day is a proper compromise to prevent urine leak in the absence of an increasing incidence of urinary tract infection. What's more, acute vascular rejection usually occurs one week after transplantation, a dwelling catheter is helpful for the patients to detect the early sharp reduction of urine output, a usual signal of acute rejection.

There always remains considerable controversy over the necessity and duration of perigraft drains. Some authors suggested non-drains closure if the heamostasis is satisfactory because drain tubes increase the infection risk in immunosuppressive patients. But most others support placing a closed suction retroperitoneal drain at the time of transplant and a considerable majority of them suggest removal of drains in 48 hours in case of infection. However some authors argue the rationality of prolonged drainage, as reported, the median day of drain removal was 18 days in individual center. (Tiong et al, 2009). Based on our preference, we suggest a "two-drain policy" routinely for every transplant patients. The incidence of postoperative hematomas and lymphoceles in renal transplantation is dramatically higher than general urological surgeries' for various reasons. So the principle of drain placing can not simply mimic the pattern of general surgery. In the early posttransplant period, bleeding is commonly from the operative bed, it is usual to record 100 to 200 mL of heavily blood-stained drainage in the first few hours of transplantation. After that, even a week later, the spontaneous bleeding of graft can also develop a problematic hematoma. Moreover, most lymphoceles formations and urine leak occur approximately one week after transplantation, too early removal of drains increase the risk. The reason of two drains is based on the fact that there are two isolated dead space created by the allograft, over the upper pole and under the lower pole of the transplant kidney; one lower drain often can not drain the bleeding from the upper pole. We place one additional drain onto the upper pole of graft and the other one down to prevesical space, centimeters away from the renal vessels and ureter. The upper drain usually is removed 4 to 5 days posttransplant or until drainage is less than 20 mL daily, the lower drain is routinely removed one day after the catheter removal if there is no evidence of urine leak or lymphorrhea, which significantly diminishes the incidence of postoperative hematomas, lymphoceles and urinomas compared with our early experiences with one-drain policy, but no increase of wound related infection.

3. Surgical considerations in pediatric recipient

In children, the standard surgical approach in adult carries two disadvantages. First, there is a size mismatch between the available extraperitoneal space and the adult sized donor kidney. Secondly, the recipient artery may be small compared with the artery of the graft that make the vascular anastomosis more difficult and may jeopardize the blood pressure and blood flow which is required for the donor kidney to survive. The conventional view is that the transplant procedure is same as for adults if their weight is more than 20 kg. If weight less than 20 kg, the right Gibson incision can be carried up to the costal margin to increase exposure of the right extraperitoneal space or using a transperitoneal approach. Some centers usually perform transperitoneal kidney transplantation in children below 5 years. However some advocated extraperitoneal renal transplantation technique in children who weigh less than 15 kg, which limits potential gastrointestinal complications and allows the confinement of potential surgical complications, such as bleeding and urinary leakage (Furness et al, 2001). When a transperitoneal approach used, it is generally done through a midline incision from the xyphoid to the pubis, the posterior peritoneum is incised lateral to the ascending colon. Ligating and dividing two to three lumbar veins posteriorly is often necessary to facilitate the application of vascular occluding clamp. The terminal aorta is dissected free at its junction with the right or left common iliac artery. The donor artery is either anastomosed to the distal aorta to obtain the best arterial inflow, or with one of the common iliac arteries in an end-to-side fashion using 5-0 or 6-0 monofilament vascular suture. The selection of common iliac artery avoids a complete occlusion of the aorta which is associated with temporary acidosis of both lower extremities (van Heurn et al, 2009). The donor vessels are often amputated and may be spatulated to ensure a wide anastomosis and to avoid kinking which may lead to impaired blood flow. An aortic punch is basically used to prevent renal artery occlusion if significant hypotension occurs. The ureter of an adult size kidney is usually long and wide enough to obtain a tension free ureteroneocystostomy. The problem is the too long ureter is easy to be kinked and twisted, even causing internal hernia (Sánchez et al, 2005); therefore, sometimes the long ureter should be shortened to obtain best result. Temporary ureteral stenting is beneficial to prevent urological complications, but special care should be taken for the removing technique because standard cystoscopy in adults is not suitable for a very young child. It is a smart way to attach the stent with the indwelling bladder or reservoir catheter and removing it as the catheter is withdrawn. An antireflux procedure is imperative for pediatric patients. Because a large number of recipients are a result of obstructive uropathy due to outflow obstruction, small capacity or poor function of the bladder, which all predisposes to vesicoureteral reflux of the transplanted kidney.

4. Dual kidney transplantation

As a result of the shortage of kidneys for transplantation and the increasing demand for transplantable grafts, the option for using organs from expanded criteria donors has become widely accepted. One option for using organs from donors with a suboptimal nephron mass is dual kidney transplantation (DKT). Dual kidney transplantation is the deceased renal transplantation using two marginal kidneys simultaneously either from the donors older than 60 years old, or from solitary pediatric donors age younger than 5 years or small (< 21 kg). The paired kidneys from solitary pediatric donors are recovered and transplanted as en bloc, known as "en bloc kidney (EBK)". The double kidneys from old donors can be also used as en bloc, but mostly in a split individual implantation technique, bilaterally or ipsilateral. Clinical kidney transplants using solitary paired deceased donor kidneys were reported in the early 1960s, followed by increasing interest in the use of paired pediatric deceased donor kidneys as en bloc with the first case to a pediatric recipient and thereafter, to adult recipients showing possible advantage of more renal reserve and technical feasibility. One recent report shows EBK pediatric donor transplants had the best long-term outcomes among deceased donor transplants (Bhayana et al, 2010). Various strategies have improved the outcome of EBK pediatric donor transplants, including changes in techniques.
For an adult recipient, the paired kidneys usually also placed extraperitoneally in the iliac fossa via a Gibson incision. Commonly, the aorta and the inferior vena cava of EBK are anastomosed to the external iliac artery and vein with 5-0 or 6-0 monofilament vascular suture in an end-to-side technique. Sometimes, the end-to-side anastomosis is applied to the aorta and inferior vena cava to prevent kinking of renal vessels and ureters. For the same purpose, the upper pole of the grafts sometimes fixes to the iliopsoas muscle. Double ureteroneocystostomies of the native contracted bladder are performed separately, or the ends of the two ureters are reconstructed into a conjoined ureter and then one ureteroneocystostomy is performed. Sometimes ureteroureterostomies are performed. Kato and collages, in 2008, developed the urinary tract reconstruction technique with a vascularized "bladder patch" including the vesical trigone from the same donor, which precludes the challenging ureteral reconstruction and ureteroneocystostomy, and excludes the risk of anastomotic strictures and postoperative reflux, significantly reduces the incidence of urine leak. In the mean time, the donor bladder wall served a purpose of bladder augmentation as well. (Kato et al, 2008).
Since first report of DKT from an adult deceased donor in the United States was revealed in 1996, many centers now perform DKT using various organ selection criteria and surgical techniques, including the extra- or intraperitoneal bilateral placement of the two kidneys through two separate Gibson incisions or one midline incision. In 1998, Masson et al. were the first to transplant both adult donor kidneys unilaterally into the same iliac fossa. Their reasoning was that this would reduce the surgical trauma and thus facilitate the immediate postoperative recovery of the patient, and also leave the contralateral iliac fossa intact for a further transplantation procedure in the event of graft loss. However, extraperitoneal unilateral placement through a single Gibson incision presents several technical hurdles, such as more extensive vessel dissection and a higher risk of renal vein thrombosis due to compression by the two kidneys. A comparison between 29 unilateral and 29 bilateral DKT

procedures in an initial series has showed both techniques are safe, with no differences in surgical complication rates. In brief, the procedure begins with the classic Gibson incision, preferably on the right side. After creating an adequate extraperitoneal space, the right donor kidney is preferably placed superiorly because its renal vein can be lengthened by a segment of inferior vena cava. Another reason to position the right kidney superolaterally in the right flank is because the right kidney has a longer artery. If necessary, the internal iliac vein is dissected to mobilize the external iliac vein and thus facilitate renal vein anastomoses to the external iliac vein of the recipient. The extended renal vein and renal artery of the right kidney are anastomosed end-to-side to the iliac vessels of the recipient; these anastomoses are often to the external iliac vessels. After revascularization of the right kidney, vascular clamps are placed immediately below the venous and arterial anastomoses. The left donor kidney is transplanted distally, allowing the transplanted right kidney to continue to be perfused. The left kidney is positioned inferomedially to the right kidney. The renal artery and vein of the left kidney are anastomosed end-to-side to the external iliac vessels. Extravesical ureteroneocystostomies are performed separately, with a double J stent for each ureter, leaving the ureter of the upper transplanted kidney lateral to the lower one.

5. Orthotopic kidney transplantation

Orthotopic kidney transplantation (OKT) is seldom performed due to its complicated procedure and high related morbidity. However an increasing percentage of patients with end-stage renal disease currently are not candidates for a heterotopic kidney transplant because of associated severe vascular pathology, obesity, or retained iliac fossae from a former graft. In such situations, where heterotopic transplant is not appropriate, an orthotopic kidney transplant is an alternative.

The surgical technique consists of a retroperitoneal approach to the splenic hilus via lumbotomy. To preserve its entire length, the vein is ligated close to the renal parenchyma including its bifurcation. The renal artery is often narrow and cannot be used in most cases. The recipient's urinary tract is always carefully dissected and preserved. In most of the reported cases, renal graft revascularization was performed using the recipient's splenic artery and left renal vein. Types of artery revascularization include end-to-end anastomoses between graft renal artery and native splenic artery, renal artery or inferior mesenteric artery or end-to-side anastomoses between graft renal artery and Aorta. Types of vein revascularization include end-to-end anastomoses between graft renal vein and native renal vein or splenic vein or end-to-side anastomoses between graft renal vein and inferior vena cava. The excretory system is reconstructed using pyelo-pyelic anastomoses in most cases, and uretero-ureteral anastomoses, uretero-pyelic anastomoses, ureterocalicostomy in the others.

The reported overall vascular complication rate is about 5.4%, and total urological complication rate is about 8.1%. Musquera et al. in their recent report demonstrated that no statistically significant differences are observed between orthotopic and heterotopic transplant series when comparing overall patients and graft survival. OKT is a feasible alternative for selected patients who are considered unsuitable for heterotopic kidney transplant.

6. Minimally invasive kidney transplantation

During the past decade, the use of minimally invasive surgical procedures has increased in popularity among surgeons and patients. The introduction of minimally invasive techniques in the transplant field is expanding the number of living-related donor nephrectomies. The minimally invasive approach allows a significant reduction of postoperative pain, decreased length of hospital stay, shorter recovery time, and enhanced cosmesis, representing a significant advantage for the patient. However, the renal transplant surgery is always the forbidden zone of minimally invasive techniques because of the formidable technical barriers. The pioneers initially attempted the laparoscopic techniques in the renal autotransplantation of experimental animals, establishing the basis for clinical performance of autotransplantation and other complex urologic vascular procedures laparoscopically. Then the laparoscopic autotransplantation for patients with ureteral lesions or renovasular hypertension have been reported in few cases. In 2002, Hoznek and associates presented their initial experience on robotic assisted kidney transplantation, Operative time was 178 minutes. Robotic assistance made anastomosis possible by its unique ability of stereoscopic magnification and ultra-precise suturing techniques due to the flexibility of the robotic wristed instruments. Renal perfusion was excellent with immediate diuresis. The study demonstrates that robotic assisted kidney transplantation is feasible. However, technical and cost hindrances limit the routine use of robots. Until 2010, another robotic transabdominal kidney transplantation has been reported in a morbidly obese patient (BMI $41Kg/m^2$) with 4 trocars and a 7 cm midline incision. The operative time was 223 min, and the blood loss was less than 50 ml. The kidney had immediate graft function. No perioperative complications were observed, and the patient was discharged on postoperative day 5 with normal kidney function. In 2011 the first European case of robotic renal transplantation was accomplished using 3 trocars and a 7 cm suprapubic incision. The suprapubic incision used for introduction of the kidney and also the uretero-vescical anastomosis. Besides the robotic renal transplantation, Rosales et al presented the first laparoscopic renal transplantation, without robotic assistance, using 4 trocars, a hand-access device and a 7 cm Pfannenstiel incision. In this case the ureterovesical reimplantation was done laparoscopically using a modified Taguchi technique. In view of the rapid progresses in laparoscopic vascular and urological reconstruction technique, we have reason to believe that minimally invasive kidney transplantation would have a bright future.

7. Surgical complications of kidney transplantation

Surgical complications of kidney transplantations have always been received considerable attention in the literature, because they can lead to morbidity, graft loss and mortality. As with other surgical cases, postoperative hemorrhage, wound complication may be seen in kidney transplant operation. However, there are some transplant-related surgical complications are special issues unique to kidney transplantation recipients, which can be categorized as vascular, urologic or lymphatic.

7.1 Wound complications

As with other types of surgery, wound complications are probably the most common surgical complication after a kidney transplant, with an approximate incidence of 5%. The general risk factors of wound complications is similar to other sorts of surgery, including systemic factors (e.g. increased age, obesity, diabetes and malnutrition), wound features (e.g. hematoma and dead space) and operative characteristics (e.g. poor surgical technique, lengthy operation (>2 h) and intraoperative contamination). In the transplant setting, the graft creates two natural dead spaces at the either pole of the kidney, and the formation of hematoma and lymphoceles is more frequent than general urological procedure.

Furthermore, the inevitable immunocompromising medications have significant adverse effect on wound healing and resistance to infection. Besides the well-known impairment of steroids on wound healing, the commonly used immunosuppressant, mycophenolate mofetil (MMF), has been defined as a significant risk factor of wound complications. Recently, the mammalian target of rapamycin (mTOR) inhibitors, sirolimus and everolimus, believed not to be nephrotoxic, have showed the strong association with problematic lymphoceles and impaired wound healing attributed to their powerful antiproliferative, anti-inflammatory, antiangiogenesis and antilymphangiogenic activity, which are essential for the healing and repair of wounds. Interestingly, although patients undergoing transplantation are at an elevated risk for poor wound healing and infection, the incidence of wound complications are not significantly higher in kidney recipients compared with that in nontransplant patients undergoing similar types of surgery. But wound complication often incurs patient dissatisfaction and increasing cost, moreover, in certain situations, wound complications may also be associated with graft loss and mortality. In general, wound complications can be broadly categorized into infectious and noninfectious complications.

7.1.1 Wound Infections

Wound infections can be divided into superficial wound infections and deep wound infections.

Superficial wound infections: Diagnosed within 30 d of operation, limited to skin or subcutaneous tissue, and at least one of the following should be present:

a. purulent drainage from the superficial incision;
b. a sign or symptom of infection, such as pain, tenderness, heat, or swelling, and the incision is deliberately left open by a surgeon, unless culture becomes negative;
c. the diagnosis of superficial wound infection is confirmed by the surgeon.

Deep wound infections: Diagnosed within 30 d of operation, involvement of the fascial or muscular layers, and at least one of the following should be present:

a. purulent drainage from the deep incision;
b. spontaneous dehiscence while the patient has fever (>38℃), localized pain, or tenderness;
c. An abscess is found on direct examination, on reoperation, or by radiologic examination; the content contains pus, and the culture yielded one or more micro-organisms;
d. the diagnosis of deep incisional infection is confirmed by the surgeon.

The treatment of wound infections should follow the universal principals of general surgery including application of broad-spectrum antibiotic and surgical care, such as opening the wound, evacuating pus, cleansing the wound and dressing changes. But for kidney transplant patients, the aggressively higher doses of immunosuppressors in recipients should be lowered; the sirolimus-based immunosuppressive regimen might be converted to tacrolimus or cyclosporine-based scheme according to conditions of surgical site. On the other hand, the timing and dosage of broad-spectrum antibiotic should be investigated systematically for prolonged duration of antibiotic administration in immunocompromised patients usually incurs opportunistic infection.

7.1.2 Noninfectious wound complications

Noninfectious wound complications generally refer to all of the wound problems except infections including wound dehiscence, perigraft sterile fluid collection and incisional hernias. Although noninfectious, each of them is important risk factor of wound infections. Perigraft sterile fluid collections mainly involve the seroma and lymphocele, which we will expatiate on later. Herein, we chiefly discuss the clinical characteristics of wound dehiscence and incisional hernias.

Wound dehiscence is defined as an incision prematurely bursting open or splitting along surgical suture lines in the absence of documented infection. Similarly, it can be categorized into superficial and deep wound dehiscence. Incisional hernias refer to a protrusion of a portion of an organ or tissue through the incision, which is a result of deep wound dehiscence. The majority of incisional hernias developed in the first three months after kidney transplantation.

Generally, superficial wound dehiscences are treated as superficial wound infection excluding antibiotic therapy. For an anergic wound the healing process can be electively stimulated with the vacuum sealing method, which has shown promising results. Conversely, deep wound dehiscence, as well as symptomatic incisional hernias, requires operative repair. The open surgical procedure varies according to the surgeon's preference. Routinely, small defects undergo primary fascial repair, and large or recurrent defects are repaired with mesh.

7.2 Vascular complications

Vascular complications during and after kidney transplantation are usually uncommon with an incidence of less 10%. But they are important causes of graft dysfunction. According to the location of affected vessels, vascular complications can be grouped into graft vessels complications and recipient vessels complications. Actually, the lesion often affected the both.

7.2.1 Graft vessels complications

7.2.1.1 Renal Artery Thrombosis

Occlusion of renal artery by thrombus is a rare event occurring in 0.2-3.5% of renal transplantations. Though uncommon, it is a transplant emergency that often results in graft loss. The exact cause of renal artery thrombosis has remained obscure. The aetiology is multifactorial. Technical factors are the important causes, but not always. Other possible contributory factors may be concluded as thrombophilic state, history of previous thrombosis, lupus anticoagulants, atherosclerosis, poor cardiac output, ATN or acute rejection. Vessel kinking, torsion, intimal injuries are the frequently reported technique errors resulting in renal artery thrombosis, which should be avoided. Adequate training on techniques of vascular anastomosis and graft recovery is essential, to reduce the occurrence of repeated reanastomosis and iatrogenic vascular injury. Renal artery thrombosis can occur at any time, but commonly occurs in the early postoperative period. The typical clinical presentation is a sudden onset of oliguria or anuria with deterioration of graft function, usually painless, which demands a differential diagnosis with acute rejection and urologic complications. Helical computerized tomography (CT) may be more diagnostic than ultrasound for that it can directly depict renal artery thrombosis when ultrasound studies are inconclusive. Angiography is warranted in confusing cases. Prompt reoperation is crucial to salvage such a graft when diagnosis is suspected, because irreversible cortical necrosis can occur within minutes. That is why it could be responsible for more than one-third of early graft losses. Actually, transplant nephrectomy is usually the rule. Since the extremely bad prognosis of graft survival, prevention is of utmost importance especially in high-risk patients.

7.2.1.2 Renal Vein Thrombosis

Renal vein thrombosis (RVT) is an unusual but disastrous complication, reported to occur with an incidence of 0.3-3%, more frequent than renal artery thrombosis. Pathogenesis of RVT is still controversial, the multiple factors conducing to renal artery thrombosis discussed earlier also contribute here, moreover, technique reasons seem to play an invariable role. A long renal vein is considered a contributory thrombogenic factor by some studies, some center even routinely shorten the left renal vein at the time of surgery to prevent thrombosis. So an immoderately prolonged right renal vein using the inferior vena cuff should be avoided during the back table preparation. Small vein and multiple veins may also predispose to thrombosis. Unlike artery, wall of vein is subtle and fragile, more inclined to be damaged, compressed and twisted, meticulous surgical techniques on renal retrieval, renal vein repair and anastomosis and positioning of kidney may prevent most avoidable occurrence of RVT. In contrast to the renal artery thrombosis, the clinical presentation of RVT is more evident and perilous, sometimes, life-threatening. Majority of RVT occurs during the early period after transplantation, particularly due to technique problems. Rare late RVT even occurring years after operation mainly results from thrombophilic states, secondary thrombosis from ipsilateral DVT or de novo nephropathy. For most early acute cases, besides the typical sudden onset of oliguria or anuria with deterioration of graft function, severe pain and swelling over the graft is definite, an unstable haemodynamics status and decreasing concentration of haemoglobin is present if incurring rupture of graft. Clinical presentation of late RVT may be gentle, especially for the kidneys with partial occlusion of the renal vein, sometimes, only present a deteriorating dysfunctional graft. On Ultrasound images, the allograft may appear swollen and hypoechoic. At Doppler ultrasound examination, venous flow is absent, and the arterial waveform shows reversed, plateauing diastolic flow. A perinephric fluid collection or huge hematoma can be seen if graft rupture occurs.

After an early diagnosis is made by clinical presentation and ultrasound examination, patient should be underwent emergent exploration as soon as possible, which is the sole chance to salvage the graft. There are two ways to save the allograft, thrombectomy or retransplantation. Firstly, patient needs to be heparinized before any procedure, if no obvious evidence of technique error, a thrombectomy of renal vein may be attempted, fresh clot should be removed and flushed out completely, and the transplant renal artery might be clamped to control the bleeding if the graft is ruptured, accompanying with a repair of rupture. A routine vein tissue biopsy is essential to identify the cause. Removal of the kidney and reperfusion with preservation solution may be the last option especially if encountering the short right renal vein from live donor. The iliac vein has to be mobilized to a maximal extent to facilitate the reanastomosis. Besides the open surgical technique, percutaneous chemical and mechanical thrombolysis has been showed a feasible method but with a risk of leading to pulmonary embolism. It may be possible to treat a partial RVT with heparin. We have been associated with three cases of late partial RVT, revascularization of renal vein in all three cases has been achieved by subcutaneous low molecular weight heparin injection combing with intravenous infusion of thrombolytics for 2-3 weeks, no graft loss occurs.

7.2.1.3 Transplant Renal Artery Pseudoaneurysm and Transplant Renal Artery Rupture

Transplant renal artery pseudoaneurysm and transplant renal artery rupture are two extremely rare but potentially devastating vascular complications after kidney transplantations, with an incidence rate of less than 1%. Transplant renal artery pseudoaneurysm is a major risk factor of transplant renal artery rupture. Related data are limited in isolated case reports, but some essentials can be concluded from them. Transplant renal artery pseudoaneurysm can be extra-renal or intra-renal. Extra-renal pseudoaneurysm are usually located at the anastomotic site, and are commonly caused by poor surgical technique, vessel wall ischemia or arterial dehiscence caused by perivascular infection, especially fungi infection. Patients with pseudoaneurysm after their renal transplant are usually asymptomatic and diagnosed incidentally. Few are reported to present with fever, anemia, hypertension, functional impairment, graft loss and life-threatening hemorrhage due to acute rupture. From the review of literature, there are no specific physical findings to predict the risk of rupture. Ultrasound doppler and scanning can readily recognize them. CT angiography, Magnetic resonance (MR) angiography or catheter directed conventional angiography can be used to confirm the diagnosis. The indications for repair of pseudoaneurysm and management options remain controversial. Life-threatening hemorrhage due to acute rupture needs an urgent intervention, the allograft is definitely jeopardized and transplant nephrectomy might inevitably be needed. Recent reports advocate that symptomatic false aneurysms, large size (larger than 2.5 cm), presence of infection, progressive enlargement and impending rupture are indications for repair. Some authors suggest positive surgical repair so long as the pseudoaneurysm is found regardless of if it is symptomatic. Asymptomatic small pseudoaneurysms can be managed conservatively with regular monitoring, but with a risk of acute transplant renal artery rupture. Open surgical repair, endovascular repair and ultrasound-guided percutaneous thrombin injection are the current reported treatment options for managing extra-renal pseudoaneurysm complicating renal transplantation.

7.2.1.4 Transplant Renal Artery Stenosis

Transplant renal artery stenosis (TRAS) is the most common vascular complication following renal transplantation. Depending upon the criteria used for diagnosis its incidence varies from 1 to 23%. It accounts for approximately 1 to 5% of cases of posttransplant hypertension and at least 75% of all posttransplant vascular complications. TRAS is a potentially curable cause of refractory posttransplant hypertension and graft dysfunction. There are three main types of renal transplant artery stenosis: (1) stenosis at the anastomosis; (2) localized stenosis, and (3) multiple or diffuse stenoses. It can occur at any times, usually becomes apparent between 3 mo and 2 yr after renal transplantation. Different locations and timings of disease onset may reflect different etiologies. The most common causes of stenosis are technical resaons. The stenosis due to defective surgical technique, usually located at the anastomosis and especially at the end-to-end anastomosis. The other technical causes reported were vessel lesions during preservation or intimal trauma due to vascular clamps and torsion, kinking or angulation of the artery. Stenosis can be also a result of donor or recipient atherosclerosis. Immunological injury is also proposed as the possible cause, especially in diffuse and multiple stenoses. TRAS resulting from technical resaons usually arises early after transplantation. Stenoses occurring later, sometimes several years posttransplant, usually reflect atherosclerotic disease either of the transplant renal artery or of the adjacent proximal iliac artery. In subtle TRAS postglomerular resistances are usually increased to sustain intracapillary pressure despite the low renal perfusion pressure. Thus, the glomerular filtration rate may be normal or only slightly depressed. When hemodynamically significant stenoses occur, hypertension and progressive kidney dysfunction are common, without treatment, irreversible graft loss is the rule. TRAS is usually manifested as intractable hypertension, with deterioration of renal function. A vascular murmur in the iliac fossa can often be present but significant stenosis can also occur in the absence of the audible bruit. The gold standard for diagnosing TRAS still remains renal angiography, but it is only electively indicated when a stenosis is suspected on the basis of non-invasive tests. Doppler ultrasound, with many advantages has become the imaging modality to enable the diagnosis and follow-up of TRAS.

A TRAS could be treated conservatively or by revascularization. Stenosis can be treated successfully pharmacologically provided that allograft perfusion is not jeopardized. Revascularization can be by percutaneous transluminal angioplasty (PTA) or by surgical correction. PTA is the preferred initial mode of therapy. Technical success has been reported at greater than 80% with clinical success, the restenosis rates are reported to be 10% to 60%. Surgical techniques include resection and revision of the anastomosis, saphenous vein bypass graft of the stenotic segment, patch graft, or localized endarterectomy. The success rate ranges from 63 to 92%, and the recurrence rate is close to 12%. A prompt intervention is mandatory in stenosis exceeding 70%.

7.2.2 The recipient vessels complications

7.2.2.1 Iliac Artery Stenosis

Iliac artery stenosis is a rare complication after renal transplantation, though unusual it can be the cause of hypertension and renal dysfunction. The stenosis can occur at proximal or distal to the anastomosis site or both, also can be bilateral or multilevel occlusive disease. Usually the lesion is located proximal to the transplant anastomosis site, known as" stenosis of the iliac segment proximal to the transplant renal artery (Prox-TRAS)". The incidence for Prox-TRAS was reported to be 2.4%. The causes inducing TRAS are also predisposing factors of iliac artery stenosis, such as technical errors and atherosclerosis. The iliac artery stenosis is usually suspected by the clinical manifestations including bruits, lower extremity claudication, hypertension and renal allograft dysfunction. But it may be asymptomatic and discovered incidently. Surgeons have paid much more attention to Prox-TRAS not only because of the higher incidence but it can cause ischemia of allograft and ipsilateral lower extremity at the same time compared with the distal stenosis. The diagnosis is established based on direct and indirect evidences, because visualization of the stenosis proximal to the transplant artery could not be achieved with the duplex sonography method in all the patients due to the depth of the common iliac artery or an unfavorable angle of the Doppler beam. The criteria for diagnosing isolated Prox-TRAS are summarized as follows (Voiculescu et al, 2003):

1. Decrease in low pulsatility index when compared with data obtained before
2. Low low pulsatility index (<1.0)
3. Pulsus parvus et tardus
4. No TRAS
5. V max within the iliac artery proximal to the graft greater than 200 cm/sec
6. Monophasic flow profile within the iliac artery distal from the transplant artery

PTA with stents for short iliac artery occlusions or stenosis has showed profitable short- and long-term outcomes in most patients. In patients with multilevel occlusive or bilateral lesions, particularly with atherosclerotic disease, endarterectomy or bypass surgery could be taken into consideration.

7.2.2.2 External iliac Artery Pseudoaneurysms

External iliac artery pseudoaneurysms following renal transplantation are very uncommon, with an incidence rate of <1%. Its etiology is similar with that of the transplant renal artery pseudoaneurysm, usually a result of vascular injury due to defective surgical technique or perivascular infection. On ultrasound the diagnosis is straightforward. However, the surgical management is somewhere different. Besides the transplant nephrectomy and pseudoaneurysm excision, arterial reconstruction is recommended to prevent lower limb ischemia. During the past decade, endovascular repair has become the first-choice treatment of posttransplant iliac pseudoaneurysms even in emergent setting in some centers. As the end-to-side arterial anastomosis has been becoming the standard fashion, the incidence of internal iliac artery pseudoaneurysms is exceedingly rare regardless of the biopsy-induced complications.

7.2.2.3 Deep Venous Thrombosis

Deep venous thrombosis (DVT) is a well-recognized complication in patients undergoing any type of surgery. Its occurrence after general surgical procedures is well characterized. However, the real incidence of DVT after kidney transplantation is uncertain, varying from 0.8% to 25%. In our center the incidence of symptomatic posttransplant DVT is less than 1%. Some authors feel it occurs with greater frequency, comparing with patients underwent other types of major surgery. Possible resaons include a pelvic dissection, venous anastomosis with clamping of the vein, decreased venous emptying secondary to the position of the kidney, mechanical compression by hematoma or lymphoceles, and the higher proportion of diabetic patients. The opponents advocate the reasons of a decreased risk of DVT, including bleeding tendency of uremic patients and lower hematocrit levels. Theoretically, the position of the graft adjacent to the iliac vein could affect venous outflow from the lower limb. But in previous studies, no statistically significant difference of posttransplant DVT was found on the side of the graft versus the contralateral side. One study suggested the recipients with severe early renal insufficiency should be regarded as high risk patients for late DVT after renal transplantation. Other well defined risk factors of DVT, such as age >40 years, obesity, history of venous thromboembolism, bed rest >5 days also contribute to DVT after kidney transplantation. Purely clinical signs and symptoms of pain, swelling and calf tenderness cannot be used to diagnose DVT, but they alert one to obtain further testing to exclude or confirm the diagnosis. Actually, majority of the DVT patients are asymptomatic and some present as acute pulmonary embolism alone, a potentially fatal complication. In rare occasion, DVT can be a cause of renal allograft loss due to proximal extension of ileofemoral deep venous thrombosis. Duplex ultrasonography has now replaced venography as the most widely used diagnostic test for an acute DVT with excellent sensitivity and specificity of 97% and 94% respectively, CT pulmonary angiography can be performed when excluding pulmonary embolism.

Therapeutic anticoagulation is imperative for a symptomatic posttransplant DVT patient to prevent clot extension, fatal and non-fatal pulmonary embolism and to reduce the risk of recurrent thrombosis. The current options include unfractionated heparin, warfarin and low molecular weight heparin. Graduated compression stockings should be used immediately to reduce pain and swelling and decreases the incidence of the post-thrombotic syndrome. The role and timing of venous thrombectomy for ilio-femoral vein thrombosis is pendent, especially for kidney transplant patients. Early clot removal is achieved by either mechanical thrombectomy using an open or endovascular approach, or catheterdirected thrombolysis. Permanent or retrievable inferior vena caval filters could be placed for the patients at highest risk of pulmonary embolism. The usual principles and measures of DVT prophylaxis, such as early ambulation, calf exercises or fitting of graduated compression stockings, are also important for kidney transplant patients, in particular, the high risk patients. Subcutaneous injection of low molecular weight heparin can be added for higher risk patients, such as an obese patient with a history of DVT. Of course, the corresponding bleeding risk should be taken into account as well.

7.3 Urological complications

Urological complications are quite common following renal transplant procedure associated with significant morbidity and sometimes a compromising graft function. In general, the urological complications involve any postoperative morbidity related to urinary system and male genital system, whereas the surgical complications are undoubtedly the most important, to some extent, may be prevented. Other urologic complications discussed in the literatures such as hematuria and urinary tract infection, are often a portion of symptoms or results of surgical complications; and some overlaps the surgical aspects but not the whole, for instance, urinary calculi and erectile dysfunction. Four major surgical urological complications discusses here are urine leak, ureteral obstruction, vesicoureteral reflux, and renal allograft rupture.

7.3.1 Urine leak

Urine leaks can be pyelic, vesical or ureteral in origin with a reported incidence of 1% to 4.3%. Pyelic leak is often a result of unrecognized surgical laceration of the renal pelvis during the back table preparation or transplantation. The occurrence of vesical leak is dramatically low after L-G technique fundamentally replaced the conventional transvesical ureteroneocystostomy due to escape from an additional cystic incision. But ureteral leak is constantly considered for its high incidence because the transplant ureter is by nature prone to ischemia, which is one of the two key contributing factors to ureteral leak. The blood supply of the transplant ureter only derives from the small branches of renal artery of allograft in the subtle periureteral fat and sometimes from the end arterial branches of a lower pole renal artery; thereby the more distal ureter is the more tendencies to be ischemic, which partially interprets the fact that most ureteral leak originate from the ureterovesical junction. The ischemia can be aggravated by immune injury during the course of acute rejection. The other key causative factor of leakage is surgical technical problems, most of which are technical errors that should be avoided. The leading technical error is the failure to achieve a watertight and tension-free anastomosis. Dehiscence of anastomotic site due to a full bladder from blocked Foley catheter or undetected electrocautery injury to ureter is occasionally encountered. Ureter ischemia and perforation caused by a malposed double J ureteral stent is the rare cause. The clinical presentation of ureteral leaks can be apparent or mild. Timetable of obvious symptoms have a few diagnostic significance. Leaks due to technical errors like misplacement of ureteral sutures often occur within the first 4 days, whereas leaks from necrosis usually occur within the first 14 days. The symptoms are various typically with a significant reduction of urine output but volume of perigraft drain increases dramatically, however it is not always the case. Sometimes the urine leak can not be drained due to displacement of drains or drain tubes have been removed, the urine would flow into retroperitoneal cavity or out of the wound, or even be reabsorbed into the peritoneal cavity under high pressure or from an unrecognized hole made in the transplant procedure, developing into urine ascites. Evident manifestations include lower abdominal bulge, a swollen, tender scrotum or edema of labia, abdominal and/or back pain. Fever is a frequent signs even no evidence of infection. Graft function is compromised when large volume urine leak compress the collecting system or vessels. The diagnosis can be established if the urine output recovers and collections decrease immediately after the reinsertion of catheter into the bladder. However, generally a creatinine value mensuration of collections is needed to differentiate urine from the lymphorrhea or seroma. Creatinine in lymph and serum are almost identical, whereas that in urine is prominently high. Various imaging modalities may be used to assist the diagnosis. Ultrasonography often may be applied first for its advantages of convenient and atraumatic, urinary extravasation can be found but usually impossible to identify the origin. Intravenous pyelography might have a positive finding if the graft function is normal and a cystogram may show the leak especially when it is situated at the anastomotic site. Radionuclide imaging can be diagnostic if a confusing case is presented.

Most ureteral leak may be cured simply by prolonged catheterization for at least 2 weeks if there is an indwelling ureteral stent. If there is no ureteral stent conservative treatment is still recommended as the initial management and quite a few leakages can be resolved. If conservative method fails, surgery is indicated. Endoscopic technique is fascinating but technically challenging, the ectopic ureteral orifice and unfixed irregular position of the ureter usually make the retrograde placement of ureteral stent a mission impossible. Percutaneous nephrostomy tube placement might be more practical if there is a hydronephosis as a result of the secondary ureteral obstruction. Therefore open surgery is recommended by many authors as a preferred management. Difficulty in locating the leak is often beyond our imagination due to the presence of extensive tissue edema. Filling and emptying the bladder intermittently, sometimes using the methylthioninium chloride, a dye, can help to identify the leak. Based on our experience, we do not recommend simple repair of the leak even if it is clear at the ureterovesical junction because ureteral stent can not be placed, more important, most leaks are a result of necrosis. Reimplantation of the ureter over a stent is a good option. If the visible necrosis is found, the transplant ureter should be cut back to where it is clearly healthy. After the removal of the necrotic part of ureter, if a tension-free anastomosis can be achieved reimplantation of the transplant ureter is usually sufficient, if not there are multiple options available to solve the problem. Above all native urinary tract should be considered, and ureteroureterostomy with the ipsilateral native ureter may be the best choice with many advantages. Boari bladder flaps are also useful if native ureter is unavailable. Boari bladder flaps have been used to bridge a loss of total ischemic ureter with a satisfactory result. But this technique reduces the bladder volume and should be selected cautiously for the "small bladder" patient from any reason. Sometimes, the bladder can be anastomosed directly to the kidney capsule with a nephrostomy tube for several weeks, but pyelovesicostomy often fail to perform due to an inability to mobilize the transplant kidney or bladder sufficiently. If the native urothelium can not be reached ileal substitution is a feasible alternative and has been reported successfully to salvage difficult and recurrent transplant urinary fistulae when native urinary tract could not be used. Appendix has been reported to replace complete necrotic ureter of pediatric recipient successfully. Recently a new minimally invasive technique of total ureteral replacement, initially described for the palliative treatment of ureteral obstructions has been introduced as an alternative to an open procedure to treat ureteral necrosis after renal transplantation. This technique is based on the use of a silicone-polytetrafluoroethylene -bonded tube tunnelled underneath the skin to bypass the graft and bladder.

7.3.2 Ureteral obstruction

The obstruction of the transplant ureter is another most common urological complication; the incidence would be probably 3% to 7%. Causes of the obstruction are miscellaneous, which can be broadly divided into extraureteral, ureteral and intraureteral. Extraureteral factors include compression from lymphocele, hematoma, urinoma, spermatic cord or adhesive band. Ureteral cause means a ureteral twist, ureteral narrowing from ischemia, infarction or fibrosis due to rejection or infection, an anastomotic site stenosis, congenital ureteropelvic junction obstruction in the donor ureter, or in exceptional condition, a ureteral inguinal hernia. Intraureteral factors involve stone, clot, sloughed renal papilla, fungal ball or foreign body. The clinical presentation of ureteral obstruction can occur in early postoperative period or years after the transplant depending on different causes, the symptoms commonly subtle, whereas the obstruction symptoms associated with a technical error usually occur early and obvious with a symptom of acute or subacute upper urinary tract obstruction and a climbing creatinine level. Hydronephrosis on ultrasound may be seen or not according to the extent of obstruction and timing of detection.

The emergent exploration should be considered if the symptoms are apparent and advancing. The original incision can be reopened, and some possible technique faults should be taken into consideration. One rare but serious fault is that the anterior transplant ureter is angulated by a careless stitch during closing the wound, in that situation, the suture should be removed and injured ureter should be repaired carefully. A redundant and twisted ureter usually needs correction by another ureteroneocystostomy. More frequently, the problem arises from the ureterovesical junction due to overtight muscular tunnel by an aggressive anti-reflux anastomosis. We prefer reimplantaion of the transplant ureter instead of simple loosen the suture over the seromuscular layer because the local edema and inflammation may proceed. Spermatic cord should be divided if it is suspected a cause of obstruction. Late ureteral stenosis is usually asymptomatic but gradual; the reason is complicated, and some of them have little relation to the surgery but most of the obstruction usually need surgical intervention for better long-term graft survival. Endoscopic technique is above all considered, unlike the urine leak, late ureteral stenosis basically accompany a hydronephrotic transplant kidney, the stricture can be diagnosed and managed in an antegrade fashion and approximately half of the patients can be cured. Balloon dilation, incision with a holmium:YAG laser or knife have been reported effective in treating transplant ureter stricture. Recurrent stricture is the main barrier for the technique as other percutaneous dilation surgery. A long-term stent is a compromise between redilation and open surgery. Open surgery is the standard way to manage the recurrent strictures, but painstaking and dangerous course is inevitable. A sufficient preparation is essential to identify the location of the stenosis, a preoperative temporary percutaneous ureteral stent is very benenifical for the assistance of locating the ureter. After finding and removing the unhealthy part of transplant ureter, the various reconstruction techniques discussed earlier can be used.

7.3.3 Vesicoureteral reflux

The exact incidence of posttranspant vesicoureteral reflux (VUR) is not known since most patients with VUR are asymptomatic and the gold standard for diagnosis, voiding cystourethrograms (VCUG), is not a routine item. When routinely checked in transplant patients in some series, the frequency of VUR varies from 1% to 86%; such a large variation can be attributed to different surgical techniques, time when VUR was tested, methods used to detect VUR, underlying urological condition, and selection criteria of the study groups. Surgical techniques are vital and controllable factors to reduce the occurrence of posttranspant VUR, therefore the non-antireflux techniques have been nearly abandoned in most of institutions. The association between VUR and urinary tract infection and reflux nephropathy has been well established in pediatric patients with native kidneys. However, the clinical significance of posttranspant VUR in the kidney transplant patients and the impact of postoperative VUR on short-term and long-term graft survival still remain controversial. Early, it was argued that VUR might be a cause of late deterioration in function, mimicking chronic rejection. Shortly after that, however, researchers suggested VUR is not a frequent cause of late renal allograft failure. A recent report has showed posttransplant VUR did not negatively affect graft function during short-term period after kidney transplantation. More recently, other authors described the presence of low-grade VUR did not affect long-term graft function in patients with late urinary tract infections. Therefore it is not necessary to screen the posttransplant VUR routinely. Positive management is only taken into account for a symptomatic posttransplant VUR. A VCUG is indicated if recurrent pyelonephritis or urinary tract infections are present, which show a symptomatic posttransplant VUR incidence of approximately 1%.

Administration of appropriate antibiotics is the primary and crucial treatment. Long-term continuous prophylaxis was sufficient in most cases. Surgical intervention is only considered for intractable cases because randomized trials of antibiotic prophylaxis versus surgical therapy plus antibiotic prophylaxis have not shown a difference in development of nonfebrile urinary tract infection in primay VUR studies. The surgery indications are recurrent febrile graft pyelonephritis or urinary tract infections refractory to antibiotic therapy and severe reflux (grade IV ~V) resulting in renal scarring or a compromising graft function. Open surgery is the standard approach to solve the problem. Reimplantation of the transplant ureter using the L-G technique has been proved to be effective and provides excellent long-term results for patients with VUR in combination with recurrent urinary tract infections after kidney transplantation. Endoscopic treatment has developed rapidly over the past decade along with the advancement of minimally invasive technique in the treatment of primary VUR. Endoscopic techniques mainly involve injection of a bulking substance into the muscular posterior wall of the ureterovesical junction. The resulting bulking effect compresses the ureteral lumen and provides a substitute for the normal muscular backing of the transmural ureter. However the overall success rates are lower than those reported for primary reflux or for open reconstruction.

7.3.4 Renal allograft rupture

Renal allograft rupture (RAR) was first described by Murray et al. in 1968. The reported incidence varies from 0.3 and 9.6%, although uncommon, it is an emergent and dangerous urological complication, potentially threatens graft and patient survival. The acute rejection is the most frequent cause of graft rapture. Acute tubular necrosis has been revealed another important risk factor comparable to severe acute rejection. Uncommon causes of RAR include renal vein thrombosis, ureteric obstruction, renal biopsy, heparin therapy, complete lymphatic legation, trauma, nephrostomy tubes and renal cell cancer development. RAR usually develops within 2-3 weeks after transplantation, however, the longest reported interval between clinical renal transplantation and renal allograft rupture was 4 years. Timing of the onset often indicated etiologies; rupture emerging in very early posttransplant period usually a result of renal vein thrombosis due to technique errors, for instance, twisting and kinking of the vein or intima tear; whereas rupture occurs later when caused by rejection. Clinical manifestations are commonly similar, presenting a sudden pain and swelling over the graft area, oliguria or anuria with hypotension and a drop in haematoglobin. Sometimes bleeding from the incision or haematuria can be found, fever is not uncommon. Clinical diagnosis may be confirmed by ultrasound or CT scan. On ultrasound a perinephric fluid collection or crescent of clot along the convex margin of the kidney usually can be revealed, sometimes, associated with extensive renal vein thrombosis. At the emergent exploration, a huge hematoma surrounding the convexity of the graft can usually be found, the rupture can occur along the convex border or at either renal pole. Do not hesitate to perform a prompt graft nephrectomy if there is an unsteady hemodynamic status. In other situations, the immediate decision of transplant nephrectomy is mainly depending on the condition of graft and experience of surgeon. Nephrectomy is almost the definite treatment for RAR in early age; however, surgical conservative treatment has been advocated by more authors over the past two decades, with a amazing reported salvage rate varying from 40~ 100%. Mattress suture of parenchyma over haemostyptic material as well as electrocautery haemostasis are the most commonly used and efficacious salvage techniques. The additional application of a mesh (Polyglactin absorbable mesh, lyophilized dura, fascia) wrapping the graft can improve the haemostasis and prevents the expansion and fragmentation of the parenchyma. In our opinion, transplant-preserving management could be attempted but not recommended when there is irreversible concomitant rejection, or a second RAR.

7.4 Lymphorrhea and lymphoceles

Lymphorrhea, also known as lymphorrhagia, is the large volume collection of lymph that drains from perigraft drainage tubes, which may develop into a lymphocele when the collection accumulates in the postoperative dead space. The clinical incidence of lymphorrhea and lymphocele is uncertain in large series varying from 0.6% to 18.1%, however, the actual rate of occurrence is unexpected high up to approximately 50% owing to the advent of ultrasound for routine graft surveillance, for that the majority of lymphatic collections are asymptomatic or subclinical. The major origin of the lymphorrhea has been identified by lymphangiography and radionuclide imaging as extravasation of the lymph from the lymphatics adjacent to the iliac vessels of the recipient due to an excessive dissection of lymphatic vessels and a failure to occlude all of the lymphatic vessels divided during the preparation of the operative bed. It still remains unexplained why unligated lymphatic vessels from the renal hilum and capsule of the graft contribute so little to the formation of a lymphocele. Despite of unavoidable dissection of lymphatics overlying the iliac vessels and potential dead space the allograft create the high occurrence of lymphocele after kidney transplantation is also closely related to the immunosuppressive regimen. Steroids adversely affected macrophage function, and more important, the mTOR inhibitors such as sirolimus and everolimus have a direct antilymphangiogenic effect and powerful antifibroblastic activity, which could prevent the healing of dissected lymph channels around the host iliac vessels. Another important contributing factor is acute cellular rejection. Obesity has been reported an independent risk factor for lymphocele formation. Low molecular weight heparin and excessive use of diuretics also have been implicated as contributing factors to lymphocele formation. Most lymphorrhea and lymphoceles are clinically silent and resolve spontaneously over time, but the clinical presentation can also be clinically evident, even presenting as 'acute abdomen'. Symptoms usually emerge at 2 weeks to 6 months after transplantation with the peak incidence at 6th week posttranplant. Symptoms may be primary or secondary, primary symptoms result from mechanical compression of lymphoceles to the adjacent strcutures such as abdominal bulging or mass, painless leg edema due to compression of ipsilateral iliofemoral vein, hydronephrosis as a result of compression of the ureter, urinary frequency or retention due to compression of the bladder neck. Secondary symptoms may be local or systematic, frequently misleading, such as ipsilateral DVT, deterioration of renal function, weight gain, hypertension and fever, even compartment syndrome. Ultrasonography is crucial to diagnosis, simple and effective. On ultrasound, lymphoceles appear as mostly anechoic or hypoechoic, rounded, perigraft fluid collections, they can have septations and multiple in number, Most noninfectious lymphoceles can be distinguished from hematomas and abscesses in term of distinctive homogeneity. Urinomas, usually around the ureter, have the similar appearance to a lymphocele, and may be distinguished by the irregular and indistinct margins owing to the lack of true wall. The accurate differential method is to measure the creatinine concentration of the liquid accommodating in the cysts by ultrasound-guided aspiration, also a way of treatment. This measure can also be used to differentiate lymphorrhea and urine leak when large volume of clear, weak yellow liquid collections appearing in perigraft drainage bag. Other adjunctive procedures such as CT, MR and intravenous pyelography are not routine diagnostic modality unless complicated cases happens or in preparation for a surgery.

It is unnecessary to deal with the small and asymptomatic collections for that most of them may resolve spontaneously; on the contrary, if large or symptomatic, an intervention may be necessary. The modality of treatment may be simple aspiration, percutaneous drainage placement, sclerotherapy and surgery. Percutaneous aspiration or drainage alone is sometimes curative, however, frequently the therapeutic effect is counteracted by the high recurrence rates and infection incurred. Because of the trait prone to recurrence, percutaneous aspiration or drainage combining the injection of sclerosants have been advocated by more authors as a simple, safe and efficacious minimally invasive method to manage the majority of lymphoceles due to a significantly fall of recurrence rates. Povidone-iodine is the classic and effective sclerosant, with which many novel sclerosants compare the therapeutic efficacy. Other potent sclerosants suggested in the literatures include the ethanol, diatrizoate and octreotide. Surgery is only indicated for refractory cases, the main purpose of surgery is to drain the lymph collections into the peritoneal cavity, known as "unroofing" or "fenestration". The procedure can be performed using either open or laparoscopic surgical techniques depending on its relationship with the allograft. If the cysts locate adjacent to peritoneal cavity, laparoscopic unroofing is an agreeable option. Surgeons can reach the lymphocele via transperitoneal approach; during the surgery the lymphocele wall is excised a 5cm disc and sutured to the peritoneum to keep the window open, a simultaneous omentoplasty has been recommended for a better resolvable effect. Laparoscopic procedures are least invasive but should be done meticulously to prevent the inadvertent lesions of the urinary tract to promote the advantages of laparoscopy. Open surgery is considered when the lymphoceles situates an improper position especially deep in pelvic beside vessels of graft, usually via a lower midline abdominal incision and a transperitoneal approach. In some conditions, previous transplant incision may be reopened for better access. It is important to ensure the lymphocele cavity is full and the bladder is empty before the operation. Intraoperative ultrasound is beneficial for localization when the operative finding is dubious.

8. Conclusion

Surgical operation is the first, critical step of a successful kidney transplant. A good few graft loss result from severe surgical complications, which are frequently associated with technique errors. Meticulous surgical technique during transplantation may help avoid majority of preventable surgical complications and related morbidity and mortality.

9. References

Bhayana, S.; Kuo, YF.; Madan, P.; Mandaym, S.; Thomas, PG.; Lappin, JA.; Rice, JC. & Ishihara, K. (2010). Pediatric en bloc kidney transplantation to adult recipients: more than suboptimal? *Transplantation*, Vol.90, No.3 (August 2010), pp. (248-254), ISSN 0041-1337

Boggi, U.; Vistoli, F.; Signori, S.; D'Imporzano, S; Amorese, G.; Consani, G.; Guarracino, F.; Melfi, F.; Mussi, A. & Mosca, F. (2011). Robotic renal transplantation: first European case. *Transplant International*, Vol.24, No.2 (February 2011), pp. (213-218), ISSN 0934-0874

Filocamo, MT.; Zanazzi, M.; Li Marzi, V.; Marzocco, M.; Guidoni, L.; Dattolo, E. & Nicita G. (2007). The approach by midline incision for extraperitoneal kidney transplantation. *Transplantation Proceedings*, Vol. 39, No. 10, (December 2007), pp. (3077-3080), ISSN 0041-1345

Furness, PD 3rd.; Houston, JB.; Grampsas, SA.; Karrer, FM; Firlit, CF. & Koyle, MA. (2001). Extraperitoneal placement of renal allografts in children weighing less than 15 kg. *Journal of Urology*, Vol.166, No.3 (September 2001), pp. (1042-1045), ISSN 0022-5347

Giulianotti, P.; Gorodner, V.; Sbrana, F.; Tzvetanov, I.; Jeon, H.; Bianco, F.; Kinzer, K.; Oberholzer, J. & Benedetti, E. (2010). Robotic transabdominal kidney transplantation in a morbidly obese patient. *American Journal of Transplantation*, Vol.10, No.6 (June 2010), pp. (1478-1482), ISSN 1600-6135

Hoznek, A.; Zaki, SK.; Samadi, DB.; Salomon, L.; Lobontiu, A.; Lang, P. & Abbou, CC. (2002). Robotic assisted kidney transplantation: an initial experience. *Journal of Urology*, Vol.167, No.4 (April 2002), pp. (1604-1606), ISSN 0022-5347

James, F. (2004). Transplantation of Abdominal Organs, In: *Sabiston Textbook of Surgery*, Seventeenth Edition, pp. (708-709), Elsevier, ISBN 0-7216-0409-9, Philadelphia, Pennsylvania, USA

John, M. (2002). Renal Transplantation, In: *Campbell's Urology*, Eighth Edition, pp. (358-359), Elsevier Science, ISBN 0–7216–9058–0, Philadelphia, Pennsylvania, USA

Jones JW. (1998). A new anastomotic technique in renal transplants reduces warm ischemia time. *Clinical Transplantation*, Vol. 12, No. 1, (February 1998), pp. (70-72), ISSN 0902-0063

Kato, T.; Selvaggi, G.; Burke, G.; Ciancio, G.; Zilleruelo, G.; Hattori, M.; Gosalbez, R. & Tzakis, A. (2008). Partial bladder transplantation with en bloc kidney transplant--the first case report of a 'bladder patch technique' in a human. *American Journal of Transplantation*, Vol.8, No.5 (May 2008), pp. (1060-1063), ISSN 1600-6135

Kayler, L.; Kang, D.; Molmenti, E.& Howard, R. (2010). Kidney transplant ureteroneocystostomy techniques and complications: review of the literature. *Transplantation Proceedings,* Vol.42, No. 5 (June 2010), pp. (1413-1420), ISSN 0041-1345

Mangus, RS.; Haag, BW.& Carter, CB. (2004). Stented Lich-Gregoir ureteroneocystostomy: case series report and cost-effectiveness analysis. *Transplantation Proceedings,* Vol.36, No.10 (May 2004), pp. (2959-2961), ISSN 0041-1345

Mital, D.; Foster, PF.; Jensik, SC.; del Rio, JV.; Sankary, HN.; McChesney, LP.& Williams, JW. (1996). Renal transplantation without sutures using the vascular clipping system for renal artery and vein anastomosis--a new technique. *Transplantation,* Vol. 62, No. 8, (October 1996), pp. (1171-1173), ISSN 0041-1337

Nanni, G.; Tondolo, V.; Citterio, F.; Romagnoli, J.; Borgetti, M.; Boldrini, G.& Castagneto, M. (2005). Comparison of oblique versus hockey-stick surgical incision for kidney transplantation. Transplantation Proceedings, Vol. 37, No. 6, (August 2005), pp. (2479-2481), ISSN 0041-1345

Nie, Z.; Zhang, K.; Huo, W.; Li, Q.; Zhu, F.& Jin, F. (2010). Comparison of urological complications with primary ureteroureterostomy versus conventional ureteroneocystostomy. *Clinical Transplantation,* Vol.24, No. 5 (October 2010), pp. (615-619), ISSN 0902-0063

Park, SC.; Kim, SD.; Kim, JI. & Moon IS. (2008). Minimal skin incision in living kidney transplantation. *Transplantation Proceedings,* Vol. 40, No. 7, (September 2008), pp. (2347-2348), ISSN 0041-1345

Sánchez, AS.; Tebar, JC.; Martín, MS.; Bachs, JM.; Moreno, MJ.; Navarro, HP. & Rodríguez, JA. (2005). Obstructive uropathy secondary to ureteral herniation in a pediatric en bloc renal graft. *American Journal of Transplantation,* Vol.5, No.8 (August 2005), pp. (2074-2077), ISSN 1600-6135

Stuart, M. (2008). Renal Transplantation, In: *Smith's general Urology,* Seventeenth Edition, pp. (547-548), Lange Medical Publication, ISBN 0-07-145737-2, New York, USA

Timsit, MO.; Lalloué, F.; Bayramov, A.; Taylor, M.; Billaut, C.; Legendre, C.; Kreis, H.; Badet, L.& Méjean, A. (2010). Should routine pyeloureterostomy be advocated in adult kidney transplantation? A prospective study of 283 recipients. *Journal of Urology,* Vol.184, No. 5 (September 2010), pp. (2043-2048), ISSN 0022-5347

Tiong, HY.; Flechner, SM.; Zhou, L.; Wee, A.; Mastroianni, B.; Savas, K.; Goldfarb, D.; Derweesh, I.& Modlin, C. (2009). A systematic approach to minimizing wound problems for de novo sirolimus-treated kidney transplant recipients. *Transplantation,* Vol.87, No.2 (January 2009), pp. (296-302), ISSN 0041-1337

Voiculescu, A.; Hollenbeck, M.; Plum, J.; Hetzel, GR.; Mödder, U.; Pfeiffer, T.; Sandmann, W& Grabensee, B. (2003). Iliac artery stenosis proximal to a kidney transplant: clinical findings, duplex-sonographic criteria, treatment, and outcome. *Transplantation,* Vol.76, No.2 (July 2003), pp. (332-339), ISSN 0041-1337

van Heurn, E & de Vries, EE. (2009). Kidney transplantation and donation in children. *Pediatric Surgery International,* Vol.25, No.5 (May 2009), pp. (385-393), ISSN 0179-0358

Wong, VK.; Baker, R.; Patel, J.; Menon, K. & Ahmad N. (2008). Renal transplantation to the ovarian vein: a case report. *American Journal of Transplantation,* Vol. 8, No. 5 (May 2008), pp. (1064-1066), ISSN 1600-6135

Ye, G.; Mo, HG.; Wang, ZH.; Yi, SH.; Wang, XW. & Zhang YF. (2006). Arterial anastomosis without sutures using ring pin stapler for clinical renal transplantation: comparison with suture anastomosis. *Journal of Urology,* Vol. 175, No. 2, (February 2006), pp. (636-640), ISSN 0022-5347

23

Novel Renal Transplant-Related Surgical Approaches in the 21st Century

Shih-Chieh Jeff Chueh and Bashir R. Sankari
Glickman Urological and Kidney Institute, Cleveland Clinic, and Cleveland Clinic Lerner College of Medicine, OH USA

1. Introduction

The surgical procedures of implanting a kidney graft into the extraperitoneal iliac fossa has not changed much since its inception in 1950s; whereas the other renal transplant-related surgical approaches have been dramatically updated recently, especially with the commencement of urological laparoscopic surgery. The mile-stone advancement is the laparoscopic live donor nephrectomy (LDN). Conventional open LDN technique has been alleged as a hurdle for expanding live donor programs. Minimally invasive surgery approaches, like laparoscopic LDN, have been advocated to overcome this obstacle (Boulware et al., 2002). A variety of laproscopic LDN approaches will be detailed.

1.1 Pre-operative evaluation of live kidney donor

The eligibility as a living donor is subject to the regulations of the respective local Health Authorities. In the United States the United Network of Organ Sharing (UNOS) operates Organ Procurement and Transplantation Network (OPTN) under contract with the Health Resources and Services Administration (HRSA) of the U.S. Department of Health and Human Services (HHS), which was established by the United States Congress under the National Organ Transplant Act (NOTA) of 1984 and provides policies of live kidney donors to be abided by. Under UNOS/OPTN policy, relatives, loved ones, friends, and even individuals who wish to remain anonymous may serve as live donors. Donating an organ is a personal decision that should only be made after fully informed about the possible risks and benefits. Live donors should be older than 18 years old, in good overall physical and mental health and free from uncontrolled high blood pressure, diabetes, cancer, HIV/AIDS, hepatitis, and organ diseases. Pre-operative assessments exclude incompatibility between the donor and the recipient and also confirm the proper functioning of the donor's bilateral kidneys, and ensure that the risks of surgery and anesthesia are acceptable (OPTN, 2006; UNOS, 2009).

1.2 Which kidney to harvest?

Usually left kidney is preferred for live donation because the left renal vein is longer, which makes the implantation surgery easier and safer. In specific situations like: complex vascular or ureteral structures of the left kidney, significant inferiority of the right renal function relative to the left, right renal stone, etc., right kidney will be harvested for transplantation.

2. Laparoscopic live donor nephrectomy

2.1 History of laparoscopic live donor nephrectomy

Kavoussi and Clayman performed first laparoscopic nephrectomy for a cancerous kidney (Clayman et al., 1991). Ratner and Kavoussi first reported a successful laparoscopic live donor nephrectomy (LLDN, Ratner et al., 1995). Initially there were concerns about graft function and donor's safety with such procedure, and only limited centers routinely performed such procedure (Jacobs et al., 2004; Su et al., 2004). With more experience it revealed non-inferiority of the LLDN results, as compared with those of the open LDN. The benefits of the LLDN include smaller wounds, less pain, earlier resumption of oral intake, and faster recuperation and earlier return to previous life style and to work. Nowadays, LLDN has been the surgery of choice for harvesting a kidney from a live donor (Kercher et al.,2003; Troppmannet al., 2003; Tooher et al., 2004; Velidedeoglu et al., 2002).

2.2 Techniques of laparoscopic live donor nephrectomy

2.2.1 Hand-assisted laparoscopic live donor nephrectomy

2.2.1.1 Immediate preoperative preparation

The most important pre-operative conditioning of the live donor is vigorous hydration to combat the detrimental effect of pneumoperitoneum on the kidney function. Usually before the kidney is harvested 3~6 liters of fluid has been given to the donor to ensure good renal perfusion and diuresis. The operation is carried out under general anesthesia; an oro- or nasogastric tube is necessary to decompress the stomach, and a urethral catheter drains the bladder and helps monitoring urine output. Continuous or frequent blood pressure monitoring during the surgery to ensure mean arterial blood pressure about 100 mmHg, and a central line to ensure central line pressure around 10 mmHg help the kidneys well perfused. At the initiation of renal hilar dissection and right before the transection of the renal vessels, 12.5 grams of Mannitol are given to protect the kidneys and to induce diuresis.

2.2.1.2 Left hand-assisted LLDN (Chueh et al., 2002a; Hollenbeck et al., 2004)

The donor is positioned in an oblique flank position with the operating table flexed at the waist and all the pressure points are well padded. First, around the navel a 7-cm midline incision is made, or alternately a Pfannenstiel incision, if the donor's body size allows the intra-abdominal hand to reach the kidney. The incision is deepened layer by layer into the peritoneal cavity. A hand-assisted device (HAD) is set-up at this site. With one hand in the abdomen through the HAD, the insertion sites of the ports are tented up by the operator's fingers to ensure safe insertion of the trocars. The working port is located in the anterior axillary line about the level of the umbilicus, and the laparoscopic port can be at the left lower abdomen between the umbilicus and the anterior superior iliac crest (making sure to avoid injuring the inferior epigastric artery) or in the midline (epigastrium) above the HAD. The pneumoperitoneum of the abdominal cavity was then insufflated up to 10-12 mmHg, and a 30 degree laparoscope is used for the whole procedure.

The dissection begins by taking down the descending colon along the white line of Toldt to expose the kidney and ureter. Special attention must be exercised to the tissue planes between the structures: the Gerota fascia and soft tissues in front of the ureter needs to be preserved with the ureter, whereas the Gerota fascia in front of the kidney can be taken down with the colon, so the color of the kidney can be visualized during the dissection and abundant soft tissues around the ureter can be preserved to ensure good blood supply to the

ureter. Initial series showed higher rate of ureteral complications and urine leakage when no special attention to preserve the ureteral blood supply was exerted (figure 1; Bartlett, 2002).
The take-down of the descending colon extends from its distal junction with the sigmoid colon up to its splenic flexure, and it further extends cranially up to the lateral parietal attachment of the spleen; i.e.: the phrenicocolic and splenophrenic ligaments are divided. This extensive take-down facilitates the colon, spleen and the pancreatic tail to fall off the main operative field and helps to harvest a long ureter (figure 1b). The intra-abdominal hand is used freely for retracting the colon, spleen and pancreas away from the operative field, and for some blunt dissection between the kidney and the surrounding soft tissues. Pressure on the kidney or the renal vessels, either by the intra-abdominal fingers or by any instruments, is absolutely forbidden.
Further dissections aim at the tributaries of the left renal vein: namely, the gonadal, adrenal and lumbar veins. The gonadal vein is dissected along its medial side and off the underlying psoas muscle; whereas the majority of its lateral border is kept intact to preserve the blood supply to the ureter, except near its entrance into the left renal vein where it is dissected circumferentially and transected to expose a window for further dissection of the lumbar vein(s) and the left renal artery. The gonadal vein is controlled and transected again distally near the iliac vessels. The lumbar vein(s) usually drain into the posterior surface of the left renal vein. Its dissection is facilitated by elevating the gonadal vein stump or the lower margin of the renal vein. The lumbar vein is often quite short and might be multiple. The division of the lumbar vein(s) further opens up the window to dissect the renal artery. The dissection of the upper margin of the left renal vein leads to the insertion point of the left adrenal vein into the renal vein, which is usually more medial to that of the gonadal vein. The adrenal vein is controlled and divided. The adrenal gland was dissected off the upper pole of the kidney with special attention not to interfere with upper pole branch(es) of the renal artery if there is any extra-hilar early branching of the renal artery.
The left renal vein is dissected medially beyond its anterior crossing of the aorta. The renal artery is first partially dissected without any grasping or compression of the artery to avoid arterial spasm. Then the lateral, posterior and superior surfaces of the kidney were dissected off its surrounding attachments along the plane of the renal capsule, while leaving some soft tissues attached to the capsule for further traction. The adipose and soft tissues around the renal hilum and those in the triangle between the low pole of the kidney and the ureter (golden triangle, figure 1b*) are preserved to ensure adequate blood flow to the ureter.
The posterior and superior surfaces of the renal artery are then further freed when the kidney is flipped forward. The arterial dissection is carried out proximally to include its take-off from the aorta in order to facilitate retrieving longer artery.
The ureter is dissected medial to the gonadal vein to leave abundant tissues around it all the way down to its crossing at the iliac vessels, where it is transected immediately before the division of the renal pedicle to avoid torsion of the kidney (figure 1a and 1b). Only the distal ureter is clipped, and the proximal end of the ureter is left open to observe and ensure brisk urine output. The dissection of the upper pole and posterior-upper part of the kidney sometimes might be difficult because of the limited angles of the pivot function of the laparoscopic ports. Special care must be exerted not to put pressure on the renal parenchyma during this part of the dissection.
After making sure that the kidney is attached to the body only by the renal vessels the kidney is held up gently with the intra-abdominal hand, and the renal artery is first ligated at its origin from the aorta. Then the renal vein is controlled at the point of its crossing to the

aorta or even more medially if the dissection allows. This sequence of vessel ligations prevents congestive stasis of blood in the kidney. The control of the renal pedicles have been performed with either a standard laparoscopic vascular stapler (usually 3 rows of staplers on both sides of a dividing knife), Endo TA™ 30 stapler (only a triple staggered row of titanium staples, Covidien), polymer locking clips (Hem-o-lok, Weck, Teleflex), or laparoscopic metal clips (for artery only). The Endo TA stapler and the polymer locking clips provide the advantage of preserving maximal graft vascular length, which makes the implantation vascular anastomosis easier; whereas the use of conventional laparoscopic vascular stapler sacrifices 4 mm of the graft vascular length because 3 rows of staggered staplers at the end of the vessels need to be excised before anastomosis.

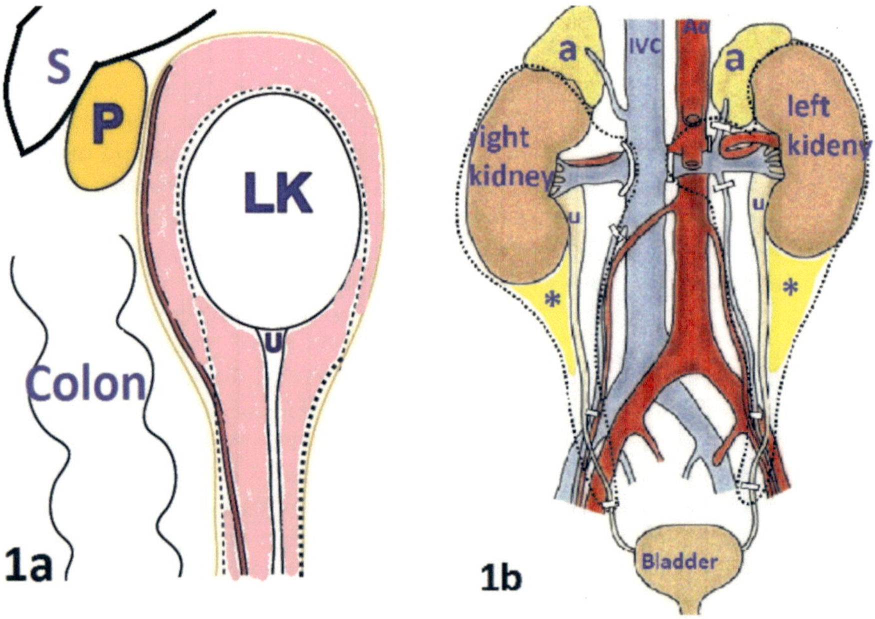

Fig. 1. Schematic planes of dissection during various nephrectomies. 1a. sagittal view. LK= left kidney, P= pancreatic tail, S= spleen, u= left ureter, painted pink area= perirenal soft tissues inside Gerota's fasia, dotted line= dissection plane during LDN, red line= anterior dissection plane during radical nephrectomy. 1b. coronal view. a= adrenal gland, Ao= aorta, IVC= inferior vena cava, u= ureter, *= Golden triangle, tubular structures painted in red= arteries, tubular structures painted in blue= veins, rectangle areas over vessels or ureter= sites of ligating vessels or ureter, dotted lines= planes of dissection during LDN.

Even though there have been several papers reporting successful applications of Hem-o-lok clips in controlling the pedicles during LLDN (Chueh et al., 2004; Ponsky et al., 2008), however, LLDN had been indicated by the manufacturer of the Hem-o-lok clip as a contraindication for the use of the polymer locking clips in 2006, and FDA announced a product recall, too (FDA, 2006), because Hem-o-lok clips may become dislodged following ligation of the renal artery after laparoscopic donor nephrectomy; and cases of delayed bleeding leading to severe morbidities or even mortality of the donor after using the Hem-o-lok clips. This issue has been further pointed out when UNOS first sent a notice to its members and FDA regarding the Hem-o-lok clip in 2008. More recently, UNOS and

American Society of Transplant Surgeon (ASTS) again sent a letter to their members to emphasize the importance of this issue, and urge the centers those perform live donor nephrectomy not use this clip for LLDN. Possible technical explanations for the complication might be related to that some harvesting surgeon just applied one Hem-o-lok clip over the artery in order to retrieve longer artery, and the Hem-o-lok clip slipped off an arterial stump that was left too short, or due to that the polymer clip(s) were weakened because of some thermal energy damage during the operation, and they fell apart in a couple days later. Hence, Endo TA™ 30 stapler is our current preference because of its ability of ensuring arterial seal and of harvesting longer vessels. Cold scissors cut of the renal pedicle vessels lateral (distal) to the stapler lines of the TA stapler completely frees the kidney, and the kidney is immediately retrieved out of the abdomen via the HAD wound to the back table for ex vivo perfusion and bench preparation in ice slush.

Once the kidney is delivered to the back table, the harvesting surgeon re-establishes the HAD and the pneumoperitoneum for meticulous hemostasis. Laparoscopic suction and irrigation are freely used to locate the bleeders. Attention is first focused on the transected ends of pedicles, and then the adrenal bed, lumbar vein stump, and lymphatic openings. The pneumoperitoneum is progressively decreased to 5 mmHg to ensure all minor bleeders are detected and securely controlled. Usually a drainage tube is not necessary.

The procedural sequences of LLDN are different from those of other types of laparoscopic nephrectomies because the renal pedicles are usually first ligated in the later circumstances, but in the former the pedicle vessels are initially dissected from the surrounding tissues, yet not ligated until the whole kidney is ready to be retrieved. This is to ensure a shortest warm ischemic time (WIT) of the harvested kidney for a better graft function after implantation.

A pinkish kidney with tense tone of the renal cortex and a well distended renal vein during the dissection indicate good perfusion of the kidney (and usually translated into immediate graft functioning after transplantation). But if the color is dusky or pale, or the tone of the kidney is floppy, or the renal vein is collapsed during the dissection, it indicates that the kidney is not adequately perfused and thus requires immediate attention and corrections of the donor's conditions by the surgeon and the anesthetic team must be executed. Maneuvers that might help include: more vigorous hydration, elevating the blood pressure and vasodilation of the renal artery with pharmaceutical agents, decrease the pressure of the pneumoperitoneum (5~8 mmHg), correction of any kinking or spasm of the renal artery, etc.

2.2.1.3 Right hand-assisted LLDN (Buell et al., 2004; Chueh et al., 2002a)

Only the procedural differences from the above-mentioned left hand-assisted LLDN are described below. The donor is placed similarly but with the right side up. The first camera port at the umbilicus is safely placed. After CO_2 insufflation to create pneumoperitoneum, a 7-cm subcostal oblique line corresponding to the level of right renal pedicle is marked on the skin. Three working ports, 2 at the ends of the marked line and 1 at the anterior axillary line between iliac bone and lower costal margin, are inserted. The ascending colon and the 2nd portion of the duodenum are taken down to expose the kidney and the inferior vena cava (IVC). After division of the right gonadal vein near its insertion into the IVC, and preliminary dissection of the renal pedicle and right ureter, the incision between the two working ports is connected to set-up the HAD and the surgeon's hand is inserted. The dissection of the right renal artery is done mainly when the kidney is flipped medially to expose its posterior surface. After all the dissections are completed, the ureter is transected. Then the hand is removed from the HAD, and the pneumoperitoneum is desufflated, while leaving the base wound retractor of the HAD still in place. This creates a window large enough for division of the vessels with traditional Satinsky vascular clamp to yield a full-length right renal vein with a partial IVC cuff. After the kidney is retrieved to the back table, the defect in the IVC is closed with 4-0 Prolene continuous sutures in 2 layers for meticulous hemostasis. Then the Satinsky vascular clamp is released. Some right renal donors might have longer renal vein, which can be measured from the Computed Tomography angiographic images preoperatively during the donor evaluation. In that case the HAD wound for the hand and for extracting the kidney can be moved down to a periumbilical, right Gibson, or Pfannenstiel incision. And the right kidney, after totally freed from the surrounding tissues, is pulled up laterally during the application of the Endo TA stapler, which is then pushed as medially as possible at the junction of right renal vein and the IVC to harvest a renal vein at its maximal length.

2.2.2 Pure laparoscopic live donor nephrectomy

The basic concept, planes of dissection, and the majority of the "pure laparoscopic" approach are very similar to those of the hand-assisted approach. The followings will only depict the differences:

2.2.2.1 Pure left LLDN

A working instrument, which usually enters into the operative field through a left subcostal port, substitutes all the functions of the intra-abdominal hand in the HAD approach. Without the HAD, the laparoscopic port can be at the umbilicus or left upper abdomen, depending on the body habitus of the donor. The port for the right-hand instrument is located at the same position. Another 15 mm port is created along the Pfannenstiel incision, which is later extended to 5-6 cm, with muscle split in the midline for the final extraction of the harvested kidney. An extra-large retrieving bag- EndoCatch II (Covidien, Mansfield, MA, USA) is employed through that port for helping traction during the dissection and for retrieving the kidney. Once all the dissections have been done and the ureter has been transected, the EndoCatch II is partially activated to "bag" the kidney and the ureter into the EndoCatch II bag while the edge of the bag and the string are still attached to its metallic ring; in this way, the renal pedicles can be tented up tight by elevating the Endocatch II ring (kidney) in the air. This tremendously facilitates the ligation of the renal pedicles and ensures long vessel length of the graft.

2.2.2.2 Pure right LLDN (Boorjian et al., 2004; Johnson et al., 2001)

Procedures are similar to those of pure left LLDN. The main differences are: 1. The ascending colon and the 2nd portion of duodenum, instead of the descending colon, pancreatic tail and the spleen, are taken down. 2. The right gonadal vein usually drains into the inferior vena cava (IVC), but it might also drain into the right renal vein directly. 3. There might be some small, thin-walled, innominate veins, which have higher chance to cause bleeding, draining into the right renal vein. 4. The wall of the right renal vein is thin, in comparison to that of the left renal vein, which is more prone to tear or bleeding during the procedures. 5. The length of the right renal vein is usually only 1-2 cm in length, which is much shorter than that of the left renal vein. 6. During the dissection of the upper pole of the right kidney, retraction of liver is usually necessary for better exposure. Once the kidney is completely dissected with only the renal vessels attached to the body, the kidney is bagged into the EndoCatch bag, and lifted high to tent up the renal pedicles. The right renal artery is stapled behind the IVC, and the renal vein is stapled at the IVC where it drains into, both with the Endo TA stapler, and then both vessels are transected immediately lateral (distal) to the staplers.

2.2.3 Retroperitoneoscopic live donor nephrectomy

Several teams (Bachmann et al., 2008; Sundqvist et al., 2004; Tanabe et al., 2005; Kohei et al., 2010) published successful series of retroperitoneoscopic LDN. Tanabe's revised technique usually employs a 3-port dissection technique combined with a Pfannenstiel 5-cm retrieving wound to accomplish the surgery.

The donor is in a lateral flank position, but the table is not bent. It requires a flexible laparoscope inserted through a mid-axillary port between the lower costal margin and the iliac crest, and a very experienced and skillful assistant as the telescope holder to collaborate with the operator. The surgeon develops the retroperitoneal working space, and dissects the kidney off the surrounding tissues with a pure retroperitoneoscopic dissection technique under a low 5-10 mmHg pressure of pneumo-retroperitoneum. After the kidney is totally freed (except the vascular pedicles), that Pfannestiel wound is deepened to the extraperitoneal space to connect to the previously dissected retroperitoneal space, then a Lapdisc (Hakko Medical, Tokyo, Japan) is setup at that incision and an Endocatch II retrieving device is inserted through the Lapdisc to harvest the kidney. Laparoscopic EndoGIA Stapler (Covidien, Mansfield, MA, USA) is used to control the renal artery and renal vein, or even larger gonadal vein or lumbar vein during the dissection.

The benefits of such an approach are early and direct dissection of the renal artery, no violation of the intraperitoneal organs, bowels, etc., and theoretically might lead to less post-operative ileus or bowel injury. The risks and challenges are that the retroperitoneal working space is much smaller and it is more technically demanding to operate in such circumstance without exerting unnecessary pressure on the kidney.

Summarizing their experiences with a total of more than 600 live donors operated via such approach shows that the chance of open conversion was low, and the complication rates were 4.9~ 7.7 %. Mean warm ischemia time was 2.2- 4.8 minutes. And the recipients' allograft function recovered smoothly. Thus, in experienced hands retroperitoneoscopic LDN seems provide similar outcome as compared with those of laparoscopic LDN.

2.3 Comments and summary of laparoscopic LDN

Evidences showed that the post-operative pain and quality of life of the donors, either operated by the hand assisted approach or the pure laparoscopic approach are similar, and both are significantly better that those of the traditional open approach (Velidedeoglu et al., 2002; Kercher et al., 2003; Troppmann et al., 2003; Mjøen et al., 2010; Leventhal et al., 2010). Laparoscopic LDN has evolved to be the surgery of choice for live kidney donors. Yet the bottom line issues are still the donor's safety and the functional integrity of the kidney graft. The donor surgeons should work in the way that they are most confident with and have very low threshold of converting to an approach with bigger incision to ensure the ultimate basic principles. For beginners it might be easier and safer to start with the hand-assisted approach, but this approach is ergonomically not friendly; and also poses some difficulty in fine handling and traction of the tissues by the left hand (fingers). Even though with the most experienced LLDN surgeon, there should always be a set of open exploration instruments immediately available in the operation suite during the LDN surgery; and the threshold of converting to a safer procedure should always be low.

3. Laparoendoscopic Single Site (LESS) live donor nephrectomy

Through the last 2 decades of developing minimally invasive surgery, urological laparoscopic surgery has gained more acceptance as a standard of care in various intra-abdominal procedures. Novel endeavors to advance this field are aimed at further mitigating morbidity and improving cosmetic outcomes. This trend has led to the development of multi-channel single-access ports, articulating instruments, and surgical techniques that could allow the laparoscopic procedures to be performed through a single small skin incision (laparoendoscopic single-site [LESS] surgery). The majority of such reports often hide the incision within the umbilicus, and transperitoneal route is typically employed. There have been reports of LESS live donor nephrectomy (LDN) in some elite transplant centers (Gill et al., 2008; Gimenez etal., 2010., Andonian et al., 2010a). We recently also successfully completed 4 cases of LESS LDN with speedy convalescence of the donors, and smooth recovery of the recipients' graft function.

3.1 Technique of LESS LDN

3.1.1 Belly-Button LESS LDN (Chueh and Sankari, submitted, 2011)

We will depict our technique of LESS LDN performed through a small incision at the belly-button. The donor is placed in a 60 degree flank position as in the pure laparoscopic LDN. A first layer transparent adhesive drape is applied over the whole abdomen after it has been prepped and draped. A 4.5 ~5-cm vertical midline incision is made around the umbilicus, and the wound is deepened layer by layer until the peritoneum cavity is entered. A GelPort® hand-assisted device (HAD) is setup at this wound. A second layer transparent adhesive drape is then applied over the abdomen, which also covers the whole GelPort and obliterates intra-operative gas leakage from the central pre-made entry/exit hole of the gel-cap. Thus the GelPort is used as the access platform for the following LESS LDN.

A 12-mm port is inserted through the gel-cap portion of the GelPort at its periphery part, but not right at the margin of its rigid ring. Pneumoperitoneal insufflation is started and a 30-degree 5 or 10-mm laparoscope is used to examine the peritoneal cavity. Another 2 laparoscopic ports, one 5-mm and one 12-mm in size, are inserted through the gel-cap portion of the GelPort under direct vision; again at the periphery of the gel-cap, forming a triangular relationship with the first port, and each port stays away from the others as far as possible. Then with a grasper in the non-dominant hand, and a cutting device in the dominant hand, the colon is taken down to expose the kidney. Most of the time two straight instruments can be used at the same time, or a grasper with a flexible angled tip and a straight cutting instrument might work better at some situations.

Then the other following procedures are very similar to those of the pure laparoscopic LDN described above. In case of difficulty dissections (e.g.: distended colon obscuring clear visualization of the renal hilum, or some bleeding requiring efficient suction to localize the bleeder), a third 5-mm working port can be inserted through the Gel-cap at a point away from the other ports for a 3rd instrument to provide effective traction or suction. The dilemma of adding the 3rd or more instruments is that although it might provide better operative field, the sword-fighting limited angles of the crowded instruments through the LESS incision might also make smooth progression of the procedures difficult. Hence the decision of how many ports necessary should be evaluated individually.

When the kidney is only attached to the body by the renal pedicles, and the ureter has been transected at its crossing of the iliac vessels, an extra-large EndoCatch II (Covidien) is separately inserted through the gel-cap either directly or through a 15-mm port for retrieving the kidney. The EndoCatch II is opened to "bag" the kidney and its proximal ureter into the retrieval bag while the edge of the bag and the string are still attached to its metallic ring. Thus, the renal pedicles can be tightly tented up by elevating the Endocatch II ring in the air. This significantly opens up the space of the renal vessels with their body attachments (aorta and IVC) and facilitates the ligation of the renal pedicles and ensures long vessel length of the graft. The ligation of the renal artery and the renal vein is performed by applying the laparascopic Endo TA stapler (Covidien), and then the vessels are transected distal to the staple lines with scissors. If there are 2 or more renal arteries, they can be controlled separately by Endo TA staplers, or the smaller artery can ligated with Hem-o-lok or metal clips (at least 2 to 3 clips are necessary). The smaller artery is ligated first to shorten the warm ischemic time of the major portion of the kidney.

At this point, the kidney is totally freed, and the string of the EndoCatch is pulled to detach the retrieval bag from the metallic ring to keep the kidney in the bag, the 2nd layer of the transparent adhesive drape is cut around the external ring of the GelPort, and the gel-cap is released from its base fascial retractor to harvest the kidney easily without squeezing it.

Then the GelPort device is quickly assembled again, and the pneumoperitoneum is re-insufflated for meticulous hemostasis. The pressure of pneumoperitoneum is decreased to 5 mmHg to detect even mild venous or lymphatic oozing. Usually no drain tube is necessary. The GelPort devise is removed, and the wound is closed in a standard fashion.

3.1.2 Pfannenstiel LESS Live Donor Nephrectomy (Andonian et al., 2010a)

This technique is pioneered by Kavoussi et al. Their main benefit is to hide the skin incision line low in the supra-pubic area, instead of via the belly-button. Through a 5-cm Pfannenstiel incision, three 5-mm ports are placed in a triangular manner (2 at the midline [5 cm apart], and 1 at the ipsilateral rectus mucle 5 cm from the inferior port in the midline). A 5 mm flexible-tip laparoscope (EndoEye, Olympus, Japan), along with other long bariatric laparoscopic instruments, is used to perform laparoscopic donor nephrectomy in the fashion similar to the pure laparoscopic LDN. Before ligating the renal hilum, the superior midline trocar is exchanged for a 12-mm trocar to allow for an Endo-GIA stapler. After the kidney is placed in the entrapment sac, the anterior rectus fascia between the 2 midline ports is incised and the kidney is removed. After closure of the fascial defects, the Pfannenstiel incision is closed in a subcuticular manner.

Its initial outcomes are successfully in 6 patients without standard laparoscopic or open conversion; and no additional needlescopic instruments used. The median operative time, median warm ischemia time (5 minutes), and median hospital stay are similar to those of the case-matched standard laparoscopic (SL) approach. Although VAS (visual analog pain scale) scores were lower in the LESS versus SL group at each of post-operative day (POD) #2 (1.5 vs. 4) and discharge (0 vs. 2), this did not reach statistical significance (Andonian et al., 2010b).

3.2 Comments and summary of LESS LDN

The benefit of using the GelPort® as the access platform for the LESS LDN in our series is its feasibility of conversion to a standard multiple-port laparoscopic LDN or even a hand-assisted LDN in case any difficult dissections or significant bleeding occur during the procedure of LESS LDN. This offers an immediate 'exit strategy', because considerable and difficult-to-control bleedings might suddenly happen anytime during the procedure, and endangers the safety of the donor or the function of the graft. No matter what approach of

LDN is performed, cannot the bottom-line principles of ensuring the safety of the live donor and good quality of the kidney harvested be over-emphasized. Only when these 2 basic important principles can be strictly upheld, can we pursue the smaller incision and smoother recovery of the live donors. Thus, during the procedure of LESS LDN the threshold of conversion to a conventional laparoscopic LDN (either pure-laparoscopic or hand-assisted approach) should be kept low to protect the donor and the kidney. In case of a significant bleeding that cannot be adequately secured or a situation that endangers function of the kidney (e.g.: prolonged warm ischemic time), instead of continuing struggles with the LESS approach it is recommended to compress or grasp the bleeder with a grasper, and then add one or more ports outside the LESS platform, or even insert a hand into the operating field to control the situation. Use of a GelPort™ as the LESS platform during LDN gives the flexibility of different degrees of speedy conversions.

Even though there have been multiple reports demonstrating the feasibility of LESS LDN, one important basic question not well-answered so far is how many benefits or disadvantages to the live donors this technique provides in comparison to the conventional laparoscopic LDN. The answer to this question can only be achieved by an adequately powered multi-center prospective randomized comparison using tools designed to detect subtle differences in morbidity and to assess cosmetic satisfaction. The other issue is regarding the cost of the surgery. A recent report by Lunsford et al concludes that Single-site laparoscopic living donor nephrectomy offers comparable perioperative outcomes to conventional laparoscopic living donor nephrectomy at a higher cost. (Lunsford et al., 2011) More reports with detailed economic analyses are required to answer this question.

4. Other renal transplant-related laparoscopic procedures

Besides laparoscopic donor nephrectomy there are other laparoscopic or novel procedures feasible among ESRD patients with a transplant kidney (Fornara et al., 1997). These procedures aim at either problems related to the transplanted kidneys (e.g.: lymphocele, tumor in transplant kidney); or problems related to the native kidneys (e.g.: polycystic kidneys, renal cell carcinomas). Their respective details are described as follows:

4.1 Laparoscopic marsupialization of lymphoceles

Lymphocele development after renal transplantation is a well-recognized possible complication that occurs with the incidence of 0.6-26%. Lymphoceles may originate either from the lymphatic system of the recipient or the transplanted kidney. Before the laparoscopic era, the standard treatment of symptomatic lymphoceles is first puncture aspiration to differentiate between urinoma/lymphocele and to test for bacterial infection; then percutaneous drainage, with or without the injection of sclerosing solution; and finally, open marsupialization if initial approaches fail. With the advent of laparoscopic surgery, laparoscopic approaches to remove an ellipse of peritoneal wall along with the adjacent lymphocele wall, to lyse all internal lymphocele loculations, and even tuck in a piece of omentum by laparoscopic suture allow for the free flow of lymph into the peritoneal cavity and remove the pressure effect of the lymphocele on the transplant kidney, graft ureter, and even venous drainage can be achieved (Parra et al., 1992; Khauli et al., 1992).

There are many caveats in performing such procedure. Several cases of graft ureter transaction have been reported. Thus, pre-operative stenting the graft ureter should be performed whenever possible. (Abou-Elela et al., 2006; Shokeir et al., 1994). Multiple septa and loculations of the lymphoceles might lead to early recurrence or failure of the surgery. Tricks to deal with this circumstance includes transcutaneous staining of the lymphocele lining with methylene blue, and use of intraoperative ultrasonography (Schilling et al., 1995; Matin & Gill, 2001). Other tips for anatomically difficult lymphoceles lateral or inferior to the transplant kidney, which without a common wall between the lymphocele and peritoneal cavities has been reported by placing a cable of 2 internalized peritoneal dialysis catheters between the lymphoceles and the peritoneal cavity for maintaining permanent lymphoperitoneal drainage (Matin & Gill, 2000). Other potential problems associated with laparoscopic marsupialization of lymphoceles consist of injury to other organs (6%), and open conversion (6%) (Atray et al., 2004; Gruessner et al.,1995).

4.2 Laparoscopic nephrectomy for renal cell carcinoma or polycystic kidneys in native kidneys

Laparoscopic nephrectomy has been shown effective in removing diseased kidneys with tumors, even tumors larger than 7-cm in diameter. (Berger et al., 2008; Steinberg et al., 2004) Long-term oncologic outcomes (overall, cancer-specific, and recurrence-free survivals) of laparoscopic radical nephrectomy, either with pure laparoscopic or HAD technique, or with trans-peritoneal or trans-retroperitoneal approach, for renal cell carcinoma (RCC) are comparable to those of its open counterpart, with the obvious benefits of less pain, less blood loss and earlier recuperation (Colombo et al., 2008; Chung et al., 2007; Venkatesh et al., 2007; Desai et al., 2005; Nambirajan et al., 2004).

Patients with ESRD are known to have higher surgical risks (higher American Society of Anesthiologists score, higher comorbidity index, higher incidence of previous abdominal surgery, and higher incidence of hypertension), and yet they also have higher incidence of renal tumors and which does not decrease even after renal transplantation because of maintenance immunosuppression (Chueh SC et al., 2011a; Melchior et al., 2011; Navarro et al., 2008; Tollefson et al., 2010). Laparoscopic radical nephrectomy among this special patient group, even though more challenging and might be associated with slightly longer admission and higher perioperative risks, is well recognized as feasible and safe (Bird et al., 2010). Recently, there was even report of successful LESS radical nephrectomy among these patient groups (Greco et al., 2010; Chueh et al., 2011b).

Technically, laparoscopic radical nephrectomy is similar to that of the previously mentioned LDN, with their main differences depicted are as follows: 1). The sequence/ timing of pedicle ligation: during LDN in order to shorten the warm ischemic time the renal artery and renal vein are ligated right before retrieving the kidney; whereas during radical nephrectomy in order to decrease the chance of tumor cell seeding along the vessels, renal artery and vein are controlled as early as possible and before further mobilization of the whole kidney. 2). The plane of dissection (figure 1a): during LDN peri-renal fat and soft tissues are not necessary and Gerota's fascia is opened to reveal the color and tone of the kidney during the dissection; whereas during radical nephrectomy dissection is made along outside the Gerota's fascia to encompass all the soft tissues around the kidney to ensure enbloc resection. Adrenal gland is spared during LDN but it is excised during radical nephrectomy if the tumor is in the upper pole or no clear plane between the tumor and adrenal gland discerned on the images (Siemer et al., 2004). Abundant soft tissues around the ureter are mandatory during LDN; whereas ureter can be stripped during radical nephrectomy unless urothelial carcinoma is suspected preoperatively. 3). Method of specimen extraction: Some urologists morcellate the kidneys for cancerous renal specimen of radical nephrectomy to achieve key-hole wounds, whereas at least a 5-cm incision needs to be made to harvest the LDN kidney. 4). Laparoscopic setting: during LDN the pressure of the pneumoperitoneum is kept as low as possible (usually around 10-12 mmHg or less) to avoid interfering the renal perfusion and subsequent graft function; whereas during radical nephrectomy a pneumoperitoneum of 15 mmHg is usually employed.

Polycystic kidney disease (PCKD) might lead to ESRD, and renal transplant is a well-known therapy for those patients. Indications for native nephrectomies among those PCKD patients include severe fullness and early satiety, abdominal pain, recurrent urinary tract infections, recurrent hematuria, poorly controlled hypertension, need space for future transplant; and suspicion of malignancy in the enlarged kidneys. Laparoscopic nephrectomy for PCKD kidneys has been shown as a viable alternative of its open counter-part. Either transperitoneal or retroperitoneoscopic approach is feasible. Retroperitoneoscopic approach provides quicker and direct access to the renal hilum, but requires separate port wounds on each side of the body. And many papers reported the use of HAD facilitate the dissection and excision of the diseased PCKD kidneys. When compared to open surgery, the laparoscopic approach results in significantly shorter hospital stay, decreased morbidity and quicker recovery (Rehman et al., 2001; Gill et al., 2001). The use of Vacuum Curettage System (Berkeley VC-10, ACMI, Southborough, MA) to morcellate and aspirate the kidney was reported to provide a significant decrease in the overall size and allow easy extraction through the midline incision (Whitten et al., 2006).

As to when is the best timing to do the surgery, and whether simultaneous bilateral or staged surgery is safer for the patients are still in dispute. Some articles reported 60% complication rate if performed simultaneously, and thus recommend staged operation. Another report mentioned renal transplantation and ipsilateral native PCKD nephrectomy carry no significant additional morbidity compared to that of renal transplantation alone (Ismail et al., 2005; Lucas et al., 2010).

4.3 Laparoscopic nephroureterectomy and bladder cuff eecision for localized urothelial carcinomas in native upper urinary tract

Standard treatment for localized urothelial carcinoma (UC) of the upper urinary tract (UUT) is nephroureterectomy with resection of the ipsilateral distal ureter and bladder cuff. Since Clayman et al. reported in 1991 the initial case of laparoscopic nephroureterectomy (LNU), there have been reports demonstrating that LNU decreases pain and accelerates convalescence of patients (Jarrett et al., 2001). It can be done either with pure laparoscopic approach or with the help of a hand-assisted device (McNeill et al., 2000; Gill et al., 2000; Shalhav et al., 2000; Chen et al., 2001).

Operative technique of a hand-assisted nephroureterectomy (HALNU; Chen et al., 2001): The patient is placed in a 60° oblique position with no change in posture during the entire procedure. The operating table can be rotated from side to side to facilitate exposure during different parts of the surgery. Via a 7-cm lower abdominal Gibson incision, distal ureterectomy with bladder cuff resection was done according to the classic open maneuver. If this is on the side of the transplant kidney cautions need to be exerted to prevent interfering with the transplant ureter. The bladder is closed so that it is watertight with 2-0 absorbable sutures. The end of the distal ureter was double ligated, wrapped with a 4 x 4 gauze, tied up, and left in the retroperitoneum. Then a hand-assisted device (HAD) is set up at this incision, and pneumoperitoneum is insufflated. Two laparoscopic ports are inserted, under the guidance of the intraperitoneal hand and telescope. A 30° telescope is used.

Nephroureterectomy is then performed similarly to those described. The surgeon and the assistant, both facing the patient's abdomen, stand side by side. For a left HALNU, if the surgeon is ambidextrous, he/she inserts his/her right hand intraperitoneally, and operates the laparoscopic instrument with his/her left hand. If he/she is right-handed, the operator's left hand is placed intraperitoneally. For a right HALNU, the surgeon inserts his/her left hand into the HAD. After the colon is taken down, the renal vessels are first identified, dissects, then ligated and transected. An adrenalectomy is performed only when the tumor involved the upper pole parenchyma of the kidney in image studies. Then the kidney and the entire length of the ureter with the surrounding tissues are excised and removed en-bloc from the lower abdomen incision made for the HAD.

4.4 Simultaneous laparoscopic bilateral nephroureterectomy (nephrectomy) without changing body position

The incidence of UC is higher in patients with ESRD, especially in some Asian countries and countries with Balkan Nephropathy and the carcinomas are often multifocal (Liao et al., 2004). When there is UC in either one or both sides of the upper urinary tract in ESRD patients, the treatment of choice usually is simultaneous bilateral nephroureterectomy. Traditionally, open simultaneous bilateral nephroureterectomy is usually done via a long midline incision extending from the xyphoid to the symphysis pubis. To perform unilateral LNU smoothly, the patient has to be positioned at 60° oblique to a full lateral flank position for better exposure and easier dissection because the surrounding organs are displaced downward by gravity (Jarrett et al., 2001; McNeill et al., 2000; Gill et al., 2000; Shalhav et al., 2000). For laparoscopic bilateral nephroureterectomy (LBNU) to be completed in one session with the above-mentioned approach, one needs to do additional position changes to perform the nephroureterectomy on the contralateral side. This is cumbersome and prolongs operation time, and patients need to be re-sterilized and re-draped. The following is an easy and convenient maneuver to facilitate and speed up the operation.

Operative technique (Chueh et al., 2002): Two 6-inch-wide inflatable cuffs (an air tourniquet device originally used for damping blood flow during orthopedic surgery on extremities), one on each side of the back, are placed underneath the patient. The patient is placed in a supine position with his/her chest, shoulders, and thighs loosely secured by straps to the operation table, so that there is some room for the air cuff to lift the patient upwards when it is inflated. And thus the patient would not slide off the table when the table is maximally rotated to its side. Possible pressure-bearing areas (when the table is rotated and the cuff is inflated) like both sides of the thighs, hips, axillae, and shoulders and other bony prominences were well padded with soft gel pads (Action Product, Hagertown, MD, USA) to avoid neuromuscular injuries.

To begin the operation, a 7 cm infra-umbilical midline incision is made for the HAD, and a telescopic port is created immediately supra-umbilically to hide this scar. The operator and the assistant stand on the contra-lateral side of the kidney to be operated first. Then the air cuff on the ipsilateral side of the target kidney is inflated (up to 400 mmHg), and the operation table is rotated completely to the contra-lateral side (facing the operator). This brought the patients into a ~60° oblique position which make dissection of the ipsilateral kidney, ureter, and especially the renal pedicles much easier because the surrounding organs will slide down due to gravity after they are taken down from their original attachments. A 12-mm port was inserted in the ipsilateral abdomen at the midclavicular line slightly higher than the level of the umbilicus. If there is difficulty during dissection, another 5-mm port (optional) can be inserted at the sub-xyphoid midline. For hand-assisted laparoscopic nephroureterectomy (HALNU) on the left side, the surgeon inserts his/her left hand into the HAD, stands caudal to the assistant, and operates the laparoscopic instruments with his/her right hand.

For a right HALNU, if the surgeon is ambidextrous, he/she inserts his/her right hand intraperitoneally, stands caudal to the assistant and operates the laparoscopic instrument with his/her left hand. If he/she is right-handed, the assistant stands caudal to him/her, and the surgeon's left hand is placed intraperitoneally (the main 12-mm working port is moved to the right upper quadrant in this circumstance). The middle to lower ureter is first dissected and ligated (without cutting) with clips distal to the tumor to avoid squeezing tumor cells into the bladder during dissection. Then the hand-assisted laparoscopic nephrectomy is performed similarly to those described. The adrenal gland is not excised unless preoperative studies strongly suggested invasion of the tumor into the upper-pole parenchyma of the kidney. After transecting the renal pedicles and freeing the kidney and upper ureter, the specimen could be placed down to the ipsilateral pelvic cavity for later en bloc removal at the final stage of the surgery.

After completing the first side, the 12-mm working port wound on that side is closed in an air-tight manner, and the table is tilted completely to the other side. The air cuff on the first side is deflated, and insufflation of the cuff underneath the other side of the patient proceeds. The surgical team moves to the other side of the table (the side on which the kidney has been excised), inserts a new 12-mm port, and the nephroureterectomy on the second side is performed similarly. In patients with a functional renal graft, a 5-Fr. ureteral catheter was inserted into the graft ureter cystoscopically before the entire laparoscopic procedure to assist identification and protection of the graft kidney and ureter during later dissection.

After the above-mentioned procedures are done, in order to ensure complete resection of the distal ureter and bladder cuff, the operative table is brought back to a neutral position and both air cuffs are deflated. Traditional bladder cuff resection and bladder closure on both sides are performed in an open fashion through the lower midline wound originally made for the HAD. When a transplant kidney is present, dissection of the native lower ureter stays just medial to the lateral border of the native ureter on that specific side. If difficult dissection is encountered (e.g.: a heavy patient with a deep pelvic cavity and/or a patient with a stage T2-T3 lower ureteral tumor), the wound can be extended further towards the symphysis pubis to provide a clearer operative field, and two complete sets of nephroureterectomy specimens are subsequently brought out of the wound.

An intermediate term (median 35 months) follow-up of a total of 40 patients who were identified to have pathologically confirmed urothelial carcinoma of upper urinary tract, either operated by HALBNU (n=25) or by its open counterpart (OBNU, n=15) revealed that the HALBNU group was associated with less blood loss, earlier bowel recovery, less narcotic use, shorter hospital stay, and earlier convalescence. The operative time and complication rate were comparable between the two groups. There was no open conversion in the HALBNU group. The overall, cancer-specific, and bladder-recurrence-free survival were all equivalent between the HALBNU and OBNU group (Tai et al., 2009).

5. Partial nephrectomy for transplanted kidneys

Development of tumors in renal allograft represents a challenging opportunity to both urologists and transplant surgeons. We report our experience with a recent case and present our innovative approach to this problem.

5.1 Case presentation (Sankari and Chueh, submitted, 2011)

The patient has a simultaneous tumor in the native right kidney and a tumor in the transplanted kidney located in the right lower quadrant. The native right kidney was removed with a transperitoneal laparoscopic approach through an incision over the right lower quadrant. Then transplanted kidney was dissected intraperitoneally via the same incision. This allowed us to reflect the colon and avoid any intraperitoneal injury. The iliac artery above and below the kidney was encircled with vessel loops in case we needed to temporarily occlude the blood inflow. The tumor was located over the lateral mid aspect of the kidney and was intrarenal. Following dissection and exposure of the kidney, the tumor could not be palpated or visually identified. Intraoperative ultrasound was used to locate the tumor and markers was made 1 cm above and below the tumor margin. We believe a zero warm ischemia time is more favorable for kidney function outcome, particularly in solitary kidneys. Resection then proceeded quickly with circumferential resection of the tumor all the way down to the underlying renal sinus. Suturing of the deeper collecting system tissue was performed with 3:0 chromic running suture. Floseal hemastatic agent was used to control the exposed small renal vessels. And cupsular sutures with 2:0 chromic interrupted sutures were done. Blood loss was 300 ml. Resection time was 25 minutes without any warm ischemia time. Kidney function remained unchanged post operatively.

5.2 Comments on partial nephrectomy for transplanted kidneys

Kidney transplant recipients are at increased risk for malignancies (Chueh SC et al., 2011a; Navarro et al., 2008; Tollefson et al., 2010). Development of cancer depends on the duration and type of immunosuppression or association with viral infection. Renal cell carcinoma (RCC) in renal transplant recipients is the most common urologic cancer in both native kidneys and transplanted kidneys (Melchior, et al., 2011). The development of tumors in the renal allograft represents a very challenging task for the urologist and transplant surgeon to treat these malignancies, especially when the allograft kidney is still functioning. The overall incidence of de novo malignancies after renal transplant is 4-5 times higher than that of the general population (Penn I, 1998). Malignancy can arise from unnoticed transmission of tumor cells or metastasis within the graft, or they can originate from the recipient.

Transplanted and native kidneys should be screened for tumors by yearly ultrasound after transplant (Kalble T, et al., 2005). Thus tumors can be diagnosed at an early stage. If a tumor is detected in a functionless native kidney, radical nephrectomy is the treatment of choice. RCC within the renal allograft itself is a less frequent event and accounts for approximately 10% of the cases (Kalble T, et al., 2005; Melchior, et al., 2011; Penn I, 1998). Once RCC in the transplanted kidney is diagnosed, it is crucial to determine the genetic origin of the tumor by means of DNA analysis. Thus the potential transmission of tumor cells to other recipients from the same donor can be assessed (Boix, et al., 2009).

There is no consensus on treatment of RCC in the transplanted kidney. Available treatment options include ablative techniques, nephron sparing surgery and allograft nephrectomy. Nephron sparing surgery in the allograft can be a challenging procedure even for experienced urological surgeons (Chambade, et al., 2008). We applied the same surgical principles for partial nephrectomy in the non-transplant patient.

Modification of the immunosuppressive regimen for renal transplant recipients in whom the tumor developed is a matter of debate. But most centers would recommend adjustment of the medications. The mammalian target of Rapamycin (mTOR) inhibitor which is used to prevent acute rejection after renal transplant does not increase the risk of malignancy

(Campistol, 2009). This is in contrast to calcineurin inhibitors (CNI; tacrolimus and cyclosporine) and antimetabolites (mycophenolic acid and azathioprine). Consideration should be given to switch transplant recipients with RCC to mTOR inhibitor (sirolimus or everolimus) and discontinue CNIs and antimetabolites. Prednisone has no effect on tumor progress and can be continued to provide prophylaxis against renal allograft rejection. mTOR inhibitor is a growth factor inhibitor and will affect wound healing and its use should be delayed till after surgical wounds have healed.

In most cases partial nephrectomy requires temporary occlusion of the renal artery to allow for tumor resection and renal reconstruction in a relatively bloodless field (Uzzo and Novick, 2001). This is supplemented with surface cooling if warm ischemia time is expected to exceed more than 30 minutes. The risk of vascular injury though uncommon remains a potential risk of vascular occlusion (Thompson,et al., 2007). Renal artery occlusion can be avoided during open surgery in selected peripheral renal masses based on the rapidity with which hemostasis and renorraphy is possible. Vascular clamping has the potential to lead to renal ischemia and reperfusion injury which are associated with adverse outcome. Vascular clamping during open partial nephrectomy in patients with solitary kidney was associated with greater risk of renal failure and temporary dialysis than partial nephrectomy without ischemia (Wszolek et al., 2010). Duration of ischemia is found to be the strongest modifiable risk factor for decrease renal function after partial nephrectomy (Lane, et al., 2011).

Libertino described his technique for partial nephrectomy without vascular occlusion essentially achieving a 0-ischemia time (Smith, et al., 2010). The renal vessels are dissected all the way to the level of the intrarenal branches. Both renal arteries and renal veins are secured with vessel loops but not occluded. Hemostasis of the resected parenchyma is achieved with electrocautary for small vessels and suture ligation for large vessel. Pediatric clamps are used to occlude the larger vessels prior to ligation with a figure of eight 4:0 vicryl sutures. Opening in the collecting system is closed with absorbable sutures, and a JJ stent is inserted antegradely as needed. Renal parenchyma is then approximated with absorbable sutures. Throughout the procedure an assistant provides exposure with a Frazier suction tip and a Penfield neurosurgical spatula. The percentage change in estimated GFR was higher in the clamped group; yet, the transfusion rate was higher for the unclamped group.

Partial nephrectomy in transplanted kidney represents a unique opportunity to apply techniques developed in partial nephrectomies for solitary kidneys. Modification of the operation is necessary. Anatomically, the transplanted kidney is encased in a bed of scar tissues. Dissection of the renal hilum is tedious and risks injury to the renal vasculature. The dissection of the kidney is aided by performing the operation intraperitoneally. This will allow avoiding inadvertent injury to the intraabdominal organs. Proximal and distal control of the iliac artery above and below the level of the renal artery anastomosis will allow for temporary occlusion in the event of excessive bleeding. We recommend performing the operation without vascular occlusion if possible to avoid any ischemic injury to the transplant kidney.

6. Conclusions

Implantation of a kidney graft into the extraperotineal iliac fossa has not changed much surgically since its inception from 1950s; whereas the other renal transplant-related surgical approaches have dramatically been updated for the past ten more years, especially with the commencement of urological laparoscopic surgery.

The most important mile-stone advancement is the laparoscopic live donor nephrectomy. Since its original report in 1995, in spite of the initial concerns regarding the quality of the graft function and the safety issue for the live donor, laparoscopic live donor nephrectomy has been recently well recognized academically and practically as the surgery of choice for harvesting live donor kidney; which in fact was driven both by the donors' preference and by the surgeons' competence in performing this surgery. It can be performed either via a pure laparoscopic approach, in which a wound is extended at the end of the procedure to harvest the kidney; or it can also be performed via a hand-assisted approach, in which the graft is harvested from the hand-assisted incision.

More recently a newer variant of the laparoscopic surgery—laparoendoscopic single site (LESS) surgery has been evolved to the field of live donor nephrectomy in certain elite transplant centers. This technique creates a smaller and single incision to accomplish the procedure under the same surgical principles with a much steeper learning curve, and some special equipments are necessary to facilitate such operation. The ultimate value of LESS live donor nephrectomy still warrants further proof with prospective randomized data even though it is surgically feasible.

Besides the donor nephrectomy, laparoscopic surgery has also been applied to a variety of procedures related to the renal transplant recipients. Recurrent lymphoceles resistant to repeated aspiration and drainage can be managed with laparoscopic marsupilization (internal drainage into the peritoneal cavity). Incidence of renal cell carcinomas (RCC) in the native kidneys has been shown higher in the transplant recipients than that of the general population. If the RCC is still localized at diagnosis, it can be treated with laparoscopic radical nephrectomy. In certain areas around the world the incidence of urothelial carcinoma in the native upper urinary tract (ureters, renal pelvis and calyses) has also been reported much higher in the transplant recipients. With proper equipment laparoscopic bilateral nephroureterectomy with bladder cuff resection can be performed in one session through several small incisions without changing the patient's position.

Very rarely, tumor in the transplant kidneys might be found during follow-up. If the graft is still functioning, and the tumor is localized, partial nephrectomy of the transplant kidney can be used to excise the tumor while preserve the graft function.

The surgical procedures of each mentioned above have been detailed in this chapter.

7. References

Abou-Elela, A.; Reyad, I.; Torky, M.; Meshref, A. & Morsi, A. (2006) Laparoscopic marsupialization of postrenal transplantation lymphoceles. *J Endourol.* Vol. 20, No. 11, pp. 904-909.

Andonian, S.; Herati, AS.; Atalla, MA.; Rais-Bahrami, S.; Richstone, L. & Kavoussi, LR. (2010a) Laparoendoscopic single-site pfannenstiel donor nephrectomy. *Urology.* Vol. 75, No. 1, pp. 9-12.

Andonian, S.; Rais-Bahrami, S.; Atalla, MA.; Herati, AS.; Richstone, L. & Kavoussi, LR. (2010b) Laparoendoscopic single-site Pfannenstiel versus standard laparoscopic donor nephrectomy. *J Endourol.* Vol. 24, No. 3, pp. 429-432.

Atray, NK.; Moore, F.; Zaman, F.; Caldito, G.; Abreo, K.; Maley, W.& Zibari, GB. (2004) Post-transplant lymphocele: a single centre experience. *Clin Transplant.* Vol. 18, Suppl. 12, pp. 46-49.

Bachmann, A.; Wyler, S.; Wolff, T.; Gürke, L.; Steiger, J.; Kettelhack, C.; Gasser, TC. & Ruszat, R. (2008) Complications of retroperitoneoscopic living donor nephrectomy: single center experience after 164 cases. *World J Urol.* Vol. 26, No. 6, pp. 549-554.

Bartlett, ST. (2002) Laparoscopic donor nephrectomy after seven years. *Am J Transplant.* Vol. 2, No. 10, pp. 896-897.

Berger, AD.; Kanofsky, JA.; O'Malley, RL.; Hyams, ES.; Chang, C.; Taneja, SS. & Stifelman, MD. (2008) Transperitoneal laparoscopic radical nephrectomy for large (more than 7 cm) renal masses. *Urology.* Vol.71, No. 3, pp. 421-424.

Bird, VG.; Shields, JM.; Aziz, M.; De Los Santos, R.; Ayyathurai, R. & Ciancio, G. (2010) Transperitoneal laparoscopic radical nephrectomy for patients with dialysis-dependent end-stage renal disease: an analysis and comparison of perioperative outcome. *Urology.* Vol. 75, No. 6, pp. 1335-1342.

Boix, R.; Sanz, C.; Mora, M.; Quer, A.; Beyer, K.; Musulen, E.; González, C., Bayona, S.; Saladié, JM. & Ariza, A. (2009) Primary renal cell carcinoma in a transplanted kidney: genetic evidence of recipient origin. *Transplantation* Vol. 87, No. 7, pp. 1057-1061.

Boorjian, S.; Munver, R.; Sosa, RE. & Del Pizzo, JJ. (2004) Right laparoscopic live donor nephrectomy: a single institution experience. *Transplantation.* Vol. 77, No. 3, pp. 437-440.

Boulware, LE.; Ratner, LE.; Sosa, JA.; Tu, AH.; Nagula, S.; Simpkins, CE.; Durant, RW. & Powe, NR. (2002) The general public's concerns about clinical risk in live kidney donation. *Am J Transplant.* Vol. 2, No. 2, pp. 186-193.

Buell, JF.; Abreu, SC.; Hanaway, MJ.; Ng, CS.; Kaouk, JH.; Clippard, M.; Zaki, S.; Goldfarb, DA.; Woodle, ES. & Gill, IS. (2004) Right donor nephrectomy: a comparison of hand-assisted transperitoneal and retroperitoneal laparoscopic approaches. *Transplantation.* Vol. 77, No. 4, pp. 521-525.

Campistol, JM. (2009) Minimizing the risk of posttransplant malignancy. *Transplantation.* Vol. 87, Suppl. 8, S19-22.

Chen, J.; Chueh, SC.; Hsu, WT.; Lai, MK. & Chen, SC. (2001) Modified approach of hand-assisted laparoscopic nephroureterectomy for transitional cell carcinoma of the upper urinary tract. *Urology.* Vol. 58, No. 6, pp. 930-934.

Chueh, S.; Sankari, B.; Chung, SD. & Jones, JS. (2011a) Retroperitoneoscopic laparoendoscopic single site nephrectomy. *Br J Urol Intl* [Epub, in press]

Chueh, SC.; Chen, J.; Hsu, WT.; Hsieh, MH. & Lai, MK. (2002b) Hand assisted laparoscopic bilateral nephroureterectomy in 1 session without repositioning patients is facilitated by alternating inflation cuffs. *J Urol.* Vol. 167, No.1, pp.44-47.

Chueh, SC.; Flechner, S.; Goldfarb, D.; Sankari, B. & Campbell, S. (2011b) Re: Tollefson et al.: Surgical treatment of renal cell carcinoma in the immunocompromised transplant patient (Urology 2010;75:1373-1377). *Urology.* Vol. 77, No. 1, pp. 254-255.

Chueh, SC.; Lai, MK.; Lee, PH. & Chen, J. (2002a) Technical considerations in hand-assisted laparoscopic live donor nephrectomy: initial Taiwan experience from National Taiwan University Hospital. *J Formos Med Assoc.* Vol. 101, No. 1, pp. 76-79.

Chueh, SC.; Wang, SM. & Lai, MK. (2004) Use of Hem-o-lok clips effectively lengthens renal vein during laparoscopic live donor nephrectomy *Transplant Proc.* Vol. 36, No. 9, pp. 2623-2624.

Chung, SD.; Huang, KH.; Lai, MK.; Huang, CY.; Pu, YS.; Yu, HJ. & Chueh, SC. (2007) Long-term follow-up of hand-assisted laparoscopic radical nephrectomy for organ-confined renal cell carcinoma. *Urology.* Vol. 69, No. 4, pp. 652-655.

Clayman, RV.; Kavoussi, LR.; Soper, NJ.; Dierks, SM.; Merety, KS.; Darcy, MD.; Long, SR.; Roemer, FD.; Pingleton, ED. & Thomson PG. (1991) Laparoscopic nephrectomy. *N Engl J Med.* Vol. 324, No. 19, pp. 1370-1371.

Colombo, JR. Jr.; Haber, GP.; Jelovsek, JE.; Lane, B.; Novick, AC. & Gill, IS. (2008) Seven years after laparoscopic radical nephrectomy: oncologic and renal functional outcomes. *Urology.* Vol. 71, No. 6, pp. 1149-1154.

Desai, MM.; Strzempkowski, B.; Matin, SF.; Steinberg, AP.; Ng, C.; Meraney, AM.; Kaouk; JH. & Gill, IS. (2005) Prospective randomized comparison of transperitoneal versus retroperitoneal laparoscopic radical nephrectomy. *J Urol.* Vol. 173, No. 1, pp.38-41.

FDA, 2006 http://www.fda.gov/Safety/Recalls/EnforcementReports/2006/ucm120409.htm

Fornara, P.; Doehn, C.; Fricke, L.; Hoyer, J. & Jocham, D. (1997) Laparoscopy in renal transplant patients. *Urology.* Vol. 49, No. 4, pp. 521-527.

Gill, IS.; Canes, D.; Aron, M.; Haber, GP.; Goldfarb, DA.; Flechner, S.; Desai, MR., Kaouk, JH. & Desai, MM. Single port transumbilical (E-NOTES) donor nephrectomy. *J Urol.* Vol. 180, No. 2, pp. 637-641.

Gill, IS.; Kaouk, JH.; Hobart MG.; Sung, GT.; Schweizer, DK. & Braun, WE. (2001) Laparoscopic bilateral synchronous nephrectomy for autosomal dominant polycystic kidney disease: the initial experience. *J Urol.* Vol. 165, No. 4, pp. 1093-1098.

Gill, IS.; Sung, GT., Hobart, MG.; Savage, SJ.; Meraney, AM.; Schweizer, DK.; Klein, EA. & Novick, AC. (2000) Laparoscopic radical nephroureterectomy for upper tract transitional cell carcinoma: the Cleveland Clinic experience. *J Urol.* Vol. 164, No. 5, pp. 1513-1522.

Gimenez, E.; Leeser, DB.; Wysock, JS.; Charlton, M.; Kapur, S.; Del Pizzo, JJ. (2010) Laparoendoscopic single site live donor nephrectomy: initial experience. *J Urol.* Vol. 184, No. 5, pp. 2049-2053.

Greco, F.; Wagner, S.; Hoda, MR.; Weigand, K.; Inferrera, A. & Fornara, P. (2010) Single-Portal Access Laparoscopic Radical Nephrectomy for Renal Cell Carcinoma in Transplant Patients: The First Experience. *Eur Urol.* 2010 Oct 15. [Epub]

Gruessner, RW.; Fasola, C.; Benedetti, E.; Foshager, MC.; Gruessner, AC.; Matas, AJ.; Najarian, JS. & Goodale, RL. (1995) Laparoscopic drainage of lymphoceles after kidney transplantation: indications and limitations. *Surgery.* ;Vol. 117, No. 3, pp. 288-295.

Hollenbeck, BK.; Seifman, BD. & Wolf, JS. Jr. (2004) Clinical skills acquisition for hand-assisted laparoscopic donor nephrectomy. *J Urol.* Vol. 171, No. 1, pp. 35-39.

Ismai;, HR.; Flechner, SM.; Kaouk, JH.; Derweesh, IH.; Gill, IS.; Modlin, C.; Goldfarb, D. & Novick, AC. (2005) Simultaneous vs. sequential laparoscopic bilateral native nephrectomy and renal transplantation. *Transplantation.* Vol. 80, No. 8, pp. 1124-1127.

Jacobs, SC.; Cho, E.; Foster, C.; Liao, P. & Bartlett, ST. (2004) Laparoscopic donor nephrectomy: the University of Maryland 6-year experience. *J Urol.* Vol. 171, No. 1, pp. 47-51.

Jarrett, TW.; Chan, DY.; Cadeddu, JA. & Kavoussi, LR. (2001) Laparoscopic nephroureterectomy for the treatment of transitional cell carcinoma of the upper urinary tract. *Urology.* Vol. 57, No. 3, pp. 448-453.

Johnson, MW.; Andreoni, K.; McCoy, L.; Scott, L.; Rodegast, B.; Friedman, E.; Thomas, S.; Salm, J.; Gerber, DA. & Fair JH. (2001) Technique of right laparoscopic donor nephrectomy: a single center experience. *Am J Transplant.* Vol. 1, No. 3, pp. 293-295.

Kälble, T; Lucan, M.; Nicita, G.; Sells, R.; Burgos Revilla, FJ.; Wiesel, M. & European Association of Urology. (2005) EAU guidelines on renal transplantation. *Eur Urol.* Vol. 47, No. 2, pp. 156-166.

Kerche, KW.; Heniford, BT.; Matthews, BD.; Smith, TI.; Lincourt, AE.; Hayes, DH.; Eskind, LB.; Irby, PB. & Teigland, CM. (2003) Laparoscopic versus open nephrectomy in 210 consecutive patients: outcomes, cost, and changes in practice patterns. *Surg Endosc.* Vol. 17, No. 12, pp. 1889-1895.

Khauli, RB.; Mosenthal, AC. & Caushaj, PF. (1992) Treatment of lymphocele and lymphatic fistula following renal transplantation by laparoscopic peritoneal window. *J Urol.* Vol. 147, No. 5, pp. 1353-1355.

Kohei, N.; Kazuya, O.; Hirai, T.; Miyauchi, Y.; Iida, S.; Shirakawa, H.; Shimizu, T.; Ishida, H. & Tanabe, K. (2010) Retroperitoneoscopic living donor nephrectomy: experience of 425 cases at a single center. *J Endourol.* Vol. 24, No. 11, pp. 1783-1787.

Lane, BR.; Russo, P.; Uzzo, RG.; Hernandez, AV.; Boorjian, SA.; Thompson, RH.; Fergany, AF.; Love, TE. & Campbell, SC. (2011) Comparision of cold and warm ischemia during partial nephrectomy in 660 solitary kidneys reveals predominant role of nonmodifiable factors in determining ultimate renal function. *J Urol.* Vol. 185, No. 2, pp. 421-427.

Leventhal, JR.; Kocak, B.; Salvalaggio, PR.; Koffron, AJ.; Baker, TB.; Kaufman, DB.; Fryer, JP.; Abecassis, MM. & Stuart, FP. (2004) Laparoscopic donor nephrectomy 1997 to 2003: lessons learned with 500 cases at a single institution. *Surgery.* Vol. 136, No. 4, pp. 881-890.

Leventhal, JR.; Paunescu, S.; Baker, TB.; Caciedo, JC.; Kocak, B.; Gallon, L.; Friedewald, J.; Luo, X.; Kaufman, DB.; Fryer, JP. & Abecassis, MM. (2010) A decade of minimally invasive donation: experience with more than 1200 laparoscopic donor nephrectomies at a single institution. *Clin Transplant.* Vol. 24, No. 2, pp. 169-174.

Liao, CH.; Chueh, SC.; Lai, MK. & Chen, J. (2004) Transitional cell carcinoma in renal transplant recipients. *Transplant Proc.* Vol. 36, No. 7, pp. 2152-2153.

Lucas, SM.; Mofunanya, TC.; Goggins, WC. & Sundaram, CP. (2010) Staged nephrectomy versus bilateral laparoscopic nephrectomy in patients with autosomal dominant polycystic kidney disease. *J Urol.* Vol. 184, No. 5, pp. 2054-2059.

Lunsford, KE.; Harris, MT.; Nicoll, KN.; Collins, BH.; Sudan, DL.; Kuo, PC. & Vikraman, D. (2011) Single-Site Laparoscopic Living Donor Nephrectomy Offers Comparable Perioperative Outcomes to Conventional Laparoscopic Living Donor Nephrectomy at a Higher Cost. *Transplantation.* Vol. 91, No. 2, pp. e16-17.

Matin, SF. & Gill, IS. (2000) Laparoscopic marsupialization of the difficult lymphocele using internalized peritoneal dialysis catheter. *J Urol.* Vol. 163, No. 5, pp. 1498-1500.

Matin, SF. & Gill, IS. (2001) Laparoscopic ultrasonography. *J Endourol.* Vol. 15, No. 1, pp. 87-92.

McNeill, SA.; Chrisofos, M. & Tolley, DA. (2000) The long-term outcome after laparoscopic nephroureterectomy: a comparison with open nephroureterectomy. *Br J Urol Intl.* Vol. 86, No. 6, pp. 619-623.

Melchior, S.; Franzaring, L.; Shardan, A.; Schwenke, C.; Plümpe, A.; Schnell, R. & Dreikorn, K. (2011) Urological de novo malignancy after kidney transplantation: a case for the urologist. *J Urol.* Vol. 185, No. 2, pp. 428-432.

Mjøen, G.; Holdaas, H.; Pfeffer, P.; Line, PD. & Øyen, O. (2010) Minimally invasive living donor nephrectomy - introduction of hand-assistance. *Transpl Int.* Vol. 23, No. 10, pp. 1008-1014.

Nambirajan, T.; Jeschke, S.; Al-Zahrani, H.; Vrabec, G.; Leeb, K. & Janetschek, G. (2004) Prospective, randomized controlled study: transperitoneal laparoscopic versus retroperitoneoscopic radical nephrectomy. *Urology.* Vol. 64, No. 5, pp. 919-924.

Navarro, MD.; Lopez-Andreu, M.; Rodriguez-Benot, A.; Agüera, ML.; Del Castillo, D. & Aljama, P. (2008) Cancer incidence and survival in kidney transplant patients. *Transplant Proc.* Vol. 40, No. 9, 2936-2940.

OPTN, (2006) http://optn.transplant.hrsa.gov/ContentDocuments/Guidance_ProgramSpecificLivingKidneyDonorMedEvalProtocols.pdf

Parra, RO.; Jones, JP. & Hagood, PG. (1992) Laparoscopic intraperitoneal marsupialization: report on a new treatment for lymphoceles. *Surg Laparosc Endosc.* Vol. 2, No. 4, pp. 306-311.

Penn, I. (1998) Occurrence of cancers in immunosuppressed organ transplant recipients. *Clin Transpl.* 147-158.

Ponsky, L.; Cherullo, E.; Moinzadeh, A.; Desai, M.; Kaouk, J.; Haber, GP.; Chen, D.; Ng, C.; Fuchs, G.; Singh, D.; Finelli, A.; Frank, I. & Matin, S. (2008) The Hem-o-lok clip is safe for laparoscopic nephrectomy: a multi-institutional review. *Urology.* Vol. 71, No. 4, pp. 593-596.

Ratner, LE.; Ciseck, LJ.; Moore, RG.; Cigarroa, FG.; Kaufman, HS. & Kavoussi, LR. (1995) Laparoscopic live donor nephrectomy. *Transplantation.* Vol. 60, No. 9, pp. 1047-1049.

Rehman, J.; Landman, J.; Andreoni, C.; McDougall, EM. & Clayman, RV. (2001) Laparoscopic bilateral hand assisted nephrectomy for autosomal dominant polycystic kidney disease: initial experience. *J Urol.* Vol. 166, No. 1, pp. 42-47.

Schilling, M.; Abendroth, D. & Kunz, R. (1995) Treatment of lymphocele in renal transplant recipients by laparoscopic fenestration after transcutaneous staining. *Br J Surg.* Vol. 82, No. 2, pp. 246-248.

Shalhav, AL.; Dunn, MD.; Portis, AJ.; Elbahnasy, AM; McDougall, EM. & Clayman, RV. (2000) Laparoscopic nephroureterectomy for upper tract transitional cell cancer: the Washington University experience. *J Urol.* Vol. 163, No. 4, pp. 1100-1104.

Shokeir, AA.; Eraky, I.; el-Kappany, H. & Ghoneim, MA. (1994) Accidental division of the transplanted ureter during laparoscopic drainage of lymphocele. *J Urol.* Vol. 151, No. 6, pp. 1623-1625.

Siemer, S.; Lehmann, J.; Kamradt, J.; Loch, T.; Remberger, K.; Humke, U.; Ziegler, M. & Stockle, M. (2004) Adrenal metastases in 1635 patients with renal cell carcinoma: outcome and indication for adrenalectomy. *J Urol.* Vol. 171, (6 Pt 1), pp. 2155-2159, discussion 2159.

Smith, GL.; Kenney, PA.; Lee, Y. & Libertino, JA. (2010) Non-clamped partial nephrectomy: techniques and surgical outcomes. *Br J Urol. Intl.* online publication Oct 29, 2010. doi:10.1111/j.1464-410X.2010.09798.x[Epub ahead of print]

Steinberg, AP.; Finelli, A.; Desai, MM.; Abreu, SC.; Ramani, AP.; Spaliviero, M; Rybicki, L.; Kaouk, J.; Novick, AC. & Gill, IS. (2004) Laparoscopic radical nephrectomy for large (greater than 7 cm, t2) renal tumors. *J Urol.* Vol. 172, (6 Pt 1), pp. 2172-2176.

Su, LM.; Ratner, LE, Montgomery, RA.; Jarrett, TW.; Trock, BJ.; Sinkov, V.; Bluebond-Langner, R. & Kavoussi, LR. (2004) Laparoscopic live donor nephrectomy: trends in donor and recipient morbidity following 381 consecutive cases. *Ann Surg.* Vol. 240, No. 2, pp. 358-363.

Sundqvist, P.; Feuk, U.; Haggman, M.; Persson, AE.; Stridsberg, M. & Wadstrom, J. (2004) Hand-assisted retroperitoneoscopic live donor nephrectomy in comparison to open and laparoscopic procedures: a prospective study on donor morbidity and kidney function. *Transplantation.* Vol. 78, No. 1, pp. 147-153.

Tai, HC.; Lai, MK.; Chung, SD.; Huang, KH.; Chueh, SC. & Yu, HJ. (2009) Intermediate-term oncological outcomes of hand-assisted laparoscopic versus open bilateral nephroureterectomy for dialysis and kidney transplant patients with upper urinary tract urothelial carcinoma. *J Endourol.* Vol. 23, No. 7, pp.1139-1144.

Tanabe, K.; Miyamoto, N.; Tokumoto, T.; Yamamoto, H.; Ishida, H.; Kondo, T.; Okuda, H.; Shinmmura, H.; Shirakawa, H.; Shimizu, T.; Ishikawa, N. & Toma, H. (2005) Retroperitoneoscopic live donor nephrectomy: extended experience in a single center. *Am J Transplant.* Vol. 5, (4 Pt 1), pp. 739-745.

Thompson, RH.; Frank, I.; Lohse, CM.; Saad, IR.; Fergany, A.; Zincke, H.; Leibovich, BC.; Blute, ML. & Novick, AC. (2007) The impact of ischemia time during open nephron sparing surgery on solitary kidneys: a multi-institutional study. *J Urol.* Vol. 177, No. 2, 471-476.

Tollefson, MK.; Krambeck, AE.; Leibovich, BC.; Blute, ML. & Chow, GK. (2010) Surgical treatment of renal cell carcinoma in the immunocompromised transplant patient *Urology* Vol. 75, No. 6, pp. 1373-1377.

Tooher, RL.; Rao, MM.; Scott, DF.; Wall, DR.; Francis, DM; Bridgewater, FH. & Maddern, GJ. (2004) A systematic review of laparoscopic live-donor nephrectomy. *Transplantation.* Vol. 78, No. 3, pp. 404-414.

Troppmann, C.; Ormond, DB. & Perez, RV. (2003) Laparoscopic (vs open) live donor nephrectomy: a UNOS database analysis of early graft function and survival. *Am J Transplant.* Vol. 3, No. 10, pp. 1295-1301.

UNOS, 2009, http://www.unos.org/docs/Living_Donation.pdf

Uzzo, R. & Novick, AC. (2001) Nephron-sparing surgery for renal tumors. Indications, techniques and outcomes. *J Urol.* Vol. 166, No. 1, pp. 6-18.

Velidedeoglu, E.; Williams, N.; Brayman, KL.; Desai, NM.; Campos, L.; Palanjian, M.; Wocjik, M.; Bloom, R.; Grossman, RA.; Mange, K.; Barker, CF.; Naji, A. & Markmann, JF. (2002) Comparison of open, laparoscopic, and hand-assisted approaches to live-donor nephrectomy. *Transplantation.* Vol. 74, No. 2, pp. 169-72.

Venkatesh, R.; Belani, JS.; Chen, C.; Sundaram, CP.; Bhayani, SB.; Figenshau, RS. & Landman, J. (2007) Prospective randomized comparison of laparoscopic and hand-assisted laparoscopic radical nephrectomy. *Urology.* Vol. 70, No. 5, pp. 873-877.

Whitten, MG.; Van der Werf, W. & Belnap, L. (2006) A novel approach to bilateral hand-assisted laparoscopic nephrectomy for autosomal dominant polycystic kidney disease. *Surg Endosc.* Vol. 20, No. 4, pp. 679-684.

Wszolek, MF.; Kenney, PA.; Lee, Y. & Libertino, JA. (2010) Comparison of hilar clamping and non-hilar clamping partial nephrectomy for tumours involving a solitary kidney. *Br. J Urol. Intl.* 2010 Nov 11. doi: 10.1111/j.1464-410X.2010.09713.x. [Epub ahead of print]

24

Minimally Invasive Renal Transplantation

Ole Øyen
Oslo University Hospital Rikshospitalet
Clinic for Specialised Medicine and Surgery,
Norway

1. Introduction

During the last 20 years minimally invasive surgery (MIS) has replaced many open, conventional operations and is now important in almost every facet of abdominal surgery (Harrell & Beniford, 2005). Benefits regarding postoperative pain, convalescence, return to normal activities, and cosmetic results have been proven for a wide range of MIS procedures.

Within the field of transplantation, laparoscopic fenestration of lymphoceles in kidney recipients was first described in 1991 (McCullough et al.). Furthermore, laparoscopic living donor nephrectomy (L-LDN) has gained widespread acceptance, since the first procedure was performed in Baltimore, USA in 1995 (Ratner et al., 1995).

Reduction of tissue trauma seems particularly appropriate in the immunosuppressed population, with significantly delayed wound healing and a high "background" complication rate. Due to the immunosuppressive theraphy, the incidences of lymphoceles, wound dehiscence and incisional hernia are distinctly higher in kidney-Tx (KTx) - recipients. On this background it is rather surprising that MIS techniques for the renal transplant procedure itself, first have been reported during recent years. Possible explanations for these seemingly conservative attitudes, may include the urge for safe handling of the kidney through sufficient access, for total control during revascularization; and the present unfeasibility of automating the vascular anastomoses.

In 2002, however, a french case report on robotic-assisted (da Vinci system) kidney transplantation, from a deceased donor, was presented (Hoznek et al., 2002). Thereafter, no further cases/series of robotic-assisted KTx seem to have been published.

In 2006 a minimally invasive KTx (MIKT) technique was described in Transplantation and Transplantation Proceedings (Øyen et al., 2006); using a minimal skin incision (7-9 cm) and still giving optimal access to the anastomotic area of the iliac vessels - mostly without using scopic aid. Twentyone consecutive MIKT procedures, performed by a single surgeon was compared to a control group subjected to conventional KTx. Since then, a South Korean group has published two reports (Seong-Pyo et al., 2007; Park et al., 2008) on a video-assisted MIKT technique.

Another MIKT report was contributed by a spanish group (Rosales et al., 2010); a case report describing a laparoscopic KTx technique, without robotic assistance.

Furthermore, in 2010 a minimally invasive technique for renal auto-transplantation was reported (Øyen et al., 2010); by combining 'hand- assisted laparoscopic nephrectomy'' and

'MIKT, using the same incision (7–8 cm) for hand-assistance, kidney harvesting, and transplantation.
The MIKT procedure have so far not gained widespread acceptance and still seem to be at a "pioneer stage". However, considering the rapid evolution of MIS during the last two decades, there is little reason to believe that KTx and Auto-KTx in future will be excluded from this development.

2. The minimally invasive surgical revolution

During the last 20 years minimally invasive techniques have revolutionised surgery in general, and in particular have laparoscopic procedures replaced most conventional operations, including advanced surgery on liver, pancreas and intestines. Benefits regarding postoperative pain, convalescence, return to normal activities, and cosmetic results have been proven for a wide range of MIS procedures. The development has been facilitated by improvements in optical and hemostatic equipment (High definition imaging, Ultracision, LigaSure), miniaturization, and the introduction of robotic technology (da Vinci robot system).
The revolutionary MIS development was started by a French gynecologist, with experience from simple laparoscopic procedures like sterilisation, and he actually invented laparascopic cholecystectomy (Dubois et al., 1991). This invention, started in 1987, has indeed turned out to be the greatest revolution in surgical technique during the last 2000 years. In fact, our conventional instruments for open, conventional surgery (scalpel, scissors, forceps etc) have no further subtleties than those found in archeological findings from Pompei (to be seen in the Archeological Museum of Napoli). The great achievements in surgery during the last part of the 19th century and first part of the 20th century was actually due to developments in anesthesia and bacteriology/septicemiae - not in surgical technique.
During the last two decades of rapid MIS evolution, an almost linear correlation between incisional/tissue trauma and postoperative morbidity has been demonstrated.
Within the field of transplantation, laparoscopic fenestration of post-KTx lymphoceles was first described in 1991 (McCullough et. al.). This MIS technique has in recent years taken over as the standard treatment option for lymphoceles, replacing the traditional deroofing by laparotomy. Furthermore, laparoscopic living donor nephrectomy (L-LDN) has gained widespread acceptance, since the first procedure was performed in Baltimore, USA in 1995 (Ratner et al.). Many centres have adopted hand-assisted L-LDN techniques, because this is perceived to be faster, easier and safer than with the strictly laparoscopic technique (Wolf JSJ et al., 1998). By any method, a 6-9 cm incision is required for decent kidney extraction. With hand-assistance/handport the incision must usually be extended to 8-12 cm.

3. Robotic surgery: The da Vinci robot in renal transplantation; a case report from France (2002)

3.1 Method: The da Vinci surgical system

The *da Vinci* surgical system (Intuitive Surgical, Inc., Mountain View, California), based on robotic technology and introduced during the first years of this millennium, enabled surgeons to perform delicate and complex MIS operations, without extensive laparoscopic experience - affording excellent vision, precision, dexterity and control. The key components of the *da Vinci* surgical system included: an ergonomically designed console where the surgeon was seated while operating, , four interactive robotic arms, a high-definition 3D vision system, and proprietary so called *EndoWrist*® instruments. The.*da Vinci* system was powered by state-of-the-art robotic technology that allowed the surgeon's hand movements to be scaled, filtered and translated into precise movements of the *EndoWrist* instruments working inside the patient's body.

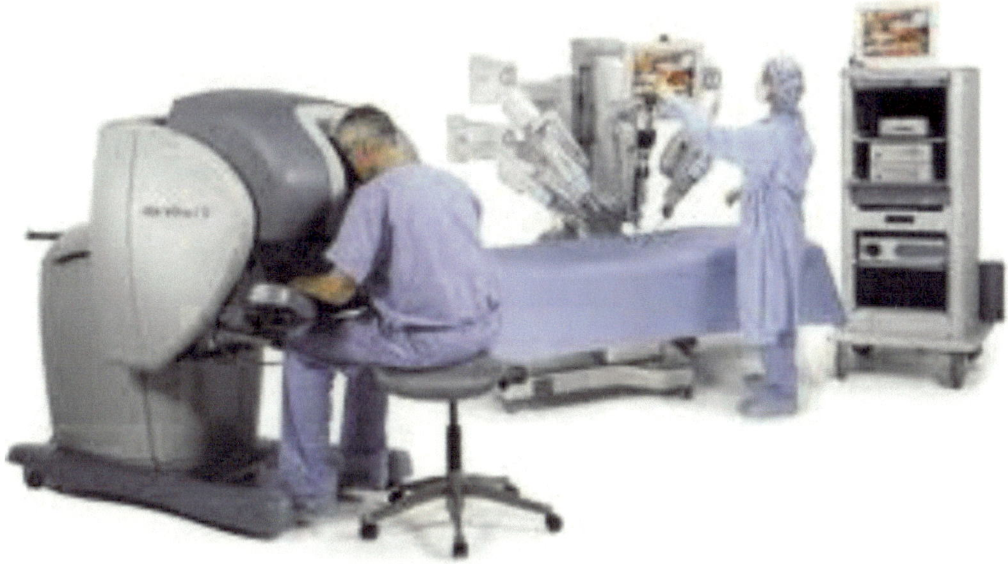

Fig. 1 The da Vinci robotic system.

During the last decade , the da Vinci system has particularly made progress within the field of laparoscopic urology, including radical prostatectomy, simple nephrectomy (not living donor nephrectomy) and pelvic lymph node dissection.
A great prospective feature of robotic surgery is the ability to dissociate the surgeon from the operative field. Specialised operations may be executed at remote hospitals, by a centralized surgeon.

3.2 Case report on 'da Vinci' KTx

The paper from 2002 (Hoznec et. al.) described a right cadaveric kidney transplanted into a 26-year-old male recipient, who had been on hemodialysis for 11 years. Surgery was done with the help of the da Vinci robot, by a "locally remote" surgeon, who completely performed vascular dissection and anastomoses, as well as ureterovesical anastomosis. The role of the assistant by the side of the patient was limited to access creation, exposure, hemostasis and maintaining traction on the running sutures performed by the robot. Operative time was 178 minutes. Robotic assistance made the vascular anastomoses feasible by stereoscopic magnification and ultraprecise visuality and manuvering. Renal perfusion was reported to be excellent with immediate diuresis. Nevertheless, postoperative acute tubular necrosis was first resolved one week post-Tx.

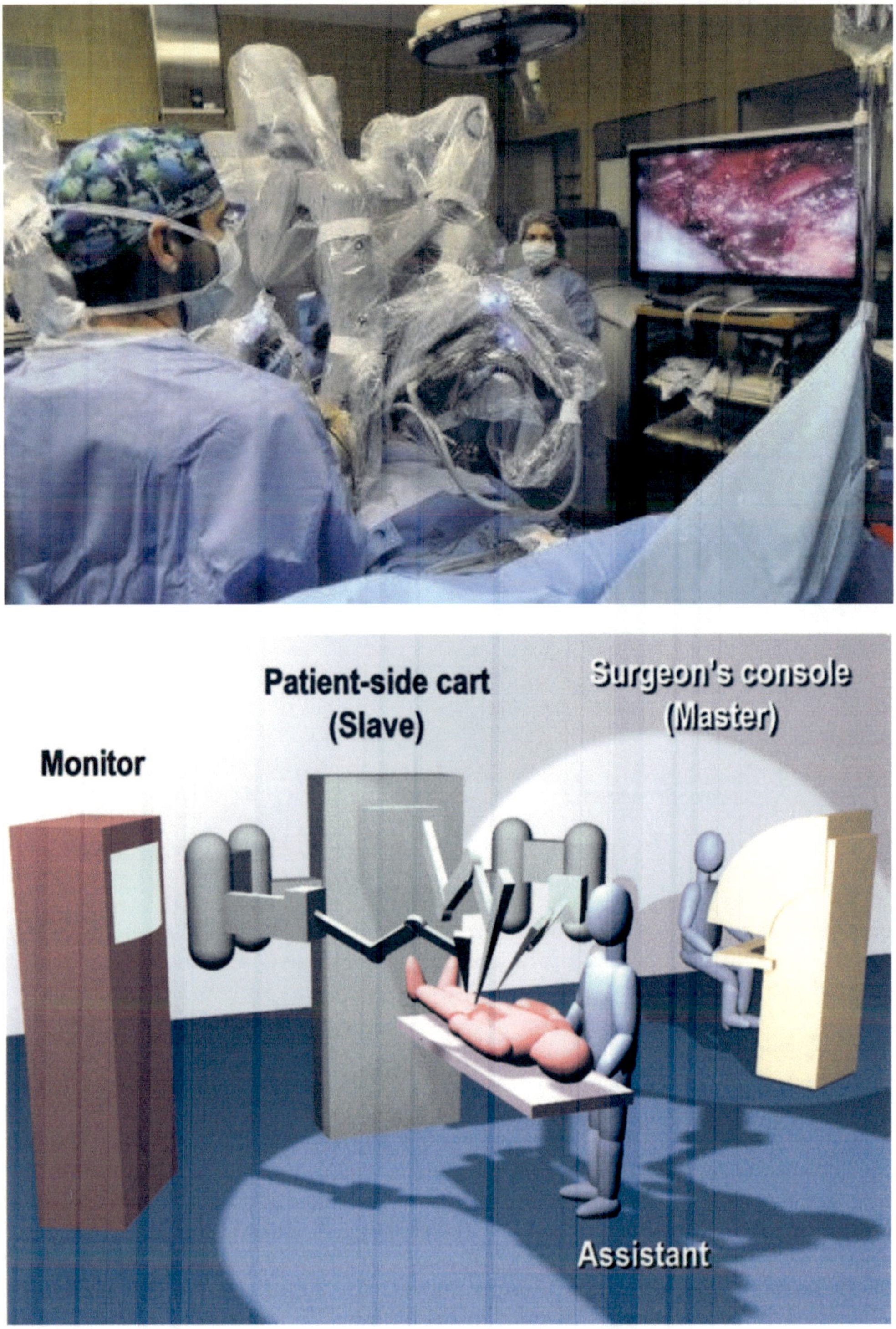

Fig. 2. The da Vinci robot system: Positioning of patient and surgeon. (Hoznek et al., 2002).

According to the authors, the case demonstrated that robotic assisted kidney transplantation was feasible. However, at that time, technical and cost hindrances was suspected to retard routine use of robots in future.

3.3 Further course/evolution of the 'da Vinci surgical system' in KTx

During recent years, the main application of the 'da Vinci robotic system' has been radical prostatectomy. In most other fields of laparoscopy, refined suturing has not been necessary, because ot the evolutionary development in stapling/clipsing devices, Ultracision and LigaSure. This is the main reason why the 'da Vinci system' has not taken over in other laparoscopic fields.

By close literature searches, the French group (nor any other group) does not seem to have reported any further 'da Vinci KTx' cases during the last decade. For the sake of completeness; the 'da Vinci KTx' case was mentioned in a review article about 'Robotic renal surgery' by the same authors (Hoznek et. al., 2004).

In the 'da Vinci KTx' paper, the size of the incision used for kidney introduction, is not indicated. The fact that a 6-9 cm incision is nevertheless required for decent implantation, and 3 hours 'da Vinci KTx' operating time, may explain why this method for KTx was not found worthy to pursue. In addition to the 6-9 cm implantation incision, the 'da Vinci' method is dependent on 2-3 laparoscopic ports (10-12 mm each), which are not necessary in the MIKT setting.

In a recent publication (Khanna & Horgan, 2011) a laboratory training and evaluation technique for robot assisted ex vivo KTx was demonstrated.

4. Minimally invasive KTx (MIKT); mostly without scopic aid – The Oslo experience (2006)

In 2005, a MEDLINE search for recent publications (years 2000-2005) containing both 'Kidney transplantation' and 'MIS' yielded 227 hits. However, a careful look at these references revealed that the great majority was about L-LDN, a few presented various MIS procedures in transplanted patients, but none of them were concerned with the transplantation procedure itself. The french da Vinci robot KTx report was not detected by our searches, because 'MIS'/'Laparoscopy' had not been included as key words..

The lack of MIKT publications in the literature was a bit surprising, for several reasons. Firstly, because MIS procedures had been described for all kinds of abdominal surgery, including sophisticated procedures, such as liver and pancreas resections. Secondly, because the potential advantages of reducing incisions/tissue trauma are probably of greater benefit in immunosuppressed patients, with significantly impaired wound healing. Possible explanations might include the urge for safe handling of the kidney through sufficient access, for total control during revascularization; and the present unfeasibility of automating the vascular anastomoses.

4.1 Developing MIKT: Method/technique

During the first years of the 21th century a MIKT technique was developed in Oslo, restricting to an appendectomy-like, approximately 8 cm long incision and with division only of the conjoined tendon (Øyen et al., 2006).

A careful and meticulous "back table" preparation of the kidney prior to transplantation was essential for MIKT, because of limited access to the parenchyma/hilus after revascularization. All redundant fatty tissue outside the "hilus-plane" was removed, to get undisturbed access for "complete" hemostatic control. All minor blood vessels, including capsular vessels, were secured by ligation or diathermy. Furthermore, the lymphatic vessels, mostly located alongside the artery, were ligated. The short right renal vein was extended by reconstruction using part of the caval tube caudally.

In the recipient, a 7-9 cm transverse incision was placed 3-5 cm above the inguinal ligament, with the medial end 2-3 cm from the midline. Only the 'conjoined tendon' and hardly any muscular tissue was divided. The iliac vessels were dissected free extraperitoneally, in a minimalistic fashion. A self-retracting system (Omnitract®) was introduced, giving medial, vascular exposure while allowing space for the kidney lateral/cranial to the skin incision. The meticulously prepared kidney was then placed in a small/fitting, lateral, retroperitoneal pouch, which has been precooled by ice sludge. All three anastomoses were performed with the kidney in this final "in situ" position. The renal vein was anastomosed to the external iliac vein ('end-to-side'). Therafter, the renal artery was anastomosed to the external iliac artery ('end-to-side'), or in most living donor cases (no aortic cuff) to the internal iliac artery ('end-to-end'). The MIKT access made it necessary to suture the back wall of the vascular anastomoses from the inside. Clamping of the vessels was done in a simplified, one-stage manner, using a Key-Lambert® clamp.

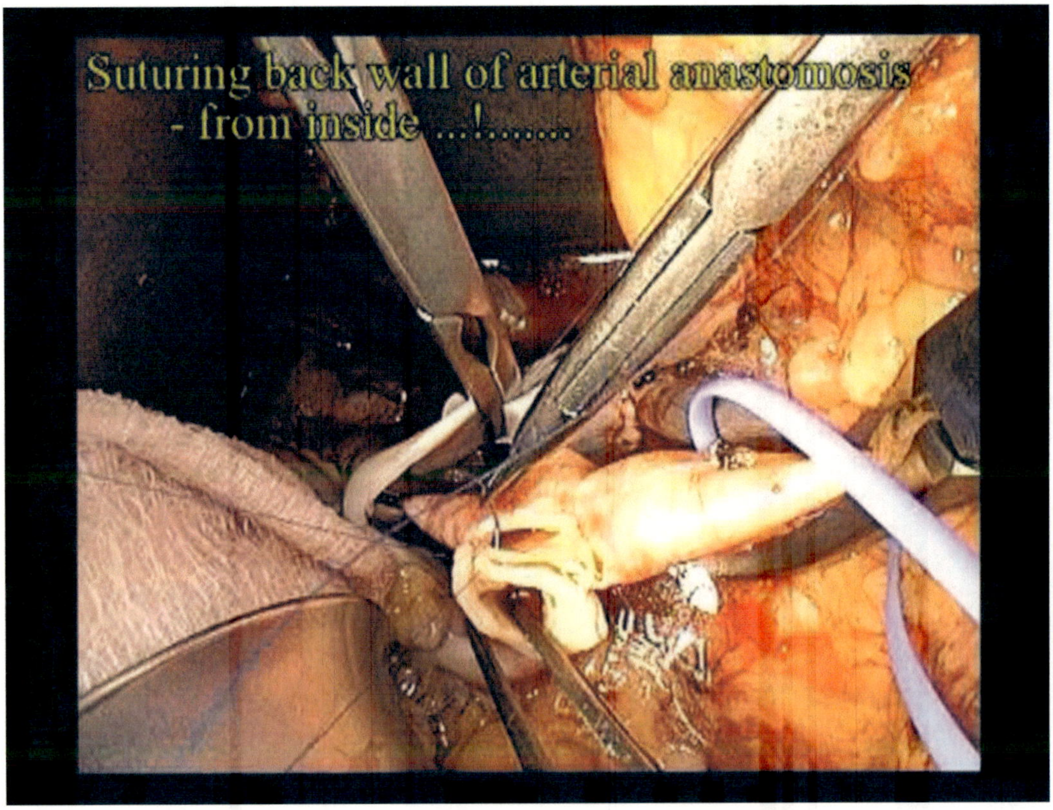

Fig. 3. Suturing the renal artery end-to-side to the external iliac artery (Clamp on renal vein).

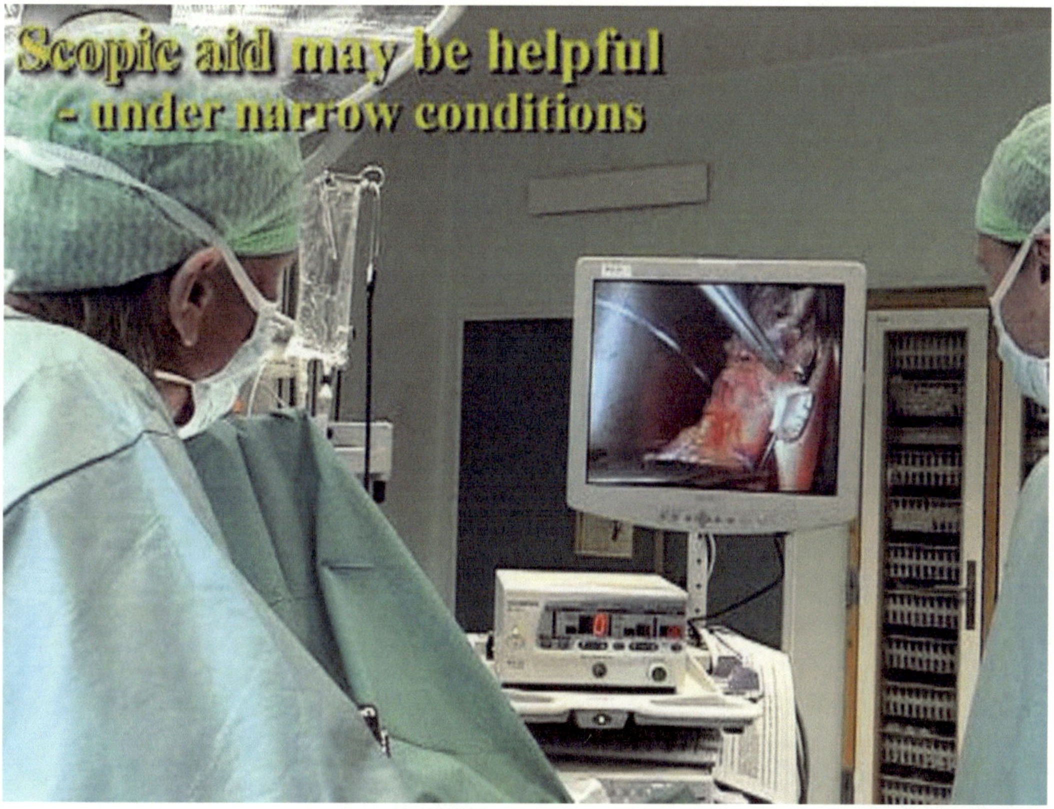

Fig. 4. MIKT scopic aid during the arterial end-to-side anastomosis.

In most cases the kidney was not moved from the neatly fitting retroperitoneal pouch after revascularization. Reimplantation of the ureter was performed by extravesical technique a.m. Lich-Gregoir, with minimal bladder dissection.
Scopic aid was only found necessary in a few cases under very deep, narrow circumstances. The scope was then simply introduced through the same incision, alongside the instruments, giving a "close up" of the anstomotic area.
A simplistic approach, with minimal dissection/tissue trauma was attempted at all stages.

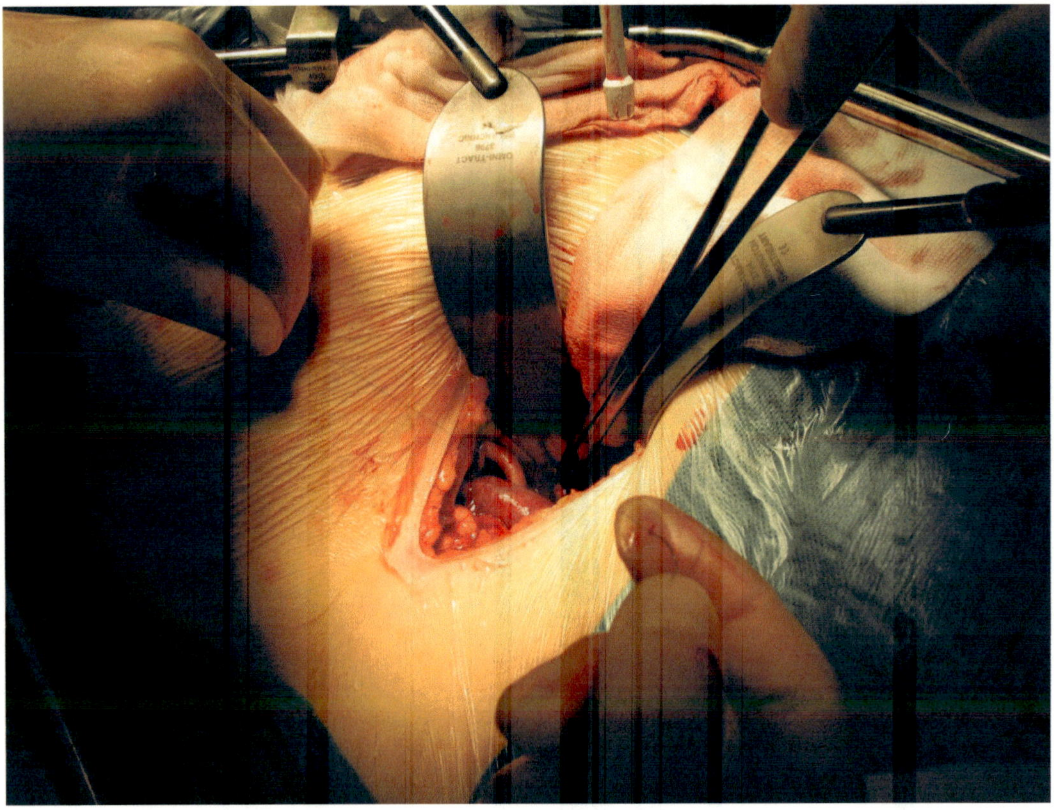

Fig. 5. After revascularisation: The perfused renal artery and vein are seen, while the kidney lies lateral to the skin incision.

4.2 MIKT: Results

A series of patients, transplanted by strict MIKT technique was then compared with matched controls subjected to conventional surgery. From December 2004 to July 2005, 21 kidney recipients were subjected to the new, minimally invasive technique. The MIKT patients constituted a consecutive series of transplantations performed by a single surgeon. A control group, subjected to conventional KTx (n=21) had been concurrently selected to match the MIKT group regarding age, sex, donor source, and primary-/retransplant status. No MIKT procedures were interrupted or converted to COKT. The results have been summarized in Table 1.

RESULTS *[mean (range)]*	MIKT n=21	Conventional Tx **n=21**	**Student t-test p-value**
Skin incision length (cm)	8,1* (7 - 9)	20,5 (17-23)	p<0,01
Operative time (min)	118* (95-140)	187 (130-270)	p<0,01
Analgesic requirementsPostop. days 0 + 1+ 2 (Morphine Equiv.; mg)	35 (3-86)	56 (20-173)	n.s. (p=0,053)
Hospitalization (days in hospital postop.)	8,2* (6-13)	12,4 (7-29)	p=0,02
Delayed graft function	10 % (2)	14 % (3)	
Measured GFR 10-12 weeks post-Tx (Cr-EDTA- Clearance; mean [range]; ml/min/1,73 m^2)	57,4 (35 – 81)	51,2 (26 – 72)	n.s. (p=0,053)
Peroperative incidents	No major	No major	
Surgical complications/reinterventions			
- Lymphocele: Reop.	2 (10 %)	3 (14 %)	
- Wound dehiscence: Reop.	0	1 (5 %)	
- Urinary obstruction: Reop.	0	1 (5 %)	
- Perirenal hemorrhage: Reop.	1 (5 %)	1 (5 %)	
- Bladder hemorrhage	0	2 (10 %)	
- *Total*	*3 (14 %)*	*8 (38 %)*	

Table 1. MIKT results. (extracted from Øyen et al., 2006)

Naturally, the MIKT skin incision was very much shorter. There were significant differences in favour of MIKT regarding operative time and postoperative stay in hospital. Furthermore, the analgesic requirements, expressed as morphine equivalents during postoperative days 0+1+2 were less in the MIKT group, however at non-significant levels. There were less complications and reinterventions in the MIKT recipients, totally 3 (14 %) - versus 8 (38 %) in the open KTx group. Because of the high complication rate in the control group, the total complication/reintervention rate of open KTx outside the study during the inclusion period (n = 97) were investigated and found to be 30-40 % (data not shown).

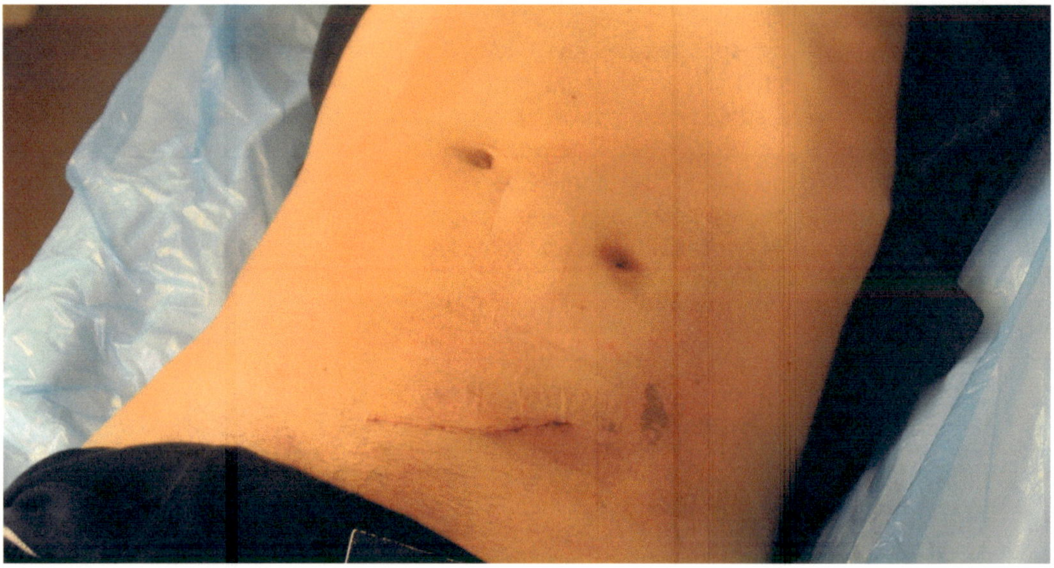

Fig. 6. Exterior result after left-sided MIKT in a slim patient, through a 7,5 cm incision.

4.3 MIKT: Discussion

Compared with L-LDN employing a 6-9 cm skin incision for kidney harvesting, the MIKT incision was only faintly larger (7-9 cm), and besides the L-LDN was dependent on 2-3 additional laparoscopic ports (5-12 mm each).

The first MIKT results were good, compared with the open, conventional KTx group and indicated that the procedure might be executed fast (because of its simplicity) and safe. By reducing incision, extent of dissection and thereby tissue trauma, the wound complications would be suspected to be reduced accordingly. Potentially it may also reduce hospitalization, and thereby the risk for nosocomial infections.

A major point about the MIKT approach (also when disregarding the results), was that reduction of tissue trauma appeared particularly appropriate in these patients, with significantly delayed wound healing and a high "background" complication rate. Due to the immunosuppressive theraphy, the incidences of wound dehiscence and incisional hernia were distinctly higher in Tx recipients, in particular after the introduction of Sirolimus/Everolimus. For simple reasons, a significant reduction of the abdominal wall incision would be anticipated to reduce these wound-related problems. Potentially, the MIKT procedure might also counteract the huge lymphocele/lymph leakage problem, by minimizing the dissection cavity and leaving less space available for fluid expansion.

Except from the single MIKT surgeon's extensive Tx experience , the distinctly shorter MIKT operating time might be explained by the simplified/minimalistic handling of the vessels, the extravesical reimplantation technique, and fast closure of a small incision.

Our data did suggest the same beneficial effects on postoperative pain/analgesia and recovery, that had been documented for a wide range of MIS procedures.

During recent years, Tx surgeons in Oslo have in part adopted the MIKT technique, by significantly reducing the size of the incision, even though not conforming strictly to MIKT. A significant reduction in overall KTx complication rates has been observed during 2008-2011, which may be partly attributed to reduced incision size and thereby tissue trauma.

5. Minimally invasive video-assisted KTx (MIVAKT) - The South Chorean experience (2007)

In 2007 a minimally invasive, partly video-assisted KTx technique (MIVAKT) was described by a South Chorean group (Seong-Pyo et al., 2007, Park et al., 2008) - obviously quite independent of the previous 'da Vinci robot' and MIKT reports.

5.1 MIVAKT: Method/Technique

The MIVAKT pocedure was carried out in 20 patients. Clinical variables were compared with the conventional KTx method. A 7-8 cm skin incision was employed. By means of a scopic balloon instrument a retroperitoneal space was created for the kidney. The vascular anastomoses and ureteroneocystostomy were performed under both direct vision and video-assisted aid.

5.2 MIVAKT: Results/Conclusion

The average length of the wound incision was 7-8 cm, placed below the belt line. The average operating time were 186 min. Less analgesics was given compared with conventional methods. There was one postoperative complication, a mild lymphocele. All patients showed normalized serum creatinine levels within 4 days post-Tx and normal findings on postoperative ultrasound and renal scintigraphy.
MIVAKT was shown to be technically feasible and might offer benefits in terms of better cosmetic outcomes, less pain, and quicker recuperation, compared with conventional KTx.

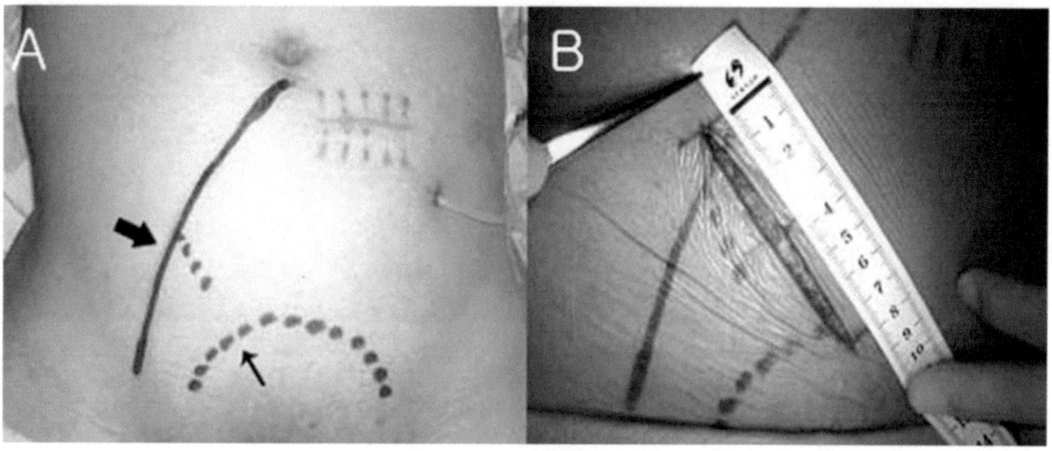

Fig. 7. (A) The location and course of the external iliac vessels (thick arrow) and the contour of the urinary bladder (thin arrow), marked preoperatively using ultrasound. (B) The 7–8 cm oblique incision. (Seong-Pyo et al., 2007)

5.3 MIVAKT: Discussion

We consider the transverse (horizontal) MIKT incision to offer better access to the iliac vessels, than the oblique MIVAKT incision. Furthermore, it is not at all necessary to use a laparoscopic balloon dissector to create the retroperitoneal space. A kidney-fitting retroperitoneal pouch is easily and safely made by hand/retractors through a minimal incision.

The video-assisted MIVAKT approach is interesting. Though, in the MIVAKT series, it seems like the vascular anastomoses for the most part were carried out under direct vision. In the MIVAKT discussion it is stated that "The grafted kidney was hung over the skin incision during the vascular anastomosis because the procedure is nearly impossible after the placing of the grafted kidney in the retroperitoneal space." This is not at all 'impossible'; but exactly what the MIKT technique is all about. Both the venous and arterial MIKT anastomoses were performed with the kidney in its final retroperitoneal position, suturing the back walls from the inside.

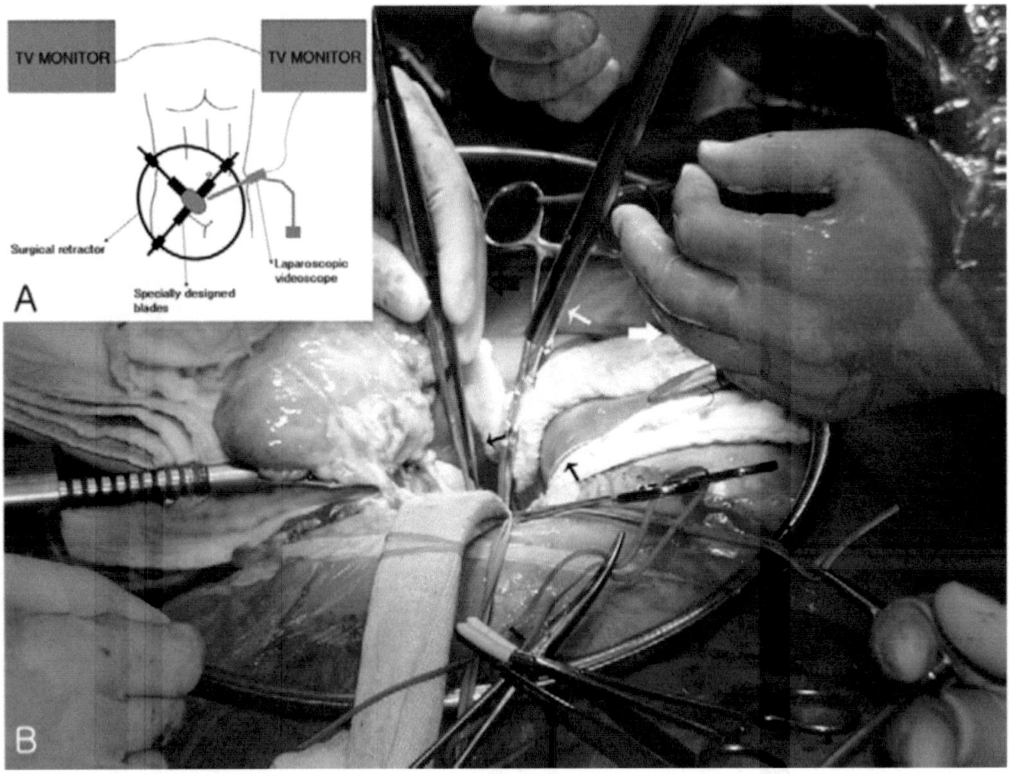

Fig. 8. (A) The circular retraction system and video-assisted TV monitoring. (B) The kidney was placed just above the skin incision during the vascular anastomoses. The laparoscope (thin white arrow) was found useful for visualisation and illumination. (Seong-Pyo et al., 2007)

6. Laparoscopic KTx – A case report from Barcelona (2010)

In 2010 a spanish group presented a case report on KTx by means of regular laparoscopic access, using 4 trocars and a Pfannenstiel incision (Rosales et al.).

6.1 Laparoscopic KTx: Method/Technique

With the recipient in the left lateral decubitus position, a hand-port was placed into a 7 cm Pfannenstiel incision. One trocar was put through the hand-port, while three more trocars were introduced in the right hemiabdomen.

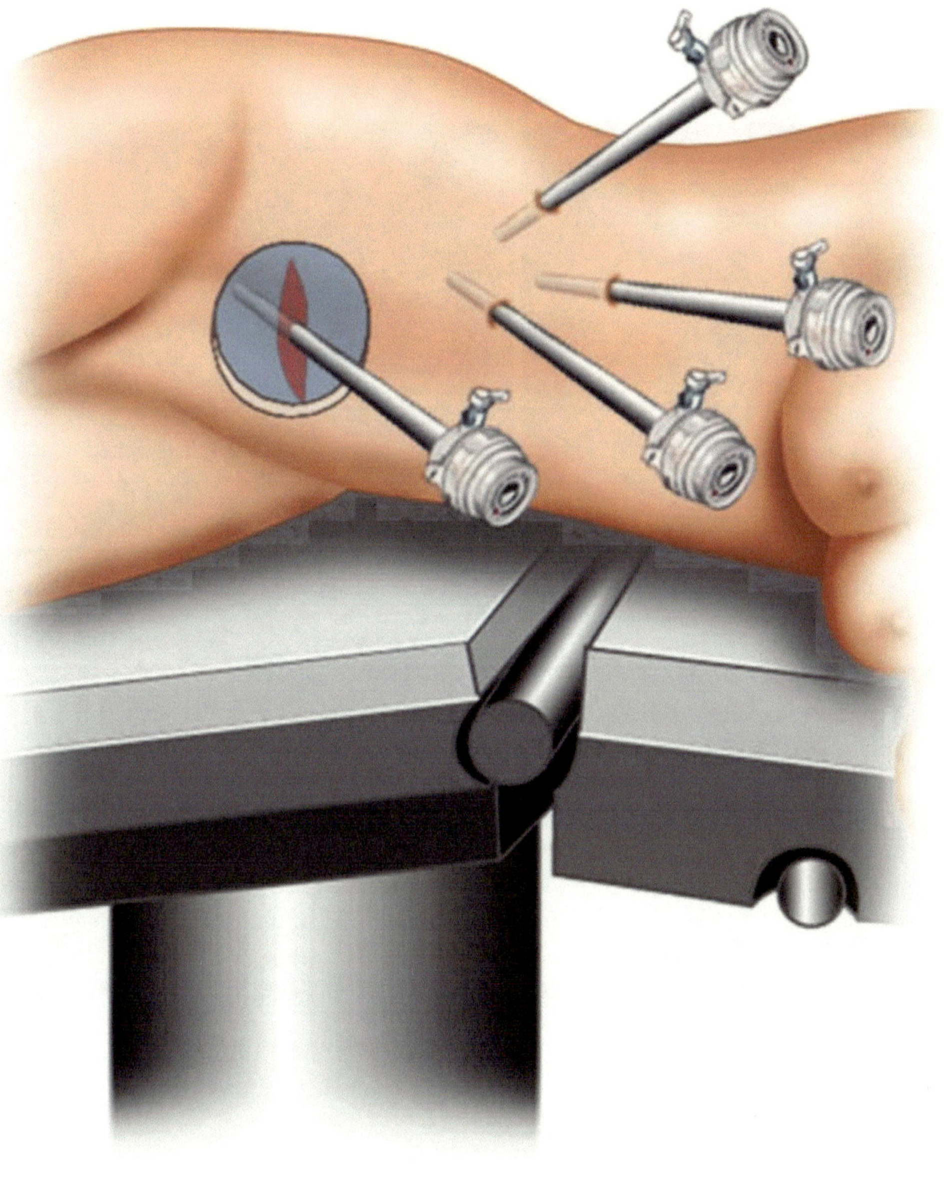

Fig. 9. Trocar positioning. Pfannenstiel incision. (Rosales et al., 2010)

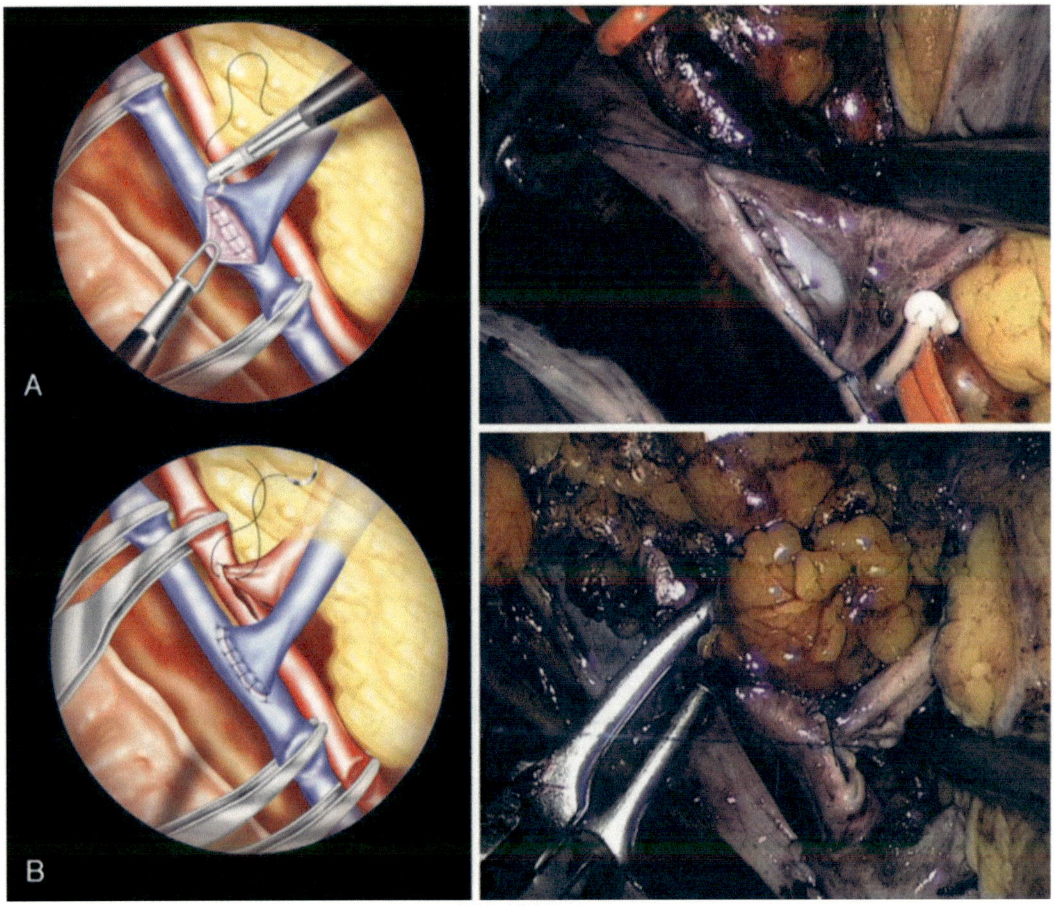

Fig. 10. Laparoscopic venous and arterial end-to-side anastomoses (Rosales et al., 2010).

By making a retroperitoneal, pelvic window ,the right external iliac vessels were dissected free. The kidney was introduced through the hand-port, and end-to-side anastomoses were performed by bulldog clamping through the hand-port and continous suture.
The ureterovesical anastomose was done by a modified Taguchi technique. Finally, the kidney graft was placed extraperitoneally by continuous suture of the peritoneal window.

6.2 Laparoscopic KTx: Results

Surgical time was 240 min, with 300 cm^3 bleeding. Cold ischemia time was 182 min. The postoperative course was uneventful and functionally satisfactory. Serum creatinine decreased progressively, to 73 µmol/l on the day of discharge. Stay in hospital was 14 days.

6.3 Laparoscopic KTx: Discussion

A laparoscopic KTx operating time of 4 hours seems too much, when MIKT can be executed in 2 hours, and with a total incision size that is probably smaller, when taking into account the 3 additional laparoscopic ports. The transverse (7-9) cm MIKT incision in the iliac fossa offers excellent direct access to the anastomotic area of the external iliac vessels. And regarding safety towards vacular incidents, the laparoscopic approach must be considered inferior.
Altogether, it seems unnecessary to perform the vascular anastomoses by laparoscopic technique - when these can be performed openly by an incision that is nevertheless needed for decent introduction/transplantation of the kidney.

7. Minimally invasive renal auto-transplantation (MI-Auto-KTx) (2010)

By combining "hand- assisted laparoscopic nephrectomy" and MIKT – using the same incision (7-9 cm) for hand-assistance, kidney harvesting, and transplantation – we have during 2009-2011 conducted "Minimally invasive renal auto-transplantation" (MI-Auto-KTx) in 6 patients. The first two MI-Auto-KTx cases have allready been documented and published (Øyen et al., 2010).

7.1 MI-Auto-KTx: Method

Laparoscopic hand-assisted nephrectomy: The handport incision (7-8 cm) was made medially in the right iliac fossa; displaced laterally compared with the usual Pfannenstiel L-LDN incision.
Extracorporeal 'back bench' preparartion: In the first case (female 38 years; renal artery aneurysm) it was possible to maintain a single arterial stem, after resection of the 16 mm aneurysm. In the second case (female 55 years; ureter lesion) three renal arteries had to be reconstructed.
MIKT: We utilized the handport incision, targeted on the iliac vessels, without extension. The meticulously prepared kidney was placed in a small/fitting, retroperitoneal pouch; and anastomosed to the iliac vessels. Reimplantation of the ureter was performed by extravesical technique.

7.2 MI-Auto-KTx: Results

Total operative times were 335 min and 434 min, respectively. In both cases the postoperative course was uneventful, and the patients were transferred to the local hospital

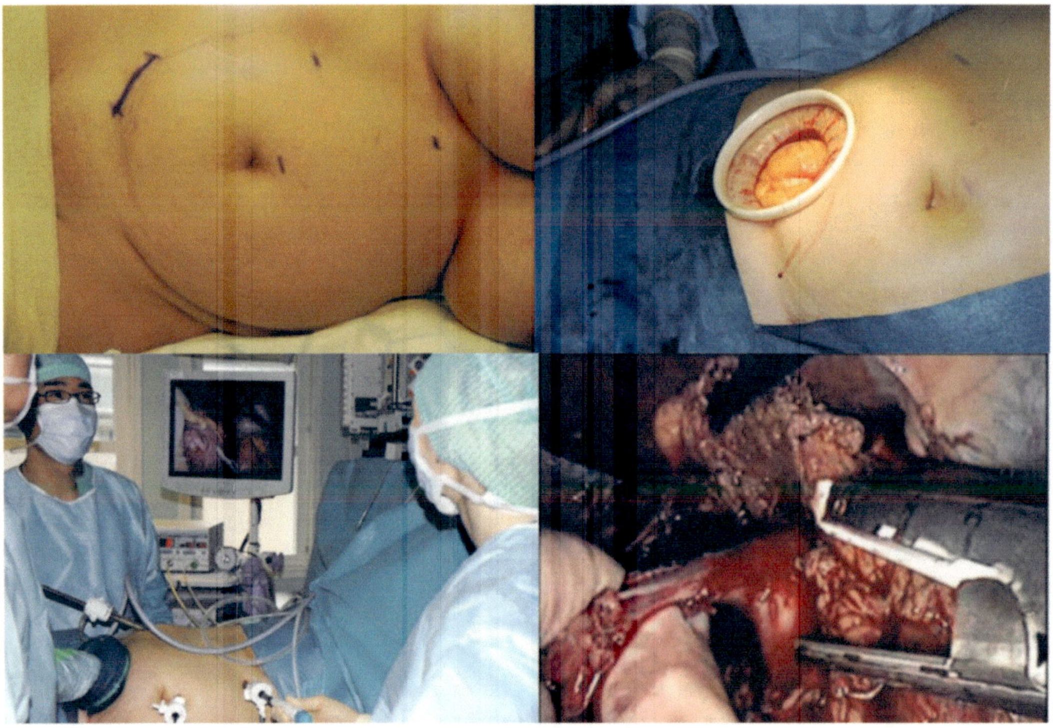

Fig. 11. MI-Auto-KTx: Laparoscopic, right-sided, hand-assisted nephrectomy; by a 7-8 cm medial "transplant incison", using GelPort and 3 trocars. The right renal vein is stapled and divided flush with the caval vein. (Øyen et al., 2010)

at day 4/day 5. When examined 3 mts postoperatively, both auto-transplants were shown to have excellent function by renal scintigraphy.

7.3 MI-Auto-KTx: Discussion

Our first two MI-Auto-KTx cases have demonstrated that a traditionally major surgical procedure, with extensive incisions/tissue trauma, can be made minimally invasive, by a similar incision as that used for L-LDN. Taking into regard the highly traumatic conventional incisions, we expect the generally proven minimally invasive benefits to be considerable.

8. Considerations about the future

The minimally invasive KTx procedures have so far not gained widespread acceptance and still seem to be at a "pioneer stage". However, considering the rapid evolution of MIS during the last two decades, there is little reason to believe that KTx and Auto-KTx in future will be excluded from this development.
Since a ≥ 6 cm incision will anyway be needed for decent introduction of the kidney (except for the possibilty of introduction through natural orifices) , we think the MIKT procedure is the most suited for further developments in this field.

9. References

Dubois F, Icard P, Berthelot G & Levard H (1991). Coelioscopic cholecystectomy: preliminary report of 36 cases. *Ann Surg*, 211: 60-2.

Harrell AG, & Beniford BT. (2005). Minimally invasive abdominal surgery: lux et veritas past, present, and future. *Am J Surg*, Vol 190, No 2, pp 239-43.

Hoznek A, Zaki SK, Samadi DB, Salomon L, Lobontiu A, Lang P & Abbou CC (2002). Robotic assisted kidney transplantation: an initial experience.. *J Urol*, Vol 167, pp 1604–06.

Hoznek A, Hubert,J, Antiphon, Gettman MT, Hemal AK & Abbou CC (2004). Robotic renal surgery. *Urol Clin N Am*, Vol 31, pp 731-76.

Khanna A & Horgan S (2011). A laboratory training and evaluation technique for robot assisted ex vivo kidney transplantation. *Int J Med Robot*. Vol 7, No 1, pp 118-122.

McCullough CS, Soper NJ, Clayman RV, So SSK, Lendrisak MD, & Hanto DW (1991). Laparoscopic drainage of a post-transplant lymphocele. *Transplantation*, Vol 51, No 3, pp 725-27.

Øyen O, Scholz T, Hartmann A & Pfeffer P (2006). Minimally invasive kidney transplantation: The first experience.. *Transpl Proc* , Vol 38, pp 2798-2802.

Øyen O, Scholz T, Hartmann A & Pfeffer P (2006). Minimal invasive kidney transplantation - The first experience. *Transplantation*, Vol 82, Suppl 2, pp 930-31.

Øyen O, Lien B, Line P-D, & Pfeffer P (2010). Minimally invasive renal auto-transplantation: The first report (2010). *J Surg Res*, Vol 164, pp e181-84.

Park SC, Kim SD, Kim JI, & Moon IS (2008). Minimal skin incision in living kidney transplantation. *Transpl Proc*, Vol 40, pp 2347-48.

Ratner LE, Ciseck LJ, & Moore RG.(1995) Laparoscopic live donor nephrectomy. *Transplantation;*, Vol 60, No 9, pp 1047-49.

Rosales A, Salvador JT, Urdaneta G, Patino D, Montllo M, Esquena S, Caffaratti J, Ponce de Leon J, Guirado L & Villavicencio H (2010). Laparoscopic kidney transplantation. *Eur Urol*, Vol 5 7, pp 164-67.

Seong-Pyo M, Jeong-Whan C, Kuyong-Jong K, Gui-Ae J, Min-Woo C, Young-Joon A & Seong-Whan K (2007). Minimally invasive video-assisted kidney transplantation (MIVAKT) (2007). *J Surg Res* Vol 141, pp 204-10.

Wolf JSJ, Tchetgen MB & Merion RM (1998). Hand-assisted laparoscopic live donor nephrectomy. *Urology*, Vol 52, No 5, pp 885-87.

25

Surgical Complications of Renal Transplantation

Marcelo Ferreira Cassini, Murilo Ferreira de Andrade and Silvio Tucci Junior
Ribeirão Preto Medical School, São Paulo University
Brazil

1. Introduction

In the early era of kidney transplant, surgical complications were a major cause of graft loss. Between 1960 and 1980, the estimated incidence was around 20%. With the improvement of surgical techniques, the frequency of these complications has dropped significantly and this subject until then common in the medical literature came to be seldom discussed (Botto V, 1993; Hernandez D, 2006). Currently, it is estimated that in large transplant centers the incidence of surgical complications is less than 5%. In general, the results of renal transplantation have improved primarily as a consequence of advances in medical and immunosuppressive therapy and progress in surgical techniques. Posttransplant urologic complications are unusual, with the range of 2.5% to 27% in most series, and can cause significant morbidity and mortality (Zargar MA, 2005; Dalgic A, 2006) Results have improved over the past decade as a direct application of less invasive endourologic diagnostic and therapeutic techniques of the surgical complications (Streem SS, 1994).

However, the etiologies are the most common technical problems and association with immunological complications. Surgical complications after renal transplantation can be classified mainly as vascular (arterial and venous thrombosis, renal arterial stenosis, lymphocele, hemorrhage) and urologic (ureteral obstruction, vesicoureteral reflux, urinary fistula), although other types of complications are not uncommon, like graft's rupture and hematoma. These complications can occur early in the intra-operative, immediate postoperative period or later, and imply in increase morbidity, hospitalization and costs (Humar A, 2005).

Urologic complications are the most common surgical complication after renal transplantation, causing significant morbidity and mortality. Recently, the incidence of urologic complications after renal transplantation has decreased to 2.5% to 12.5% (Emiroglu R, 2001). Unfortunately, there is a still higher incidence of technical complications in pediatric recipients, reaching approximately 20% with an associated 58% and 74% graft survival rates for cadaveric and living-related transplantation (Salvatierra O Jr, 1997; US Renal Data System, 1996). Urologic complications represent an important cause of morbidity, delaying normal graft functioning, and in some cases leading graft loss and/or patient death (Beyga ZT, 1998; Colfry AJ Jr, 1974; Mundy AR, 1981; Hakim NS, 1994).

The most frequent urological complications after kidney transplantation involves the ureterovesical anastomosis (fistula, stenosis and reflux), with a frequency ranging from 5% to 10% in different séries.

2. Urologic complications

2.1 Urinary fistula

This is the leakage of urine from the collecting system. It can occur at the level of the bladder, ureter or renal calices. The leakage of urine can be collected around the graft, move to the retroperitoneum, scrotum or may manifest through the incision. His average prevalence in many studies is around 5.7%. In general, most urinary leaks are the results of ureteral problems, failure of ureterovesical anastomosis or ischemia and necrosis of the distal ureteral stump.

Like the majority of surgeons now employ an extravesical ureteroneocystostomy technique for implantation of the ureter, there are shorter ureter and decreased likelihood of ischemia, and a limited cystostomy that rarely leads to leakage from the bladder (Gibbins WS, 1992; Thrasher JB, 1990).

Clinical presentation:

In most cases, there is constant discharge of clear liquid (yellow citrus) through the drain, in the immediate postoperative period, and sometimes the flow through the drain can even surpass the diuresis the urinary catheter.

When later, after removal of the tubular drain, there may be bulging store kidney with extension into the perineum and scrotum or decreased urine output with maintenance of renal function. Unexplained graft dysfunction, pelvic fluid collection, fever, graft tenderness, an lower extremity edema can also occur (Streen SB, 1994).

Early urinary leaks can be divided into two types: the first usually occurs within the first 1 to 4 days and is almost always related to technical problems with the implantation. In this case, the ureter has usually pulled out of a tunnel caused by excessive tension at the anastomosis. This complication appears to be more common with the extravesical ureteroneocystostomies (Streen SB, 1994). Some authors have recommended use of a ureteral stent to lessen the likelihood of this complication (Gibbins WS, 1992). The second type of early ureteral leak, usually presents between 5 and 10 days, is associated with distal ureteral ischemia, which may be a consequence of injury during the donor nephectomy, technical causes such as tunnel hematoma or distal stripping of the blood supply (Rosenthal JT, 1994).

Diagnosis:

For being the most common surgical complication of kidney transplantation, urinary fistula is easily diagnosed. In doubtful cases, where there is need to exclude the lymphocele as main differential diagnosis, biochemical analysis of the liquid is characterized by having elevated levels of creatinine, urea and potassium. In the lymphocele, creatinine should be similar of blood. Urinary leak are often suspected because of increased drainage from the wound. Radiographic tests of help include an abdominal ultrasound and nuclear renal scan. The ultrasound is nonspecific for evaluating patients with suspected urinary fistula after kidney transplantation. It will only reveal a fluid collection (anechoic image) around the graft. A renal scan demonstrating extravasation (figures 1.1, 1.2) is the most sensitive method to differentiate a urine leak from other fluid collections such lymphoceles or hematomas (Bretan PN Jr, 1989). A cystogram should be performed if a bladder leak is suspected.

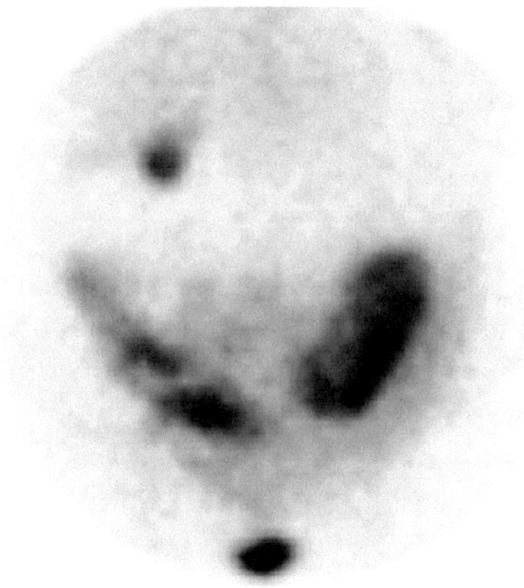

Fig. 1.1. Renal scan with contrast early extravasation (urinary fistula).

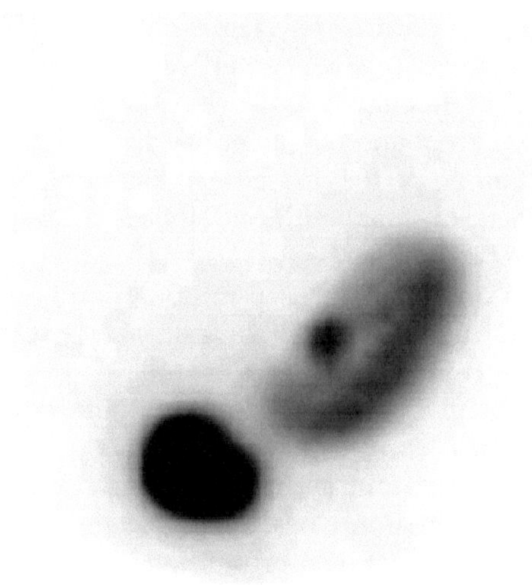

Fig. 1.2. Late renal scan without contrast extravasation (no fistula).

In the evaluation of transplant patients, nuclear medicine can contribute in the earliest complications that may arise in the period immediately following transplantation, as in the late complications and complications of surgical nature. A landmark study, conducted an initial assessment within the first 72 hours of surgery, is important so that we can better assess possible changes in the course of evolution. Studies with DTPA or MAG3 are the ones who will advise on the vascular phase and functional phase, and excretory phase, all parameters of the utmost importance in the evaluation of the graft (Kahan BD, 1989; Luk SH, 1999).
As surgical complications of kidney transplantation, the urinary fistulas are observed by scintigraphy an accumulation of the radiotracer outside the kidney (Luk SH, 1999). In cases of hematoma, other surgical complication, shows an area of low concentration of the tracer near the kidney, which may cause displacement of large structures such as vessels, ureter,

bladder and collecting system obstruction. The diuretic renogram may help elucidate this issue, because the transplanted kidney has the same performance as a native kidney scintigraphy.

Management of the urinary fistula:

Disruption of urinary tract in a renal transplant patient or graft dysfunction requires rapid diagnosis and treatment. Ureteral leakage needs careful and accurate diagnosis of the exact cause and site. It is important to know if the problem has a physical cause such a leak or an obstruction and is not associated with an acute rejection episode that required specific treatment (Streen SB, 1994; Rosenthal JT, 1994).

Surgical treatment has to be performed in all patients except those presenting with minimal extravasation at the ureteral reimplantation site and clinically stable. This group was initially treated by urinary drainage. In cases of unfavorable outcome after clinical treatment, surgery is indicated. Surgery is the initial aproach for big extravasation or when leaks arising from the mid or upper ureter were suspected. We use the same incision of the transplant to access the fistulae. The type of surgical reconstruction is based on the intraoperative evaluation of the extent of the ureteral necrosis and local and systemic condition of the patient at the time of surgery. Primary reconstruction with the ureter of the recipient or a new ureteral reimplantation are performed preferentially when local and systemic condition allowed; if local or systemic infection are present and the patient is clinically unstable an ureteral ligature associated to a nephrostomy can be performed. Ureteral stenting alone is used exceptionally. All patients received prophylactic or therapeutic antibiotic according to the antibiogram of the collected fluid (Mazzucchi E, 2006).

The need for immediate open operative surgical intervention has been replaced, to a large extent, by early endourologic intervention (Banowsky LHW, 1991). The placement of a percutaneous nephrostomy can divert a leak or relieve obstruction and allow more definitive diagnosis. As described by Streem et al., endourologic management can select patients for whom the likelihood of successful nonoperative management is good. In a few cases, percutaneous access can offer long-term treatment with chronic stent management. Percutaneous techniques like nephrostomy associated to antegrade ureteral stenting works in 40% of a much selected group of patients presenting with small fistulae from the distal ureter (Campbell SC, 1993).

Early open surgery is our preferred approach. Our policy is to perform primary urinary tract reconstruction whenever local and systemic condition allows. Termino-lateral anastomosis of the graft ureter or pelvis with the ureter of the recipient can be used as technique for the correction of urinary leaks. Some groups use termino-terminal anastomosis with the ureter of the recipient (Salomon L, 1999) with good results but can results in ureterohydronephrosis of the native kidney after ureter ligation for reconstruction. Ureteroneocystostomy "de novo" is used for reimplantation defects or for small distal ureteral necrosis and can fail in many cases due to necrosis extension or incomplete ureteral and bladder wall resection during surgery. Ureteral reimplantation remains an important option for urinary fistulae management. Ureteral ligature and nephrostomy is performed when there is gross infection of the fossa or when the patient presents in sepsis. There is also described, in cases of infected urinary fistulas and to prevent distal ureteral ligature and nephrostomy, the introduction of a Foley's catheter throught the bladder wall. The catheter's balloon is inflated at the transplanted renal pelvis to occlude the pyeloureteral junction and dry the region of the fistula (Suaid HJ, 2010).

Recurrences are due to insufficient ureter resection, leaving an ischemic stump extension of the process after the surgery or inadequate anastomosis. We recommend always leaving a double J stent in these cases in order to reduce recurrences but stents do not work if the necrosis extends. Recurrences were always managed surgically and an anastomosis with the ureter of the recipient was the first choice. Some patients can need a third procedure due to a new recurrence showing that the necrosis can extend after surgery and that extensive resection of the ureter is frequently necessary.

Mortality directly related to the fistula or to its correction was high in the early transplantation era (Dreikom K, 1992) and nowadays is reported to range from 0 to 8% (Salomon L, 1999). These better results are due to an earlier and more aggressive approach, reduction in the amount of corticosteroids in the immunosuppressive regimen and to better antibiotics and clinical support. The increase in the experience with these cases can still improve such results.

Routine ureteral stenting, to avoid urinary fistula, does not reduce significantly your incidence and its use is recommended only in special cases (contracted bladder, difficult anastomosis) (Campbell SC, 1993; Salomon L, 1999). In our center the modified Gregoir technique has been the procedure of choice in the last 35 years and the incidence of ureteral complications has been low.

2.2 Ureteral obstruction

Ureteral obstruction and ureteral leakage are the most common urinary complication after renal transplantation (Azhar, Hassanain et al. 2010). The incidence related in literature varies from 3 to 8% (Fontana, Bertocchi et al.; Smith, Windsperger et al.; Kaskarelis, Koukoulaki et al. 2008). Obstruction may occur during the early postoperative course due to blood clots, ureteral malrotation or kinking, tight submucosal tunnel, unsuspected donor calculus (Poullain, Devevey et al. 2010) or perigraft fluid collection (Kahan and Ponticelli 2000; Campbell, Wein et al. 2007). Late ureteral obstructions generally after the first month or even at years posttransplant are secondary to chronic ischemia which leads to chronic fibrosis and strictures. Other cause includes compressive limphoceles or pelvic masses, ureteral lithiasis and rarely obstruction by ureteral carcinoma (Huurman, Baranski et al. 2008) or fungus ball (Vuruskan, Ersoy et al. 2005).

The clinical presentation includes pain over the surgical site, decreased urine volume leading to oligoanuria and rise in blood pressure secondary to impaired renal function. Diagnostic tests shows gradual rise in serum creatinine. The ultrasound demonstrates pyelocaliectasis (fig. 2.1) or ureteropyelocaliectasis (fig. 2.2) in most of cases. Nuclear scintigraphy is less sensitive because the obstructed kidney also displays impaired radionuclide uptake, a sign often present in allograft rejection. When the diagnosis is unclear the antegrade pyelogram must be performed, because is an accurate method to define anatomically the site, degree of obstruction (Kahan and Ponticelli 2000).

The treatment must be instituted as early as possible to avoid loss of renal graft function. Initially the nephrostomy by puncture must be done to ensure the patency of the kidney and restore renal function to normal. The definitive treatment of the obstruction is oriented according to the etiology. Stenosis ureteral at the site of bladder reimplantation is more common and can be addressed by several endourology techniques such as ureteral meatotomy or percutaneous ureteral dilation with balloon followed by angioplasty and implant of stent at the ureters. Such techniques are at acceptable levels of success especially

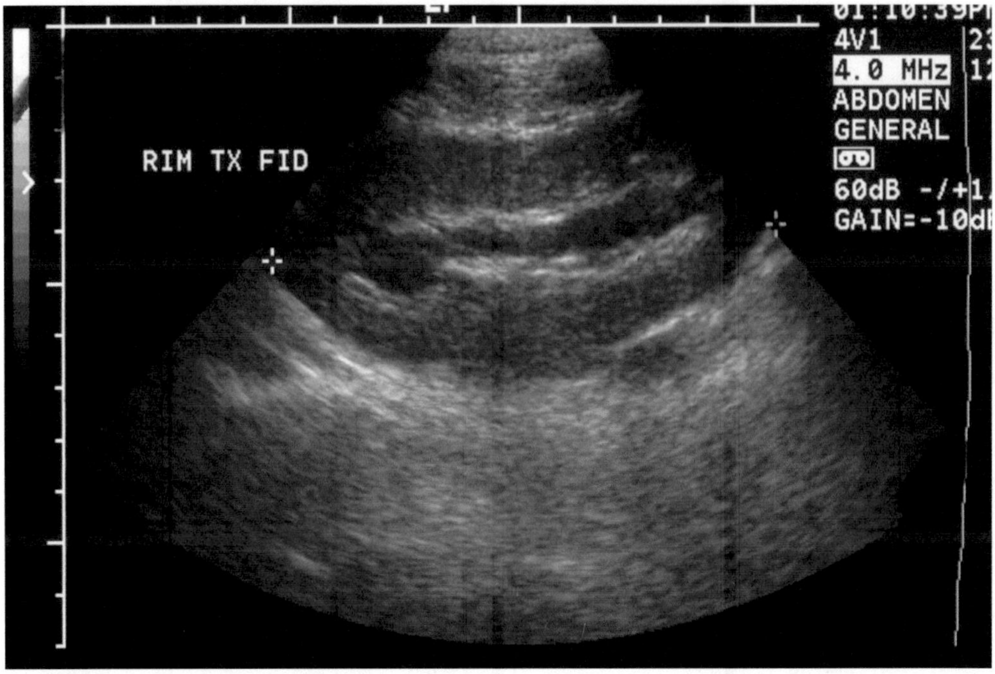

Fig. 2.1. Ultrasound with moderate hidronefrosis.

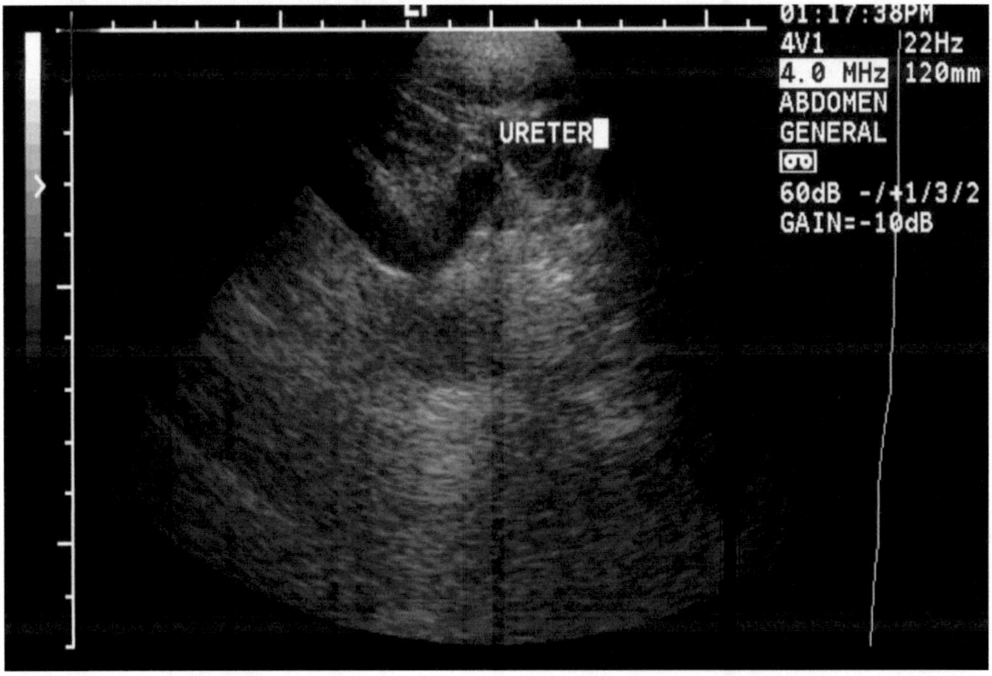

Fig. 2.2. Ultrasound of transplant kidney with ureteroectasis secundary to distal ureteral obstruction.

when treat small lesions (Burgos, Bueno et al. 2009). However, open surgery with reconstruction of the excretory pathway is still considered the gold standard. In distal ureteral obstructions or when there is redundant ureter, we can review the ureteroneocystostomy by extravesical Lich-Gregoir modified techniques (Campos Freire, de Goes et al. 1974) or intravesical (Politano-Leadbetter, 1958).
When there are multiple, long stenosis of the ureter or even poor vascularization, it is necessary to perform the anastomosis of the renal pelvis with the host ureter (ureteropyelostomy) or the ureter with the host ureter (ureteroureterostomy). However, the last technique has a higher rate of stenosis. When the native ureters cannot be used, the "Boari flap" should be done joining the short ureteral stump or the renal donor pelvis, allowing an adequate distance to the bladder. This allows tunneling the flap under the ureter, decreasing reflux and bacterial contamination during episodes of infection at the lower urinary tract. Extreme situations may require a pyelovesicostomy with anastomosis the donor urinary pelvis directly to the bladder. In this circumstance there is direct transmission of voiding pressure to the urinary collecting system as well as any urinary infection, leading to chronic pyelonephritis and deteriorating renal graft (Kahan and Ponticelli 2000).

3. Vascular complications

Although theoretically there is greater risk of surgical complications associated with living donors and recipients of kidneys with multiple arteries, in actuality it has not been considered more as a problem in laparoscopic (VLP) or open nephrectomy. This, indeed, is standard procedure in many transplant centers, (Wilson CH, 2005; Hsu TH, 2003) showing no significant adverse effects on the function and graft survival in VDL nephrectomies without or with hand assistance which may lead to higher vascular extension. (Saidi R, 2009; Hoda MR, 2010; Hoda MR, 2011) However, there is need for close attention to the anatomy of the donor due to the possibility of having two or more arteries and veins, or early arterial bifurcation (Benedetti E, 1995; Mazzucchi E, 2005; Harper JD, 2010). Furthermore, knowledge of microsurgical techniques for careful arterial graft reconstruction with multiple arteries and is essential for the reduction of vascular complications in these situations (Saidi R, 2009; Beckmann JH, 2008).

4. Arterial renal thrombosis

The most worrisome of vascular complications, it occurs in about 1% of all kidney transplants (Penny MJ, 1994; Bakir N, 1996) arterial thrombosis can reach values lower or higher in different series (Salehipour M, 2009).
Usually results from technical difficulties in removing the organ or implant. In nephrectomy and perfusion injury may occur in the endothelial layer, facilitating the process of thrombosis. The anastomoses of small vessels or of very different sizes or twisting or bending pressure are other predisposing factors for thrombosis, making demand for assessing the floor space of the kidney as well as proper positioning of the graft at surgery. With some frequency, there is a need to adjust the length of the renal artery to avoid kinking of the same. A technical care is obliquely sectioning the end of the renal artery (espatulating), which can reduce the risk of thrombosis and stenosis. Another factor to consider is the quality of the receiver because the arterial embolization of atheromatous

plaques predispose to thrombosis. Lesions in the endothelial artery caused by vascular clamp during anastomosis should also be considered (Gang S, 2009). Other situations of greater risk for vascular complications are patients receiving three or four kidney transplants, hyperacute rejection, and antiphospholipid antibodies (Gang S, 2009; Baños JLG 2005).

In children, either as donors or as recipients, renal transplantation deserves special attention, or some authors recommend the exclusion of donors under the age of 3 years and the best use of infusion solutions to reduce vascular complications and increase survival rates graft (Irtan S, 2010).

Clinical presentation and diagnosis:

The hallmark of renal artery thrombosis is the absence of blood perfusion of the parenchyma, which can still be identified intra-operatively. In the postoperative period the most common clinical presentation is the sudden interruption of urinary flow, without pain in the graft. Obstruction should be excluded from the catheter by blood clots. The renal perfusion should be evaluated by DMSA renal scintigraphy, by ultrasound Doppler, and even with arteriography, if needed (Nezami N, 2007).

The immediate surgical exploration may allow in a few cases, revascularization and recovery of the graft, especially if the diagnosis of arterial thrombosis is done before closing the incision. The loss of the graft is the most common consequence and nephrectomy should be performed (fig. 3.3).

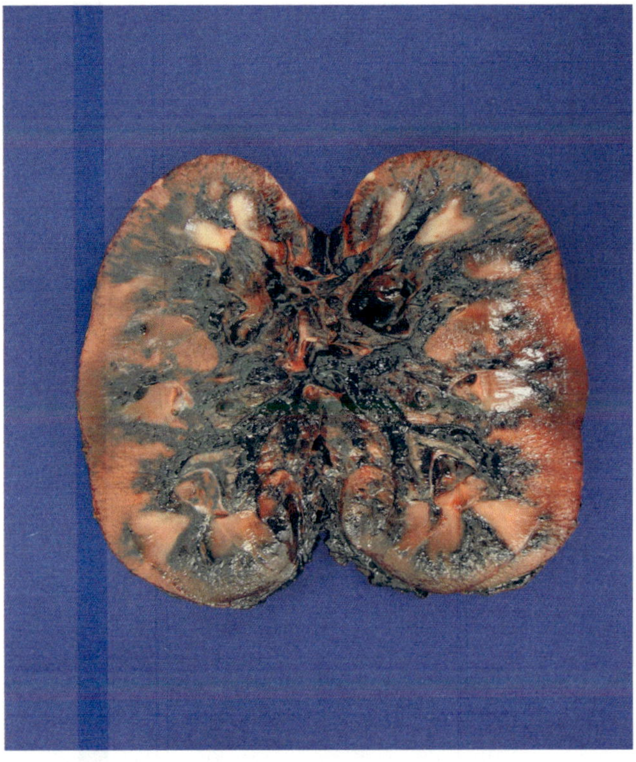

Fig. 3.3. Nephectomy: Arterial Renal Thrombosis.

5. Renal artery stenosis

The prevalence of renal artery stenosis is around 2% to 10% (mean 3.7%) (Benoit G, 1990). Clinical picture is suggested by onset severe hypertension post-renal transplant, dysfunction or presence of acute renal failure with prolonged NTA. With a peak onset at six months, renal artery stenosis can manifest itself as early as two days and as late as two years after transplantation. Stenoses located in the line of anastomosis, especially in termino-terminal anastomosis, the most frequent etiologic factor is technical failure. Other etiologic factors are largely the same that lead to arterial thrombosis, but acting with less intensity.

Clinical picture and diagnosis:

The suspicion must always occur when a transplant patient started with a progressive decline of renal function, heart murmur audible (or increasing its intensity) in the graft site and hypertension refractory to medical treatment. The diagnosis may be suggested by non-invasive techniques such as ultrasound associated with (color) Doppler (sensitivity 87 to 94%, specificity 86 to 100%). Doppler ultrasound is useful as screening and may show an increased blood flow velocity > 6 kHz12 (Nezami N, 2007).

The arteriography still remains the gold standard for diagnosis of arterial stenosis renal (Rengel M, 1998) The degree of stenosis is considered significant when more than 50% of the arterial lumen. Recently, gadolinium-enhanced MRI has allowed a noninvasive and efficacy comparable to that of renal arteriography convencional (Thornton MJ, 1999). The test with captopril, with plasma renin may be a method in the diagnosis of renal artery stenosis of kidney transplantado (Glicklich D, 1990).

The therapy depends on the location and degree of stenosis. Conservative treatment can be used in cases of mild stenosis in which blood pressure is controlled with medication and serum creatinine level remained stable.

Invasive procedures are indicated when blood pressure is not controllable by medication, there is progressive worsening of renal function or when noninvasive tests suggest the progression of stenosis. In this situation, diagnostic arteriography is indicated in combination with transluminal angioplasty and "stenting" (fig. 4.1, 4.2) (Leertouwer TC, 2000). This technique allows restoring renal perfusion in most cases and its effectiveness is confirmed immediately by a second angiography (Ghaffari S, 2009).

Intraluminal balloon dilatation with stenting is the preferred therapy for most patients, especially recommended in cases of localized stenosis and distant > 1 cm of the anastomosis. Surgery is reserved for lesions involving the anastomosis, or the surrounding area, and in cases of early artery stenosis renal (Benoit G, 1990). Other surgical procedures are indicated when the stenosis is severe and unsuitable for angioplasty or else, in this failure. Surgical techniques include reviewing local resection of the stricture and reanastomosis, may or may not be used autologous grafts (saphenous vein) or heterologous (Teflon) in the form of a patch graft or bypass, with success rates ranging between 63 to 92% (Bruno S, 2004), (fig. 4.3).

6. Renal vein thrombosis

The renal vein thrombosis is uncommon but serious complication, with incidence ranging between 0.9 and 4.5%, usually occurring in the first week after transplantation and with great potential for graft loss (Giustacchini P, 2002). Because the transplanted kidney does not have collateral circulation, venous stasis causes impairment of blood flow and consequent loss of function.

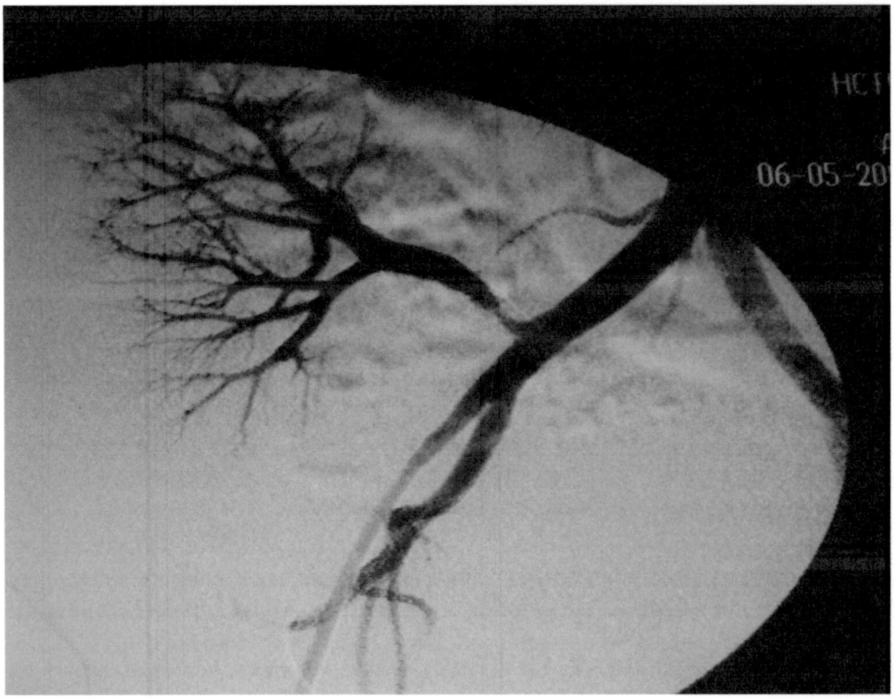

Fig. 4.1. Arteriography (post-transplant) showing a renal stenosis artery.

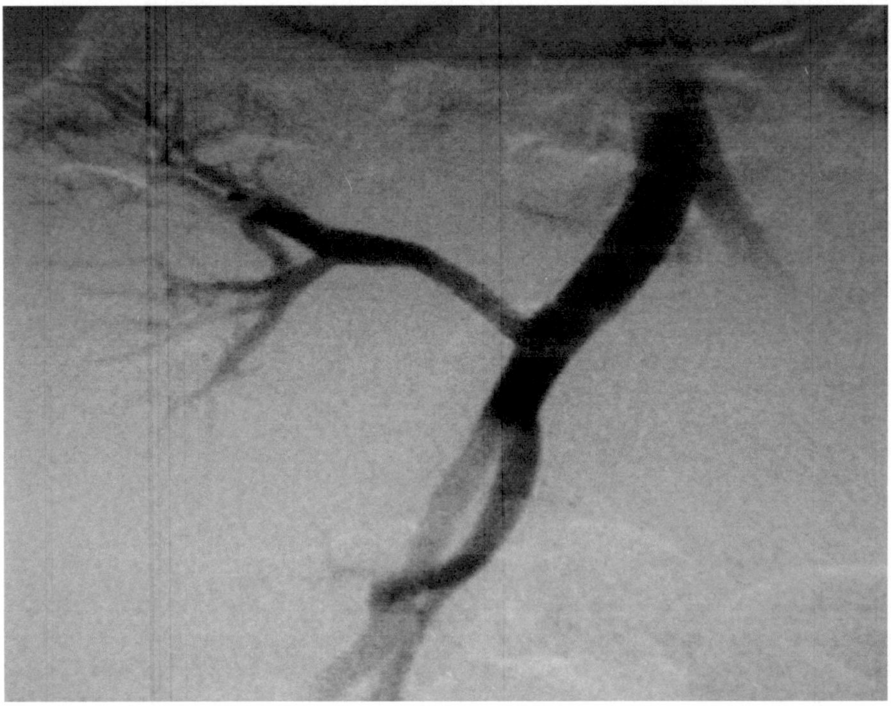

Fig. 4.2. Result after "stent" angioplasty.

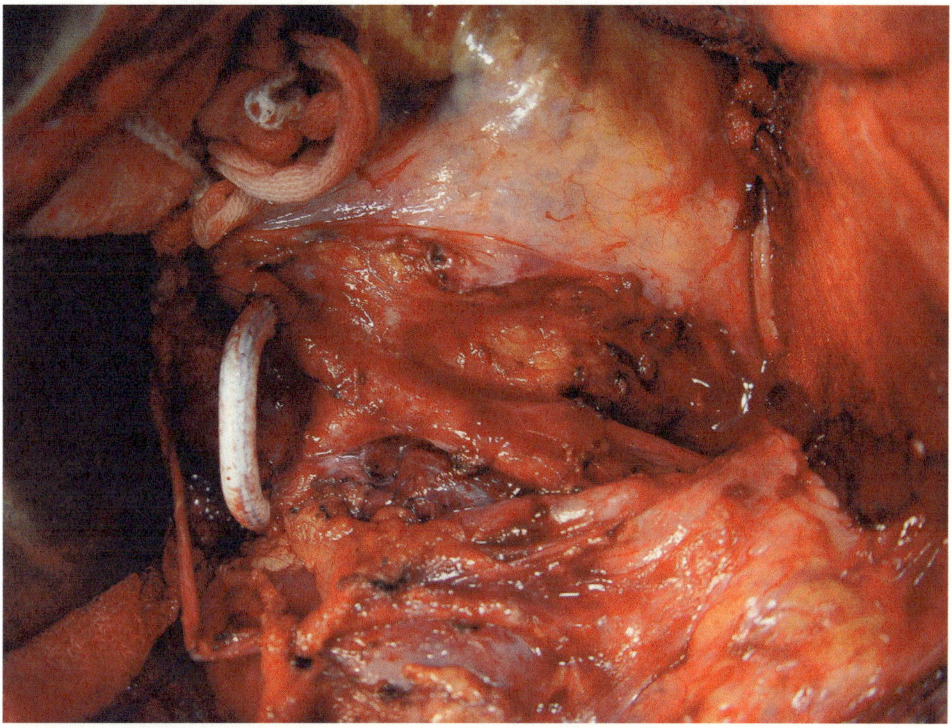

Fig. 4.3. Bypass iliac-renal arteries.

As causative agents related are: angulation of the renal vein or anastomotic stricture, dehydration, venous compression by lymphocele or hematoma, progression of ipsilateral iliofemoral thrombophlebitis should also be considered. Late cases of renal vein thrombosis have been associated with recurrence of membranous nephropathy, (Carrasco A, 2008).

Clinical presentation and diagnosis:

The symptoms is nonspecific as the sudden onset of hematuria, oliguria or anuria, accompanied by local pain and swelling of the graft. There may also increase the diameter of the ipsilateral lower limb deep venous thrombosis associated. The evaluation of renal Doppler ultrasound confirms the increase in renal volume and absence of venous flow. In the arterial can be seen reverse diastolic flow. Although it has been reported that early surgical exploration and thrombectomy allow the preservation of the graft in cases with renal vein thrombosis, but usually the kidney is no longer viable at the time of surgical exploration due to the spread intrarenal venous thrombus and prolonged hypertension. In most cases the nephrectomy is performed (Fathi T, 2007).

A complication associated with renal vein thrombosis is the rupture of the graft, which may cause hemorrhage and large hematoma perinephric (confirmed by ultrasonography), together with signs of hypovolemia and circulatory shock. Physical examination usually reveals bulging at the site. Nephrectomy is also standard procedure (figures 5.1, 5.2, 5.3).

However, in cases of rupture of the graft without thrombosis, should be attempted to suture the parenchyma and preservation of the graft (Gang S, 2009).

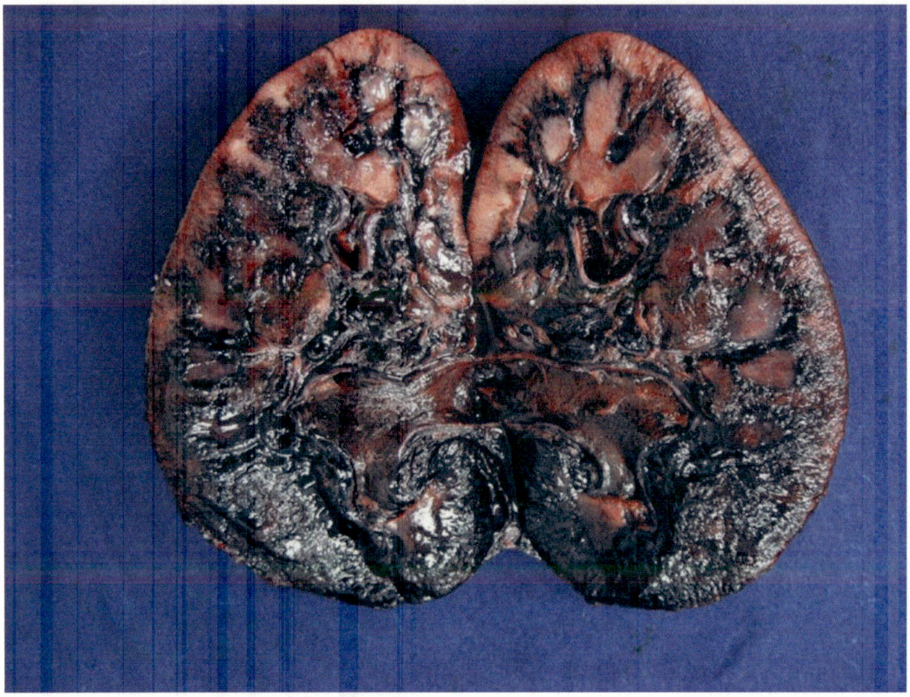

Fig. 5.1. Nephrectomy: Renal vein thrombosis.

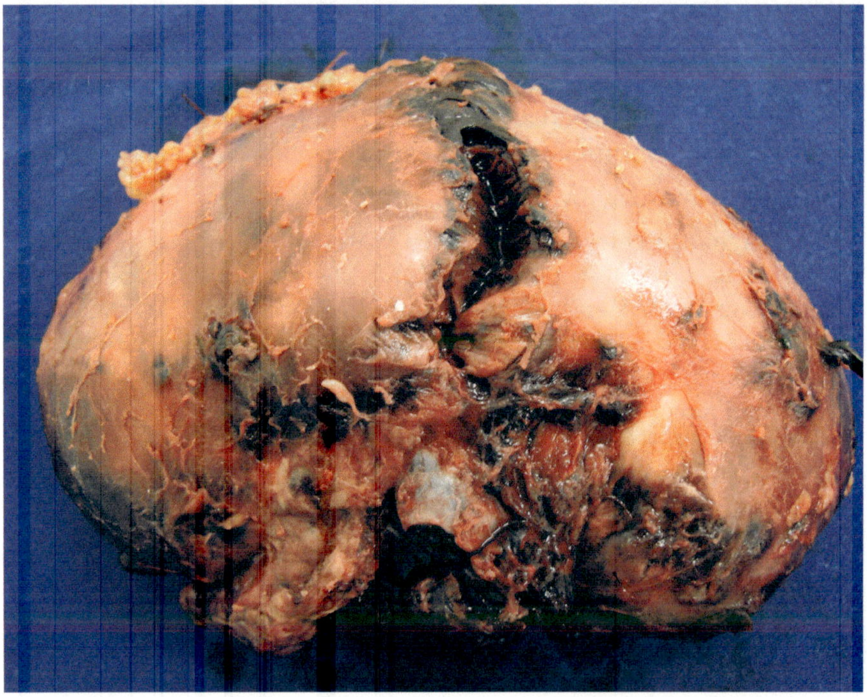

Fig. 5.2. Renal vein with thrombus inside and graft's rupture.

7. Lymphocele

Lymphocele is a lymph collection from the iliac lymphatic vessels of recipient or graft hilum that accumulates between the transplanted kidney and bladder. The average incidence of lymphocele in the literature ranges from 0.6 to 16% (Adani, Baccarani et al. 2007; Zargar-Shoshtari, Soleimani et al. 2008; Iwan-Zietek, Zietek et al. 2009). The etiology has been attributed to inadequate ligation of the delicate lymph vessels overlying the iliac vessels or present in the hilum. The method of renal uptake also appears to influence the appearance of lymphatic complications. The removal of the kidney by laparoscopy may prolong the lymphatic leak requiring drain for a longer period (Saidi, Wertheim et al. 2008). The small lymphoceles are more frequent but usually asymptomatic (Krol, Kolonko et al. 2007).
However, larger collections are manifested clinically in a few weeks to months after transplantation, bulging can occur in the surgical wound (Fig. 6.1) with or without cutaneous extravasation of lymph. In severe cases, there may be edema of lower limb ipsilateral to the graft, frequent urination due to bladder compression and ureteral obstruction leading to hydronephrosis and loss of renal graft function (Kahan and Ponticelli 2000)

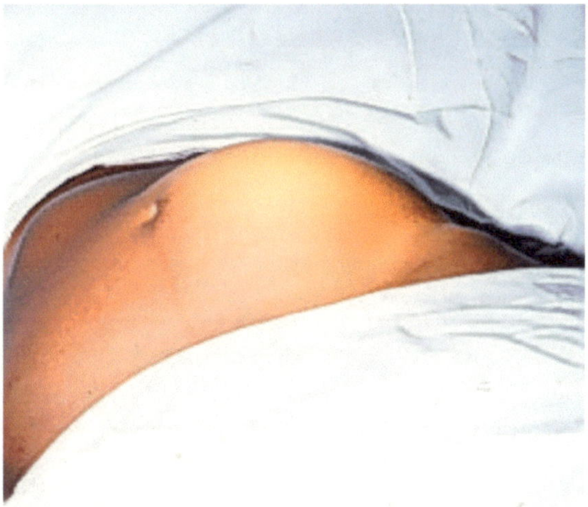

Fig. 6.1. Abdominal bulging secondary to lymphocele.

The diagnosis is confirmed by ultrasound which may show hydronephrosis, altered vascular flow by Doppler and quantify the lymphocele or the presence of other collections such as hematoma (Fig. 6.2) or urinoma (Fig. 6.3)(Krol, Kolonko et al. 2007). In cases of doubt about the etiology, a computerized axial tomography (CT) (Fig. 6.4) can be performed following puncture of the collection guided by CT or ultrasound (US) with biochemical dosages of the liquid obtained.
The treatment can be divided into expectant, puncture and drainage or surgery. As previously mentioned, small volumes of lymphocele with less than 140ml and asymptomatic, tend to resolve spontaneously without any renal graft damage. Larger collections or lymphoceles with clinical manifestations can be punctured and drained, under strictly aseptic techniques and guided by US or CT. In this case you should aim for total disappearance of the collection. If there is clinically significant recurrence, a sclerotherapy with povidone-iodine 5% ethanol or antibiotics can be performed (Chandrasekaran, Meyyappan et al. 2003; Hamza, Fischer et al. 2006; Zomorrodi and Buhluli 2007).

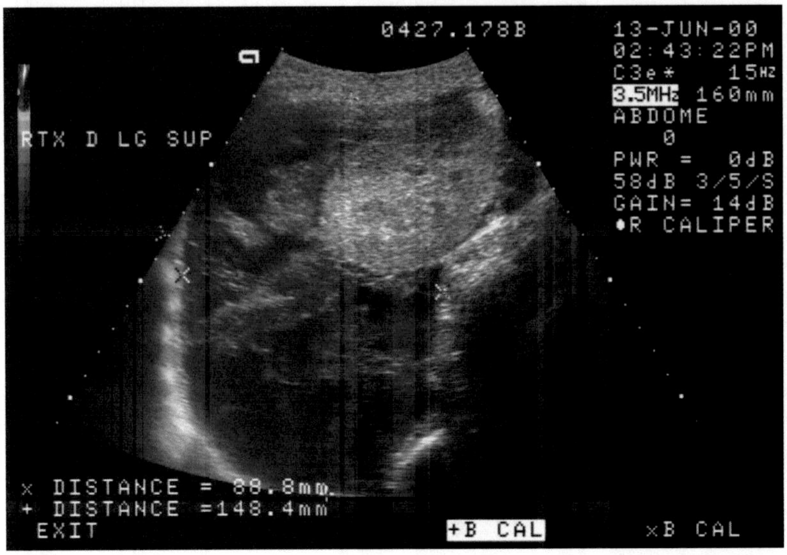

Fig. 6.2. Perinephric hematoma

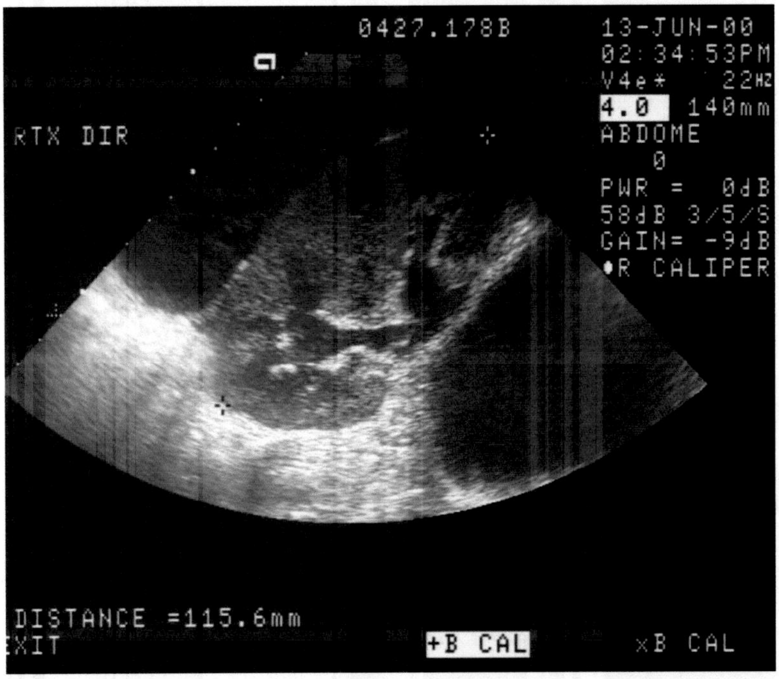

Fig. 6.3. Urinoma.

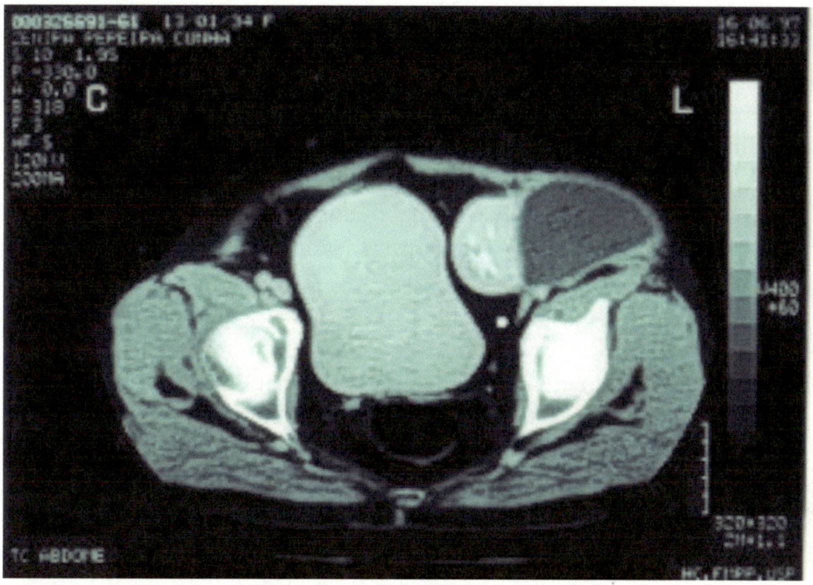

Fig. 6.4. Computerized axial tomography showing a lymphocele.

In lymphoceles larger than 500 ml, punctures, drainages and sclerotherapy are usually not effective. In cases refractory or complicated, the laparoscopic lymphocele fenestration (Marsupialization) is the procedure of choice in many centers. The laparoscopic technique reduces the risk of injury to the ureter or infection and demonstrates high rate of success. It is important to create a window sufficiently large to ensure patency of the ureter (Kahan and Ponticelli 2000).

When the location is not favorable to laparoscopy or in recurrent cases, the approach by open surgery should be performed, especially when the lymphocele is located posterior and lower to the transplanted kidney or behind the bladder (Fuller, Kang et al. 2003; Hamza, Fischer et al. 2006). In both techniques is recommended to perform the peritoneocystostomy with an oval window of at least 2.5 x 5.0 cm in width associated with interposition of short segment of omentum, allowing a good peritoneal absorption of lymphocele and avoiding internal hernias of the bowel segments (Kahan and Ponticelli 2000).

Recently was reported the treatment of recurrent and symptomatic lymphocele by inserting a Tenchoff catheter at the site of lymphocele tunneled to the abdomen, allowing the intraperitoneal drainage. This procedure offers as advantages the possibility of being performed in outpatient clinics, without general anesthesia, with good efficacy and safety, although the number of cases reported is still small (Adani, Sponza et al. 2007) (Adani, Baccarani et al. 2007).

In conclusion, the treatment of lymphoceles should begin by less invasive techniques. If there is recurrence or failure proceed to marsupialization by laparoscopy or open surgery.

8. References

Adani, G. L., U. Baccarani, et al. (2007). "Treatment of recurrent symptomatic lymphocele after kidney transplantation with intraperitoneal Tenckhoff catheter." Urology 70(4): 659-61.

Adani, G. L., M. Sponza, et al. (2007). "Intraperitoneal Tenckhoff catheter for the treatment of recurrent lymphoceles after kidney transplantation: our early experience." Transplant Proc 39(6): 1851-2.

Azhar, R. A., M. Hassanain, et al. (2010). "Successful salvage of kidney allografts threatened by ureteral stricture using pyelovesical bypass." Am J Transplant 10(6): 1414-9.

Bakir N, Sluiter WJ, Ploeg RJ. Primary renal graft thrombosis. Nephrol Dial Transplant.1996; 11:140-147.)

Baños JLG, Calabia ER, Rodrigo MHL, Martín JAP, Edreira AR, Gómez MAC, Schaan JIV, Tubet CA, Izquierdo FR, Diego RB, García RM. Aspectos quirúrgicos en los terceros y cuartos retrasplantes renales. Actas Urol Esp. 2005; 29 (2): 212-216.

Banowsky LHW. Surgical complications of renal transplantation. In: Glenn JF,ed Urologic Surgery, 4th ed. Philadelphia: JB Lippincott, 1991;252-266.

Beckmann JH, Jackobs S, Klempnauer J. Arterial reconstruction in kidney transplantation. Tx Med. 2008; 20:7-12.

Benedetti E, Troppmann C, Gillingham K, Sutherland DER, Payne W, Dunn DL, Matas AJ, Najarian JS, Gruessner RWG. Short-and long-term outcomes of kidney transplants with multiple renal arteries. Ann Surg. 1995; 221 (4):406-414.

Benoit G, Moukarzel M, Hiesse C, Verdelli G, Charpentier B, Fries D. Transplant renal artery stenosis: experience and comparative results between surgery and angioplasty.Transplant Int.1990;3:137-40.

Beyga ZT, Kahan BD: Surgical complications of kidney transplantation. J Nephrol 11:137, 1998.

Botto V, Cortese F, Baroni B, et al. Surgical complications in renal transplantation. Minerva Chir. 48(21 -22): 1341 -1346, 1993.

Bretan PN Jr, Hodge E, Streem SB, et al. Diagnosis of renal transplant fistulas. Transplant Proc 21:1962-1966, 1989.

Bruno S, Remuzzi G, Ruggenenti P. Transplant Renal Artery Stenosis. J Am Soc Nephrol. 2004; 15: 134–141.

Burgos, F. J., G. Bueno, et al. (2009). "Endourologic implants to treat complex ureteral stenosis after kidney transplantation." Transplant Proc 41(6): 2427-9.

Campbell, M. F., A. J. Wein, et al. (2007). Campbell-Walsh urology / editor-in-chief, Alan J. Wein ; editors, Louis R. Kavoussi ... [et al.]. [Philadelphia], W.B. Saunders.

Campbell SC, Streem SB, Zelch M, Hodge E, Novick AC. Percutaneous management of transplant ureteral fistulas: patient selection and long-term results. J Urol. 1993; 150:1115-1117.

Campos Freire, J., G. M. de Goes, et al. (1974). "Extravesical ureteral implantation in kidney transplantation." Urology 3(3): 304-8.

Carrasco A, Diaz C, Flores JC, Briones E, Otipka N. Late renal vein thrombosis associated with recurrence of membranous nephropathy in a renal allograft: a case report. Transplant Proc. 2008 Nov; 40(9):3259-60.

Chandrasekaran, D., R. M. Meyyappan, et al. (2003). "Instillation of povidone iodine to treat and prevent lymphocele after renal transplantation." BJU Int 91(3): 296.

Colfry AJ Jr, Schlegel JU, Lindsey ES, et al: Urological complications in renal transplantation. J Urol 112:564, 1974.

Dalgic A, Boyvat H, Karakayali G, et al: Urologic complications in 1523 renal transplantations: the Baskent University Experience. Transplant Proc 38:543, 2006.

Dreikom K. Problems of the distal ureter in renal transplantation. Urol Int. 1992;49: 76-89.

Emiroglu R, Karakayali H, Sevmis S, et al: Urologic complications in 1275 consecutive renal transplantations. Transplant Proc 33:2016, 2001.

Fathi T, Samhan M, Gawish A, Donia F, Al-Mousawi M. Renal allograft venous thrombosis is salvageable. Transplant Proc 2007 May; 39:1120-1.

Fontana, I., M. Bertocchi, et al. "Late ureteral stenosis after kidney transplantation: a single-center experience." Transplant Proc 42(4): 1174-5.

Fuller, T. F., S. M. Kang, et al. (2003). "Management of lymphoceles after renal transplantation: laparoscopic versus open drainage." J Urol 169(6): 2022-5.

Gang S, Rajapurkar M. Vascular complications following renal transplantation. JNRT. 2009; 2(1): 122 - 132.

Ghaffari S, Hakim H, Ahmadpoor P. Transplanted Renal Artery Stenosis: a Case Report and Review of Literature. J Cardiovasc Thorac Res. 2009; 1(2): 45-48.

Gibbins WS, Barr JM, Hefty TR. Complications following un-stented parallel incision extravesical ureteroneocystostomy in 1,000 kidney transplants. J Urol 148:38-40,1992.

Giustacchini P, Pisanti F, Citterio F, De Gaetano AM, Castagneto M, Nanni G. Renal vein thrombosis after renal transplantation: an important cause of graft loss. Transplant Proc. 2002; 34: 2126–2127.

Glicklich D, Tellis VA, Quinn T, Mallis M, Greenstein SM, Schechner R, et al. Comparison of captopril scan and Doppler ultrasonography as screening tests for transplant renal artery stenosis. Transplantation. 1990;49:217-8.

Hakim NS, Benedetti E, Pirenne J, et al: Complications of ureterovesical anastomosis in kidney transplant patients: the Minnesota experience. Clin Transplant 8:504, 1994.

Hamza, A., K. Fischer, et al. (2006). "Diagnostics and therapy of lymphoceles after kidney transplantation." Transplant Proc 38(3): 701-6.

Harper JD, Breda A, Leppert JT, Veale JL, Gritsch HA, Schulam PG. Experience with 750 consecutive laparoscopic donor nephrectomies—is it time to use a standardized classification of complications? J Urol. May 2010; 183, 1941-1946.

Hernández D, Rufino M, Armas S, Gonzáles A, Gutiérrez P, Barbero P, Vivancos S, Rodríguez C, de Vera JR, Torres A. Retrospective analysis of surgical complications following cadaveric kidney transplantation in the modern transplant era. Nephrol Dial Transplant. 21: 2908–2915, 2006.

Hoda MR, Greco F, Reichelt O, Heynemmann H, Fornara P. Right-sided transperitoneal hand-assisted laparoscopic donor nephrectomy: is there an issue with the renal vessels? J Endourol. 2010 Dec;24(12):1947-52.

Hoda MR, Greco F, Wagner S, Heynemmann H, Fornara P. Prospective, nonrandomized comparison between right- and left-sided hand-assisted laparoscopic donor nephrectomy. Transplant Proc. 2011; 43(1):353-356.

Hsu TH, Su LM, Ratner LE, Trock BJ, Kavoussi LR. Impact of renal artery multiplicity on outcomes of renal donors and recipients in laparoscopic donor nephrectomy. Urology. 2003; 61: 323-7.

Humar A, Matas AJ. Surgical Complications After Kidney Transplantation. Seminar in Dyalisis 2005; 18(6):505-510.

Huurman, V. A., A. G. Baranski, et al. (2008). "Transfer of ureteral carcinoma in a transplanted kidney presenting by early stenosis of the proximal ureter." Clin Transplant 22(6): 847-50.

Irtan S, Maisin A, Baudouin A, Nivoche Y, Azoulay R, Jacqz-Aigrain E, El Ghoneimi A, Aigrain Y. Renal transplantation in children: critical analysis of age related surgical complications. Pediatr Transplant. 2010 Jun; 14(4):5123-9.

Iwan-Zietek, I., Z. Zietek, et al. (2009). "Minimally invasive methods for the treatment of lymphocele after kidney transplantation." Transplant Proc 41(8): 3073-6.

Kahan, B. D. and C. Ponticelli (2000). Principles and practice of renal transplantation. [London], Martin Dunitz.

Kahan BD. Cyclosporine. N Engl J Med. 1989;321:1725-38.

Kaskarelis, I., M. Koukoulaki, et al. (2008). "Ureteral complications in renal transplant recipients successfully treated with interventional radiology." Transplant Proc 40(9): 3170-2.

Krol, R., A. Kolonko, et al. (2007). "Did volume of lymphocele after kidney transplantation determine the choice of treatment modality?" Transplant Proc 39(9): 2740-3.

Leertouwer TC, Gussenhoven EJ, Bosch JL, van Jaarsveld BC, van Dijk LC, Deinum J, et al. Stent placement for renal arterial stenosis: Where do we stand? A meta-analysis. Radiology. 2000; 216: 78–85.

Luk SH, Chan JH, Kwan TH, Tsui WC, Cheung YK, Yuen MK. Breath-hold 3D gadolinium-enhanced subtraction MRA in the detection of transplant renal artery stenosis. Clin Radiol. 1999;54:651-4.

Mazzucchi E, Souza AA, Nahas WC, Antonopoulos IM, Piovesan AC, Arap S. Surgical complications after renal transplantation in grafts with multiple arteries. Int Braz J Urol. 2005; 31 (2): 125-130.

Mazzucchi E, Souza GL, Hisano M, Antonopoulos IM, Piovesan AC, Nahas WC, Lucon AM, Srougi M. Primary reconstruction is a good option in the treatment of urinary fistula after kidney transplantation. Int Braz J Urol, 2006, 32(4):398-404.

Mundy AR, Podesta ML, Bewick M, et al: The urological complications of 1000 renal transplants. Br J Urol 53:397, 1981.

Nezami N, Tarzamni MK, H Argan, M. Doppler ultrasonographic indexes Nourifar in kidney transplant recipients. Its relationship with kidney function. Iran J Kidney Dis. 2007; (1) 2:82-87.

Penny MJ, Nankivell BJ, Disney APS. Renal graft thrombosis. Transplantation. 1994; 58: 565-569.

Poullain, J., J. M. Devevey, et al. (2010). "[Management of lithiasis of kidney transplant]." Prog Urol 20(2): 138-43.

Rengel M, Gomes da Silva G, Inchaustefgul L, Lampreave JL, Robledo R, Echenagusia A, et al. Renal artery stenosis after kidney transplantation: diagnostic and therapeutic approach. Kidney Int Suppl. 1998;54:S99-606.

Rosenthal JT. Surgical management of urological complications after kidney transplantation. Semin Urol XII(2):114-122, 1994.

Saidi, R. F., J. A. Wertheim, et al. (2008). "Impact of donor kidney recovery method on lymphatic complications in kidney transplantation." Transplant Proc 40(4): 1054-5.

Saidi R, Kawai T, Kennealey P, Tsouflas G, Elias N, Hertl M, Cosimi AB, Dicken S. C. Ko. Living donor kidney transplantation with multiple arteries. Arch Surg. 2009; 144(5):472-475.

Salehipour M, Salahi H, Jalaeian H, Bahador A, Nikeghbalian S, Barzideh E, Ariafart A, Malek-Hosseini SA. Vascular complications following 1500 consecutive living and cadaveric donor renal transplantations: a single center study. Saudi J Kidney Dis Transpl. 2009; 20(4):570-572.

Salomon L, Saporta F, Amsellem D, Hozneck A, Colombel M, Patard JJ, et al.: Results of pyeloureterostomy after ureterovesical anastomosis complications in renal transplantation. Urology, 1999; 53:908-912.

Salvatierra O Jr, Tanney D, Mak R, et al: Pediatric renal transplantation and its challenges. Transplant Rev 11:51, 1997.

Smith, K. M., A. Windsperger, et al. "Risk factors and treatment success for ureteral obstruction after pediatric renal transplantation." J Urol 183(1): 317-22.

Streem SS: Endourological management of urological complications following renal transplantation. Semin Urol 22:123, 1994.

Streen SB. Endourological management of urological complications following renal transplantation. Semin Urol XII(2):123-133, 1994.

Suaid HJ, Cassini MF, Tucci S Jr, Reis RB, Rodrigues AA Jr, Cologna AJ, Martins AC. Therapeutic option for infected urinary tract fistulas in renal transplantation. Transplant Proc. 2010 Mar; 42(2):479-482.

Thornton MJ, Thornton F, O'Callaghan J, Varghese JC, O'Brien E, Walshe J, et al. Evaluation of dynamic gadoliniumenhanced breath-hold MR angiography in the diagnosis of renal artery stenosis. AJR Am J Roentgenol.l 1999;173:1279-83.

Thrasher JB, Temple DR, Spees EK. Extravesical versus Leadbetter-Politano ureteroneocystostomy: a comparison of urological complications in 320 renal transplants. J Urol 144:1105-1109, 1990.

US Renal Data System: 1996 Annual Data Report. Bedhesta MD: National Institutes of Health, NIDDKD; 1996.

Vuruskan, H., A. Ersoy, et al. (2005). "An unusual cause of ureteral obstruction in a renal transplant recipient: ureteric aspergilloma." Transplant Proc 37(5): 2115-7.

Wilson CH, Bhatti AA, Rix DA, Soomro NA. Comparison of laparoscopic and open donor nephrectomy: UK experience. BJU Int. 2005; 95: 131-5.

Zargar MA, Shahrokh H, Fallah MMR, et al: Comparing Taguchi and anterior Lich-Gregoir ureterovesical reimplantation techniques for kidney transplantation. Transplant Proc 37:3077, 2005.

Zargar-Shoshtari, M. A., M. Soleimani, et al. (2008). "Symptomatic lymphocele after kidney transplantation: a single-center experience." Urol J 5(1): 34-6.

26

Vascular Complications in Kidney Transplantation

Alexandros Giakoustidis, Nikolaos Antoniadis and Dimitrios Giakoustidis
Division of Transplantation, Department of Surgery, Medical School
Aristotle University of Thessaloniki and Hippokration General Hospital, Thessaloniki
Greece

1. Introduction

Kidney transplantation evolved as the treatment of choice for end-stage renal disease. Accumulated expertise and experience along with refined surgical techniques resulted in excellent patient and graft survival. Despite the improvements in surgical techniques vascular complications consists a significant and sometimes life-threatening problem that occurs in 10-20% of patients. Vascular complication can be divided in general in three main categories. Graft renal artery thrombosis and stenosis, graft renal vein thrombosis and stenosis and arterial injury.

2. Transplant renal artery stenosis

Transplant renal artery stenosis (TRAS) is a very common vascular complication following kidney transplantations. It is reported in a wide range of frequency occurring in 3-12% of patients (in some reports even up to 20% depending on the awareness and the available imaging means especially MDCT-angiography) (Akbar 2005, Sebastia, 2001)]. It is very difficult to have the definitive true incidence of TRAS by looking at the literature and this discrepancy is due to the different definitions, the surgeon's experience and technical skills in avoiding or preventing the TRAS and different peri-operative management. If we try to classify all arterial stenosis in kidney transplantation, we could divide it into two main categories; TRAS and proximal or pseudo-TRAS. TRAS can be categorised by the level of stenoses and this includes anastomotic stenoses, stenoses of the proper transplant renal artery and finally segmental renal artery stenoses. Proximal-TRAS refers to pre-existing or developing atherosclerotic inflow stenoses in the native iliac arteries of the transplant recipient. The incidence of proximal-TRAS has been reported to be 0%-2.4% and may become more prevalent with increasing age. Predisposing factors for transplant renal artery stenosis, are cadaveric transplant, end-to-end anastomosis, surgical clamp injury, intimal dissection, and inadequate suturing technique, long or kinking artery, prolonged cold ischemia time, acute cellular rejection, and cytomegalovirus (CMV) infection (Audard, 2006).

Patients with TRAS in the immediate post-transplant period, present oliguria or anuria and are dialysis dependent. After the first week, patients with TRAS usually present with severe renovascular hypertension. Even though severe renovascular hypertension could be attributed to TRAS we should always keep in mind and all other causes like chronic rejection, steroid use, cyclosporine toxicity, recurrent glomerulonephritis and disease of native kidneys (Mangray, 2011, Tutone, 2005). If TRAS is not managed properly in due time, it could lead to renal dysfunction and graft deterioration. Non-invasive imaging is mandatory in the immediate post-transplant period to evaluate for possible transplant renal artery stenosis. Doppler ultrasound should be the initial diagnostic modality used because of its ability to reveal the location, length, and gross appearance of a stenosis. In addition, it is widely available, cost-effective, and does not use ionizing radiation and the nature of the transplanted renal arteries makes Doppler ultrasound an ideal screening modality (Baxter, 1995, Irshad, 2008, 2009). Whilst Doppler ultrasound is ideal in recognizing a possible lesion, categorisation and better characterisation of TRAS would be using magnetic resonance angiography with or without contrast medium (especially gadolinium-enhanced), MDCT-angiography, Radionuclide imaging that includes the administration of an angiotensin-converting enzyme inhibitor (captopril scan) shows findings similar to those of renovascular hypertension in native kidneys (Sebastia, 2001). Catheter-based angiography is the gold standard technique for diagnosing TRAS. The use of low- or iso-osmolar contrast material is recommended to reduce the risk of contrast material–induced nephropathy. When renal insufficiency is present, carbon dioxide may be substituted for an iodinated contrast agent during preliminary angiography to minimize the use of iodinated agents.

2.1 Definition and natural history

Unfortunately there is no consensus definition of TRAS and it would be difficult to have one in the future. Usually there is the classic presentation with refractory hypertension, deteriorating renal function, and congestive cardiac failure secondary to fluid retention. It is very impressive that marked reversal of symptoms occurs when stenosis is successfully treated (Garovic, 2005, Mangray, 2011). The timeline of TRAS usually begins at 2 months to 2 years after transplantation and hypertension is due to activation of the renin-angiotensin system (Basso, 2001, Mangray, 2011). Another important issue concerns asymptomatic normotensive patients with Doppler examination of at least 50% without evident graft dysfunction. The problem with those patients is the potential risk carrying from a procedure to treat a clinically insignificant TRAS in the short to medium term. It is unclear whether treating a non-clinically significant TRAS would have an impact in long term survival of renal grafts but since hypertension is an independent risk factor for long term renal graft survival, anything that could contribute to this direction would be beneficial. Close follow up of those patients, with significant expertise and experience of the transplant centre, along with availability of vascular interventional techniques is of paramount importance in decision making. Nevertheless, there are no reports of the long-term safety of this line of management, and the natural history of a 50% TRAS is unknown, and that conservative treatment is safe provided that there is no deterioration of kidney function (Audard, 2006, Buturovic-Ponikvar, 2003). This may not be the case for other causes, such as intimal hyperplasia, and the indication for angiography is strong when graft deterioration is revealed in the absence of other causes of graft dysfunction or chronic allograft nephropathy (CAN). Increased awareness with follow up observation should be in case of a stenosis of 80% on ultrasound examination, even in cases without suspicion of a hemodynamically significant TRAS. Due to increased susceptibility to occlusion in the presence of dehydration or cardiovascular instability, and in this case intervention should be considered.

2.2 Pathophysiology

Since Goldplatt et al published their study on the hypertensive role of partial reduced renal perfusion of the kidney back in 1934; there has been subsequent identification by various investigators of the role of the renin-angiotensin system, with renin being the hormone released in elevated blood levels from the ischemic kidney (Goldplatt, 1934). Angiotensin is being released enzymatically from angiotensinogen, and has various properties, including vasoconstriction, aldosterone secretion, renal sodium retention, and myocardium hypertrophy (Brewster, 2003). There is evidence that when there are two kidneys the above theory has been proven probably right, however it has been showed that this is not the case for the sole kidney or the transplanted kidney. Hypertension is also present but predominantly as a balance between volume regulation depending on salt and water retention and the renin-angiotensin dependent mechanism. It is the highly circulating volume and not the pressor effect from the renin-angiotensin system that is capable to keep a normal GFR rate with normal renin blood levels. In case that ACE inhibitors are prescribed there is a subsequent reduction in kidney perfusion and finally renal function deterioration. In patients with kidney transplantation, and in order to control hypertension, it is not uncommon to establish a diagnosis of TRAS, when an ACE inhibitor is introduced.

2.3 Diagnosis

Doppler ultrasonography is considered as the best screening test TRAS assessment. There are many advantages in the use of Doppler ultrasound as initial approach over other imaging methods, especially iodine contrast media. The fact that Doppler ultrasound is a noninvasive method, does not expose the recipient to the risk of iodine contrast examination, is widely and promptly available in all hospital settings makes it an excellent first choice for TRAS evaluation. The most significant limitation of the method, as in other conditions, is the fact that ultrasonography is operator dependent.

Digital subtractive angiography (DSA), used to be the gold standard technique for establishing the diagnosis, but today tends to be replaced by MRI angiography and more recently Multi Detector CT-angiography. DSA is an invasive technique and potential complications are groin hematoma, renal artery dissection, thrombosis, perforation, and acute kidney injury caused by contrast-induced nephropathy. Doppler ultrasound can also be used to evaluate the hemodynamic changes due to TRAS. Doppler findings in TRAS include peak systolic velocity 2.0-2.5 m/s, low pulsatility index, and a parvus et tardus waveform with a systolic acceleration time of ≥ to 0.1 seconds (Snider, 1989, Irshad, 2009, Baxter, 1995). Snider et al compared Doppler ultrasonography with conventional angiography and showed 94% sensitivity and 87% specificity on US (Snider, 1989). A velocity ratio of the stenotic to pre-stenotic segments of greater than 2:1 is considered supportive of the diagnosis.

Multidetectors helical CT gives accurate assessment of the site and degree of TRAS and provides accurate and valuable imaging, requires less volume of iodinated contrast medium than DSA (Sebastia, 2001). The nature of the vascular contrast medium may be of consideration, rather than the volume. Risk of contrast nephropathy is probably not related to the volume of contrast medium or the degree of renal failure (Birck, 2003, Pannu, 2004). Protection of the allograft with sufficient volume and N-acetylcysteine is recommended when intravenous contrast medium is injected, regardless of renal function and contrast volume. The alternative is to perform MRI with gadolinium, a non-iodinated contrast medium even though there have been reports of nephrogenic systemic sclerosis.

2.4 Treatment

Treatment options for TRAS include both surgical and endoluminal options. Primary treatment for TRAS involves Percutaneous transluminal angioplasty (PTA) with or without stent placement (Audard, 2006, Bruno, 2004). The type of arterial anastomosis that is present is the deciding factor in determining the angiographic approach utilized. The technical success rate of PTA has been reported to be as high as 94%, with a clinical success rate of 82% (Patel, 2001). Recurrent stenosis may occur in more than 10%, and allograft loss has been reported in up to 30% of cases (Fervenza, 1998). There have been reports correlating TRAS with acute cellular rejection and that long term survival is significantly higher in non-TRAS patients compared with the TRAS. Surgical revascularization is now considered rescue therapy and generally has been reserved for patients with disease unsuitable for PTA

2.5 Endoluminal Interventions

Since the introduction and the evolution of the endovascular interventions there has been a shift in TRAS treatment option with Percutaneous Transluminal Angioplasty (PTA) with or without the use of stent (Beecroft, 2004) being now the gold standard and the initial option of treatment. The method is considered very efficient especially in experienced hands and technical success has been reported to be greater than 90%. However when we consider the clinical impact that has on hypertension or improvement of allograft function, this is significantly lower.

As we have already pointed out, the results in clinically insignificant TRAS can be evaluated only on the degree of the radiological success. PTA with or without stenting, is carrying a significant risk for the allograft and unless a significant pressure decrease exists across the TRAS, PTA should not be undertaken. Unfortunately there is no consensus as to the appropriate value of stenosis measurement beyond which intervention is warranted, and it would be very difficult to obtain one in the future since radiological success does not always results in clinical improvement. A cut off point proposed by Schoenberg et al (Schoenberg, 2000), could be pressure decrease at least 10 mm Hg across the stenosis.

The type of arterial anastomosis that is present is the deciding factor in determining the angiographic approach utilized. If there is an end-to-end anastomosis with the internal iliac artery, commonly done in living donor allografts, then a contralateral femoral approach is utilized to make access to the downward sloping artery as easy as possible. However, if there is an end-to-side anastomosis with the external iliac artery, then an ipsilateral femoral approach is preferred by some authors to access the cephalad sloping artery (Bruno, 2004).

Results after PTA depend largely on the radiologists or vascular surgeons experience and expertise, and should have smooth cooperation with the transplant surgeons. Most of the complications relate to puncture site, but there could be also more severe complication like hemorrhage, rupture of transplant renal artery, iliac artery and loss of the allograft, in those case there could be a need for "salvage" operation. Evolution in endovascular technology, with newer pre-mounted stents, has minimised complications especially the life threatening ones and the risk for allograft loss. Rate of re-stenosis are reported to be 10% to 50% and depends on the primary cause of the stenosis, length of follow-up, and use of stents (Voiculescu A 2005). Even though there are several reports on the topic, there are limitations provided by the retrospective nature of those manuscripts and the limited number of patients. In a french study of 29 patients with TRAS treated with PTA, the technical success rate was 93.1%, and there was 27.5% re-stenosis (Audard, 2006). In other study from the US, TRAS was found in 26 (3.1%) renal allografts, and 17 were treated with PTA with a success rate of 94%. Re-stenosis occurred in 12% of the patients [Patel NH 2001] In case of segmental branches, there is a lower success rate and the success rate is even lower for anastomotic strictures, and even though the incidence of stenosis is similar between end-to-side anastomosis to the external iliac artery and end-to-end anastomosis to the internal iliac artery, PTA in the latter situation is technically more difficult and results in a higher complication rate and more graft loss (Voiculescu, 2005).

2.6 Surgical correction

Surgical correction of TRAS is regarded as a difficult operation with graft loss rates exceeding 20% (Bruno, 2004). A couple of risks existing; to the recipient and to the allograft, the latter is not a contraindication to surgery, since severe TRAS could deteriorate the transplanted kidney, the patient proceeds to renal failure, and finally to end up in heamodialysis. Surgery is now considered as rescue therapy for cases unsuitable for PTA.
In general indications for surgery include: TRAS caused by kinking, anastomotic strictures and complex atherosclerotic disease. There are several options to treat TRAS; mostly excision of the stenosis with direct anastomosis to the external iliac artery and grafting with saphenous vein, recipient internal iliac artery, and preserved ABO blood group compatible deceased donor artery. Reported surgical success rates range from 63% to 92%, with recurrence in 12% of patients (Roberts, 1989). A study comparing PTA vs. surgical repair of TRAS showed an immediate and long-term success rate of 92.1% and 81.5% and 69% and 40.5% for surgical repair and PTA respectively [Benoit G 1990]. Limitations of surgical procedure are access to the artery and most importantly the subsequent warm ischemia time. A warm ischemia of 60 minutes might be tolerated by a kidney allograft that has been heparinised even though the risk for Acute Tubular Necrosis (ATN) and cortical necrosis is increased due to diminished blood flow. An alternative option even though rarely used, is back table reconstruction of a complex arterial problem and autotransplantation of the allograft.

3. Transplant renal artery kinks and allograft torsion

Positioning the allograft is sometimes tricky and the source of pitfalls in kidney transplantation and can result in allograft torsion. Allograft torsion can be an early or late complication. One of the main problems caused by improper positioning or torsion is the arterial kinking. Usually arterial kinks are formed due to long renal graft artery when there is a shift in the graft and/or pelvic contents that causes turn of the artery. Even though the differential diagnosis between TRAS and arterial kinking is often difficult to have, it is of paramount importance to identify an arterial narrowing due to a kink and not TRAS. Prompt diagnosis permits graft detorsion and possible salvage. The most suggestive imaging finding is a change in the axis of the transplanted kidney. CT and MR imaging can show changes in renal graft orientation and vascular pedicle kinking. Surgery remains the primary treatment for arterial kinks and only in cases where surgery is contraindicated or patients refuses surgery, we should proceed with endovascular treatment. TPA with or without stents, may increase the risk of arterial vasospasm and dissection and in addition, placing stents across kinks usually can be technically demanding.

4. Thrombophilias

The thrombophilias, also referred to as hypercoagulable states, comprise hereditary or acquired conditions that predispose individuals to thrombosis. It was the third factor of

Virchow's triad that suggested that systemic alterations in the coagulability of blood, is a critical factor in thrombogenesis (Virchow, 1856). Thrombophilias are classified as congenital (inherited), acquired (secondary), or both (mixed) conditions (Schafer, 2007).

Congenital hypercoagulable states are caused by inherited thrombotic disorders due to mutations in genes encoding plasma proteins involved in coagulation mechanisms. They can be broadly classified into two categories: 1) quantitative deficiencies or qualitative defects of the physiologic anticoagulants: antithrombin, protein C and protein S deficiency, and 2) increased levels or function of the coagulation factors: factor V Leiden, prothrombin gene mutation, elevated levels of specific coagulation factors (Schafer, 2003). Congenital abnormalities of anticoagulant or procoagulant proteins result in an increased risk for venous thromboembolism (VTE) as well as arterial thrombosis with the risk to be higher in cases with decreased levels of antithrombotic proteins than in those with increased levels of prothrombotic proteins. The overall incidence of venous thromboembolism (per 100 patient-years) is found to be 1.07 for antithrombin deficiency, 0.54 for protein C deficiency, 0.50 for protein S deficiency, and 0.30 for activated protein C resistance or factor V Leiden (Bucciarelli, 1999). Half of the patients with inherited hypercoagulable state present with venous thromboembolism before the age of 45 years, particularly in the absence of well recognized risk factors, and often have a family history of thrombosis (Anderson, 2010). The secondary hypercoagulable states encompass a variety of heterogeneous disorders that have been associated with an increased risk of thrombotic complications (Schafer, 2003). Acquired hypercoagulable states include antiphospholipid antibody syndrome, cancer, heparin-induced thrombocytopenia, pregnancy and estrogen therapy, and a prior history of venous thromboembolism. Acquired coagulation defects are particularly common in patients with endstage renal disease (Wagenknecht, 1999). The prevalence of antiphospholipid antibodies in patients awaiting renal transplantation is more than 10%, but the rate of clinical events is far less than the frequency of thrombophilic states. Hyperhomocysteinemia is the typical hypercoagulable state that occurs due to a combination of inherited and acquired factors. Elevated serum levels of homocysteine have been associated with an increased risk of arterial thrombosis (myocardial infarction, stroke, and peripheral arterial disease) and venous thromboembolism (Cattaneo, 1999).

After renal transplantation the donor kidney endothelium is conditioned to exhibit a prothrombotic state as a consequence of reperfusion injury, tissue trauma, inflammation and expression of tissue factor, in addition to the recipient immune response (Key, 1992, Irish, 1999). The combination of a conditioned endothelium and a genetic or acquired predisposition to a hypercoagulable state increase the risk of thrombosis. Factors specific for the renal transplant patients that have been suggested to contribute to this thrombotic risk include the use of calcineurin-inhibiting drugs, high levels of homocysteine, diabetic nephropathy, antiphospholipid syndrome, cytomegalovirus infection, and the presence of proteinuria or nephrotic syndrome (Kujovich, 2004).

It has been proposed that inherited risk factors of venous thromboembolism, such as factor V-Leiden, prothrombin G20210A, and methylenetetrahydrofolate reductase (MTHFR) C677T, might be associated with poorer survival rates of transplanted kidneys, attributed to the context of graft perfusion defects, venous thromboembolic complications, and acute graft loss by vascular rejection, possibly reflecting immunological injury upon the vascular wall exacerbated or induced by the prothrombotic state (Heidenreich, 2003, Wuthrich, 2001). Later study with larger number of patients, did not find a statistically significant association of polymorphisms factor V-Leiden G1691A and MTHFR C677T with renal graft survival Meyer, 2007).

Factor V-Leiden mutation or activated protein C resistance is the most common inherited thrombophilic disorder, found in 5% to 8% of the general population, in 20% of patients with a first venous thrombosis, and in up to 50% of patients with a personal or family history of recurrent thrombosis (Kujovich, 2004). In renal transplant recipients, factor V Leiden has been associated with a variety of complications after renal transplantation and a significantly higher incidence of venous thromboembolism which occurred in up to 39% of FVL carriers (Wuthrich, 2001, Irish, 1997). Also FVL carriers had 12-fold higher risk of an early graft perfusion defect (Wuthrich, 2001). A higher risk of vascular rejection was found in FVL carriers, which was linked to the presence of endotheliolitis or fibrinoid necrosis on histopathology of renal grafts lost within the first year after transplant (Ekberg, 2000).

The reported prevalence of prothrombin gene heterozygous mutation in renal transplant recipients is 3.7%, similar to that in the general population. The mutation was associated with a nearly threefold increased risk of graft failure, which was attributable to arterial, venous, or microvascular thrombosis in the majority of carriers (Fischereder, 2001, Kujovich, 2004).

A polymorphism of the methylenetetrahydrofolate reductase (MTHFR) gene coding for an enzyme that degrades the endothelium toxic product homocysteine have been associated with ESRD (Girndt, 2007). This mutation occurs in 50% to 90% of chronic dialysis patients presenting with mild hyperhomocysteinemia and have been associated with cardiovascular disease and vascular access thrombosis in this population (Mallamaci, 2005, Mallamaci, 2002). Additionally hyperhomocysteinemia can be acquired, such as in renal failure and in deficiencies of folate, vitamin B12, or vitamin B6. Even though many studies found that hyperhomocysteinemia is an independent risk factor for both first and recurrent venous thromboembolism (den Heijer, 1996, Cattaneo, 1999) and that hyperhomocysteinemia is an independent risk factor for cardiovascular disease (Ducloux D et al 2000), the effect of hyperhomocysteinemia on the risk of graft thrombosis is unknown. Antiphospholipid syndrome is the most common acquired blood protein defect associated with either venous or arterial thrombosis or both (Koniari, 2010). Antiphospholipid antibodies (APLA) are found in approximately 10% of patients awaiting renal transplantation. Since only a fraction of patients with antiphospholipid antibodies experience thrombotic complications, the description of antiphospholipid antibody syndrome (APAS), defines by the presence of antiphospholipid antibodies and a clinical history of thrombosis. Antiphospholipid antibodies include not only the lupus anticoagulant (LA) and anticardiolipin antibodies (ACLAs) but also more recently recognized subgroups of antiphospholipid antibodies (antibodies against beta-2-glycoprotein-I [B-2-GP-I]) and antibodies to phosphatidylserine, phosphatidylethanolamine, phosphatidylglycerol, phosphatidylinositol, phosphatidylcholine, and anti-annexin-V (Bick, 2003). Patients with antiphospholipid antibodies in association with other autoimmune disease, most commonly lupus, are classified as having secondary antiphospholipid syndrome. Approximately 40% of patients with SLE have an antiphospholipid (anticardiolipin) antibody (lupus anticoagulant). The presence of antiphospholipid antibodies has been recognized as an important risk factor for early allograft failure (Wagenknecht, 1999. Patients with APAS are at high risk for renovascular thrombosis and renal allograft loss was reported to be universal in the absence of anticoagulation (Vaidya, 2000). Whereas, and despite the lack of anticoagulation, no allografts were lost to thrombosis, in patients with detectable anticardiolipin antibodies but no prior history of thrombosis. In a later report all patients with antiphospholipid antibodies were successfully transplanted using postoperative anticoagulation (Morrissey, 2002).

Other prothrombotic changes that have been reported in renal transplant recipients include decreases in antithrombin, protein C and protein S levels, markedly elevated factor VIII levels and over-expression of plasminogen activator inhibitor-1 by donor epithelium (suggestive of impaired regional fibrinolysis) (Irish, 1999).

In vitro data suggest that immunosuppressive drugs like cyclosporine and OKT3 may increase the risk of thrombosis but an independent clinical association with allograft thrombosis is unproven (Gruber, 1989, Abramowicz, 1992). Specifically, the prothrombotic effects of cyclosporine include activation of monocytes to express tissue factor, increased platelet aggregation, endothelial dysfunction and activation of the intrinsic coagulation pathway, impaired fibrinolysis and impaired activation of protein C (Carlsen, 1988, Fishman, 1991, Bombeli, 1996, Evans, 1997, Levi, 1992).

Thrombotic complications after renal transplantation are usually catastrophic. Inherited and acquired hypercoagulable states have to be considered prior to kidney transplantation and proper prophylactic treatment initiated for the purpose to improve transplant outcome. Andrassy et al. provided specified screening recommendations for thrombophilia prior to kidney transplantation (Andrassy, 2004). A general screening for thrombophilia, to include factor V Leiden, prothrombin gene G20210A polymorphism, antithrombin III, protein C and S activity, antiphospholipid antibodies and lupus anticoagulant, should be performed in all children and adolescents because they have the highest risk for thrombotic complications. Adults only with history of thrombotic events should be thoroughly screened (recurrent AVC fistula thrombosis should be taken into account). When risk factors are absent, screening only for antiphospholipid antibodies and lupus anticoagulant is recommended.

There is also no consensus on the optimal management of renal transplant patients with thrombophilic disorders. Treatment strategies to reduce thrombotic risk including heparin, warfarin, and aspirin have been evaluated in several reports. While inadequate anticoagulation may place the patient at risk for thrombosis, preemptive or intense perioperative anticoagulation can result in postoperative bleeding (Morrissey, 2002, Murashima, 2010, Friedman, 2001). Morissey et al. (Morrissey, 2002) recommended management approach for renal transplant patients with thrombophilia. Patients with diagnosis or suspected to have thrombophilia is suspected, the risk for thrombotic complications should be stratified as low, intermediate or high. In high risk are patients with inherited thrombotic disorder and history of at least two thrombotic episodes. For the high risk patients indefinite oral anticoagulation has been advocated. In intermediate risk are patients with a known inherited thrombotic disorder who are asymptomatic or have experienced a single thrombotic event. They should receive adequate prophylaxis in high-risk situations such as surgery for a minimum of 6 months. For patients with no suspicion of thrombophilia, no anticoagulation or a short term postoperative anticoagulation may be given.

5. Renal vein and artery thrombosis

Renal transplantation is established as the preferred treatment for most cases of end-stage renal disease. Postoperative vascular complications include thrombosis of renal vein and artery, with a delay in the diagnosis and management of these complications leading to significant morbidity for the recipient, with a high risk of graft loss and mortality (Akbar, 2005). It consists of a rare complication that often results in graft loss, with reported incidence ranging from 0.4% to 6% (Rouviere, 2002, Giustacchini, 2002). Bakir et al reported that thrombosis represented 45% and 37% of renal allograft loss at 3 and 12 months (Bakir, 1996).

5.1 Renal vein thrombosis

Renal vein thrombosis (RVT), although an unusual event, most often has graft loss as a result (Figure 1). The causes that may lead to this serious complication include compression due to hematomas or lymphoceles, angulation or kinking of the vein, anastomotic strictures, or an underlying state of deep venous thrombosis or hypercoaguability (Penny, 1994). RVT usually occurs suddenly and towards the end of the first week of an otherwise uncomplicated kidney transplantation. Specifically it occurs in the first 2 weeks post transplant, with 80% occurring in the first month and 93% within the first year (Kobayashi, 2007). Clinical presentation is initiated by oliguria and hematuria with a tender swollen graft, which if ruptured, is accompanied by life-treatening bleeding (Kobayashi, 2007).

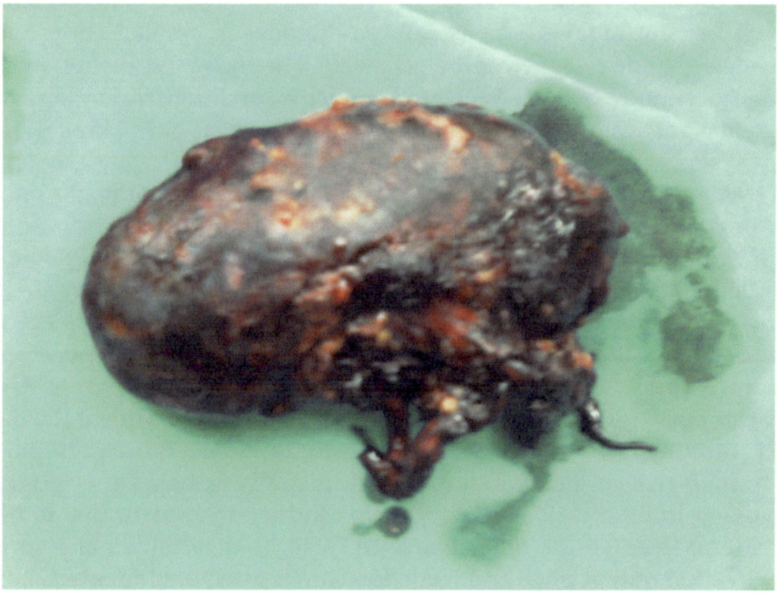

Fig. 1. Specimen of renal allograft nephrectomy due to renal vein trhrombosis

5.2 Renal artery thrombosis

This uncommon complication which may occur most often as an early but also as a late event after kidney transplantation consists a devastating clinical condition leading frequently to graft loss. Renal artery thrombosis (RAT) onset most often follows a technical problem such as intimal dissection, kinking or torsion of the vessels. Risk factors include poor cardiac output, hyperacute rejection, unresponsive acute rejection, and a hypercoagulable state. It presents with a rapid onset of oliguria. In cases of segmental infarct, there can be lack of symptomatology or a presentation of renal dysfunction and increased blood pressure. When RAT occurs as a late event, it could be attributed to renal artery stricture or its manipulation post-operatively e.g. during angiography, or usually due to graft rejection.

5.3 Diagnosis

An early clinical diagnosis is very important for both RVT and RAT, even during the morning ward round. Diagnosis of these complications is established by colour flow Doppler studies, demonstrating in RVT a swollen graft with a crescent of clot along the convex margin of the kidney. In this case it is essential that the patient is taken immediately to theatre. Under normal clinical conditions, the spectral Doppler renal arterial waveform shows high resistive index with reversal of diastolic flow. On the contrary, in RAT a lack of flow in the renal artery is demonstrated, with the presence of intraluminal filling defects. In RAT, diagnosis is set by Doppler studies or at time of surgical exploration, however by that time it is not possible for the graft to be saved due to the kidney's low tolerance to warm ischemia (Rouviere, 2002).

5.4 Treatment

Following establishment of diagnosis for RVT, the treatment of choice is urgent thrombectomy. However graft salvage may not be possible, in which case graft nephrectomy is usually required. In case thrombectomy is applied early, within 1 hour following the event, graft salvage can be achieved. The increased risk of swelling, edema and also a possible rupture of the kidney graft in such a condition, makes urgent exploration essential. Systemic anticoagulants can be applied as treatment only in cases of partial vein thrombosis.

The surgical treatment for renal graft thrombosis includes laparotomy, thrombectomy and ultimately a possible graft nephrectomy. Several authors describe endoluminal therapy for renal graft thrombosis; however the exact role of interventional radiologic treatment is not yet well-defined (Obed, 2008). The technique for percutaneous treatment involves placing the tip of a catheter within the thrombus, 1 cm distal to the surgical anastomosis, with infusion of a thrombolytic agent (Rouviere, 2002). Because transcatheter thrombolysis revascularizes arteries at a slower rate than surgical thrombectomy, patients with a heavy clot burden should be primarily offered surgical treatment (Hedegard, 2009). Transcatheter thrombolysis should be limited to low clot burden, segmental artery thrombosis, or high-risk surgical candidates. Additionally catheter-directed thrombolytics should be avoided in the first 2 weeks following kidney transplant due to the immature anastomotic suture line. On the other hand RAT can be determined as a terminal event, which can be averted only if poor graft function can be attributed to arterial inflow and in this case intervention should be immediate. By the time the diagnosis is set, the transplanted kidney is lost.

5.5 Prevention

Although in many cases of renal allograft vascular thrombosis, no cause can be identified, epidemiological studies have attempted to categorise risk factors as modifiable, including drugs and the surgical procedure among others, and nonmodifiable, including age, diabetes mellitus and vascular anomalies. Additionally studies have identified changes in coagulation or fibrinolysis promoting a more thrombotic state, as risk factors as well.

Prevention may hold an important role in avoiding the formation of vascular thrombosis. This requires of course a combination of different measures such as avoiding prolonged cold and warm ischemia. Attention to precise surgical technique, use of preservation solution such as University of Wisconsin solution and an immediate and effective management of rejection, should all be outlined as important in the prevention strategy.

Additionally identification and management of thrombophilic states could act as a preventive measure against renal vascular thrombosis, with a possible need for routine screening and directed therapy to reduce the risk of thrombosis and graft loss, however no consensus for either strategy have been introduced. Previous reports indicate a possible laboratory investigation to potential recipients with a previous history or family history of thrombotic events, such as deep and superficial vein thromboses, pulmonary emboli, fistulas having been thrombosed or incidents of multiple occlusions of central venous dialysis catheters, as well as patients undergoing preemptive transplantation with a living donor kidney (Andrassy, 2004).

The risk of thrombosis must be balanced against that of bleeding. For known thrombophilia and a history of clinical events, perioperative heparinization followed by long-term anticoagulation with warfarin has shown good results, including successful retransplantation. However since results of the few available, prospective randomized studies on heparin use in renal transplant patients, show conflicting conclusions, one understands that there is a great need for a preoperative classification of thrombotic and hemorrhagic risk among renal transplant candidates and for establishment of consensus guidelines.

6. Extrarenal pseudoaneurysm

Extrarenal arterial pseudoaneurysms in renal transplantation are rare, and their prevalence is less than 1% (Bracale, 2009). Extrarenal pseudoaneurysms are directly related to arterial anastomosis, percutaneous nephrostomy placement and infectious causes. It is usually asymptomatic and rarely can cause renal dysfunction or compression of adjacent structures (Bracale, 2009). When extrarenal pseudoaneurysms become large, there is a strong indication to be surgically removed to avoid spontaneous rupture and loss of the allograft (Figure 2).

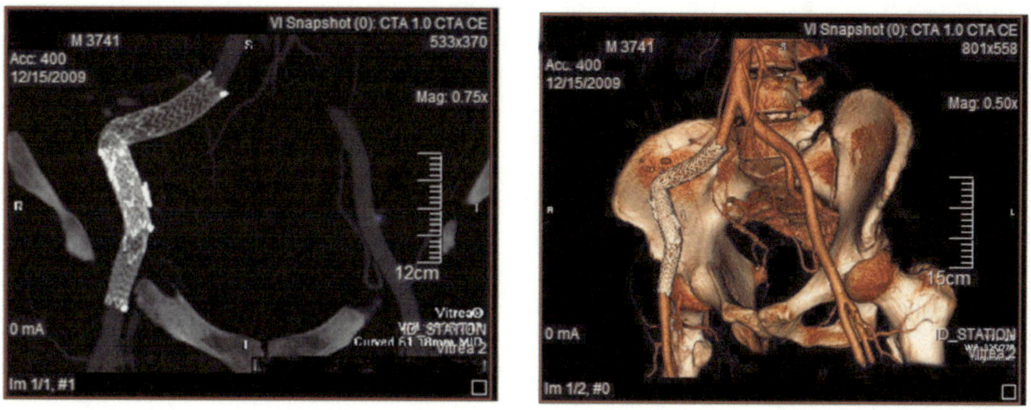

Fig. 2. External iliac artery pseudoaneurysm presented as a complication of renal vein thrombosis and allograph nephrectomy. The pseudoanurysm was formed at the stump of the arterial anastomosis due to inflammation. Preemptive treatment with double stent placement was successfully performed.

7. Arteriovenous fistula

Arteriovenous fistula (AVF) is a well-recognized vascular complication of percutaneous biopsy. The reported incidence of AVF ranges between 0.5 and 16% (Martinez, 1998). An arteriovenous fistula (AVF) may be formed when both arterial and venous walls are punched by the biopsy needle. Mostly they are asymptomatic, rarely may cause persistent hematuria or recurrence of hematuria, hypertension and deterioration of renal function. Rarely, renal graft ischemia may be the result of steal phenomenon from a large AVF (Harrison, 1994, Matsell, 1992, Cruzado, 19990. Factors that may predispose to the development of arteriovenous fistula include early postransplant period, the presence of hypertension, sclerosis and interstitial fibrosis, the formation of intrarenal hematoma (Schwarz, 2008). About 70% of AVF cases resolve spontaneously within weeks or months (Matsell, 1992).

Doppler sonography allowing noninvasive diagnosis of AVFs is the diagnostic examination of choice (Ozbek, 1995). Angiography is the reference standard as it confirms the presence of the AVF, accurately assesses its size and location, and permits endovascular treatment (Loffroy, 2008). On Doppler, the AVF shows a focal area of turbulent flow and a localized region of disorganized color that extends outside the normal vessels on color Doppler. In the area of AVF, the duplex US shows a very high velocity with low resistive index in the feeding artery with arterialization of the flow in the draining vein (Irshad, 2009).

In most cases AVFs close spontaneously within a few months, but they warrant observation to exclude the need for therapeutic intervention. The likelihood of and time to spontaneous closure in renal allografts, and the optimal time for therapeutic intervention are not predictable (Loffroy, 2008). Treatment has been recommended when bleeding persists for more than 72 h, renal function deteriorates markedly, lesion enlarges and there is suspicion of steal phenomenon. Endovascular superselective embolization is the therapeutic procedure of choice, as loss of normal parenchyma is minimal, with success rate of approximately 88% with no significant loss of allograft function (Loffroy, 2008, Tarif, 2002). In the majority of cases, successful embolization can be achieved using coils or microcoils. Schwarz et al (Schwarz,2008) proposed a hemodynamic prognostic test to predict which AVF would probably profit from AVF coiling, by comparing Doppler sonographic resistive indices of the main renal artery and the non-AVF associated segmental arteries (Schwarz, 2008). The resistive index of the main renal artery should be at least 0.05 less than that of the non-AVF-associated segmental renal arteries indicating under-perfusion of the rest renal parenchyma.

8. Conclusions

Renal transplantation is regarded as an optimal treatment for End-stage renal disease. Improvements in surgical techniques and advanced immunosuppressive drugs have resulted in remarkable survival of patients and renal grafts. However complications occur in both the immediate postoperative period and later. Awareness for early post-operative complications, like renal vein and artery thrombosis could save allografts and patients. Cardiovascular disease remains the most frequent cause of death and transplant loss after kidney transplantation, with hypertension present in vast majority of kidney transplant recipients and a risk factor for cardiovascular disease. Improvements in imagining modalities and interventional techniques resulted in earlier identification and management of TRAS. It is of paramount importance for the transplant surgeon to keep in mind that early and late vascular complications after renal transplantation could be very challenging and potentially allograft and/or life threatening

9. References

Akbar SA, Jafri SZ, Amendola MA, Madrazo BL, Salem R, Bis KG. (2005). Complications of renal transplantation. *Radiographics,*Vol. 25, No. 5, (Sep-Oct 2005), p:1335-1356,.Anderson JA, Weitz JI (2010). Hypercoagulable states. *Clinics in Chest Medine,* Vol. 31. No. 4 (December 2010), p;31:659-73.

Andrassy J, Zeier M, Andrassy K. (2004). Do we need screening for thrombophilia prior to kidney transplantation? Nephrology Dialysis Transplantation, Vol. 19, Suppl 4, p:iv-64-iv-68.

Audard V, Matignon M, Hemery F, Snanoudj R, Desgranges P, Anglade MC, Kobeiter H, Durrbach A, Charpentier B, Lang P, Grimbert P. (2006). Risk factors and long-term outcome of transplant renal artery stenosis in adult recipients after treatment by percutaneous transluminal angioplasty. *American Journal of Transplantation* Vol. 6, No. 1, (January 2006), p:95-99.

Bakir N, Sluiter WJ, Ploeg RJ, van Son WJ, Tegzess AM. (1996). Primary renal graft thrombosis. *Nephrology Dialysis Transplantation,* Vol. 11, No. 1, (January 1996), p:140-147, 1996

Basso N, Terragno NA (2001). History about the discovery of the rennin angiotensin system. *Hypertension,* Vol. 38, No 6, (December 2001) p: 1246-1249.

Baxter GM, Ireland H, Moss JG, Harden PN, Junor BJ, Rodger RS, Briggs JD. (1995). Colour Doppler ultrasound in renal transplant artery stenosis: which Doppler index? *Clinical Radiology,* Vol. 50, No. 9, (September 1995), p: 618-622.

Beecroft JR, Rajan DK, Clark TW, Robinette M, Stavropoulos SW. (2004): Transplant renal artery stenosis: outcome after percutaneous intervention. *Journal of Vascular Interventional Radiology,* Vol. 15, No 12, (December 2004), p: 1407-1413, 2004.

Benoit G, Moukarzel M, Hiesse C, Verdelli G, Charpentier B, Fries D. (1990): Transplant renal artery stenosis: Experience and comparative results between surgery and angioplasty. *Transplant International,* Vol. 3, No. 3, (October 1990), p:137-140.

Birck R, Krzossok S, Markowetz F, Schnülle P, van der Woude FJ, Braun C. (2003). Acetylcysteine for prevention of contrast nephropathy: meta-analysis. *Lancet,* Vol. 362, No. 9384, (August2003), p:598-603, 2003.

Bick RL (2003). Antiphospholipid thrombosis syndromes. *Hematology Oncology Clinics of North America,* Vol. 17, No. 1,(February 2003), p:115-47.

Bracale UM, Carbone F, del Guercio L, Viola D, D'Armiento FP, Maurea S, Porcellini M, Bracale G. (2009). External iliac artery pseudoaneurysm complicating renal transplantation. *Interactive Cardiovascular Thoracic Surgery,* Vol. 8, No. 6, (June 2009), p:654-60.

Brewster UC, Setaro JF, Perazella MA. (2003). The renin-angiotensin-aldosterone system: cardiorenal effects and implications for renal and cardiovascular disease states. *The American Journal of Medical Sciences,* Vol. 326, No. 1 (July 2003):15-24.

Bruno S, Remuzzi G, Ruggenenti P. (2004). Transplant renal artery stenosis. *Journal of the American Society of Nephrology*, Vol. 15, No. 1, (January 2004), p:134-141.

Bucciarelli P, Rosendaal FR, Tripodi A, Mannucci PM, De Stefano V, Palareti G, Finazzi G, Baudo F, Quintavalla R (1999). Risk of venous thromboembolism and clinical manifestations in carriers of antithrombin, protein C, protein S deficiency, or activated protein C resistance: a multicenter collaborative family study. *Arteriosclerosis Thrombosis and Vascular Biology*, Vol. 19, No. 4, (April 1999), p:1026-33.

Buturovic-Ponikvar J. (2003). Renal transplant artery stenosis. *Nephrology Dialysis Transplantation*, Vol. 18, No. S5, (July 2003), p:v-74-v-77.

Cattaneo M (1999). Hyperhomocysteinemia, atherosclerosis and thrombosis. *Thrombosis and Haemostasis*, Vol. 81, No. 2, (February 1999), p:165-76.

den Heijer M, Koster T, Blom HJ, Bos GM, Briet E, Reitsma PH, Vandenbroucke JP, Rosendaal FR (1996). Hyperhomocysteinemia as a risk factor for deep-vein thrombosis. *The New England Journal of Medicine*, Vol. 21, No. 334, (March 1996), p:759-62.

Cruzado JM, Torras J, Domínguez J, Sancho C, Alsina J, Grinyó JM. (1999). An unusual cause of post-biopsy oliguria in an allograft. *Nephrology Dialysis Transplantation*, Vol. 14, No. 8, (August 1999), p:2022-4.

Ducloux D, Motte G, Challier B, Gibey R, Chalopin JM (2000). Serum total homocysteine and cardiovascular disease occurrence in chronic, stable renal transplant recipients: a prospective study. *Journal of the American Society of Nephrology*, Vol. 11, No. 1, (January 2000), p:134-7.

Ekberg H, Svensson PJ, Simanaitis M, Dahlbäck B (2000). Factor V R506Q mutation (activated protein C resistance) is an additional risk factor for early renal graft loss associated with acute vascular rejection. *Transplantation*, Vol. 27, No. 69, (April 2000), p:1577-81.

Fervenza FC, Lafayette RA, Alfrey EJ, Petersen J. (1998). Renal artery stenosis in kidney transplants. American Journal of Kidney Disease, Vol. 31, No. 1, (January 1998), p:142-8.

Fischereder M, Schneeberger H, Lohse P, Krämer BK, Schlöndorff D, Land W (2001). Increased rate of renal transplant failure in patients with the G20210A mutation of the prothrombin gene. *American Journal of Kidney Diseases*, Vol. 38, No. 5, (November 2001), p:1061-4.

Friedman GS, Meier-Kriesche HU, Kaplan B, Mathis AS, Bonomini L, Shah N, DeFranco P, Jacobs M, Mulgaonkar S, Geffner S, Lyman N, Paraan C, Walsh C, Belizaire W, Tshibaka M.(2001). Hypercoagulable states in renal transplant candidates: impact of anticoagulation upon incidence of renal allograft thrombosis. *Transplantation*, Vol27, No. 72, (September 2001), p:1073-8

Garovic VD, Textor SC. (2005): Renovascular hypertension and ischemic nephropathy. *Circulation*, Vol. 112, No. 9, (August 2005), p:1362-1374.

Girndt M, Heine GH, Ulrich C, Köhler H. DialGene Consortium. (2007). Gene polymorphism association studies in dialysis: vascular access. *Seminars in Dialysis*, Vol. 20, No. 1, (Jan-Feb 2007), p:63-67.

Giustacchini P, Pisanti F, Citterio F, De Gaetano AM, Castagneto M, Nanni G. (2002). Renal vein thrombosis after renal transplantation: An important cause of graft loss. *Transplantation Proceedings*, Vol. 34, No. 6, (September 2002), p:2126-2127

Goldblatt H, Lynch J, Hanzal RE, Summerville WW. (1934). Studies on experimental hypertension, I: the production of persistent elevation of systolic blood pressure by means of renal ischaemia. *The Journal of Experimental Medicine*, Vol. 59, No. 3, (February 1934), p:347-379.

Harrison KL, Nghiem HV, Coldwell DM, Davis CL. (1994). Renal dysfunction due to an arteriovenous fistula in a transplant recipient. *Journal of the American Society of Nephrolology*, Vol. 5, No. 6, (December 1994), p:1300-6.

Hedegard W, Saad WE, Davies MG. (2009). Management of vascular and nonvascular complications after renal transplantation. *Techniques in Vascular Interventional Radiology*, Vol, 12, No. 4, (December 2009), p:240-62

Heidenreich S, Junker R, Wolters H, Lang D, Hessing S, Nitsche G, Nowak-Göttl U. (2003). Outcome of kidney transplantation in patients with inherited thrombophilia: data of a prospective study. *Journal of the American Society of Nephrology*, Vol. 14, No. 1, (January 2003), p:234-9.

Irish AB, Green FR, Gray DW, Morris PJ. (1997). The factor V Leiden (R506Q) mutation and risk of thrombosis in renal transplant recipients. *Transplantation*, Vol. 64, No. 4, (August 1997), p:604-7.

Irish A. (1999). Renal allograft thrombosis: can thrombophilia explain the inexplicable? *Nephrology Dialysis Transplantation*, Vol. 14, No. 10, (October 1999), p:2297-303.

Irshad A, Ackerman S, Sosnouski D, Anis M, Chavin K, and Baliga P. (2008). A Review of Sonographic Evaluation of Renal Transplant Complications. *Current Problems in Diagnostic Radiology*, Vol. 37, No. 2 (Mar-Apr 2008), p:67-79

Irshad A, Ackerman SJ, Campbell AS, Anis M. (2009). An overview of renal transplantation: current practice and use of ultrasound. *Seminars in Ultrasound CT and MR*, Vol. 30, No. 4, (August 2009), p:298-314.

Key NS (1992). Scratching the surface: endothelium as a regulator of thrombosis, fibrinolysis, and inflammation. *The Journal of Laboratory Clinical Medicine*, Vol. 120, No. 2, (August 1992), p:184-6.

Kobayashi K, Censullo ML, Rossman LL, Kyriakides PN, Kahan BD, Cohen AM. (2007). Interventional radiologic management of renal transplant dysfunction: Indications, limitations, and technical considerations. *Radiographics*, Vol. 27, No. 4, (Jul-Aug 2007), p:1109-30

Koniari I, Siminelakis SN, Baikoussis NG, Papadopoulos G, Goudevenos J, Apostolakis E. (2010). Antiphospholipid syndrome; its implication in cardiovascular diseases: a review. *Journal of Cardiothoracic Surgery*, Vol. 3, No. 5, (November 2010), p:101-10.

Kujovich JL. (2004). Thrombophilia and thrombotic problems in renal transplant patients. *Transplantation*, Vol. 15, No. 77, (April 2004), p:959-64.

Loffroy R, Guiu B, Lambert A, Mousson C, Tanter Y, Martin L, Cercueil JP, Krausé D. (2009). Management of post-biopsy renal allograft arteriovenous fistulas with selective arterial embolization: immediate and long-term outcomes. Clinical *Radiology*, Vol. 63, No. 6, (June 2008), p:657-65.

Mallamaci F, Zoccali C, Tripepi G, Fermo I, Benedetto FA, Cataliotti A, Bellanuova I, Malatino LS, Soldarini A. CREED Investigators. (2002). Hyperhomocysteinemia predicts cardiovascular outcomes in hemodialysis patients. *Kidney International,* Vol. 61, No. 2, (February 2002), p:609-14.

Mallamaci F, Bonanno G, Seminara G, Rapisarda F, Fatuzzo P, Candela V, Scudo P, Spoto B, Testa A, Tripepi G, Tech S, Zoccali C. (2005). Hyperhomocysteinemia and arteriovenous fistula thrombosis in hemodialysis patients. *American Journal of Kidney Diseases,* Vol. 45, No. 4, (April 2005), p:702-7.

Mangray M, and Vella JP. (2011). Hypertension After Kidney Transplant. *American Journal of Kidney Diseases,* Vol. 57, No. 2, (February 2011), p:331-341

Martinez T, Palomares M, Bravo JA, Alvarez G, Galindo P, Entrena AG, Osuma A, Asensio C. (1998). Biopsy-induced arteriovenous fistula and venous aneurysm in a renal transplant. *Nephrology Dialysis Transplantation,* Vol. 13, No. 11, (November 1998), p:2937-9.

Matsell DG, Jones DP, Boulden TF, Burton EM, Baum SL, Tonkin IL. (1992). Arteriovenous fistula after biopsy of renal transplant kidney: diagnosis and treatment. *Pediatric Nephrology,* Vol. 6, No. 6, (November 1992), p:562-4.

Meyer M, Laux G, Scherer S, Tran TH, Opelz G, Mytilineos J. (2007). No association of factor V Leiden, prothrombin G20210A, and MTHFR C677T gene polymorphisms with kidney allograft survival: a multicenter study. *Transplantation,* Vol 27, No. 83, (April 2007), p:1055-8.

Morrissey PE, Ramirez PJ, Gohh RY, Yango AY, Kestin A, Madras PN, Monaco AP. (2002). Management of thrombophilia in renal transplant patients. American Journal of *Transplantation,* Vol 2, No. 9, (October 2002), p:872-6.

Murashima M, Konkle BA, Bloom RD, Sood SL, Grossman RA, Brunelli SM, Stein SH. (2010). A single-center experience of preemptive anticoagulation for patients with risk factors for allograft thrombosis in renal transplantation. *Clinical Nephrology,* Vol. 74, No. 5, (November 2010), p:351-7

Obed A, Uihlein DC, Zorger N, Farkas S, Scherer MN, Krüger B, Banas B, Krämer BK. (2008). Severe renal vein stenosis of a kidney transplant with beneficial clinical course after successful percutaneous stenting. American Journal Transplantation, Vol. 8, No. 10, (October 2008), p:2173-2176

Pannu N, Manns B, Lee H, Tonelli M. (2004). Systematic review of the impact of Nacetylcysteine on contrast nephropathy. *Kidney International,* Vol. 65, No, 4, April 2004), p:1366-1374.

Patel NH, Jindal RM, Wilkin T, Rose S, Johnson MS, Shah H, Namyslowski J, Moresco KP, Trerotola SO. (2001). Renal arterial stenosis in renal allografts: retrospective study of predisposing factors and outcome after percutaneous transluminal angioplasty. *Radiology,* Vol. 219, No. 3, (June 2001), p:663-667.

Penny MJ, Nankivell BJ, Disney AP, Byth K, Chapman JR. (1994). Renal graft thrombosis: a survey of 134 consecutive cases. *Transplantation,* Vol. 58, No. 5, (September 1994), p:565-569.

Roberts JP, Ascher NL, Fryd DS, Hunter DW, Dunn DL, Payne WD, Sutherland DE, Castaneda-Zuniga W, Najarian JS. (1989). Transplant renal artery stenosis. *Transplantation*, Vol. 48, No. 4, (October 1989), p:580-583.

Rouvière O, Berger P, Béziat C, Garnier JL, Lefrançois N, Martin X, Lyonnet D. (2002). Acute thrombosis of renal transplant artery: Graft salvage by means of intra-arterial fibrinolysis. *Transplantation*, Vol. 73, No. 3, (February 2002), p:403-409

Sebastià C, Quiroga S, Boyé R, Cantarell C, Fernandez-Planas M, Alvarez A. (2001). Helical CT in Renal Transplantation: Normal Findings and Early and Late Complications. *RadioGraphics*, Vol. 21, No. 5, (Sep-Oct 2001), p:1103–1117

Schafer AI, Levine MN, Konkle BA, Kearon C. (2003). Thrombotic disorders: diagnosis and treatment. *Hematology American Society of Hematology Educational Program*, p:520–539

Schafer, AI. (2007). Hypercoagulable State. In *Cardiovascular Medicine*, Willerson JT, Wellens HJ, Cohn JN, Holmes DR, pp:2423-2438, Springer-Verlag, London.

Schwarz A, Hiss M, Gwinner W, Becker T, Haller H, Keberle M. (2008). Course and relevance of arteriovenous fistulas after renal transplant biopsies. *American Journal of Transplantation*, Vol. 8, No. 4, (April. 2008), p:826-31.

Snider JF, Hunter DW, Moradian GP, Castaneda-Zuniga WR, Letourneau JG. (1989). Transplant renal artery stenosis: Evaluation with duplex sonography. *Radiology*, Vol. 172, (September 1989), p:1027-30.

Schoenberg SO, Bock M, Kallinowski F, Just A. (2000). Correlation of hemodynamic impact and morphologic degree of renal artery stenosis in a canine model. *Journal American Society Nephrology*, Vol. 11, No 12, (December 2000), p:2190-2198

Tarif N, Mitwalli AH, Al Samayer SA, Abu-Aisha H, Memon NA, Sulaimani F, Alam A, Al Wakeel JS. (2002). Congenital renal arteriovenous malformation presenting as severe hypertension. *Nephrology Dialysis Transplantation*, Vol. 17, No. 2, (February 2002), p:291-4.

Tutone VK, Mark PB, Stewart GA, Tan CC, Rodger RS, Geddes CC, Jardine AG. (2005). Hypertension, antihypertensive agents and outcomes following renal transplantation *Clinical Transplantation*, Vol 19, No. 2, (April 2005), p: 181–192

Virchow R. Gesammalte Abhandlungen zur Wissenschaftlichen Medtzin. Frankfurt, Germany: *Medinger Sohn*, 1856:219– 732.

Vaidya S, Sellers R, Kimball P, Shanahan T, Gitomer J, Gugliuzza K, Fish JC. (2000). Frequency, potential risk and therapeutic intervention in end-stage renal disease patients with antiphospholipid antibody syndrome: a multicenter study. *Transplantation*, Vol. 69, No. 7, (April 2000), p:1348-52.

Voiculescu A, Schmitz M, Hollenbeck M, Braasch S, Luther B, Sandmann W, Jung G, Mödder U, Grabensee B. (2005). Management of arterial stenosis affecting kidney graft perfusion: a single-centre study in 53 patients. *American Journal of Transplantation*, Vol. 5, No. 7, (July 2005), p:1731-1738.

Wagenknecht DR, Becker DG, LeFor WM, McIntyre JA. (1999). Antiphospholipid antibodies are a risk factor for early renal allograft failure. *Transplantation*, Vol. 68, No. 2, (July 1999), p: 241–246.

Wuthrich RP, Cicvara-Muzar S, Booy C, Maly FE. (2001). Heterozygosity for the factor V Leiden (G1691A) mutation predisposes renal transplant recipients to thrombotic complications and graft loss. *Transplantation*, Vol. 72, No. 3, (August 2001), p: 549-50.